AF412447

NERVOUS SYSTEM

Cambridge Illustrated Surgical Pathology

Nervous System is the new atlas-oriented resource in nervous system pathology. As the fourth book in the Cambridge Illustrated Surgical Pathology series, it is a comprehensive text of methods utilized by pathologists to accurately diagnose diseases affecting the brain, meninges, spinal cord, peripheral nerves, skull and paraspinal soft tissues, and cerebrospinal fluid. The book is a richly illustrated guide to surgical neuropathology, including all primary brain tumors as well as others arising near the nervous system that are also within the scope of neurosurgical practice. Numerous neuroimaging examples are provided to underscore the importance of knowing the basics of radiographic studies in accurately diagnosing CNS pathology. A complete spectrum of nonneoplastic neuropathological entities is also illustrated, including infectious, inflammatory, and epilepsy-related neuropathology. Additional chapters address intraoperative consultation and frozen sections, as well as CSF cytopathology.

Hannes Vogel is a board-certified neuropathologist and the Director of Neuropathology at the Stanford University School of Medicine. He has a particular interest and expertise in the area of pediatric brain tumor pathology and biology and has written extensively on this topic and many others in the area of neuropathology.

CAMBRIDGE ILLUSTRATED SURGICAL PATHOLOGY

SERIES EDITOR
Lawrence Weiss, MD
City of Hope National Medical Center, Duarte, California

OTHER BOOKS IN THE SERIES
Peiguo Chu, MD, and Lawrence Weiss, MD, *Modern Immunohistochemistry*
Thomas Lawton, MD, *Breast*
Lawrence Weiss, MD, *Lymph Nodes*

FORTHCOMING
Margaret Brandwein-Gensler, MD, *Head and Neck*
Mahendra Ranchod, MD, *Intraoperative Consultation*
Lawrence True, MD, *Prostate*

NERVOUS SYSTEM

Cambridge Illustrated Surgical Pathology

Hannes Vogel

Stanford University School of Medicine

With a Contribution by Shawn Corey, M.D., Ph.D. (Neuroimaging)

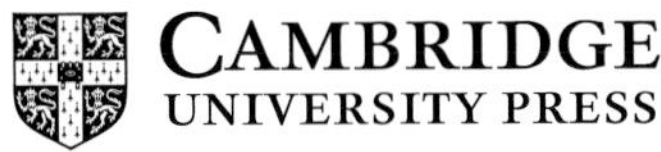

CAMBRIDGE UNIVERSITY PRESS
Cambridge, New York, Melbourne, Madrid, Cape Town, Singapore, São Paulo, Delhi

Cambridge University Press
32 Avenue of the Americas, New York, NY 10013-2473, USA

www.cambridge.org
Information on this title: www.cambridge.org/9780521881616

First published 2009

Printed in the United States of America

A catalog record for this publication is available from the British Library.

Library of Congress Cataloging in Publication Data

Vogel, Hannes, 1953–
    Nervous system / Hannes Vogel.
      p.; cm. – (Cambridge illustrated surgical pathology)
    Includes bibliographical references and index.
    ISBN 978-0-521-88161-6 (hardback)
    1. Central nervous system – Diseases – Atlases. 2. Pathology, Surgical – Atlases. I. Title. II. Series.
    [DNLM: 1. Central Nervous System – pathology – Atlases. 2. Pathology, Surgical – Atlases. WL 17 V878c 2009]

    RC361.V64 2009
    616.8′0475–dc22   2008037806

ISBN 978-0-521-88161-6 hardback

Dedicated to the persons whose conditions are depicted in this book and those who care for them.

CONTENTS

CONTRIBUTORS

HANNES VOGEL, M.D.
Professor of Pathology
Stanford University School of Medicine
Palo Alto, California

SHAWN COREY, M.D., Ph.D.
Clinical Instructor in Radiology
Stanford University School of Medicine
Palo Alto, California

MOHANPAL DULAI, M.D.
Fellow in Neuropathology
Stanford University School of Medicine
Palo Alto, California

JASON KARAMCHANDANI, M.D.
Fellow in Neuropathology
Stanford University School of Medicine
Palo Alto, California

GREGORY MOES, M.D.
Adjunct Clinical Instructor
Stanford University School of Medicine
Palo Alto, California

Attending Pathologist
Kaiser Permanente
Oakland, California

JOSEF ZÁMEČNÍK, M.D., Ph.D.
Associate Professor of Pathology
Charles University Prague
Czech Republic

PREFACE

xix

The guiding principle in this volume is the importance of knowing what pathological processes are common for a given anatomical location and age of the patient, upon a foundation of knowledge in the histology of normal and reactive processes in the nervous system. Many mistakes in surgical neuropathology may be avoided simply by maintaining an unswerving effort to determine the clinical, laboratory, and, sometimes most importantly, radiological findings in a given case. We also urge the use of standard and uniform terminology rather than idiosyncratic or descriptive diagnoses, which incorporates the World Health Organization 2007 classification for tumors along with contemporary terminology and classification schemes for nonneoplastic diseases. Unambiguous and consistent terminology is the foundation of a useful interaction primarily with neurosurgeons, but also with other allied health providers in neurooncology and radiation oncology. Our experience also dictates that diagnostic precision is required to the same degree when interacting with basic scientists who utilize tissue samples for brain tumor research.

The discipline of neuropathology is known for one of the highest discordance rates between the diagnoses of general surgical pathologists and trained neuropathologists. This book strives to underscore pitfalls in diagnostic surgical neuropathology, often due to mimicry between entirely different neoplasms or between reactive and neoplastic conditions. In the same sense, this book may be useful for general radiologists because of the detailed correlation we have sought to achieve between neuroimaging and many important neuropathological diseases.

Neuropathology, more so than other surgical pathology subspecialties, involves an extensive breadth of diagnostic entities with significant overlaps into hematopathology and the pathology of soft tissue tumors and infectious diseases. In the spirit of the Cambridge Illustrated Surgical Pathology series, this can perhaps best be approached and appreciated by a richly illustrated atlas to reinforce the vast array of pathological images the reader will encounter in the study and practice of surgical neuropathology.

Hannes Vogel, M.D.

ACKNOWLEDGMENTS

I wish to acknowledge the invaluable assistance of Anet James, Digital Imaging Specialist and Photographer in the Department of Pathology at Stanford University, for graphic art and the perfecting of photomicrographs. I also acknowledge the support and forbearance of my colleagues in the Laboratory of Neuropathology.

1 NORMAL ANATOMY AND HISTOLOGY OF THE CNS

ANATOMY

Knowledge of nervous system anatomy is essential for success in surgical neuropathology. Familiarity with native cellular elements will often predict the appearances of diverse tumors within the brain but, perhaps more importantly, recognition of normal or reactive processes will help avoid the pitfall of diagnosing malignancy when, in fact, a nonneoplastic reactive process or even normal tissue is present. Many surgical neuropathology specimens originate in the brain and spinal cord coverings, cranial and spinal nerve roots, blood vessels, and bone and soft tissue surrounding the nervous system; thus recognition of the normal brain is not enough. As with general surgical pathology, knowledge of diseases common to these locations and the ages at which they typically occur is essential.

The human brain can be described in many ways. However, for the purpose of surgical neuropathology, this description will emphasize different surgical compartments and cytoarchitectural areas that are especially associated with tumors or other pathological processes (Figure 1.1). The central nervous system (CNS) is often divided into the *supratentorial* and *infratentorial* compartments by the dural tentorium, which separates the cerebral hemispheres from the brainstem and cerebellum. The *spinal cord*, *roots*, and distalmost *cauda equina* and *filum terminale* (Figure 1.2) are often considered separately, especially in view of the paraspinal soft tissue pathology, which can affect the integrity of the spinal cord.

Brain tissue is divided into *gray* and *white matter*. This distinction may be useful in the differential diagnosis of neoplasms, but is more important in other pathological processes such as infection or neurodegeneration. The surgical neuropathologist is often interested in the relation of a tumor to the *ventricles*, including the ventricular spaces themselves and their periventricular regions. The base of the skull, including the pituitary gland-bearing *sella turcica*, is another particular region defined by the propensities of certain tumors for this region, both sellar and suprasellar.

The gross anatomy of the nervous system also reflects a level of complex and interrelated structure and function enviable to say the least of visceral organs.

Figure 1.1. Midsagittal magnetic resonance imaging of the brain with regions often associated with particular neuropathological processes.
Blue = supratentorial hemispheres with lateral and third ventricles.
Red = cerebellum.
Brainstem = midbrain (light green) pons (tan) and medulla (pink). Yellow = sella turcica and optic pathways.
Dark green = spinal cord.
Brown = pineal gland region.

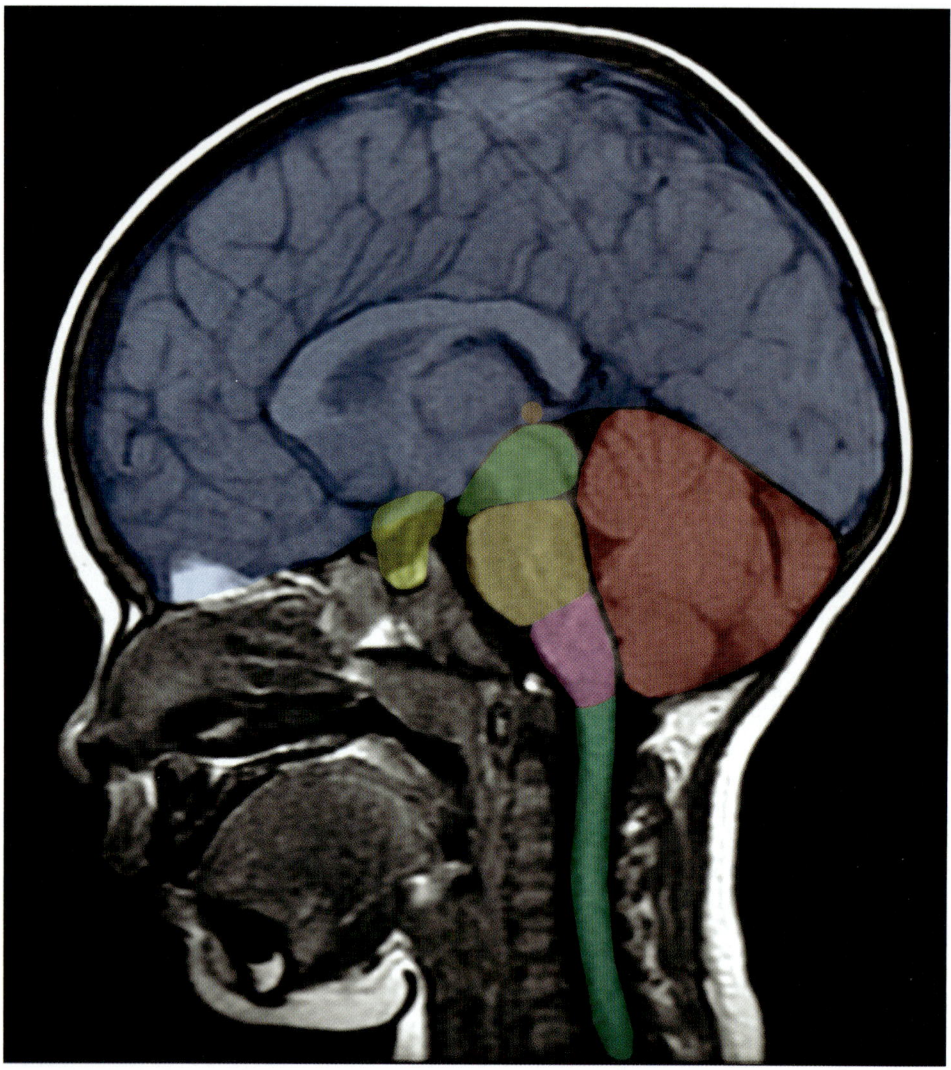

The nervous system possesses a wide array of sometimes overlapping but clinically distinct functions, thus forming the basis of a vast array of clinical symptoms attributable to the regions affected, not to mention their pace of onset. Thereby, seizures imply injury to gray matter; lesions involving given white matter tracts cause neurological deficits reflecting the normal function of the tract, including weakness, altered sensation, visual deficits, cranial neuropathies, or other motor and sensory deficits.

Mass lesions first compromise local blood supply, then intrude into ventricular spaces, sometimes causing obstruction of flow of cerebrospinal fluid at various narrow passages such as the foramina of Munro, cerebral aqueduct, or fourth ventricle, and finally compression of brain tissue via paths of least resistance. Expanding lesions are ultimately confronted by the rigid resistance of the dura and skull. These cerebral herniations cause clinical symptoms that herald the serious effects of mass lesions from the supratentorial compartment as they press the medial temporal lobes against the edge of the tentorium. A greater or diffuse swelling of the supratentorial brain will cause the brainstem to herniate downward, often resulting in hemorrhages within the pons, termed Duret hemorrhages

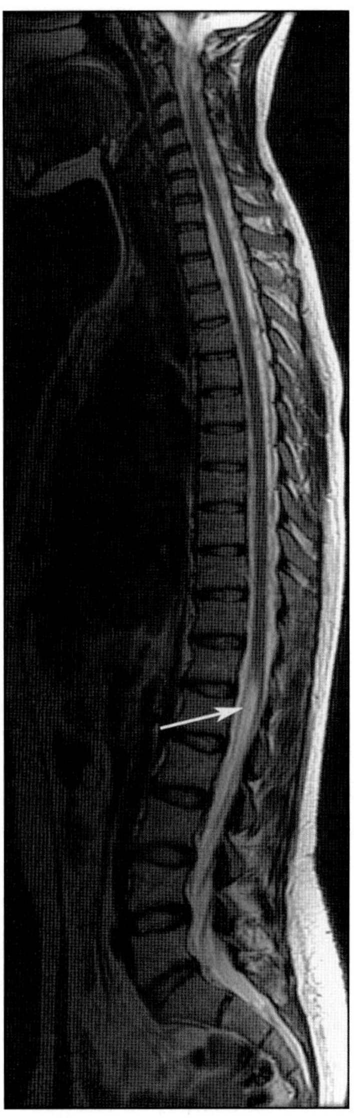

Figure 1.2. The spinal cord, roots, and distalmost cauda equina and filum terminale (arrow) are often considered separately, especially in view of the paraspinal soft tissue pathology, which can affect the integrity of the spinal cord.

representing the rupture of penetrating blood vessels that are otherwise tethered to the basilar artery. The most serious and life-threatening herniation involves downward pressure of the contents of the posterior fossa leading to compression of the medulla and vital respiratory control centers by the cerebellar tonsils.

Vascular pathology is inextricably related to virtually the entire spectrum of neuropathology. While the brain may only account for 2 percent of body weight, it accounts for 20 percent of oxygen consumption and thus normally receives 20 percent of cardiac output. The *circle of Willis* is an interconnected structure supplying arterial blood to the brain through the merging of paired sources in the carotid arteries and vertebral arteries at the base of the brain. The branching of the brain's arterial blood supply has been likened to that of an oak tree with right angles whereas that of the venous drainage is like the tapering confluence of elm branches. This is of more than botanical significance, since metastatic tumors, infections, or other arterial microemboli have a propensity to become lodged at a point of critical narrowing and angulation occurring at the grey–white junction such that this is often the location of the smallest of such lesions.

The brain is covered by successive layers. The most intimately associated is the pia mater, which tightly adheres to the entire surface of the brain and invests large penetrating blood vessels. Investing the pia mater is the arachnoid membrane, which is so intimately associated as to be combined through the term pia-arachnoid. The arachnoid membrane divests from the pia in the lower spinal canal, resulting in an expanded subarachnoid space that is amenable to lumbar puncture below lumbar vertebral body L2, which corresponds to the lower extent of the cauda equina.

HISTOLOGY

Surgical neuropathology requires the knowledge of normal histology in the immature, adult, and aged brain and how the cellular constituents vary accordingly.

Neurons are the functional unit of the nervous system and display a number of different and distinctive morphologies, which are of both functional and anatomical significance. Neurons of all types generally contain a round nucleus with a prominent nucleolus and a cell cytoplasm or perikaryon with Nissl substance. Motor neurons tend to be large trapezoidal or triangular cells (Figure 1.3) while sensory neurons have a more globular shape (Figure 1.4). A third type of neurons that are abundant in the cerebellum and dentate gyrus of the hippocampus are granular cell neurons (Figure 1.5). These are significantly smaller than most cortical neurons and do not show obvious cell processes in routine sections. The importance in recognizing normal neuronal morphology for the surgical neuropathologist lies in distinguishing normal ganglionic or neuronal cells from dysplastic or neoplastic ganglion cells, to recognize their appearance in gray matter structures or spinal or cranial nerve ganglia that are infiltrated by neoplasms, and to carefully distinguish normal granular cell neurons from "small blue cell" neoplasms or lymphocytes.

Neurons may be identified immunohistochemically with either one or a combination of three different antibodies. *Synaptophysin* is a useful marker of the neuronal cell surface or cytoplasm (Figure 1.6a), although the immunostaining results in infiltrative tumors or other processes can be difficult to interpret because of background normal staining for synaptophysin. *Neurofilament* is the characteristic intermediate filament of neurons. Antibodies to the nonphosphorylated neurofilament of the neuronal cell body (perikaryon) and to the phosphorylated neurofilament of neuronal processes can be used to distinguish these compartments accordingly. However, mixed neurofilament antibodies are commonly used in current surgical neuropathology and label both the cell body and its neurites (Figure 1.6b). A third marker of neuronal differentiation is anti-*neuN*, which offers the advantage of nuclear staining (Figure 1.6c). Not all neurons stain positively for neuN, including Purkinje cells, most neurons of the internal nuclear layer of the retina, and the sympathetic chain ganglia.

Neurons are the most quintessential cellular component of the CNS. However, *astrocytes* are the most plentiful cell type and exhibit the broadest range

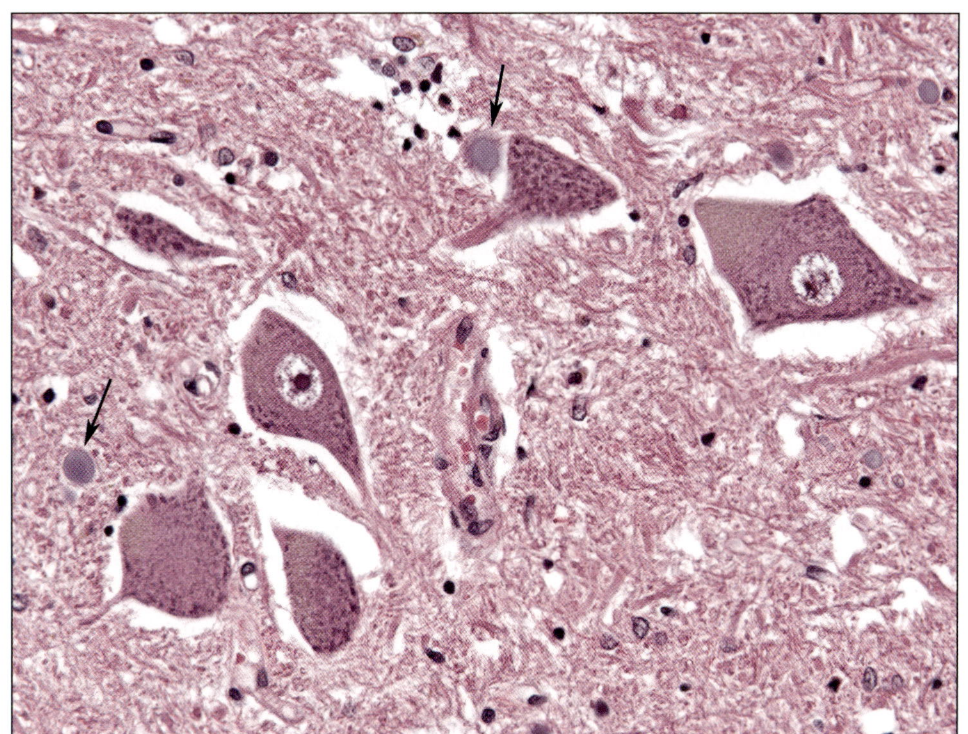

Figure 1.3. Large motor neurons tend to be large trapezoidal or triangular cells. Note cytoplasmic Nissl substance and eccentric aggregation of golden brown lipofuscin pigment. Corpora amylacea (arrows) are within slender glial cell processes not discernable in H&E sections.

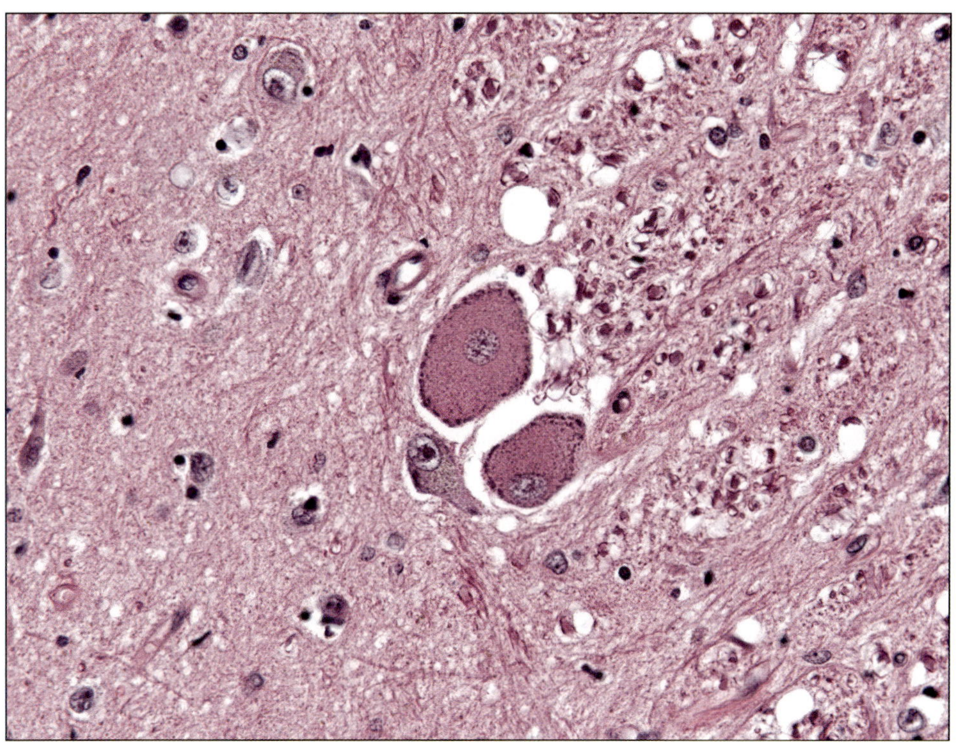

Figure 1.4. Sensory neurons have a more globular shape.

of normal and reactive morphologies. Two predominant types of astrocytes may be found in the brain: *fibrous astrocytes* in white matter and subpial and perivascular gray matter, which are detectable by glial fibrillary acidic protein (GFAP) immunohistochemistry, and *protoplasmic astrocytes* in gray matter, which contain little detectable GFAP. Reactive astrocytes often show eosino-philic cytoplasm and profusion of delicate cell processes detectable

Figure 1.5. Granular cell neurons of the cerebellum are seen in the upper field. Infiltrating neoplastic cells in this medulloblastoma are seen to be considerably larger, although cytological preparations and cryosections of cerebellar tissue in which granule cells predominate may be mistaken for a "small blue cell" tumor.

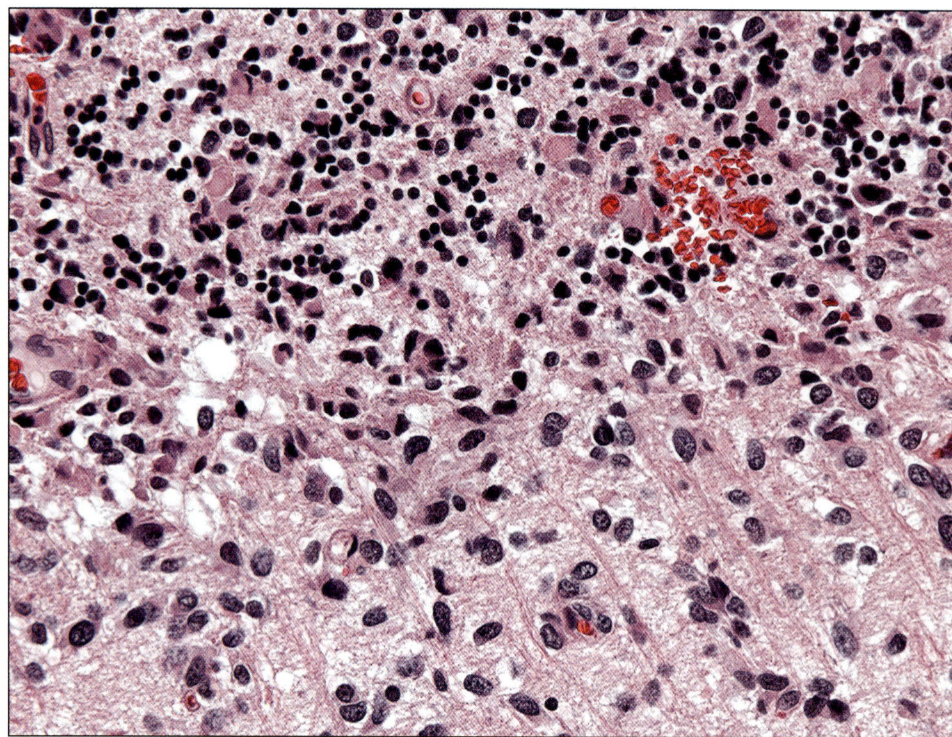

Figure 1.6. Immunohistochemistry for neuronal differentiation: (a) synaptophysin; (b) neurofilament; (c) *neuN*.

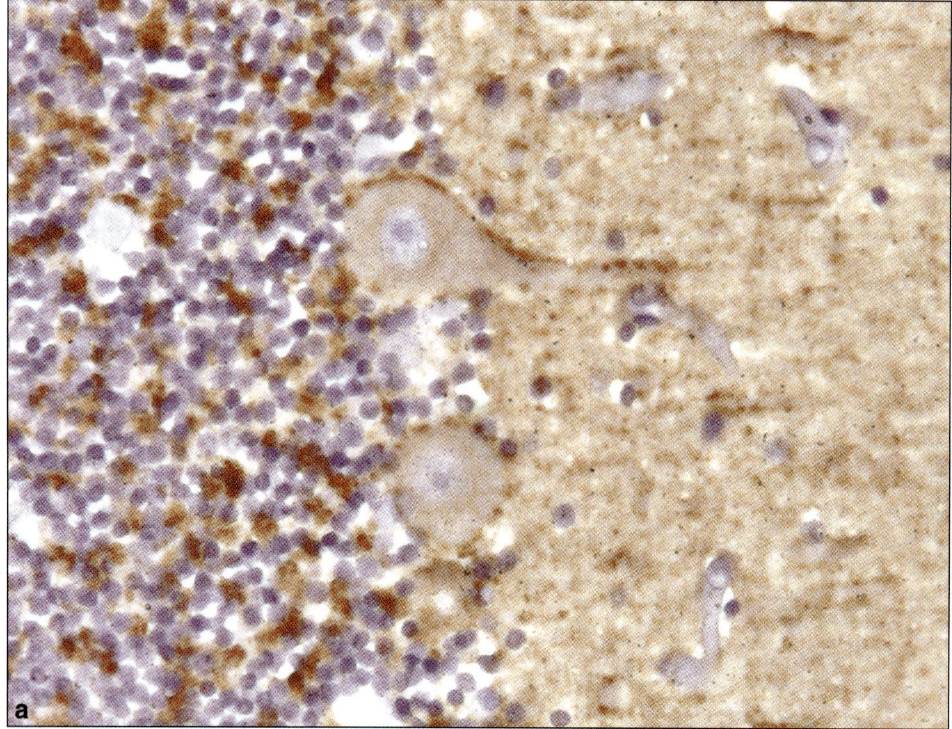

by hematoxylin – eosin defined (H&E) stain or especially by GFAP immuno-histochemistry (Figure 1.7). This may be useful in distinguishing white matter astrocytes from oligodendrocytes. A particular type of chronic gliosis is rec-ognizable as dense subpial gliosis often seen in chronic epilepsy resection specimens, known as Chaslin's gliosis (Figure 1.8). Distinguishing reactive

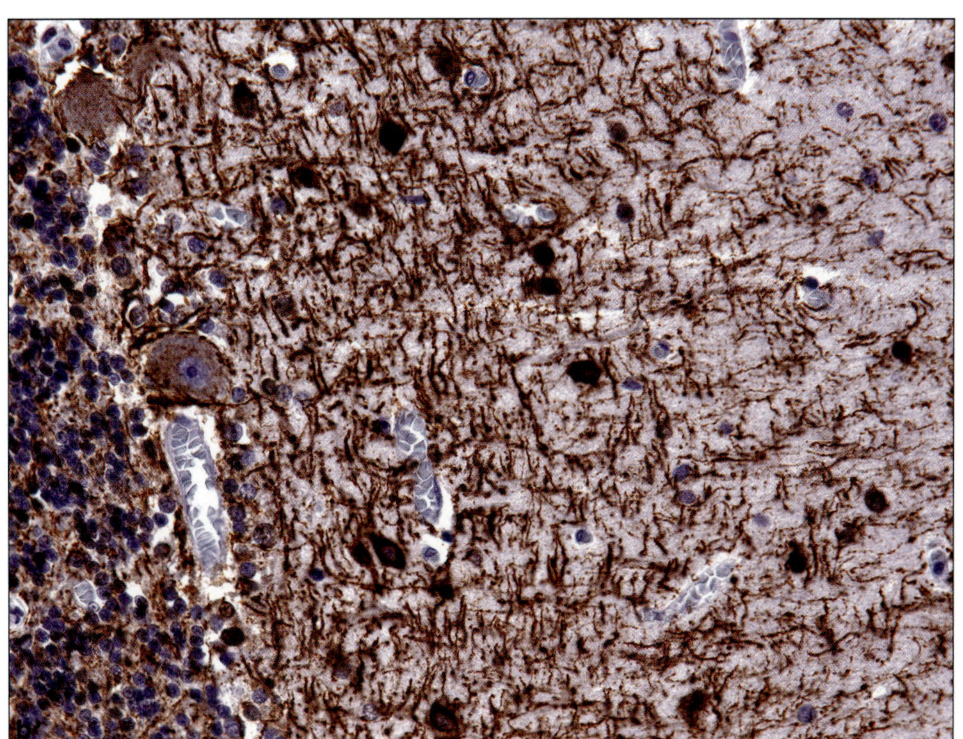

Figure 1.6. *continued.*

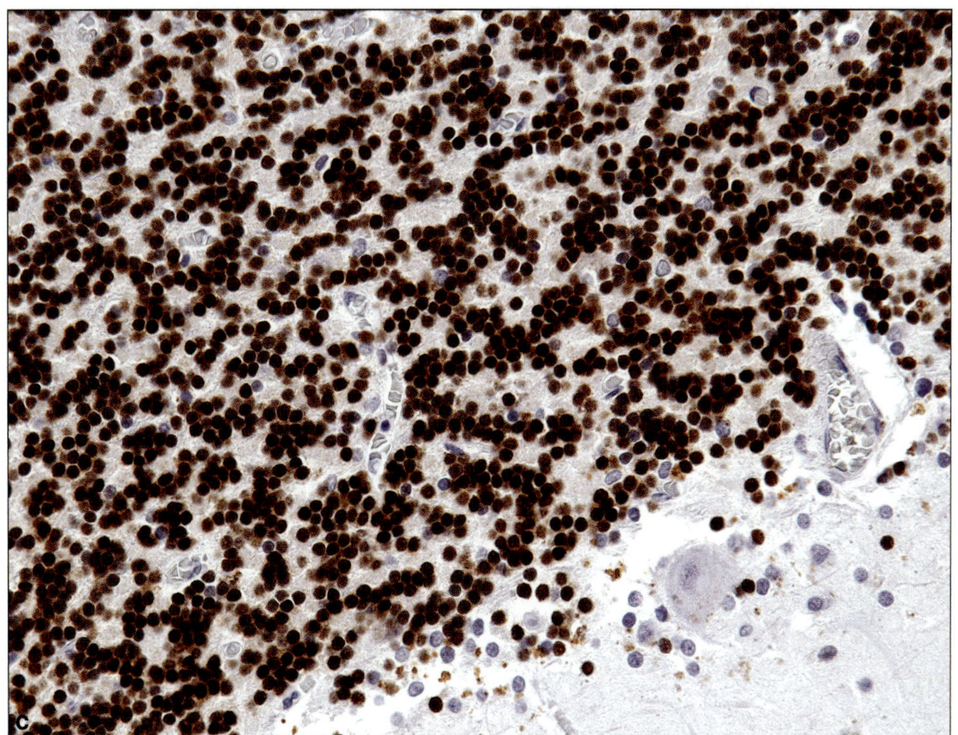

from neoplastic astrocytes may represent a significant challenge, and this challenge is discussed under "Astrocytic Tumors."

Corpora amylacea are age-related inclusions in astrocytes, which should not be confused with other pathological inclusions or microorganisms such as fungi. These are easily identified with a periodic acid – Schiff (PAS) stain and

Figure 1.7.
Immunohistochemistry for
glial differentiation:
(a) reactive fibrillary
astrocytes; (b) GFAP
immunohistochemistry.

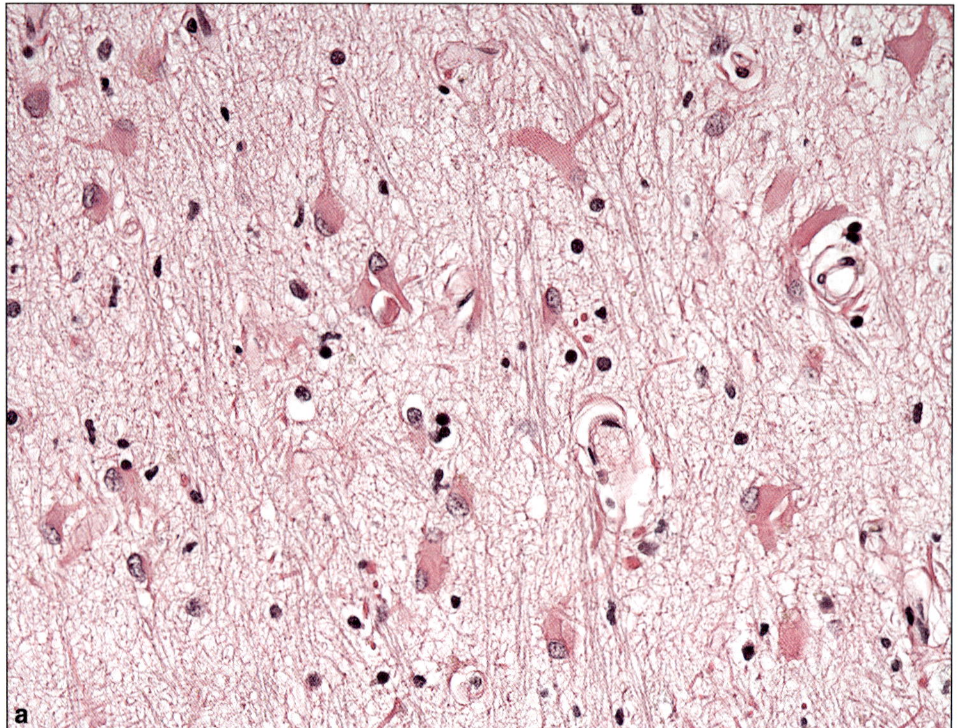

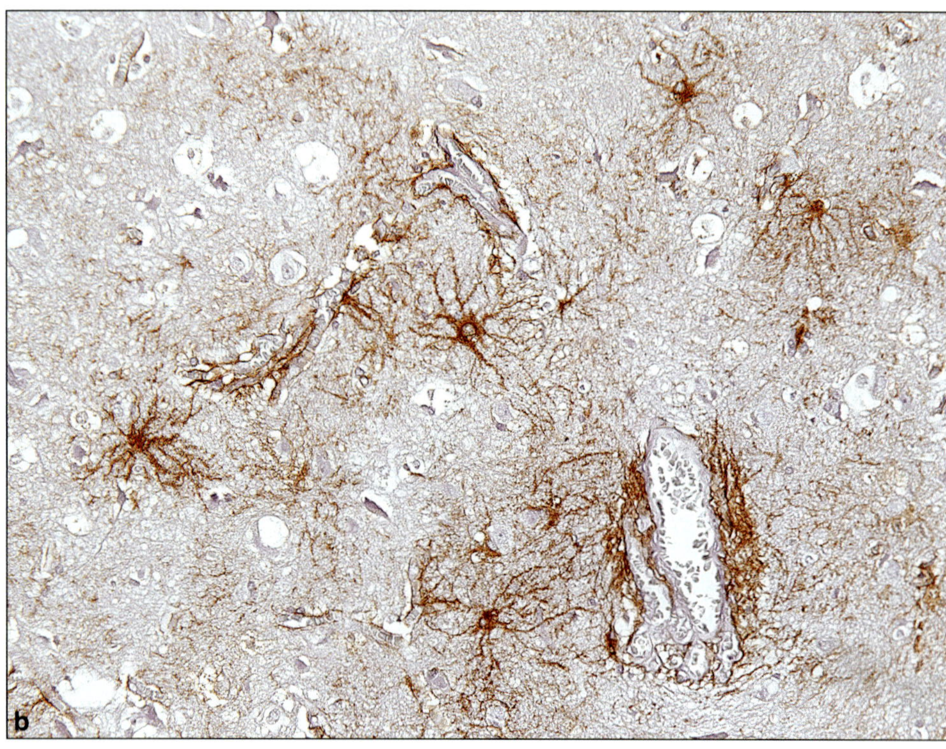

usually signify chronic gliosis (Figure 1.9). Another feature of reactive, and especially indolent and chronic gliosis are Rosenthal fibers. These are brightly eosinophilic elongated or beaded structures, which are also intracellular inclusions in astrocytes although they appear as solitary structures within the brain background (Figure 1.10).

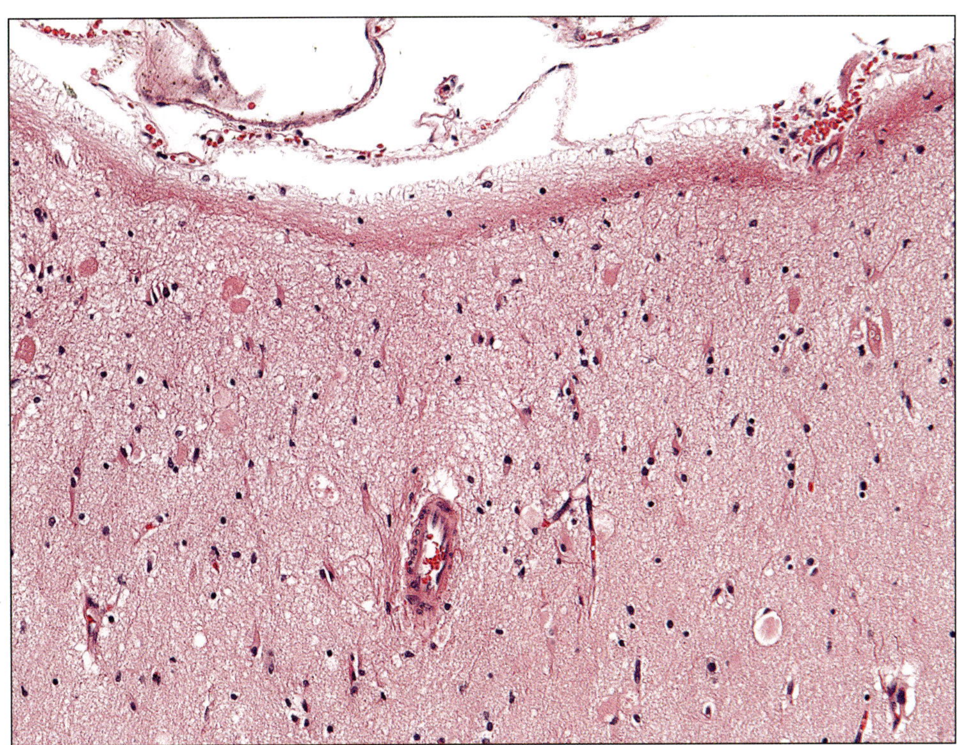

Figure 1.8. Dense subpial or interface (Chaslin's) gliosis.

Reactive astrocytes may undergo mitotic activity and one feature is the multinucleated Creutzfeldt astrocyte with its characteristic "micronuclei." These may be a conspicuous feature of demyelinating disease (Chapter 6, Figure 6.1). The *gemistocytic astrocyte* is one with abundant eosinophilic cytoplasm causing nuclear displacement. This may be a striking feature of reactive processes, such as that seen in the wall of a cerebral infarction or abscess, and is sometimes difficult to distinguish from a neoplastic gemistocytic astrocyte.

Perhaps one of the most striking examples of abnormal cellular morphologies among reactive astrocytes may be seen by the surgical neuropathologist in examples of progressive multifocal leukoencephalopathy. These are markedly enlarged cells with bizarre nuclei (Figure 1.11).

Another more subtle form of reactive astrocytosis is in the form of metabolic astrocytes, the most typical of which are designated the Alzheimer Type 2 astrocytes (Figure 1.12). This is not usually a primary diagnostic issue in surgical neuropathology; however, they should not be confused with other types of infiltrating, particularly neoplastic cells such as there in oligodendroglioma in gray matter.

Oligodendrocytes are especially plentiful in CNS white matter being the myelinating cell of the CNS, which includes the optic nerves. Their inconspicuous round nuclei are scattered evenly or in vague rows throughout white matter, a tendency that can become more pronounced in the atrophic process that affects the aged brain (Figure 1.13). This may create an unsettling degree of hypercellularity that may even be misdiagnosed as a diffuse glioma. Oligodendrocytes may also be noted in gray matter as innocuous cells loosely arranged

Figure 1.9. (a) Corpora amylacea may be inconspicuous in H&E-stained sections, but (b) are easily identified with a PAS stain.

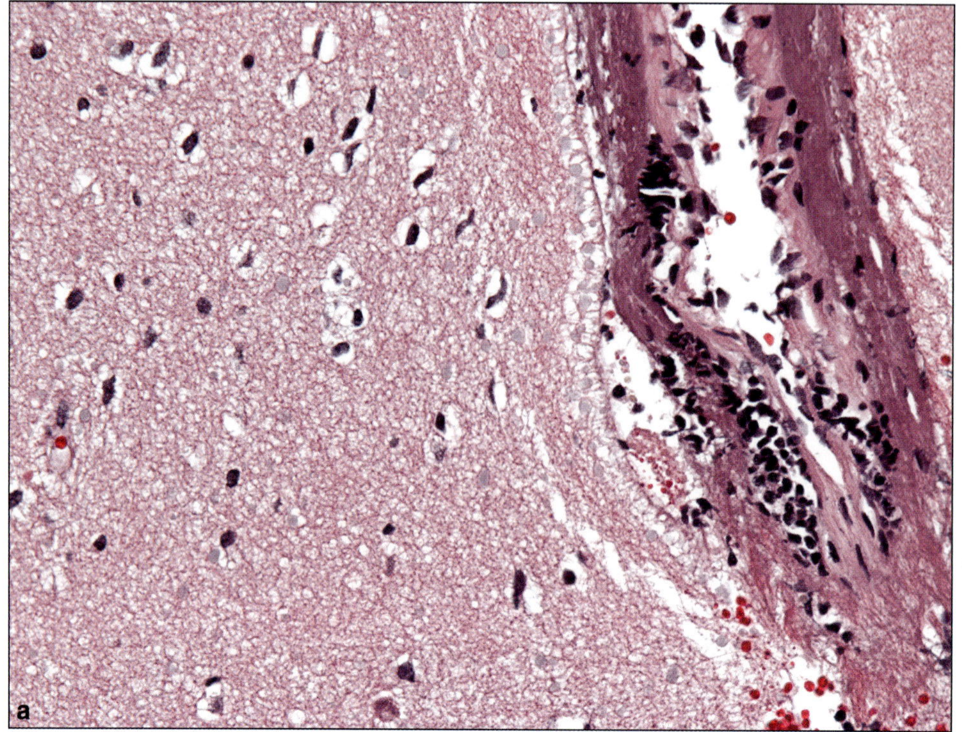

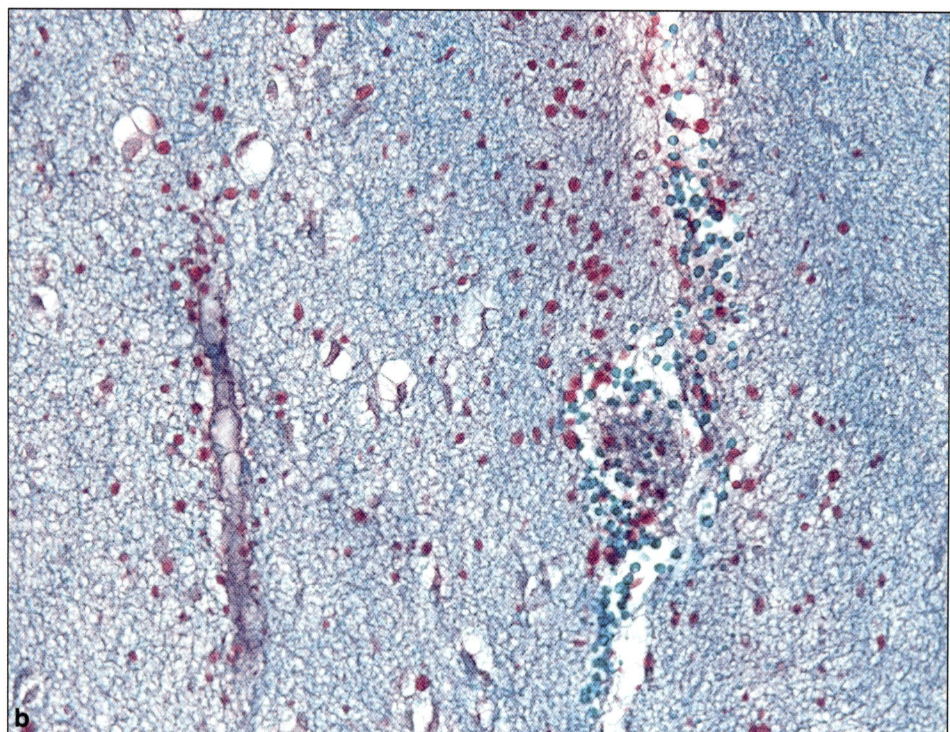

around neuronal cell bodies. Unfortunately, there are no immunostains that reliably and specifically distinguish oligodendrocytes from astrocytes.

Ependymocytes are cuboidal or columnar ciliated cells that line ventricles (Figure 1.14). *Choroid plexus epithelium* is a specialized form of ependymal cell. The hypocellular and fibrillary zone immediately subjacent to the ependymal lining is known as the subependymal plate. In this location, clusters of ependymal

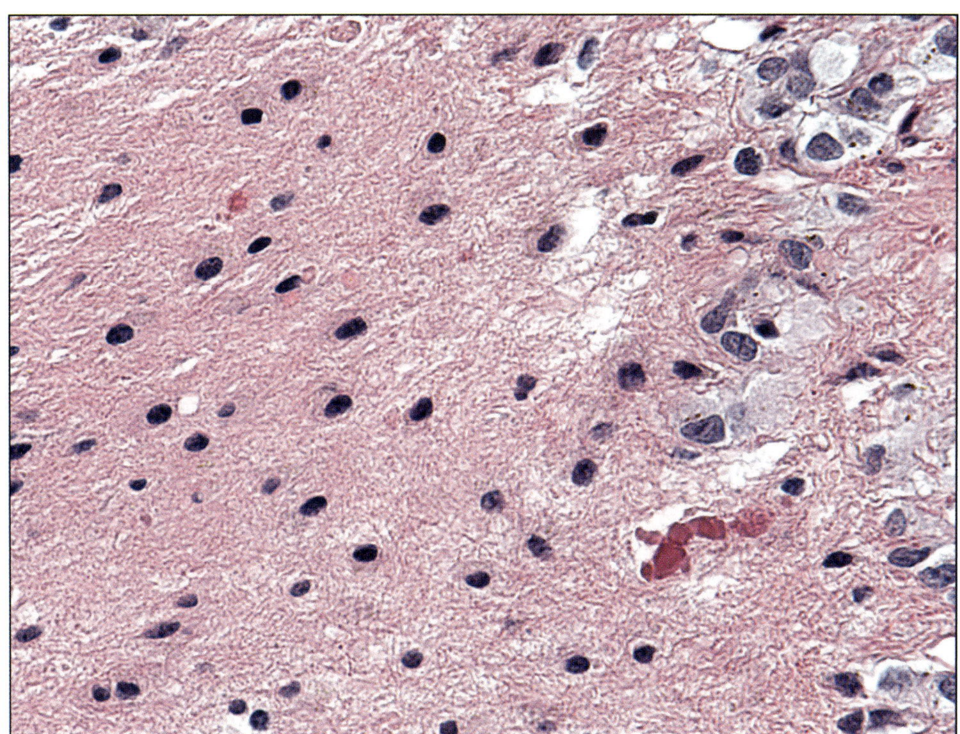

Figure 1.10. Rosenthal fibers are another feature of reactive and especially indolent gliosis.

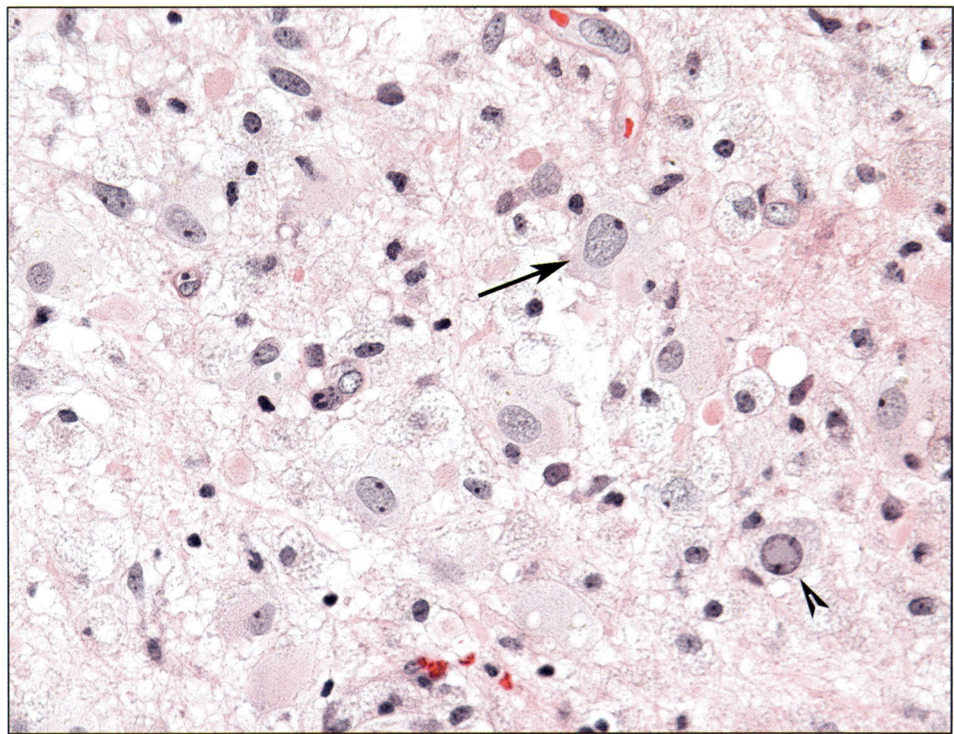

Figure 1.11. Atypical astrocytes seen in progressive multifocal leukoencephalopathy (arrow). Note the infected oligodendrocyte with nuclear chromatin margination from viral proliferation (arrowhead).

cells may be seen, particularly when overlying ependymal cells have been lost or damaged. Ependymocytes are weakly GFAP positive as are choroid plexus epithelia, which are intriguingly synaptophysin immunopositive.

Microglia, or *rod cells*, are bone marrow–derived tissue macrophages of the brain, normally residing in an almost invisible perivascular location. They

Figure 1.12. Metabolic astrocytes (arrows) should not be confused with other types of infiltrating neoplastic cells such as in oligodendroglioma in gray matter.

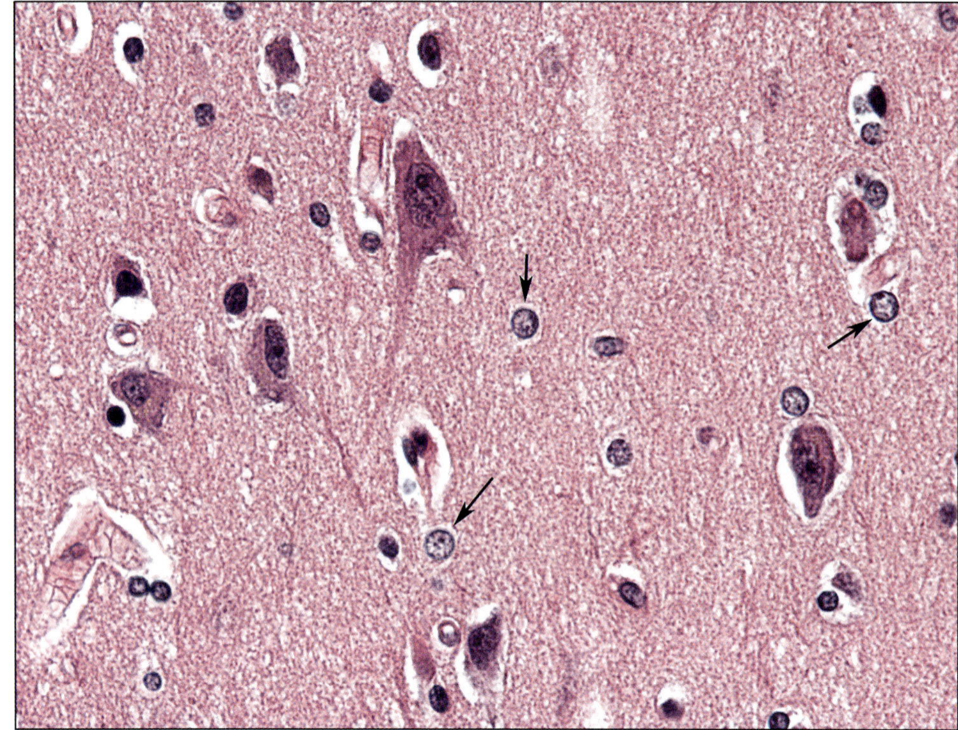

Figure 1.13. In atrophic or aged white matter, oligodendrocytes may coalesce around blood vessels or in rows, which should not be misinterpreted as perivascular or white matter spread of a glioma.

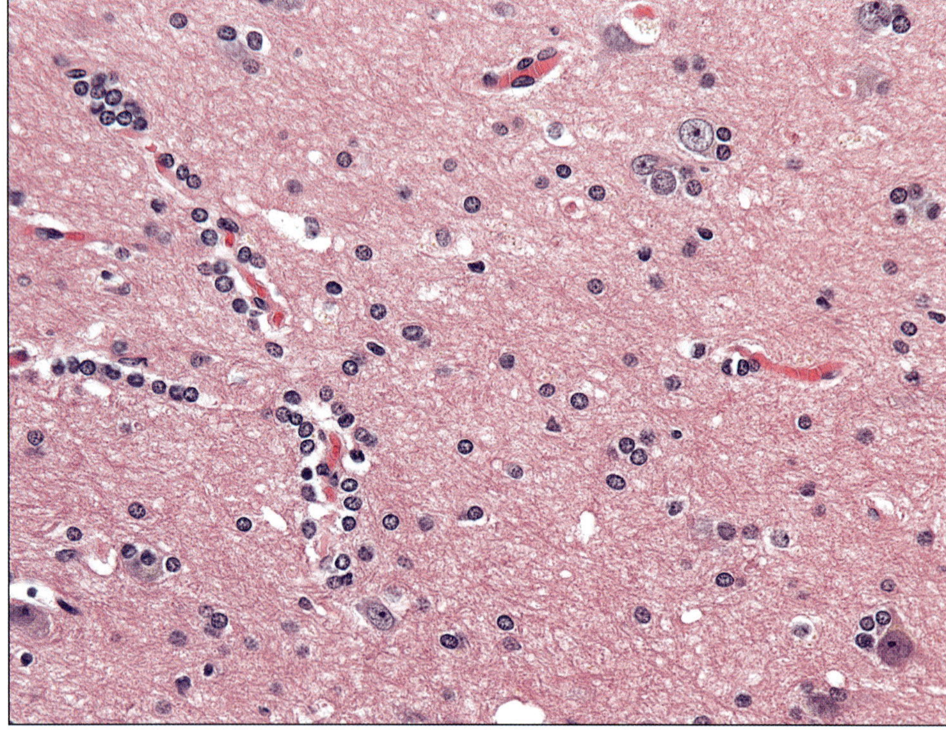

become activated by almost any injury and are recognized by their elongated shape, often with an indented or slightly crooked profile (Figure 1.15a,b), all of which reflect their ameboid motility through the brain. Microglia may be a prominent part of infiltrating glial neoplasms; thus their presence may not equate with a purely reactive lesion. Both CD68 and CD163 (Figure 1.15c) immunohistochemistry are useful in identifying microglia.

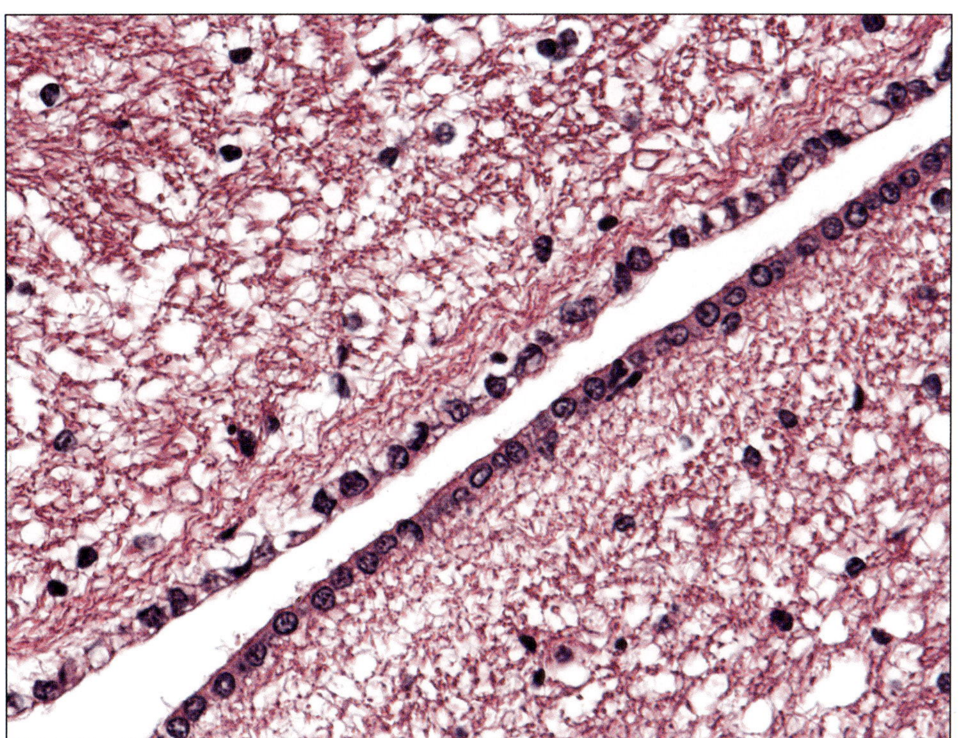

Figure 1.14. Ependymocytes.

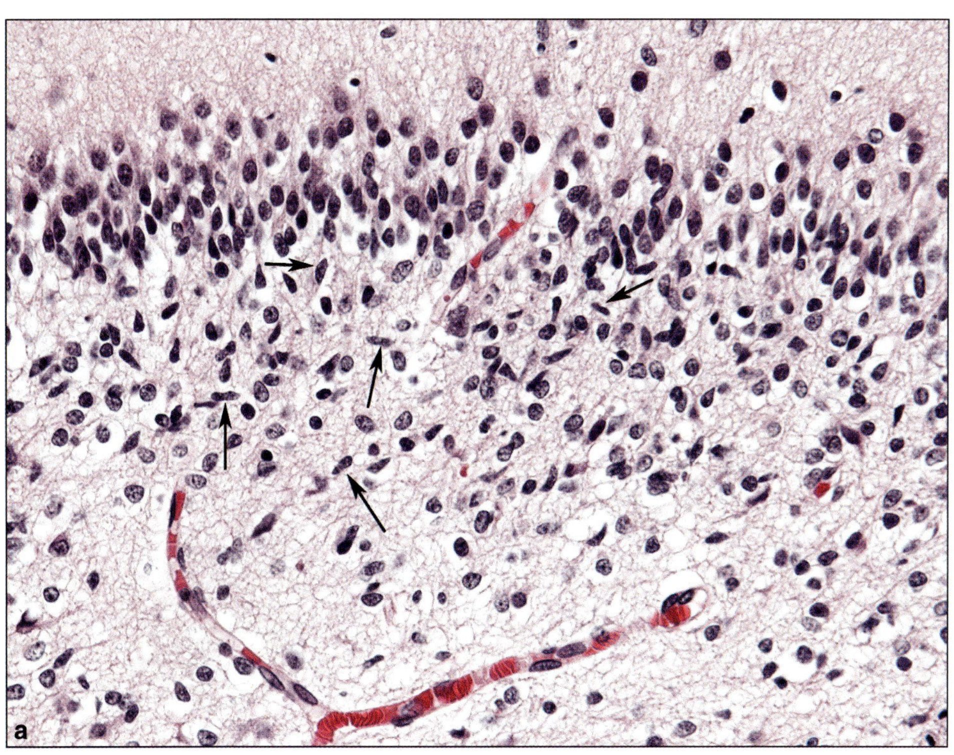

Figure 1.15. Microglia are rod-shaped cells infiltrating brain tissue in both neoplastic and nonneoplastic conditions. They are seen here in (a) a presumably physiological process within the developing hippocampus (arrows)

CNS vasculature is not significantly different from that of other tissues, except for the lack of an external elastic lamina in intracerebral arterial blood vessels. It is also important to recognize mimics of vascular malformations that arise through tangential sections of large blood vessels.

Figure 1.15. *continued*
(b) adjacent to an infarction,
and (c) immunolabeled with
anti-CD163.

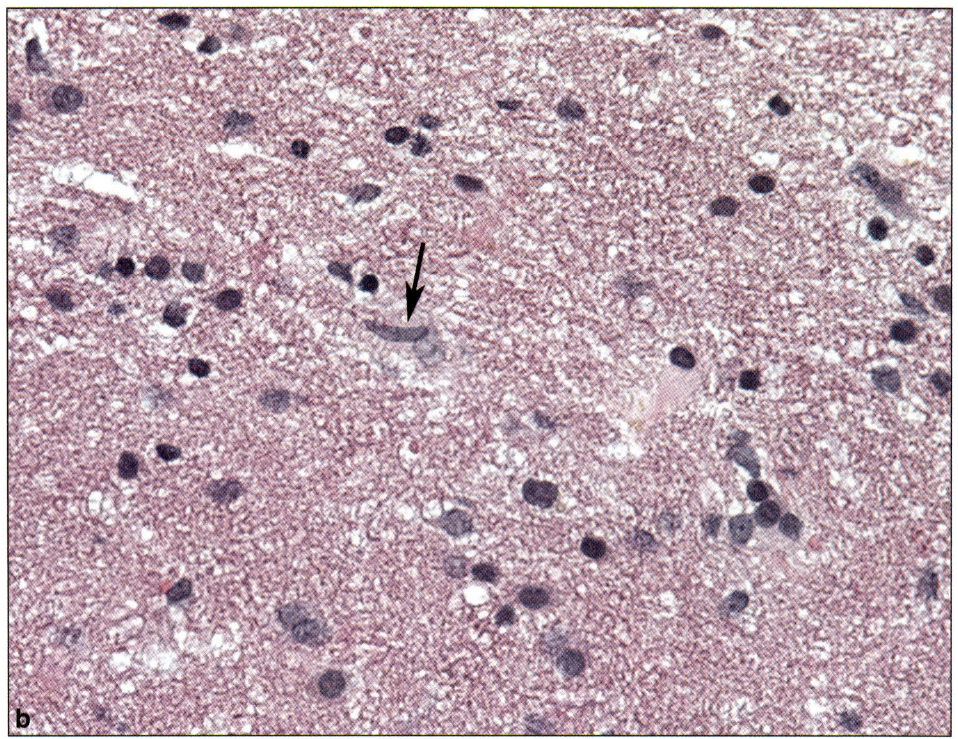

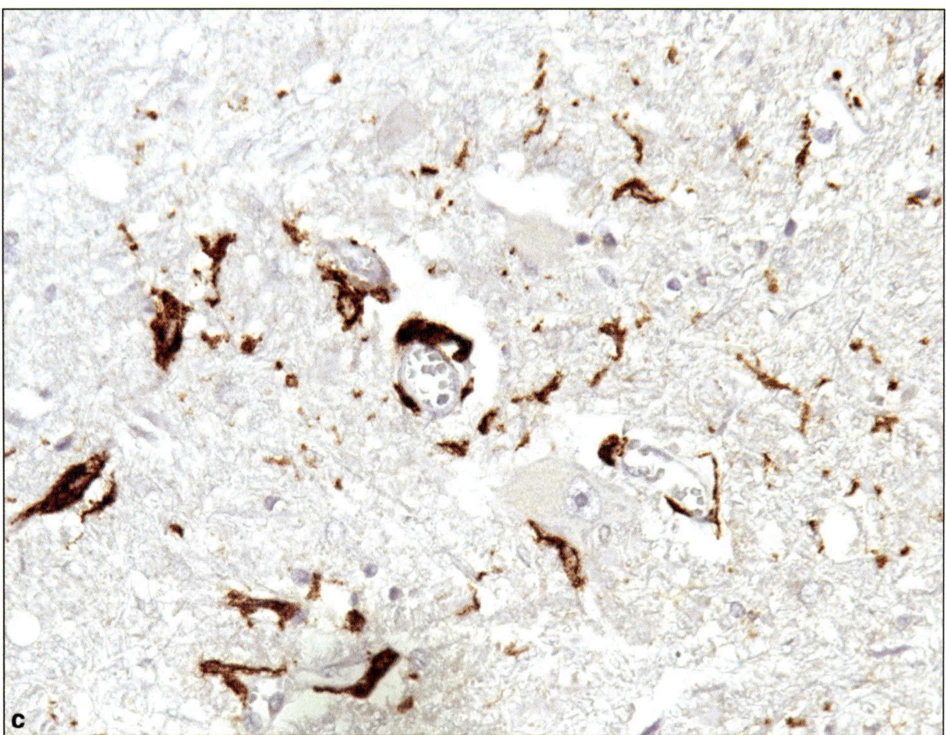

The dura mater and pia-arachnoid (leptomeninges) are of great importance
to the integrity of the CNS and may be represented in surgical neuropathology
in many ways. Dura mater and associated spinal cord ligaments are often
encountered in some spinal cord surgeries, and the ligamentum flavum has a
distinctive appearance (Figure 1.16).

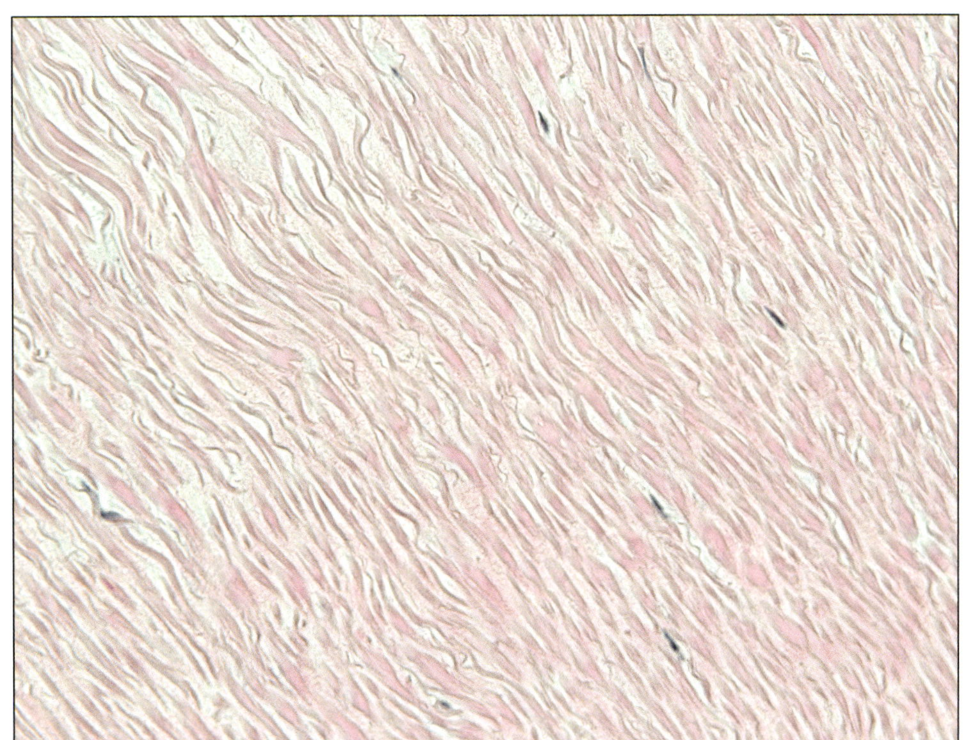

Figure 1.16. The ligamentum flavum bears a distinct microscopic appearance and is often recognizable in surgical specimens from paraspinal surgery.

Table 1.1. Common histological stains used in surgical neuropathology, cells or structures identified, and examples of pathological conditions in which they are diagnostically useful

Congo red, Thioflavin S	Amyloid	Cerebral amyloid angiopathy
		Amyloid plaques
Fontana–Masson melanin	Melanin	Leptomeningeal melanocytes
		Melanotic neoplasms
Gallyas silver impregnation	Tau inclusions	Alzheimer disease neurofibrillary tangles
		Pick bodies and tau inclusions of frontotemporal lobar degeneration
Gomori methenamine silver	Cryptococcus, coccidioides, aspergillus, etc.	Fungal infections
PAS	Corpora amylacea, fungi	Fungal infections
		Basement membrane
		Granular cell astrocytoma
		Corpora amylacea (gliosis of hippocampal sclerosis)
Perl's iron stain	Iron	Mineralization
		Hemosiderin
Reticulin	Collagen	Pericellular deposition in:
		Schwannomas
		Pleomorphic xanthoastrocytoma

continued on next page

Table 1.1. *continued*

		Gliosarcoma
		Desmoplastic infantile astrocytoma and ganglioglioma
		Loss in pituitary adenomas
		Highlights leptomeningeal invasion
Trichrome	Collagen and fibrin	Constituents of vascular malformations
Van Gieson	Vascular elastic lamina	Arteriovenous malformations
Von Kossa	Calcium	Mineralization
Ziehl–Neelsen, Fite's, and Kinyoun stains	Acid fast bacilli; Mycobacteria, Nocardia	Tuberculosis, leprosy, nocardiosis

Table 1.2. Common immunohistochemical preparations used in surgical neuropathology, cells or structures identified, and examples of pathological conditions in which they are diagnostically useful

BAF47/SNF5	Regulator of chromatin structure	Absent expression in:
		Atypical teratoid/rhabdoid tumor
		Malignant rhabdoid tumor
		Mosaic pattern in familial schwannomatosis
		Proximal epithelioid sarcoma
		Rhabdoid cells in rhabdoid glioblastoma (GBM)
β-Amyloid	Amyloid	Cerebral amyloid angiopathy
		Amyloid plaques
β-Amyloid precursor protein	Axonal spheroids	Diffuse axonal injury
		Hypoxic–ischemic encephalopathy
		Wall of infarct
CAM 5.2	Low molecular weight cytokeratin	Endothelial neoplasms
		Fibrous bodies, sparsely granulated growth hormone pituitary adenomas
CD68, CD163	Macrophages and microglial cells	Infarction
		Demyelinating processes
		Necrotic neoplasms
		White matter tract degeneration
CD1a	Langerhans cells	Langerhans cell histiocytosis
CD20	B cells	B-cell lymphoma
CD3	T cells	Reactive lymphocytes
		T-cell lymphoma

Table 1.2. *continued*

CD31	Vascular endothelium	Endothelial neoplasms
CD34	Vascular endothelium	Endothelial neoplasms
		Neurofibroma
		Epithelioid sarcoma
		Superior to CD31 for Kaposi sarcoma
CD45	All differentiated hematopoietic cells except erythrocytes and plasma cells	Lymphomas
	Also known as leukocyte common antigen (LCA)	B-cell chronic lymphocytic leukemia
		Hairy cell leukemia
		Acute nonlymphocytic leukemia
CD56	NK cells, activated T cells, the brain and cerebellum, and neuroendocrine tissues. also called neural cell adhesion molecule (NCAM)	Myeloma
		Myeloid leukemia
		Neuroendocrine tumors
		Wilms' tumor
		Adult neuroblastoma
		NK/T-cell lymphomas
		Pancreatic acinar cell carcinoma
		Pheochromocytoma
		Small cell lung carcinoma
		Ewing's sarcoma/primitive neuroectodermal tumor (PNET) is CD56 negative
Chromogranin	Secretory granules in endocrine and neuroendocrine cells	Endocrine and neuroendocrine neoplasms
		Pituitary adenoma
		Paraganglioma
CK7	54-kDa type II keratin	Non-GI carcinomas
		Most common CK7+ brain metastases are lung, breast, ovary, endometrium, bladder, or neuroendocrine system.
CK20	46-kDa low-molecular-weight keratin	Most GI carcinomas
		Mucinous ovarian carcinoma
		Biliary carcinoma
		Transitional carcinoma

continued on next page

Table 1.2. *continued*

		Merkel cell carcinomas
Cytomegalovirus (CMV)	Cytomegalovirus	CMV infection
Cytokeratin (CK) mix	"Simple" keratins	Nonspecific marker of most carcinomas
Desmin	Intermediate filament of skeletal, smooth, and cardiac muscle	Myogenic differentiation in neoplasms
		Rhabdomyoma/sarcoma; leiomyoma/sarcoma
Epithelial membrane antigen (EMA)	Normal and neoplastic epithelia; notochord; perineurial cells; arachnoidal cells; plasma cells	Carcinoma
		Meningioma
		Synovial sarcoma
		Epithelioid sarcoma
		Perineurioma
		Chordoma
		Some plasmacytomas
		Dotlike cytoplasmic positivity in ependymomas and angiocentric glioma
GFAP	Astrocytes; ependymal cells; not mature oligodendrocytes. GFAP-like protein expressed by nonmyelinating Schwann cells	Reactive fibrillary astrocytes
		Astrocytoma, except gliosarcoma
		Ependymoma
		Gliofibrillary oligodendrocytes and oligodendroglial minigemistocytes
		Some schwannomas
HMB45	Melanoma extract antigen	Melanocytic tumors, especially to distinguish metastatic melanoma from other S-100+ brain tumors.
HSV	Herpes simplex virus	Herpes encephalitis
κ and λ light chains	Immunoglobulin components	Clonal vs. mixed plasma cell proliferations
MIB-1	Ki-67 nuclear antigen associated with cell proliferation during all active phases of the cell cycle (G1, S, G2, and mitosis); absent from resting cells (G0)	Proliferation index
NeuN	Neuronal nucleus; not in Purkinje cells, neurons of the internal nuclear layer of the retina, and sympathetic chain ganglia	Neuronal and glioneuronal tumors

Table 1.2. *continued*

Neurofilament protein	Neuronal characteristic intermediate filament; nonphosphorylated in perikaryon, phosphorylated in neurites	Neuronal and glioneuronal tumors
p53	Transcription factor and TP53 tumor suppressor gene product	Abnormal nuclear staining an indirect marker of mutant TP53 gene or wild-type TP53 inactivation from hypoxia or DNA damage
		Immunopositive in some WHO Grade II–IV astrocytomas but not pilocytic astrocytoma
		Atypical pituitary adenoma and pituitary carcinoma.
S-100	Cells derived from the neural crest (Schwann cells, melanocytes, and glial cells), chondrocytes, adipocytes, myoepithelial cells, macrophages, Langerhans cells, dendritic cells, and keratinocytes	Peripheral and cranial nerve sheath tumors
		Most neuroepithelial tumors
		Chordoma
		Metastatic tumors, including melanoma
		Langerhans cell histiocytosis
Smooth muscle actin	Myogenous differentiation, including myofibroblastic and myoepithelial tissues	Myogenic differentiation in neoplasms
SV40	Simian virus 40, a polyomavirus	Surrogate for immunolabeling of JC virus-infected cells in progressive multifocal leukoencephalopathy (PML)
Synaptophysin	Synaptic vesicle protein	Neuronal, pineal, embryonal, and choroid plexus tumors
		Pilomyxoid astrocytoma
		Pituitary adenoma
		Paraganglioma
Thyroid transcription factor-1 (TTF-1)	Protein that regulates transcription of genes specific for the thyroid, lung, and diencephalon	Metastatic lung or thyroid carcinoma
		Ependymoma of the 3rd ventricle
Toxoplasmosis	*Toxoplasma gondii*	Toxoplasma infection

SUGGESTED READING

Blumenfeld H. *Neuroanatomy through Clinical Cases.* Sunderland, Mass.: Sinauer, 2002.
Fuller GN, Burger PC. Central nervous system. In: Mills SE, editor. *Histology for Pathologists.* Philadelphia: Lippincott Williams & Wilkins, 2007.

2 INTRAOPERATIVE CONSULTATION

Intraoperative consultation has always represented a significant challenge for both the general surgical pathologist and the neuropathologist alike. Most of the neurosurgeon's goals are quite similar to those of other surgeons, namely to confirm the presence of an adequate sample for diagnosis and to allow the pathologist to choose between various alternatives in processing the tissue according to the suspected diagnosis. Key aspects of the patient's neurological history should be known at the time of intraoperative consultation, including the timing of onset of symptoms, any focal features such as seizures, motor or sensory deficits, constitutional symptoms, and sometimes a history of exposures and travel.

The available radiographic studies must be examined prior to intraoperative consultation as well as previous surgical material in recurrent or metastatic lesions. As always, direct and unambiguous communication with the surgeon is of paramount importance. This includes conveying the need for cultures whenever an infectious process is suspected through intraoperative consultation.

There are also some important differences underlying the call for intraoperative consultation in neurosurgical specimens as compared with those directed at general surgical pathology. Neurosurgeons are almost never interested in determining the presence of a neoplasm at the resection margin, since complete surgical resection is not a viable option in the resection of most primary brain tumors. This is notwithstanding the fact that the extent of surgical resection is of primary importance in the prognoses of some primary brain tumors: ependymomas, some WHO Grade I tumors such as pilocytic astrocytoma, ganglioglioma or dysembryoplastic neuroepithelial tumor, meningiomas, and some metastatic lesions.

With increasing use of stereotactic biopsies, samples may be especially small and this poses a significant challenge in deciding how to divide the tissue for cryostat and smear section preparations versus retaining as much as possible for histologically superior permanent sections prepared from unfrozen tissue.

METHODOLOGY

The complete assessment of a neurosurgical specimen consists of a *gross examination, cryosectioning, cytological smear* and *touch preparations*. The gross examination of the small specimen should never be underestimated in determining the portion most likely to be abnormal when stereotactic sampling is done in a difficult or sometimes precarious situation, yielding very small samples. Gliomas will sometimes have a more obviously mucoid and looser consistency or hemorrhagic appearance.

Practices vary according to institutions and individuals in the use of cryosections and cytological preparations. It is recommended that experience be acquired in both techniques by applying them simultaneously when tissue is relatively abundant so that not only are both techniques mastered but the corresponding cytoarchitectural features best displayed in a cryosection are compared with the superior cytological detail of smear or touch preparations. The following guidelines are recommended for success in neuropathological intraoperative consultations.

1. When very small specimens are received, it may be advantageous to consider doing either a cryosection or cytological preparation, although some neuropathologists perform both as a matter of routine. In biopsies of infiltrating glioma, this calls upon considerable experience in recognizing smear preparations of essentially normal brain versus brain with infrequent infiltrating neoplastic glial cells. This difficulty is compounded by the presence of reactive astrocytes and microglia in infiltrating gliomas.

2. Either request that specimens be submitted on a slightly moistened surface or, when they are received in excessive amounts of saline, make every effort to remove excessive saline before cryosectioning, or else an unacceptably significant degree of freeze artifact will result. Drying the artifact must also be avoided.

3. Avoid the use of forceps, especially those with small grooves, in handling specimens. Small stereotactic biopsies have a tendency to adhere to the surfaces and increasingly desperate efforts to detach the specimen from the forceps may render it nondiagnostic. The edge or point of a sterile blade will often suffice.

4. The proper preparation of the cytological smear preparation is of great importance. Do not use a fragment larger than 1 mm for this purpose. The fragment must be smeared in a manner to ideally achieve a monolayer of cells that yet retains some architectural association with blood vessels or features such as papillary growth or whorls. The smearing of gliomas or cellular tumors such as some lymphomas, embryonal tumors, or metastases may create a smooth or even silky sensation in smearing the tissue. Some tumors, which are densely calcified or which contain numerous psammoma bodies, may actually impart a gritty sensation upon smearing.

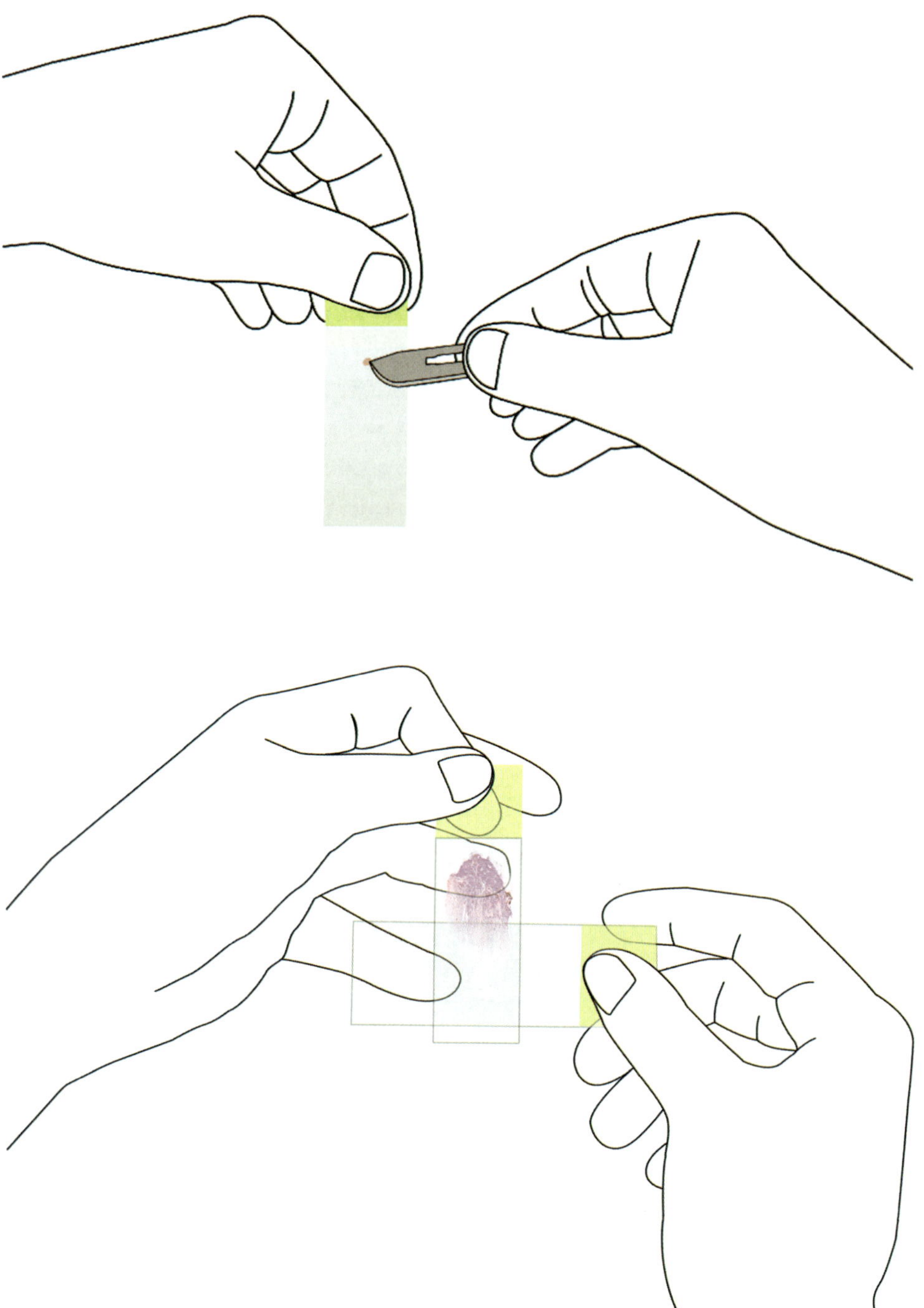

5. Other tumors are much less appropriate for cytological smears, namely those with a prominent fibrous or stromal element such as many meningiomas, schwannomas, and some parameningeal tumors. These yield clumps of distorted and crushed tissue. Nevertheless, some of these examples may lend themselves to touch preparations, especially meningiomas, whereby cytological whorls are preferentially detached. Cytological touch preparations are also diagnostic of pituitary adenomas when brisk exfoliation of cells is observed, to the extent that cryosections are superfluous in typical cases. Remember to use gloves for this procedure!

6. Be prepared for the need for electron microscopy by having fresh glutaraldehyde available. The utility of electron microscopy has been somewhat supplanted by immunohistochemistry, which however should be considered for unusual primary or metastatic tumors, particularly in the pediatric age range, viral encephalitis, and in some pituitary adenomas, particularly the sparsely granulated somatotrophic adenoma.

7. Any unusual primary brain tumor or soft tissue neoplasm, especially in children, should be considered for cytogenetic analysis whereby certain characteristic deletions or translocations may be of pivotal diagnostic importance. Therefore, culture media should be available for these eventualities.

8. Central nervous system lymphomas should be recognized through intraoperative diagnosis since bulky surgical resection is specifically avoided in most cases due to the morbidity or mortality from the resection of an hemorrhagic and necrotic infiltrative tumor in a deep location. Lymphomas usually but not always appear as dyscohesive sheets of cells without a fibrillar background. Given ample tissue, recognition of lymphomas also presents the opportunity for the pathologist to submit tissue for fluorescence-activated cell sorting analysis.

9. Demyelinating diseases carry both radiographic and histologic features that may closely mimic glial neoplasia. Whenever any of the following observations are made either singly or together, the pathologist should be highly vigilant in suggesting the possibility of demyelinating disease: a ring-enhancing lesion with incomplete C-shaped enhancement, in a periventricular or especially multiple distribution; macrophages; the histologic presence of conspicuous reactive or Creutzfeldt astrocytes; and perivascular lymphocytic cuffing.

10. It is sometimes critically important to distinguish ependymomas from other infiltrating astrocytomas or oligodendrogliomas. Since ependymomas may display a more pushing rather than infiltrative border, they are sometimes truly resectable. This has added importance since it is a major determinant of survival in patients with ependymoma. This is in contrast to infiltrating gliomas in which a surgical resection is essentially incomplete, whereby the attempted resection of any astrocytic neoplasm except the most well-circumscribed WHO Grade I tumors may cause undue surgical injury.

3 BRAIN TUMORS

continued on next page

continued on next page

BRAIN TUMORS – AN OVERVIEW

Jason Karamchandani and Hannes Vogel

Brain tumors are only the tenth most common tumor in adults, accounting for only 1.3% of cancers, but are the seventh leading cause of cancer deaths among adults in developed countries (www.cbtrus.org/reports//2007-2008/2007 supplement.pdf).

Among adults between the ages of 15 and 34 years, high-grade glial neoplasms are the third leading cause of cancer deaths. Brain tumor deaths due to cancer exceed deaths caused by melanoma, nearly equaling those of ovarian cancer (www.cancer.org/downloads/STT/caff2007PWSecured.pdf).

There has been an increase in incidence of primary brain tumors in the elderly, although increasingly sophisticated techniques in neuroimaging may have contributed to the increase in diagnoses (Legler et al., 1999).

Brain tumors are the most common solid tumor in children and the second most frequent cause of cancer death in childhood.

The following graphs depict the age-related incidence of brain tumors. They illustrate the relative rarity of pediatric brain tumors as compared with those occurring in increasing incidence with age. The diagnostician

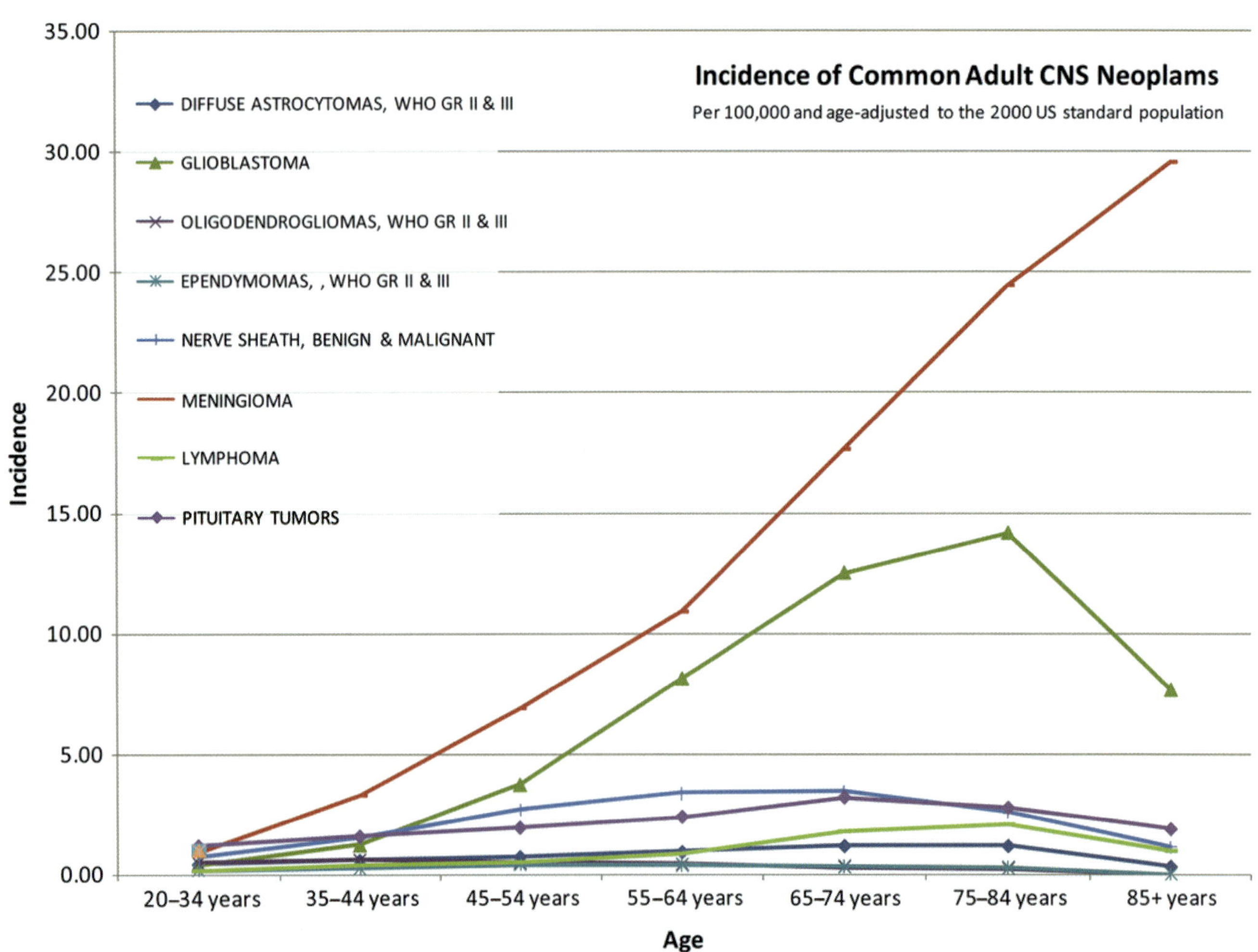

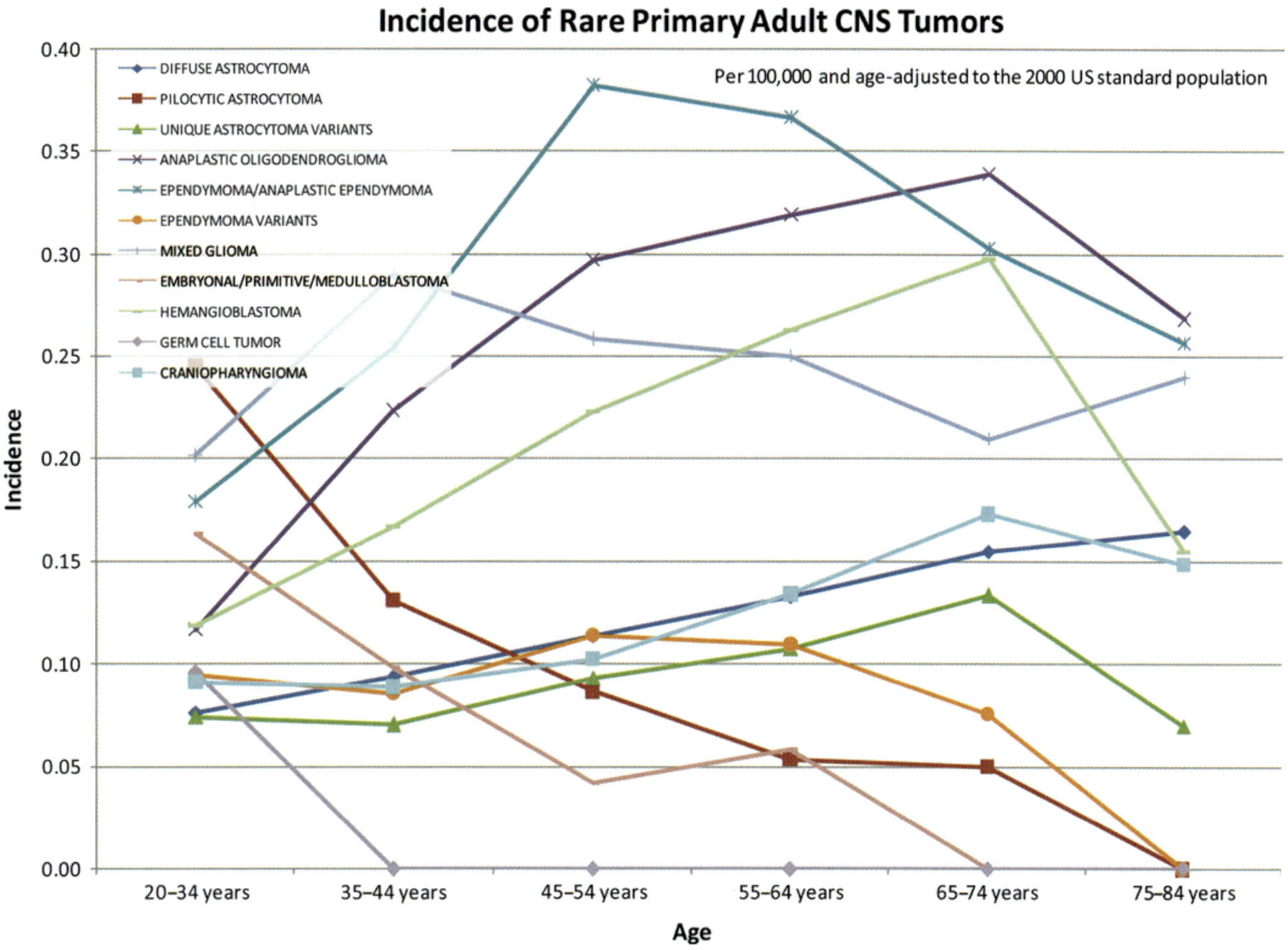

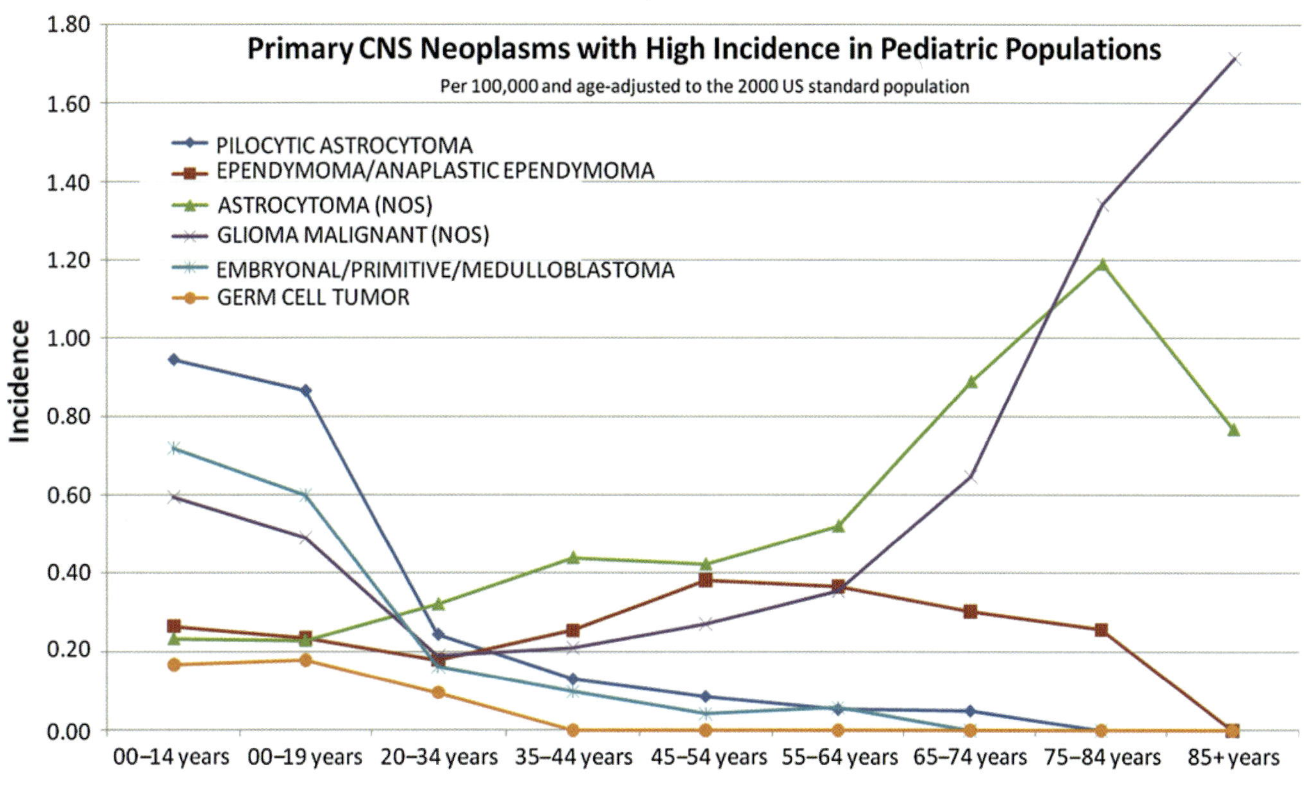
Incidence of Rare Primary Adult CNS Tumors
Per 100,000 and age-adjusted to the 2000 US standard population
DIFFUSE ASTROCYTOMA
PILOCYTIC ASTROCYTOMA
UNIQUE ASTROCYTOMA VARIANTS
ANAPLASTIC OLIGODENDROGLIOMA
EPENDYMOMA/ANAPLASTIC EPENDYMOMA
EPENDYMOMA VARIANTS
MIXED GLIOMA
EMBRYONAL/PRIMITIVE/MEDULLOBLASTOMA
HEMANGIOBLASTOMA
GERM CELL TUMOR
CRANIOPHARYNGIOMA
Incidence
0.40
0.35
0.30
0.25
0.20
0.15
0.10
0.05
0.00
20–34 years
35–44 years
45–54 years
55–64 years
65–74 years
75–84 years
Age

Primary CNS Neoplasms with High Incidence in Pediatric Populations
Per 100,000 and age-adjusted to the 2000 US standard population
PILOCYTIC ASTROCYTOMA
EPENDYMOMA/ANAPLASTIC EPENDYMOMA
ASTROCYTOMA (NOS)
GLIOMA MALIGNANT (NOS)
EMBRYONAL/PRIMITIVE/MEDULLOBLASTOMA
GERM CELL TUMOR
Incidence
1.80
1.60
1.40
1.20
1.00
0.80
0.60
0.40
0.20
0.00
00–14 years
00–19 years
20–34 years
35–44 years
45–54 years
55–64 years
65–74 years
75–84 years
85+ years
Age

Table 3.1. Supratentorial and Dural Tumors

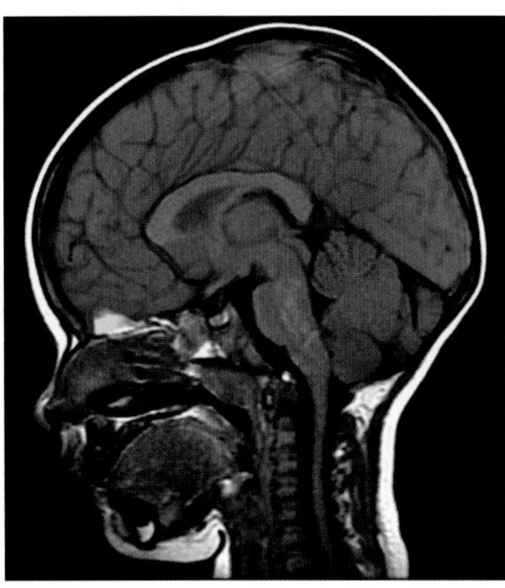

Pediatric	Adult
Parenchymal	
Pilocytic astrocytoma	Glioblastoma
Pleomorphic xanthoastrocytomas	Astrocytomas, WHO Grades II and III
Ganglioglioma	Oligodendroglioma
Ependymoma	Metastases
Astroblastoma	
Angiocentric glioma	
DNT	
Desmoplastic infantile ganglioglioma/astrocytoma (DIG/A)	
Central nervous system primitive neuroepithelial tumor (CNS PNET)	
Atypical teratoid/rhabdoid tumor (AT/RT)	
Dural	
Desmoplastic infantile ganglioglioma/astrocytoma (DIG/A)	Meningioma
	Solitary fibrous tumor/ hemangiopericytoma
Intraventricular/paraventricular	
Ependymoma	Lymphoma
Subependymal giant cell astrocytoma (SEGA)	Central neurocytoma
	Subependymoma
	Chordoid glioma (3rd)
	Colloid cyst (3rd)

Table 3.2. Cerebellar region tumors

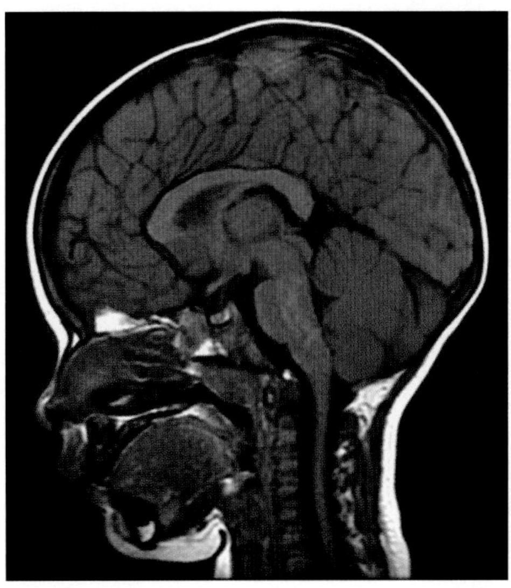

Pediatric	Adult
Parenchymal	
Medulloblastoma	Capillary hemangioblastoma
Pilocytic astrocytoma	Metastases
AT/RT	Liponeurocytoma
Cerebellopontine angle	
Choroid plexus papilloma	Schwannoma
	Meningioma
	Epidermoid cyst
	Choroid plexus papilloma

should be familiar with tumors that occur most commonly at any given age, as well as the tumors most likely to arise in different locations in the nervous system and its coverings. Please note that these data depict primary brain tumors. Overall, *metastatic brain tumors are the most commonly occurring brain tumors in adults*, being a distinct rarity in childhood, with an annual incidence four times greater than that of primary brain tumors. The cancers that most commonly metastasize to the brain are lung and breast carcinomas.

BRAIN TUMOR LOCATIONS WITH RESPECT TO AGE

The accurate radiological and pathological diagnosis of brain tumors requires a working knowledge of the fact that certain brain tumors are linked with specific

Table 3.3. Sellar and suprasellar tumors

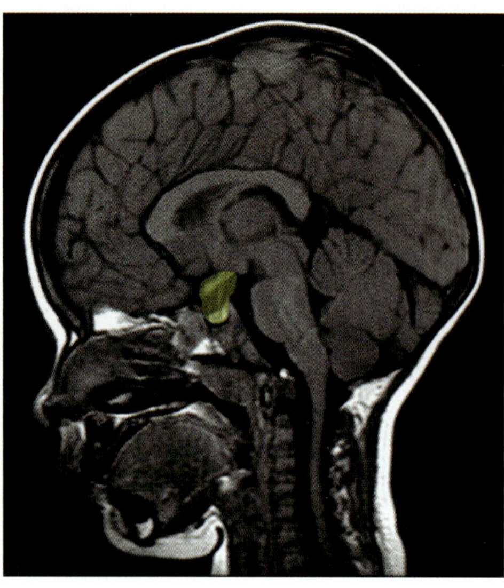

Pediatric	Adult
Sellar/infundibular	
Craniopharyngioma	Pituitary adenoma
Langerhans cell histiocytosis	Meningioma
	Metastases
Suprasellar	
Pilocytic astrocytoma/optic glioma	Papillary craniopharyngioma
Germ cell tumors	
Craniopharyngioma	

locations in the nervous system as well as a particular age range. There are exceptions to this tendency; however, the combined knowledge of the location, radiological features in the context of the age of the patient, and the associated clinical symptoms will often serve to considerably narrow the range of diagnostic possibilities and render others highly unlikely.

GRADING BRAIN TUMORS

Brain tumors are graded, not staged. The grading system is imperfect in the sense that tumors within the WHO Grade IV category may have a drastically different prognosis, such as between the relatively high five-year survival in medulloblastoma within modern therapy versus the significant short-term mortality with glioblastoma, both WHO Grade IV tumors, and both with variations in

Table 3.4. Pineal tumors

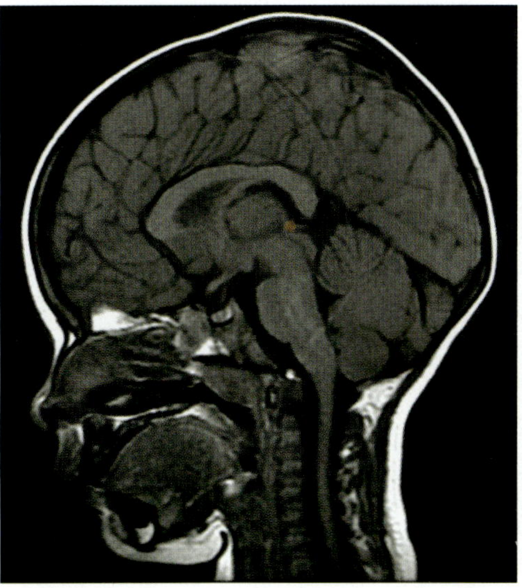

Pediatric	Adult
Germ cell tumors	Pineocytoma
Pineoblastoma	Pineal parenchymal tumor of intermediate differentiation

Table 3.5. Brainstem and fourth ventricular tumors

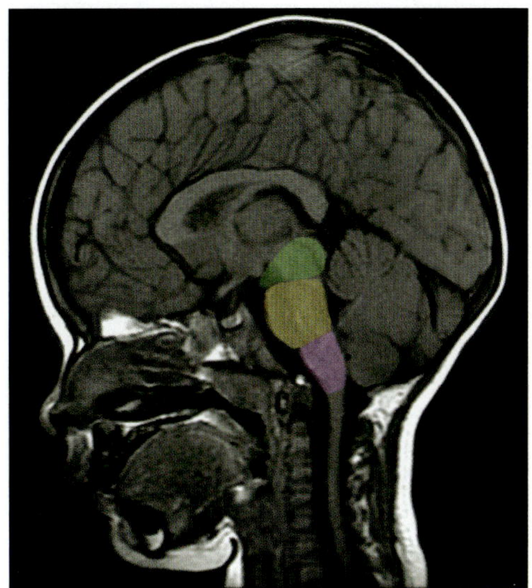

Pediatric	Adult
Brainstem	
Brainstem glioma	
Dorsally exophytic pilocytic astrocytoma	
Ganglioglioma	
Fourth ventricular	
Ependymoma	Subependymoma

Table 3.6. Spinal cord and cauda equina tumors

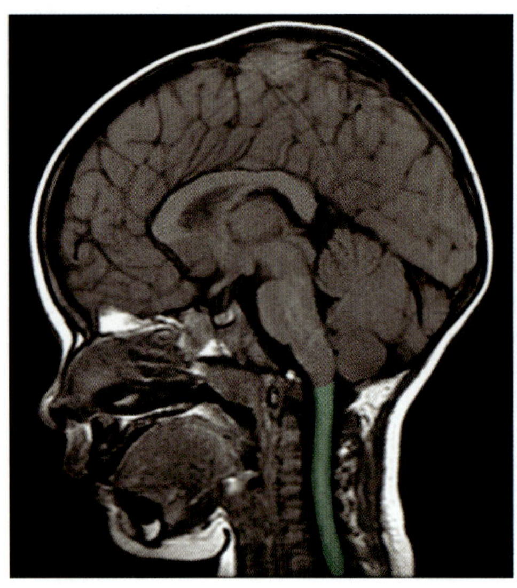

Pediatric	*Adult*
Pilocytic astrocytoma	Meningioma
Ependymoma	Schwannoma

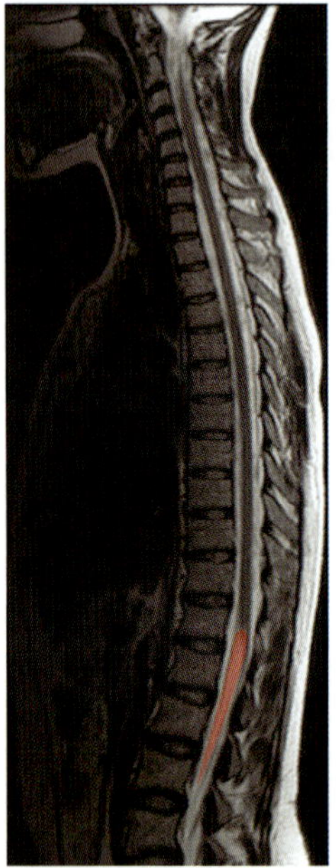

Cauda equina

Myxopapillary ependymoma	Myxopapillary ependymoma
	Schwannoma
	Paraganglioma

molecular biology and outcomes that cannot be codified within any four-tiered grading system.

Because brain tumors are comparatively infrequent as compared with the most common causes of cancer in adults, and because of the lower incidence in general among the pediatric population, it is especially important that brain tumors be included in emerging and cooperative treatment protocols involving novel and increasingly targeted treatment strategies. Many of these studies require a precise and uniform system of nomenclature, and there is nearly universal acceptance of the WHO classification system, which forms the basis for the descriptions in this text. Also, just as with an increasing number of neoplasms of all types, molecular testing is playing an increasingly important role in the assignment of a diagnosis, therapy, and prognosis in certain brain tumors.

A selection of current and authoritative references regarding brain tumors is listed.

SUGGESTED READING

Burger PC. *Tumors of the Central Nervous System*. Washington: Amer Registry of Pathology, 2007.

Burger PC, Scheithauer BW, Vogel FS. *Surgical Pathology of the Nervous System and its Coverings*. New York: Churchill Livingstone, 2002.

Ellison D, Love S. *Neuropathology: A Reference Text of CNS Pathology*. Edinburgh, New York: Mosby, 2004.

Greenfield JG, Love S, Louis DN, Ellison D. *Greenfield's Neuropathology*. London: Hodder Arnold, 2008.

Ironside JW. *Diagnostic Pathology of Nervous System Tumours*. Edinburgh: Churchill Livingstone, 2001.

Legler JM, Ries LA, Smith MA, Warren JL, Heineman EF, Kaplan RS, et al. Cancer surveillance series [corrected]: brain and other central nervous system cancers: recent trends in incidence and mortality. *J Natl Cancer Inst* 1999; 91: 1382–90.

Louis DN, International Agency for Research on Cancer. *WHO Classification of Tumours of the Central Nervous System*. Lyon: International Agency for Research on Cancer, 2007.

NEUROEPITHELIAL

Astrocytic Tumors

Astrocytoma is the general term applied to a diversity of glial tumors spanning WHO Grades I–IV showing cellular features of astrocytes. The subtypes are classified according to their similarity to certain nonneoplastic astrocytes, most commonly fibrillary, occasionally gemistocytic, and rarely protoplasmic. It is essential to recognize the similarities and differences, particularly in nuclear size and morphology between nonneoplastic cells and their neoplastic counterparts.

As with almost all gliomas, a fibrillary background is highly characteristic of astrocytomas, particularly conspicuous in cytological smear preparations as well as in histological sections. When a fibrillary background is absent, an alternative diagnosis should be seriously considered, particularly of lymphoma or metastatic tumor.

The accurate grading of astrocytomas, as in all glial neoplasia, is of paramount importance in assigning the appropriate therapy and prognosis. Grading based strictly upon histological features has been somewhat augmented by molecular and genetic markers (Louis and International Agency for Research on Cancer, 2007). WHO Grade I astrocytomas comprise a very special group within gliomas since they are associated with a distinctly better prognosis over WHO Grade II–IV astrocytomas, and the pilocytic astrocytoma exemplifies this group best. Higher grades are assigned based upon the additive criteria of

- nuclear atypia (WHO Grade II)
- conspicuous mitotic activity (WHO Grade III), and
- vascular proliferation and/or necrosis (WHO Grade IV).

Astrocytic nuclear atypia is difficult to define and requires experience and a keen awareness of the clinical circumstances for which the tissue is being examined. Nuclear atypia may be difficult to recognize when compared with reactive astrocytosis. Astrocytic nuclear atypia is characterized by a comparatively larger nuclear size and nuclear–cytoplasmic ratio, angular nuclear profile as opposed to a smoother or uniformly round or ovoid contour of benign or reactive astrocytes, and nuclear hyperchromasia.

One of the most essential features of both astrocytomas and oligodendrogliomas is their tendency to spread throughout surrounding brain tissue. Other intraaxial tumors, even metastatic tumors, may show the same tendency, but their tendency is to have a "pushing" border that is comparatively sharply demarcated from surrounding, albeit reactive brain tissue (see "Metastatic Tumors"). The pervasive ability for spread by astrocytomas and other neoplasms through gray matter may be seen as the means to overcome a dense barricade of intercellular associations in the form of synaptic and glial–dendritic associations. Infiltrating astrocytomas may be apparent at high-power magnification as single cells within otherwise remarkably intact gray or white matter, sometimes aided by the use of immunohistochemistry for proliferation markers.

Microscopic examples of infiltrating tumor cells are known as *secondary structures of Scherer* (Figure 3.1) (Peiffer and Kleihues, 1999): perineuronal malignant satellitosis, to be distinguished from reactive satellitosis and microglial neuronophagia by the recognition of atypical nuclear morphology of the infiltrating neoplastic astrocytes; as well as perivascular, subependymal, and subpial spread, reflecting the inability for the infiltrating tumor to breach the glia limitans and enter the subarachnoid space. Subarachnoid mounds of tumor are sometimes grossly recognizable to the neurosurgeon on the surface of the brain in open biopsy, thereby indicating the presence of a subjacent tumor.

Microglia have also been shown to potentiate the spread of gliomas. Thus it is not surprising that the overall volume of the most infiltrative of astrocytic tumors, the glioblastoma, may range between 10% and 34% (Badie and Schartner, 2000; Roggendorf et al., 1996).

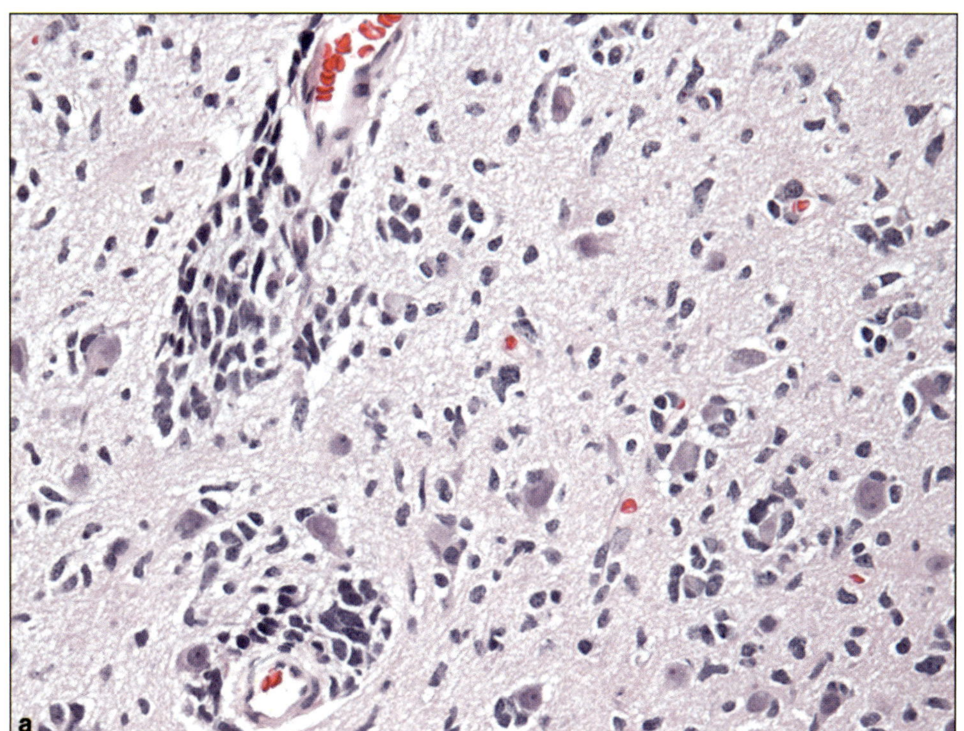

Figure 3.1. (a) Microscopic findings indicative of infiltrating tumor cells are known as *secondary structures of Scherer*, atypical astrocytic nuclei surrounding cortical neurons and microvasculature. (b) Subpial mounds of tumor develop after the neoplastic astrocytes have infiltrated the entire thickness of the cortex to the surface of the brain.

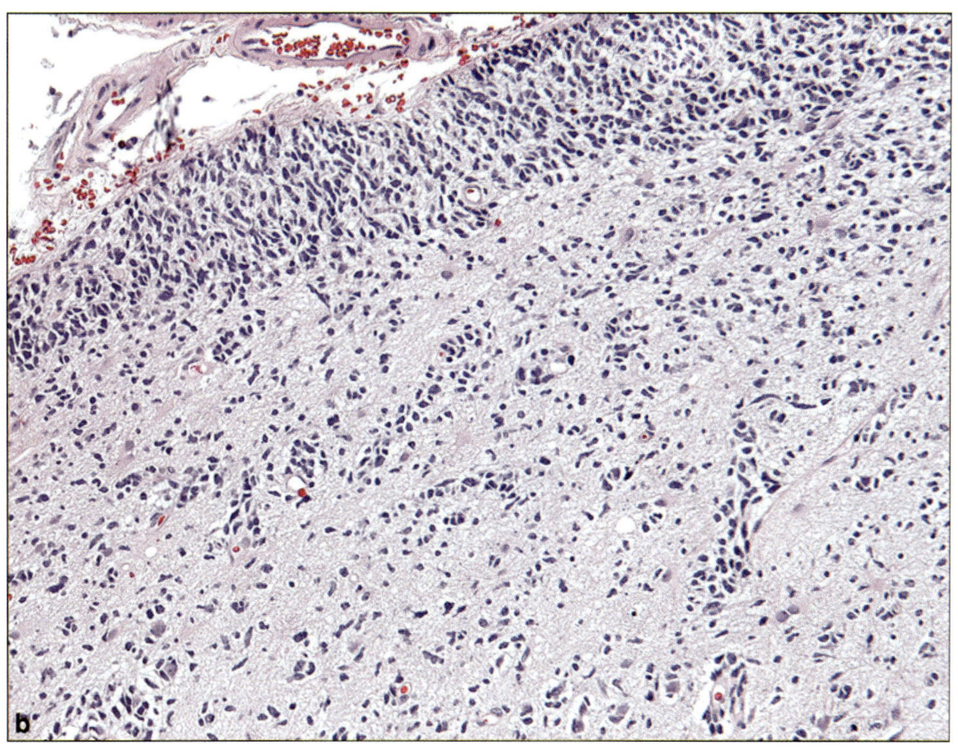

The 2007 WHO Classification of Brain Tumours (Louis and International Agency for Research on Cancer, 2007) includes nine types of astrocytoma of WHO Grades I through IV. The principal challenge that arises in assigning a diagnosis to an astrocytoma is the determination of grade and separation from reactive gliosis, mixed gliomas, oligoastrocytoma, and glioneuronal tumors in particular. The assignment of a single unifying grade may be difficult when there may be a range of cellularity and other diagnostic features within the same large resection specimen, or conversely, the lack of a clear grade when the biopsy is very small, thus not necessarily representative of the tumor as a whole. Thus, a single mitotic figure in a small biopsy may warrant the assignment of WHO Grade III anaplastic astrocytoma whereas the infrequent mitotic figure in an astrocytoma whose cellularity and lack of contrast enhancement may be more in keeping with WHO Grade II.

The WHO 2007 classification maintained a strict avoidance of the term "low grade" since a WHO Grade II diffuse astrocytoma has an entirely different prognosis from a WHO Grade I astrocytoma, epitomized by the pilocytic astrocytoma, which is often cured by surgery and amenable to surgical reresection of recurrent tumor.

WHO GRADE I

Pilocytic Astrocytoma

The pilocytic astrocytoma is one of the most enigmatic of gliomas and one that can be misdiagnosed if radiological data as well as the myriad histological appearances are not appreciated. Though once called juvenile pilocytic astrocytoma, complete awareness of this entity indicates that it is at times neither juvenile nor uniformly pilocytic, referring to the hairlike slender or "unipolar" cells often seen in the tumor.

Clinical and Radiological Features

Pilocytic astrocytomas are most common in childhood with a peak incidence in the first two decades of life and are more common in males. They may also occur well into later adulthood. They are the principal central nervous system (CNS) neoplasm associated with NF1 (Louis and International Agency for Research on Cancer, 2007).

The pilocytic astrocytoma may occur in all corners of the CNS; however, is it most common in the posterior fossa and optic–hypothalamic region. In the posterior fossa, it is frequently found as a large cerebellar cystic lesion, but solid types may arise as dorsally exophytic lesions of the brainstem. Spinal cord pilocytic astrocytomas may lack microcystic changes (Burger, 2007) and may be especially difficult to distinguish from either reactive gliosis in the setting of an adjacent ependymoma or hemangioblastoma, or a WHO Grade II fibrillary astrocytoma.

Pilocytic astrocytomas are often cystic by radiological imaging and show bright contrast enhancement (Figure 3.2a), to the extent that the pathologist should exercise considerable hesitation before diagnosing pilocytic astrocytoma in the absence of this feature. Contrast enhancement is a finding usually

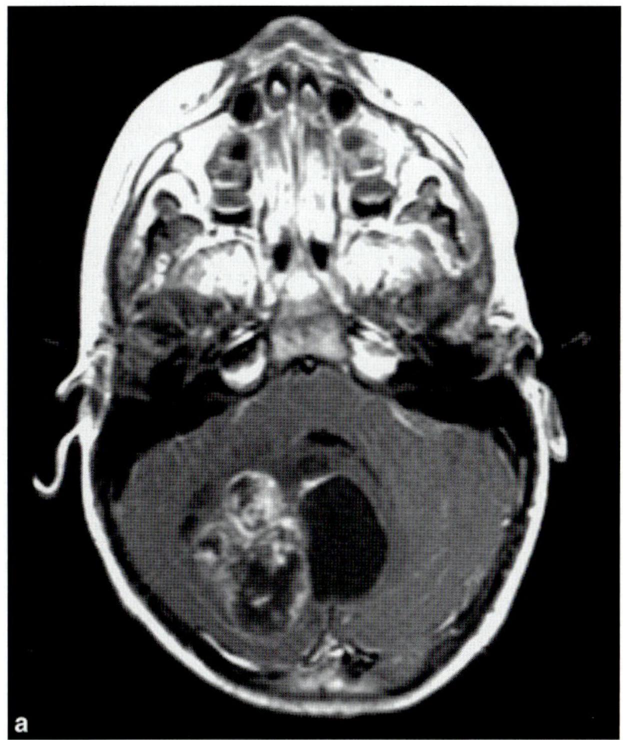

Figure 3.2. (a) Pilocytic astrocytomas are often cystic by radiological imaging and essentially always show bright contrast enhancement. Varied microscopic appearances of pilocytic astrocytomas. (b) Classic low-magnification biphasic pattern with microcysts.

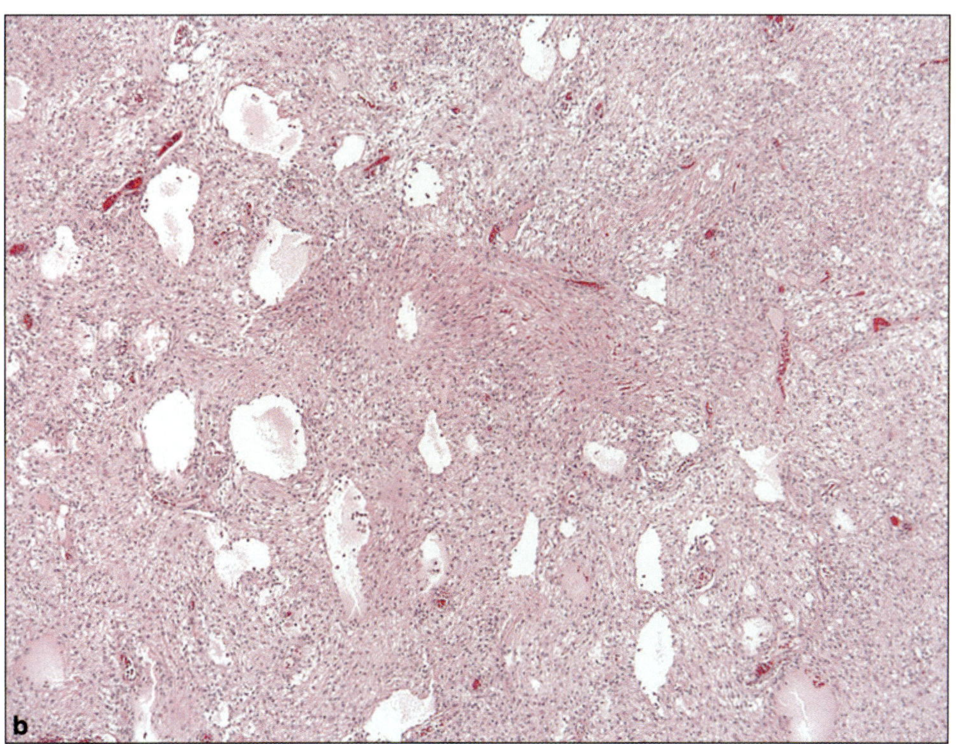

associated with increasing grade in gliomas; thus it may seem paradoxical that the most "benign" of astrocytomas shows this feature. This is most likely due to the rich vasculature seen in the pilocytic astrocytoma as well as WHO Grade I examples of the closely related ganglioglioma.

Figure 3.2. *continued*
(c) Multinucleate celsls.
(d) Clear cell differentiation.

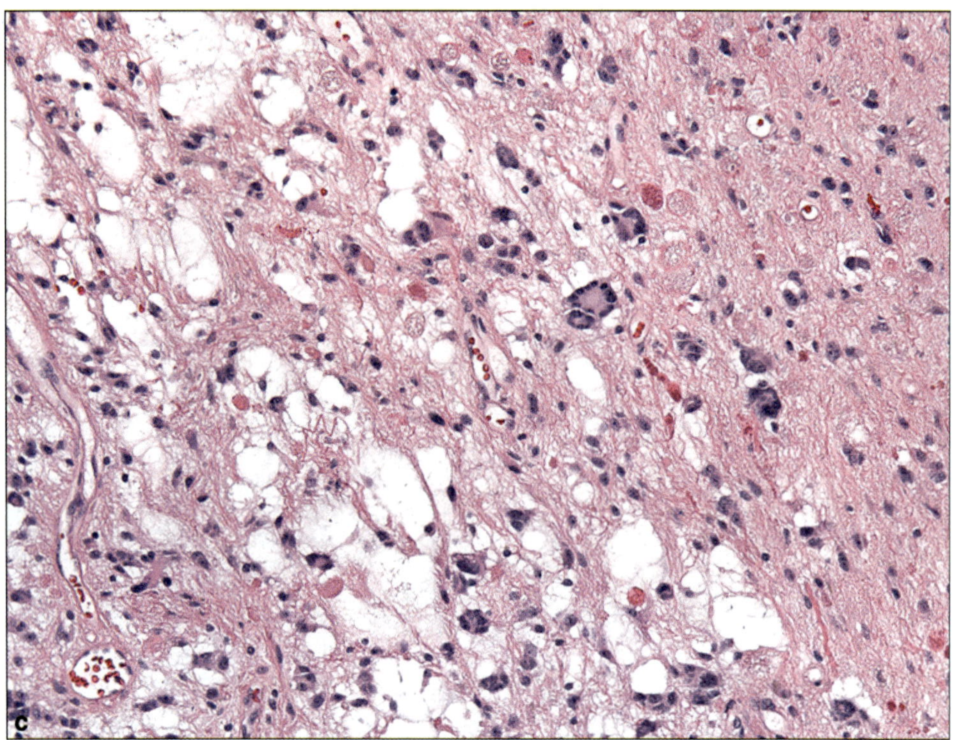

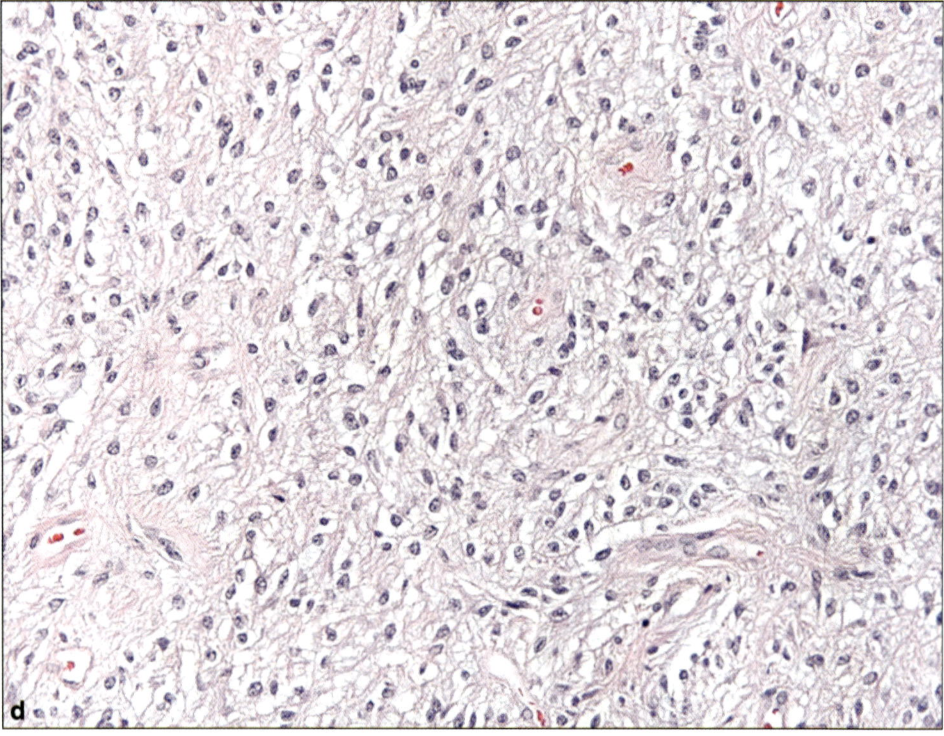

Pathology

The pilocytic astrocytoma displays a tan-pink color with a distinctly mucoid
texture, often recognizable even in the smallest specimens. Pilocytic astrocytomas
should, of course, be familiar to the diagnostician in their classical microscopic
patterns, but failure to be aware of its many and varied histological patterns can

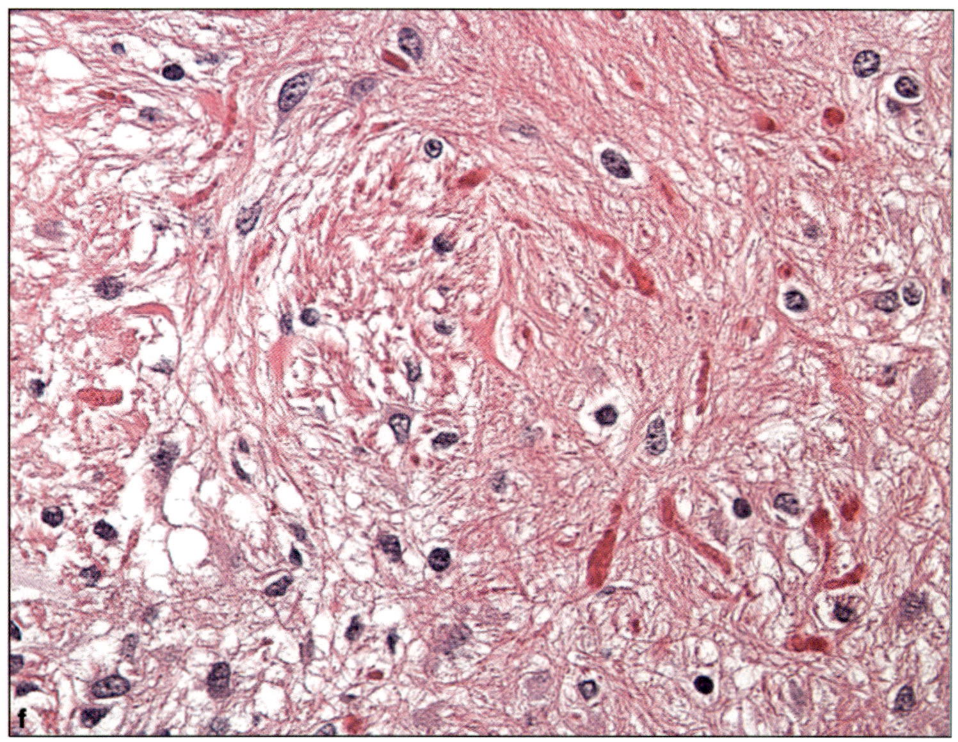

Figure 3.2. *continued*
(e) Prominent vasculature.
(f) Rosenthal fibers.

lead to misdiagnosis of a higher grade glioma. The most classic appearance of the pilocytic astrocytoma is of a microcystic tumor with a rich fibrillary background that shows a *biphasic pattern*, alternating between dense eosinophilic vasocentric regions and looser intervening areas (Figure 3.2b,c).

Figure 3.2. *continued*
(g) Eosinophilic Granular
Body (EGB) (left field).
(h) Both Rosenthal fibers in
denser areas and EGB in
looser area.

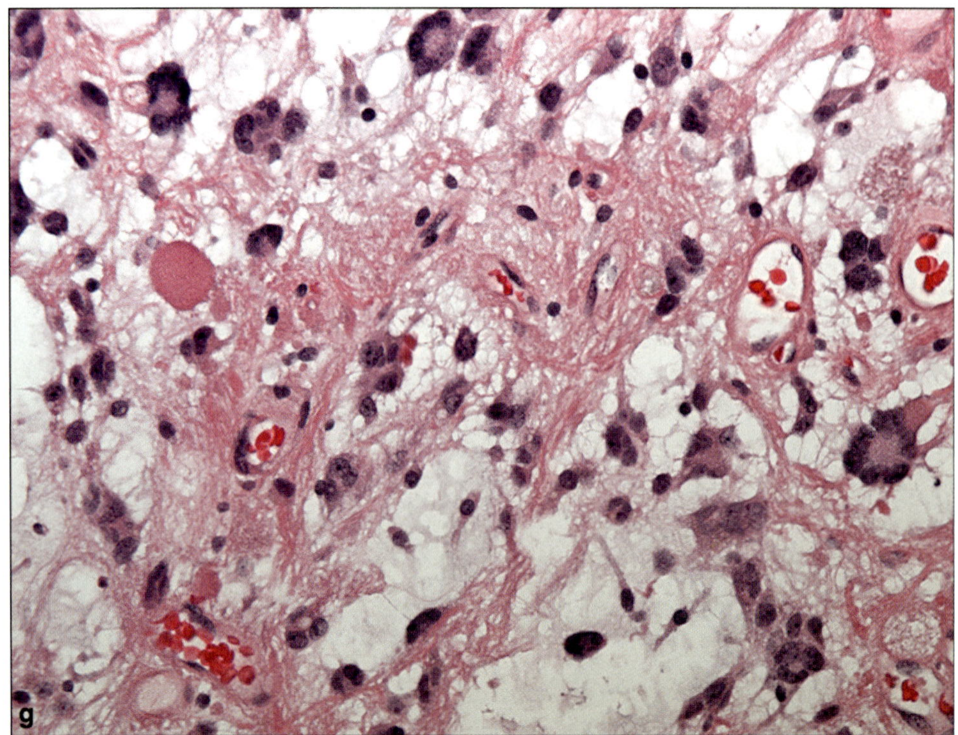

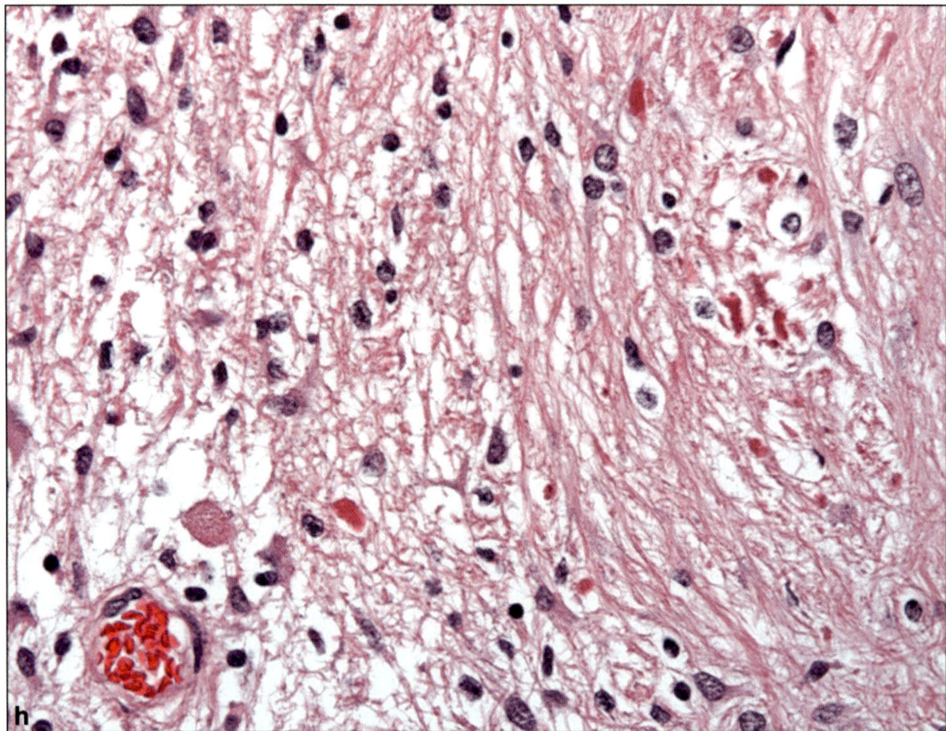

Either of the patterns may dominate the microscopic representation of the specimen; thus the dense or compact differentiation when unaccompanied by looser areas is especially prone to misdiagnosis as a diffuse fibrillary astrocytoma. At the cytological level, the classic cell is an elongated profile ("piloid" or hairlike) with a benign ovoid nucleus. *Multinucleated cells* may be prominent (Figure 3.2c). *Clear cell differentiation* may be extensive, sometimes indistinguishable

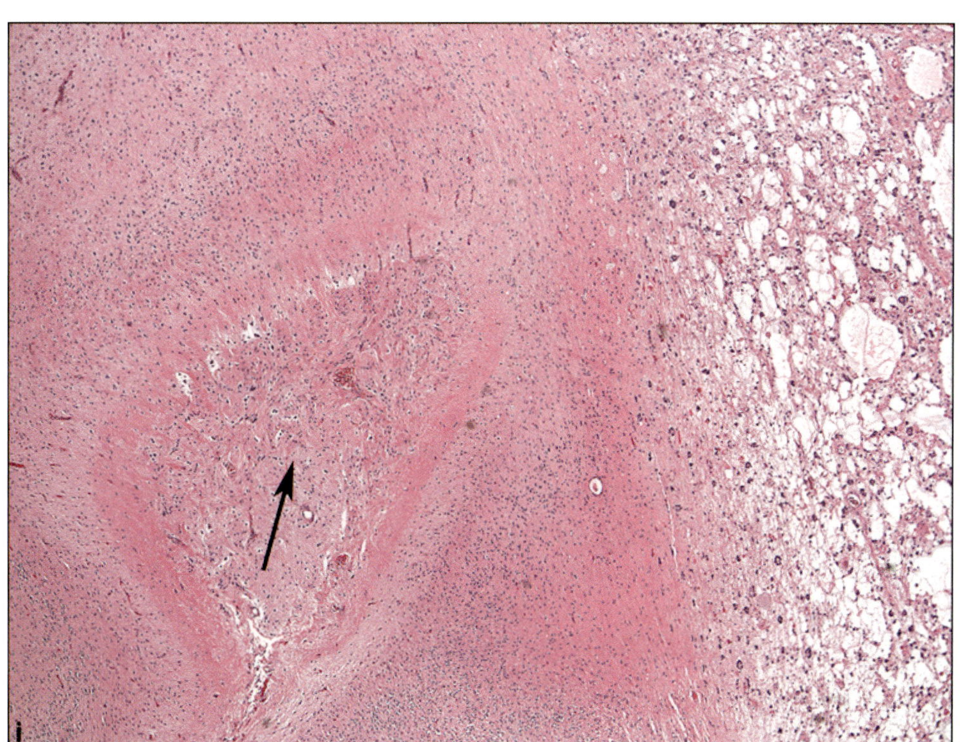

Figure 3.2. *continued*
(i,j) Subarachnoid spread
(arrows).

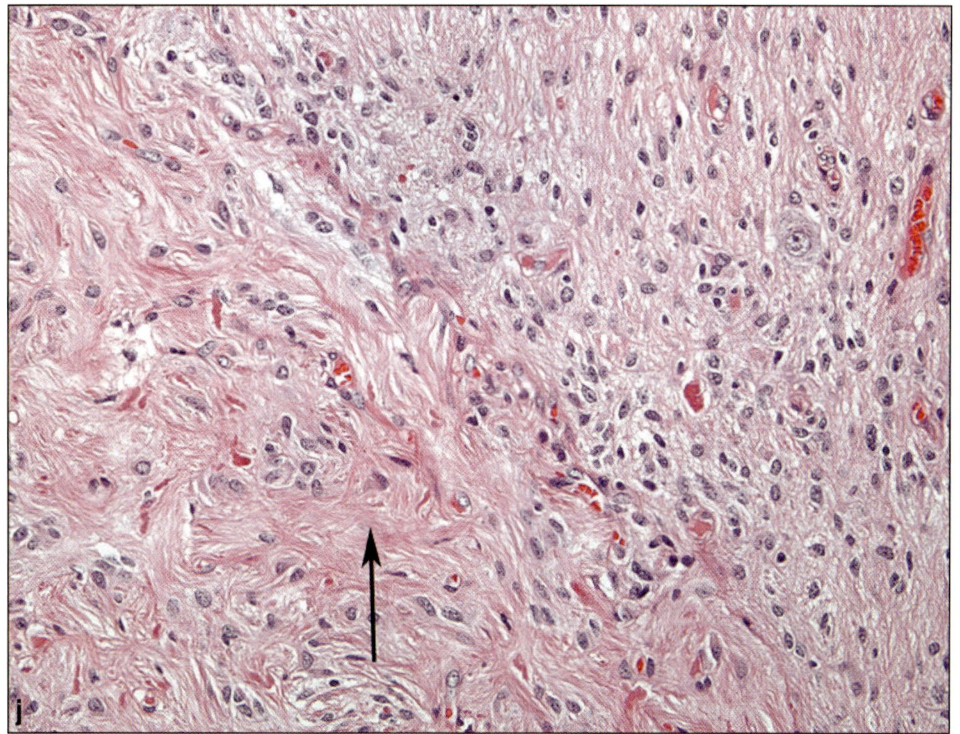

from that of oligodendrogliomas (Figure 3.2d). Considering the distinct rarity of oligodendrogliomas in the anatomic sites in which pilocytic astrocytomas most commonly occur, a clear cell tumor in the posterior fossa or optic–hypothalamic area is in fact more likely to be a pilocytic astrocytoma.

Vascular proliferation, although not identical to the glomeruloid type seen in high-grade gliomas, is characteristic and may be one of the most useful features, along with contrast enhancement, in distinguishing the pilocytic astrocytoma from a WHO Grade II diffuse astrocytoma (Figure 3.2e). Mitotic activity is very unusual, and when division figures are identified, they are often in vascular endothelial cells.

Rosenthal fibers are eosinophilic elongated or beaded structures are also quite useful in securing the diagnosis of pilocytic astrocytoma (Figure 3.2f); however, caution should be exercised since they are a frequent finding in smoldering chronic gliosis and especially in the reactive milieu within brain tissue surrounding other tumors, notably the craniopharyngioma or capillary hemangioblastoma.

Eosinophilic granular bodies (EGBs) are composed of a number of substances also found in Rosenthal fibers and are thus conceptually related to Rosenthal fibers (Figure 3.2g,h), although the former are more frequent in loose areas, while Rosenthal fibers are found in denser compact areas. Both share immunoreactivity for glial fibrillary acidic protein (GFAP), ubiquitin and αB crystallin (Murayama et al., 1992). While true eosinophilic granular bodies are an invaluable diagnostic aid in recognizing pilocytic astrocytomas (and gangliogliomas and pleomorphic xanthoastrocytomas), mimicry does occur, most often as granular cells in oligodendrogliomas or as imposters in glioblastomas (Sasaki et al., 2001).

Local *subarachnoid spread* is quite common in pilocytic astrocytomas and carries no value in predicting remote cerebrospinal fluid spread (Figure 3.2i,j). Nonetheless, the most sinister event in an otherwise typical case of pilocytic astrocytoma is remote subarachnoid spread, especially to the cauda equina.

The pilocytic astrocytoma is the quintessential WHO Grade I glioma; however, "malignant" forms apparently exist, marked by numerous mitotic figures, robust vascular proliferation, and even pseudopalisading necrosis. Notwithstanding these disconcerting features, such lesions should be designated "anaplastic" or WHO Grade III.

Pilocytic astrocytomas are GFAP positive, but this immunostain should be considered superfluous in the light of the distinctive histological features of a pilocytic astrocytoma. Staining for p53 has also been proposed as a means of distinguishing the typically p53-negative pilocytic astrocytoma from often p53-immunopositive WHO Grade II diffuse astrocytoma (Ishii et al., 1998).

Subependymal Giant Cell Astrocytoma

Clinical and Radiological Features

Subependymal giant cell astrocytomas (SEGA) have even been reported in neonates but occur more commonly into childhood and early adulthood. They are often associated with tuberous sclerosis; however, isolated examples exist without this association (Sinson et al., 1994), which may also represent a form fruste of the disease (Boesel et al., 1979). These lesions grow steadily but are usually amenable to surgical debulking.

They most commonly present as a mass originating near the foramen of Munro with protrusion into the corresponding lateral ventricle. Smaller

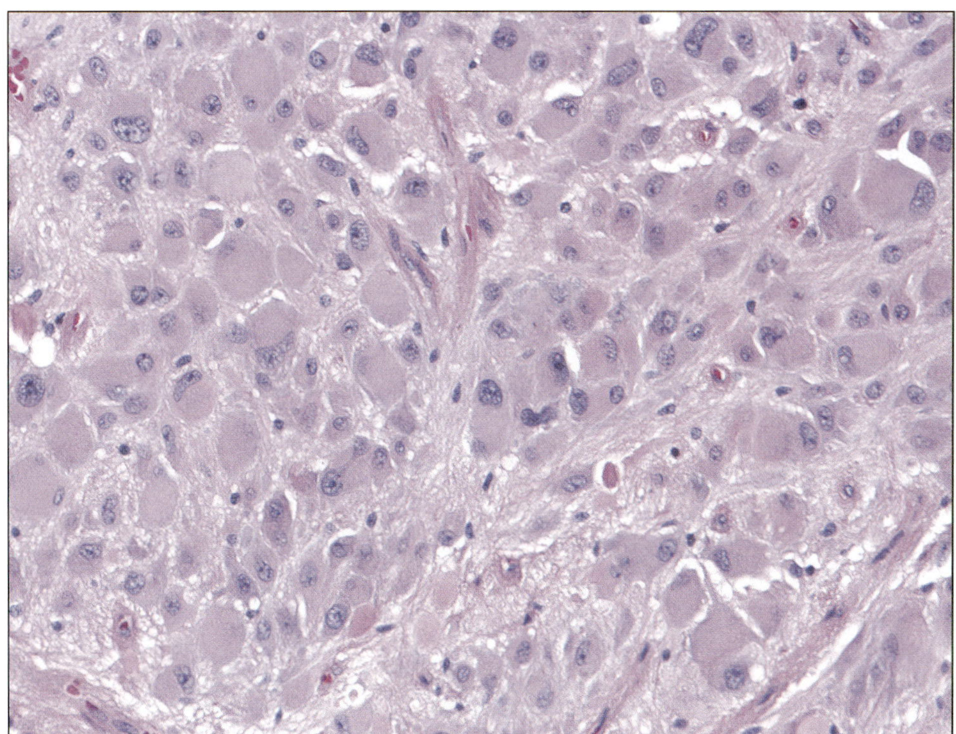

Figure 3.3. The essential feature of SEGAs is the presence of large cells with hybrid features between gemistocytic astrocytes, with eccentric eosinophilic cytoplasm, and neurons, with large round nuclei bearing prominent nucleoli.

coexistent subependymal nodules may also be detected. They show contrast enhancement and are often calcified by computed tomography (CT) scanning.

Pathology

SEGA is composed of large cells, sometimes in sheets or loose clusters, bearing hybrid features between astrocytes and neurons, with their large round nuclei and prominent nucleoli, and voluminous eosinophilic cytoplasm causing nuclear displacement (Figure 3.3). This finding can lead to a confusing similarity with gemistocytic astrocytes. Because of the hybrid astrocytic and neuronal nature of these cells, an alternative term for this lesion is *subependymal giant cell tumor* (Nakamura and Becker, 1983).

Calcification is not unusual. Vasculature is sometimes quite prominent and significant hemorrhage can herald a sudden increase in size and symptoms of ventricular obstruction (Kim et al., 2001). Mitotic activity and necrosis are distinctly rare, which, however, should not be interpreted as malignant features (Shepherd et al., 1991). The existence of malignant transformation is debatable; however, the extremely rare instance of craniospinal dissemination of a SEGA with an increased proliferative index has been reported (Telfeian et al., 2004).

BRAINSTEM GLIOMA

The brainstem, particularly in the pediatric age group, may be involved by astrocytomas in one of two dramatically different ways. Both types of tumors may cause subtle and indolent clinical signs, such as cranial nerve VI palsy, or the consequences of obstructive hydrocephalus from narrowing of the fourth ventricle (Figure 3.4). Pilocytic astrocytomas may originate in the brainstem, often from the

Figure 3.4. Brainstem glioma (diffuse fibrillary). (a) A sagittal T1 contrast-enhanced MR image of the brain shows infiltrative enlargement of the pons. The fourth ventricle is compressed, and there is no abnormal enhancement.
(b) An axial T2 image shows diffuse abnormal signal throughout the enlarged pons. The basilar artery is partially encircled. Brainstem gliomas typically minimally enhance or do not enhance and will often partially encircle the basilar artery. If there is enhancement at the time of diagnosis, it is thought to portend a poorer prognosis.
Rhomboencephalitis and demyelinating disease, which can have a similar appearance, should be carefully excluded clinically as brainstem gliomas are usually treated presumptively without biopsy.

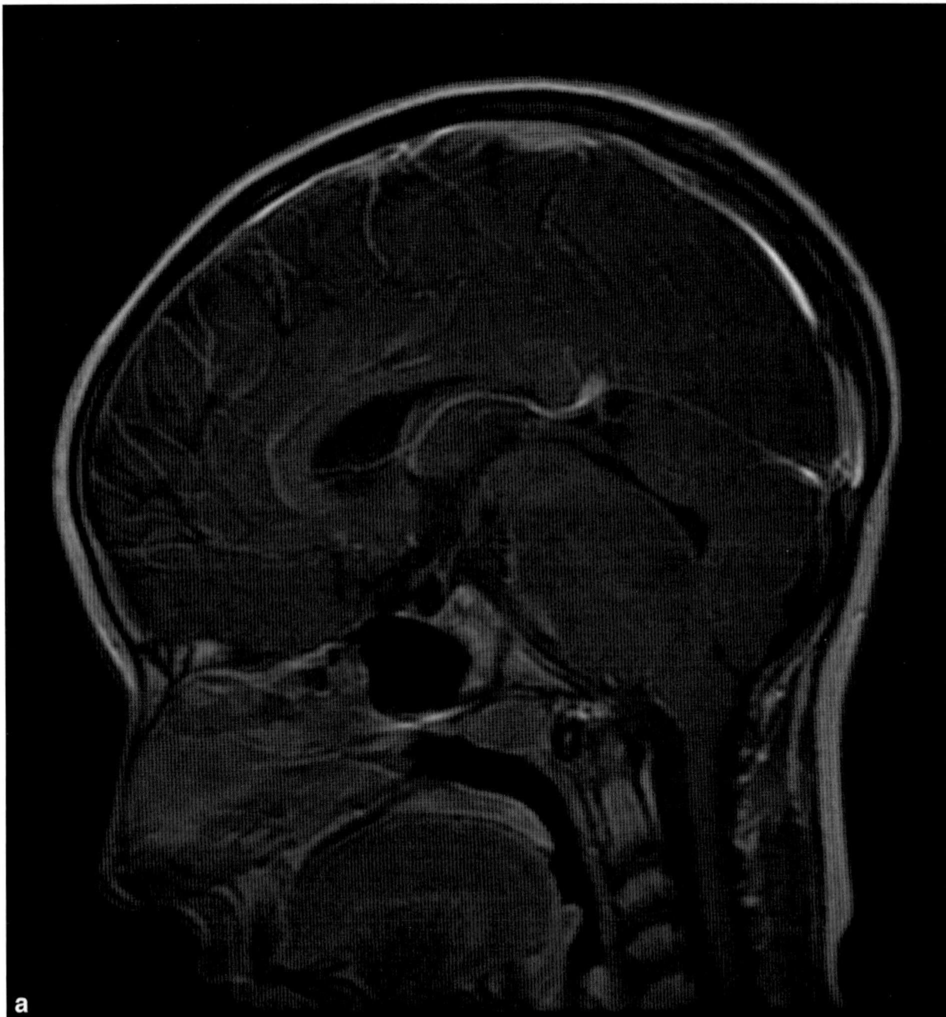

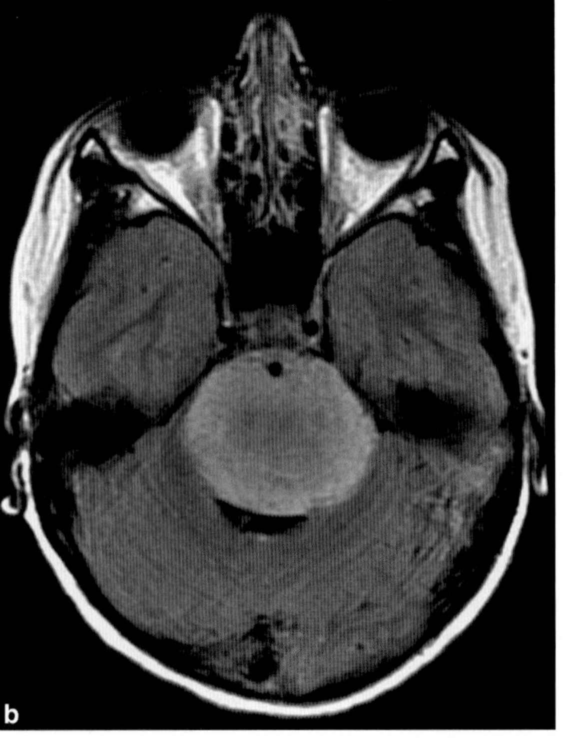

pontomedullary junction, as a dorsally exophytic tumor with the neuroimaging and histological features typical of ordinary pilocytic astrocytoma, although limited sampling may complicate the recognition of this tumor. In contrast, fibrillary astrocytomas ranging may arise within the pons and cause diffuse expansion. Pathological studies are few, owing to the rarity of biopsy, but all grades of fibrillary astrocytoma from WHO Grade II through IV may be present although the majority are probably WHO Grade II (Burger, 1996; Selvapandian et al., 1999).

Survival in cases of dorsally exophytic brainstem gliomas is comparable to that of pilocytic astrocytomas in other locations, depending upon the degree of surgical respectability. Patients with brainstem gliomas of the centrally expansile type rarely survive past two years.

WHO GRADE II

Clinical and Radiological Features

WHO Grade II diffuse astrocytomas occur predominantly in early adulthood but may occur at any age and location in the CNS (Figure 3.5a,b).

Pathology

WHO Grade II diffuse astrocytomas are wholly distinct from WHO Grade I gliomas, and thus the precaution that the term "low grade" be avoided in reference to either lesion to avoid confusion between the two. WHO Grade II diffuse astrocytomas are comprised of three types: *fibrillary*, *gemistocytic*, and *protoplasmic*. These may be at times difficult to distinguish from reactive gliosis associated with a host of nonneoplastic causes ranging from subacute conditions such as the wall of either an abscess or infarction to various chronic gliotic conditions. Mitotic activity or even a certain degree of cytological atypia and pleomorphism may not be reliable in distinguishing these astrocytomas.

All WHO Grade II astrocytomas display a degree of nuclear atypia that includes hyperchromasia, angular or irregular nuclear shapes, and an abnormal increase in nuclear–cytoplasmic ratio although this may be highly subjective. Microglial activation may also be very much a part of the microscopic appearance of any astrocytoma. The background in astrocytomas is not as likely to include neuropil except at the infiltrating border, as compared with reactive gliosis. Vascular proliferation is not a feature of WHO Grade II astrocytomas. Mitotic figures are rare, and if found in a small biopsy, should in and of itself shift the grade from II to anaplastic WHO Grade III.

Fibrillary Astrocytoma

This is the most frequent histologic type of astrocytoma overall, characterized by a delicate fibrillar background formed by an array of fibrillary neoplastic astrocytes, sometimes of a cellularity not much greater than that seen in reactive

Figure 3.5. (a) T1 MRI with contrast enhancement of a temporal lobe WHO Grade II diffuse astrocytoma example is predominantly hypointense with minimal focal contrast enhancement. Greater contrast enhancement should suggest a higher grade in at least a portion of the tumor. (b) Greater T2 signal in the same lesion.

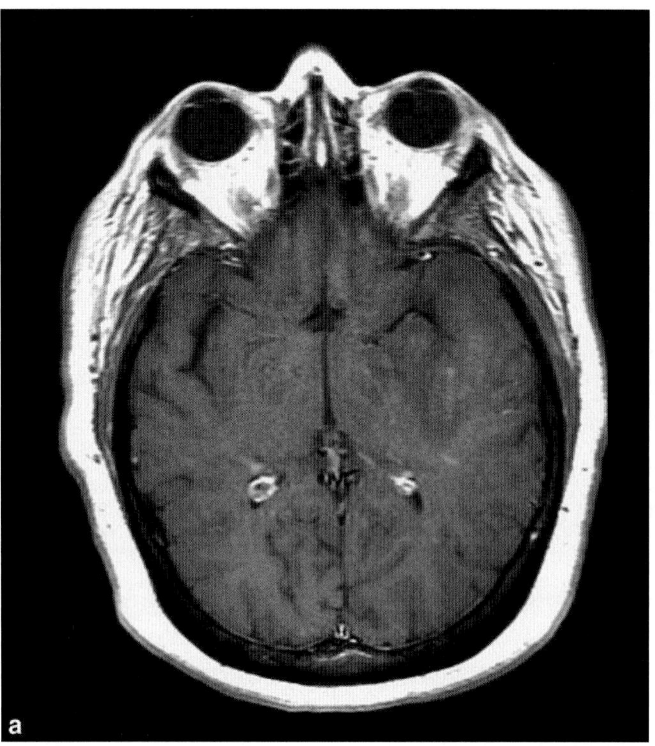

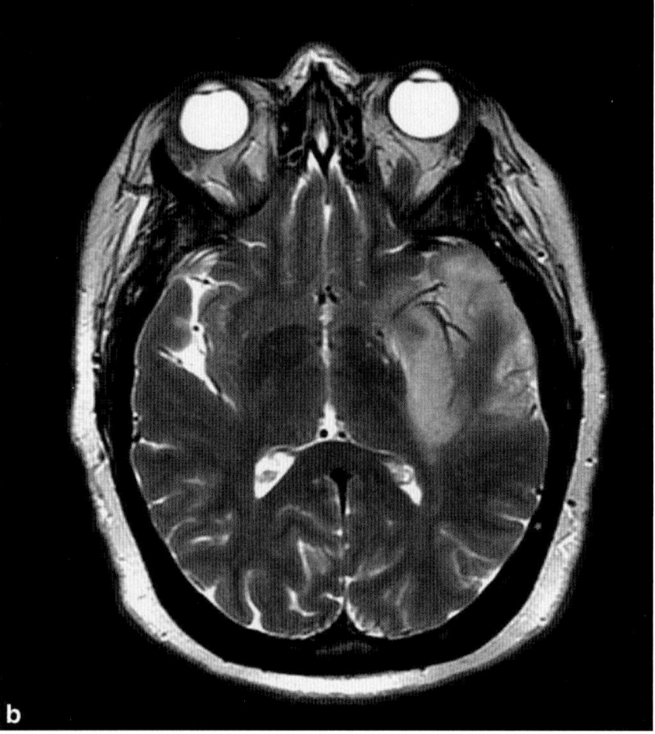

astrocytic proliferations (Figure 3.5c–i). Careful observation of nuclear features will allow these entities to be distinguished in most cases. Microcysts are common and focal gemistocytic differentiation may be seen. Mitotic figures are distinctly rare; however, large resections may show occasional examples. A MIB-1 labeling index is usually less than 5% (Jaros et al., 1992).

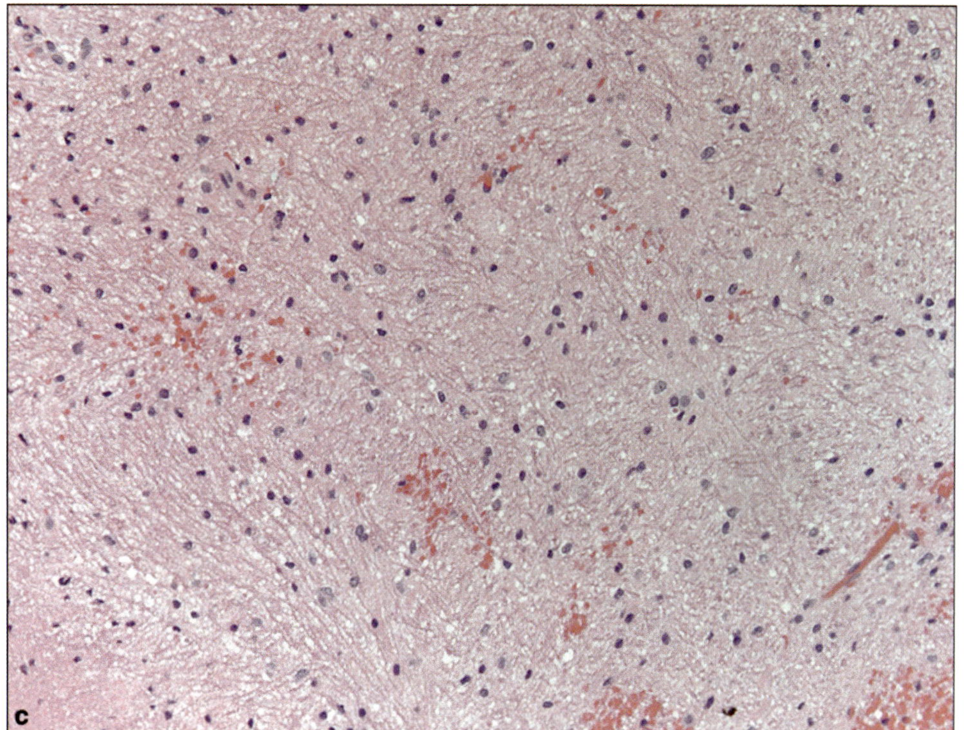

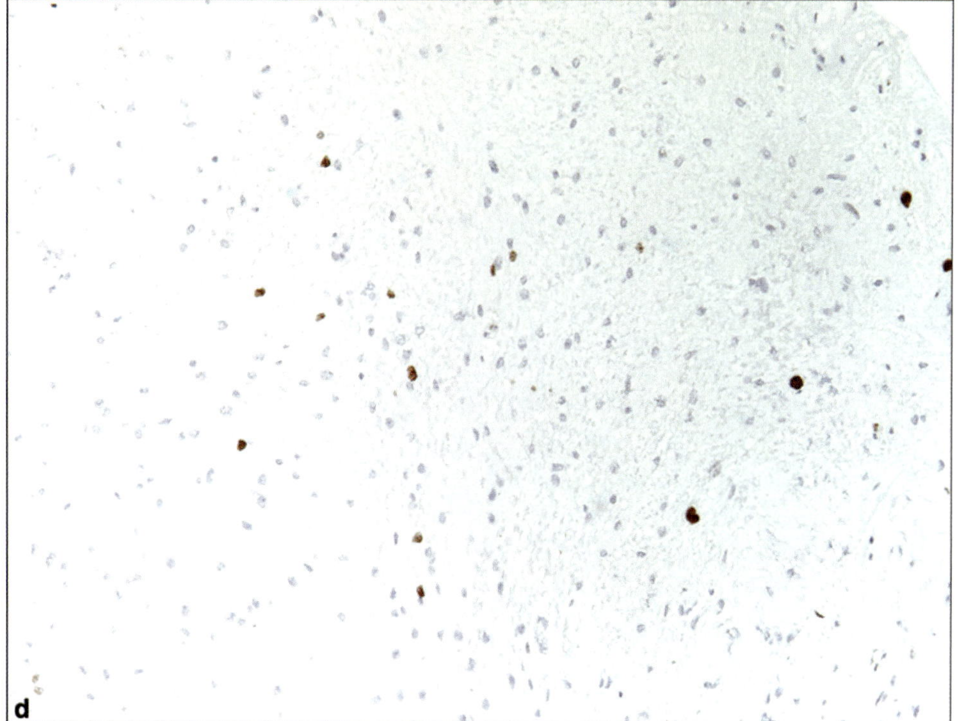

Figure 3.5. *continued*
(c) Regions with infiltrating WHO Grade II astrocytomas can represent a significant diagnostic challenge, especially in frozen sections, at which time the diagnostician is urged to avoid speculation in the face of no obvious neoplasm.
(d) MIB-1 staining for proliferating cells in the same region may highlight infiltrating cells, (e) seen at higher magnification, with enlarged atypical nuclei staining positively.
(f) Cytological squash preparation of diffuse astrocytoma, with fibrillar background and atypical nuclear features. (g) Low magnification view of WHO Grade II diffuse astrocytoma, showing disorganized array of mildly pleomorphic astrocytic cells in a fibrillar background. (h) Higher magnification shows delicate vasculature and absence of noticeable mitotic activity (i) and a tendency for microcystic change.

Fibrillary astrocytomas are uniformly GFAP positive although nuclei without prominent cytoplasm may appear immunonegative. As in all astrocytomas, care should be exercised in recognizing typically and strongly GFAP positive reactive astrocytes. It has been stated that neoplastic astrocytes possess thick or stubby processes as compared with the slender and elongated processes of reactive astrocytes, and GFAP immunohistochemistry may be useful in making this distinction.

Figure 3.5. *continued.*

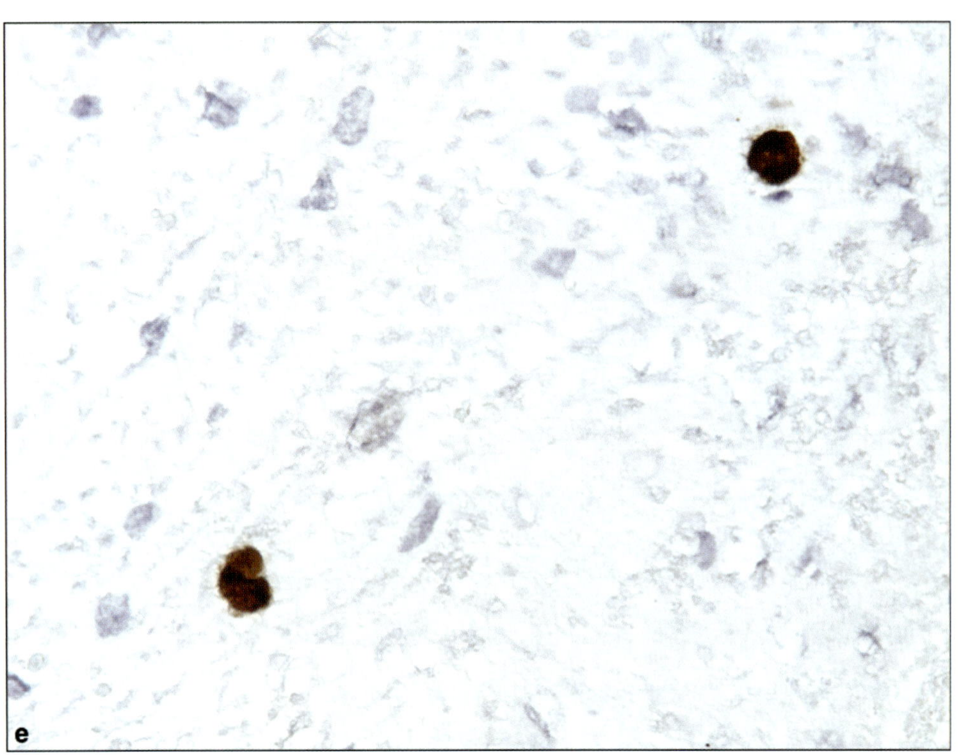

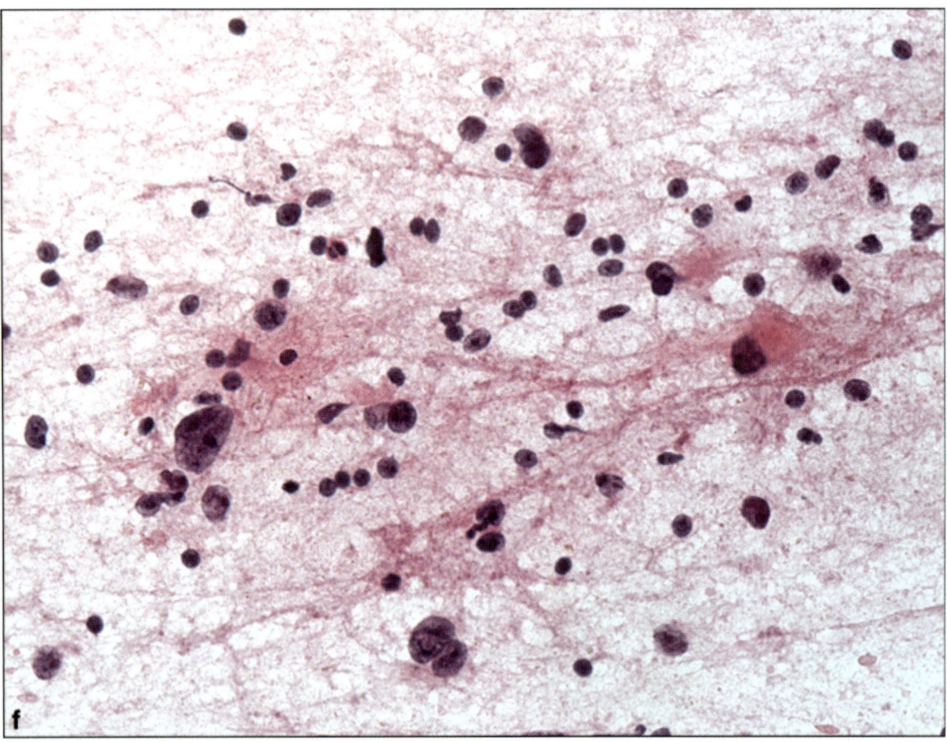

Gemistocytic Astrocytoma

The gemistocytic astrocytoma recapitulates the appearance of reactive gemistocytic astrocytes, with a large homogeneous eosinophilic cytoplasmic mass and nuclear displacement. This type of astrocytoma has traditionally carried a stigma of aggressive growth and evolution into glioblastoma (Schiffer et al., 1988). Neoplastic

Figure 3.5. *continued.*

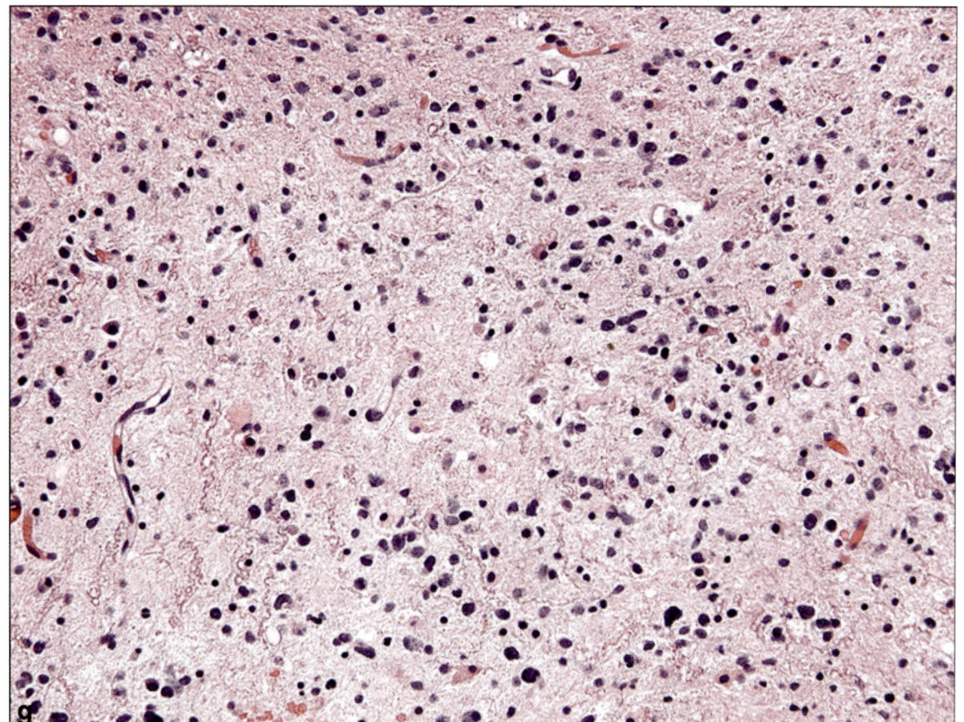

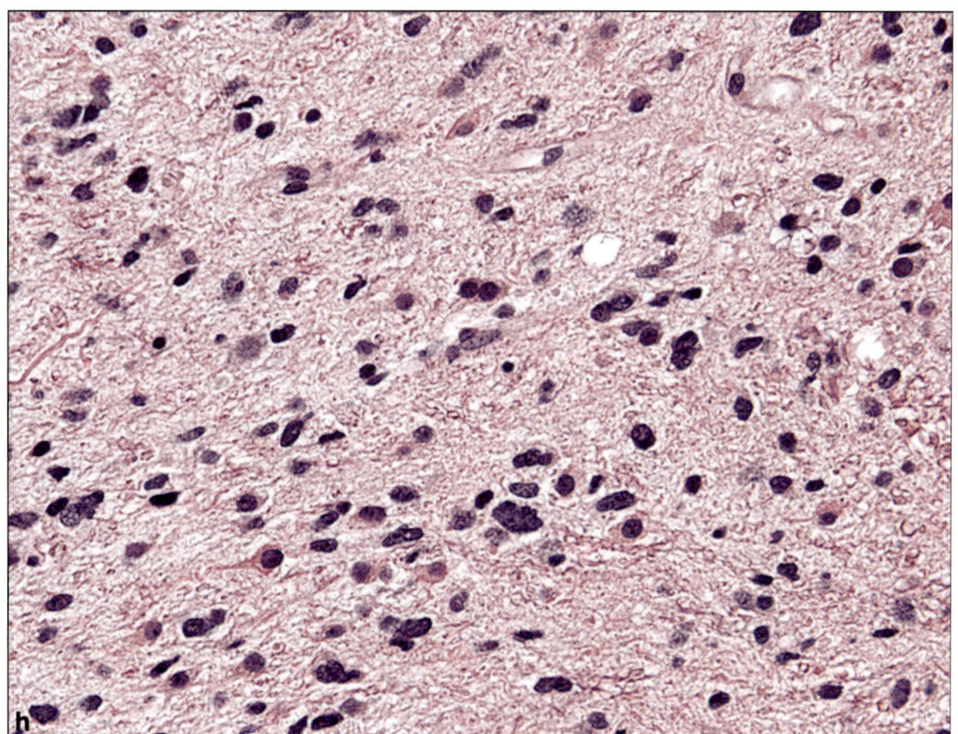

gemistocytes show the nuclear atypia typical of astrocytomas, that is, nuclear enlargement, hyperchromasia, and nuclear membrane irregularity (Figure 3.6). Mitotic activity is not necessarily a reliable criterion in distinguishing reactive from neoplastic astrocytic proliferation, unless the mitotic figure is distinctly atypical.

Figure 3.5. *continued.*

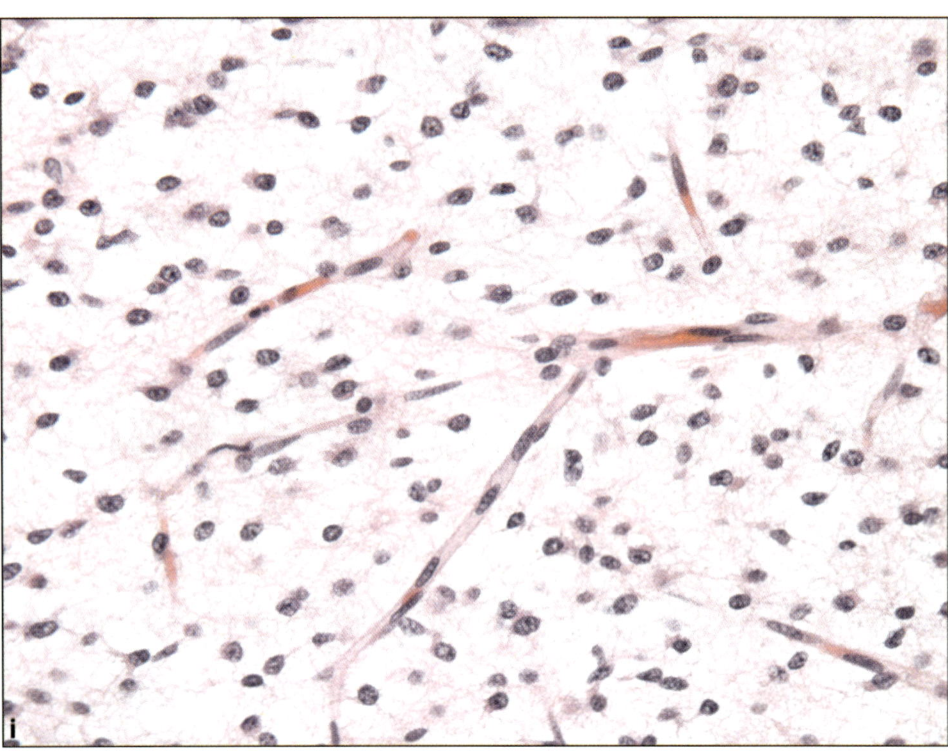

Figure 3.6. Gemistocytic
astrocytoma. (a) Cytological
preparation shows pervasive
fibrillar background common
to most gliomas.

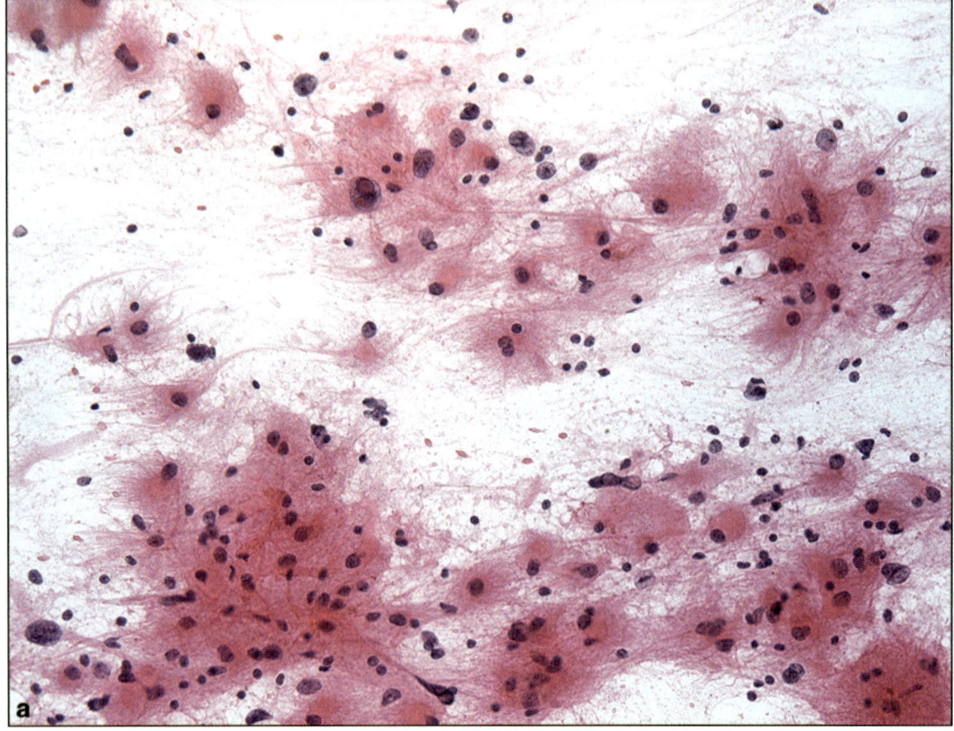

The gemistocytic astrocytoma is similar to another subtype of astrocytoma, the *granular cell astrocytoma*, in which conspicuous eosinophilic cytoplasm may show a fine granularity and is sometimes accompanied by perivascular lymphocytic infiltration. The granular cell astrocytoma also carries a poor prognosis (Brat et al., 2002).

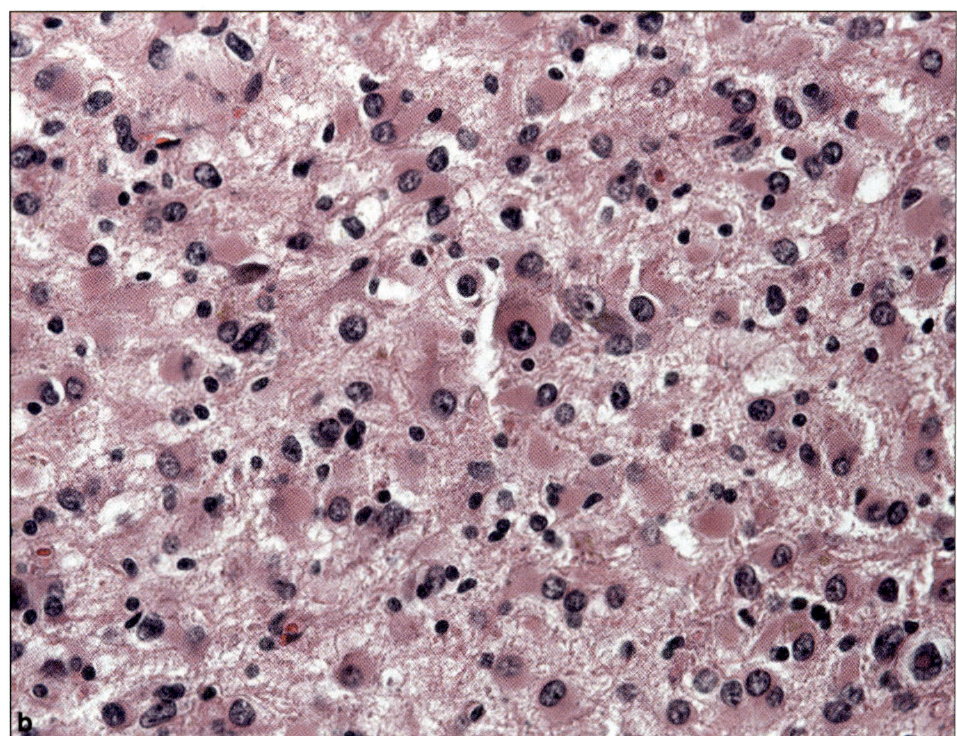

Figure 3.6. *continued*
(b) Histological section showing moderate nuclear pleomorphism and displacement by prominent eosinophilic cytoplasm.
(c) Reactive gemistocytic astrocytosis shows more diminutive nuclei and elongate slender cytoplasmic processes.

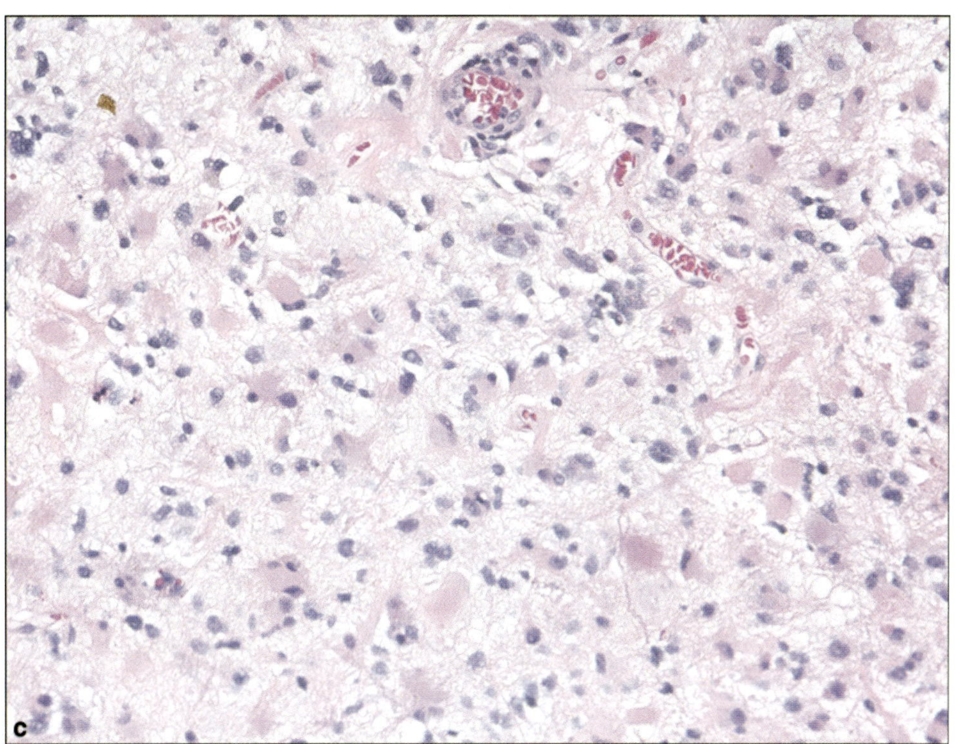

Protoplasmic Astrocytoma

This extremely rare form of diffuse astrocytoma is reportedly more common in the frontotemporal region (Prayson and Estes, 1995). They are composed of inconspicuous neoplastic astrocytes with small cell bodies and weakly GFAP-

Figure 3.7. Pilomyxoid astrocytoma, WHO Grade II. (a) Radiographic image of the characteristic appearance, although indistinguishable from pilocytic astrocytoma, a cystic and brightly contrast enhancing optic–hypothalamic region tumor in a child, mid-sagittal T1 MRI with contrast.

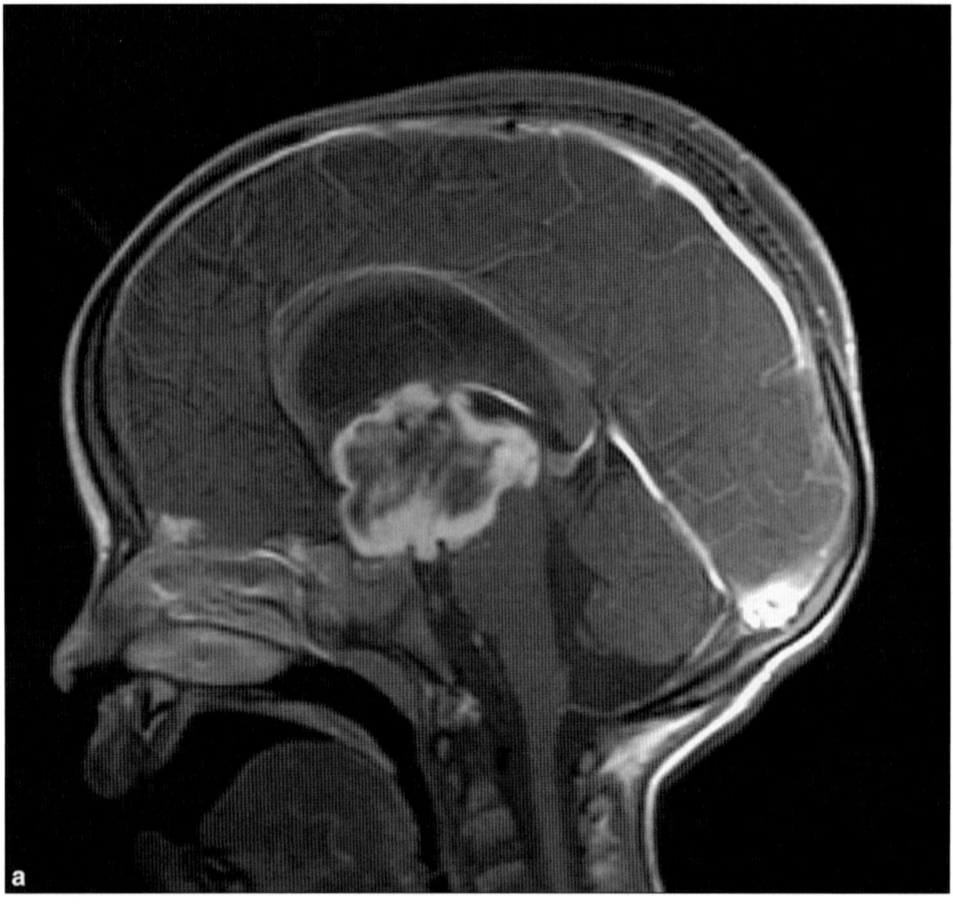

immunopositive cell processes. Microcystic change and mucoid degeneration are characteristic features.

Pilomyxoid Astrocytoma

Clinical and Radiological Features

The pilomyxoid astrocytoma was first reported to characteristically occur in the optic–hypothalamic region but have now been recognized in the posterior fossa and spinal cord (Brat et al., 2007a; Tihan et al., 1999). It appears that the pilomyxoid astrocytoma is a variant of pilocytic astrocytoma and not a wholly distinct entity, although it appears to portend a worse prognosis. Magnetic resonance imaging (MRI) imaging shows homogeneous contrast enhancement (Figure 3.7a).

Pathology

Pilomyxoid astrocytomas are solid, gelatinous masses, which may focally infiltrate regional tissues. The microscopic appearance is dominated by monotonous bipolar spindle cells in a myxoid matrix without the typical biphasic architecture of the related pilocytic astrocytoma (Figure 3.7b–e). The tumor cells are characteristically arranged perpendicularly around the large vessels. Rosenthal fibers and eosinophilic granular bodies are characteristically absent. Prominent capillary microvasculature is present, analogous to that seen in pilocytic astrocytomas. Necrosis is rare.

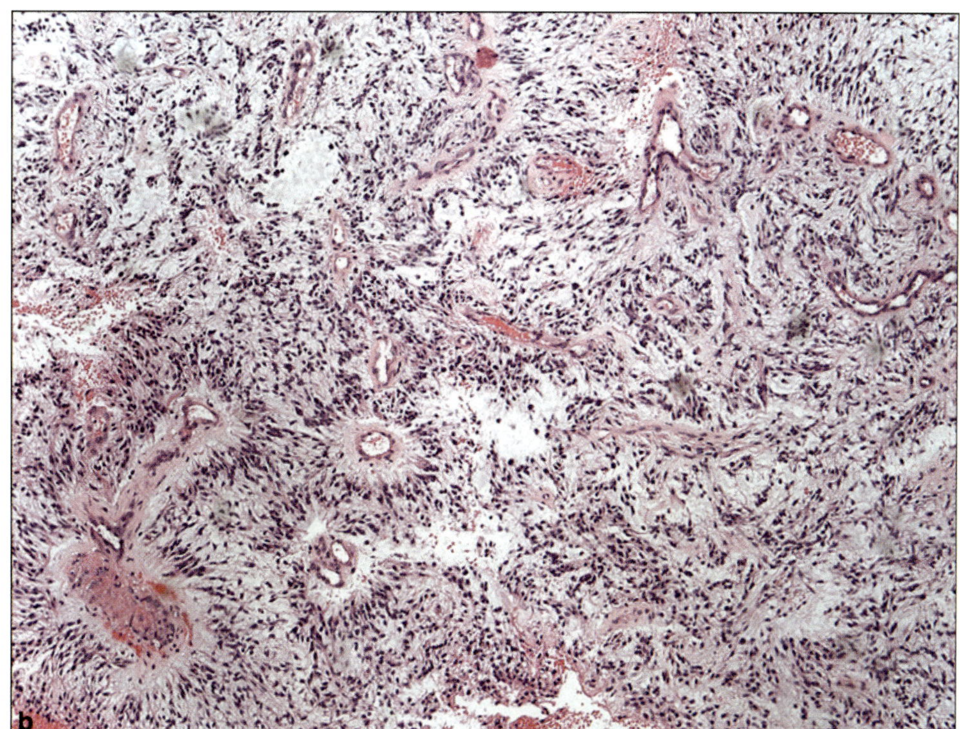

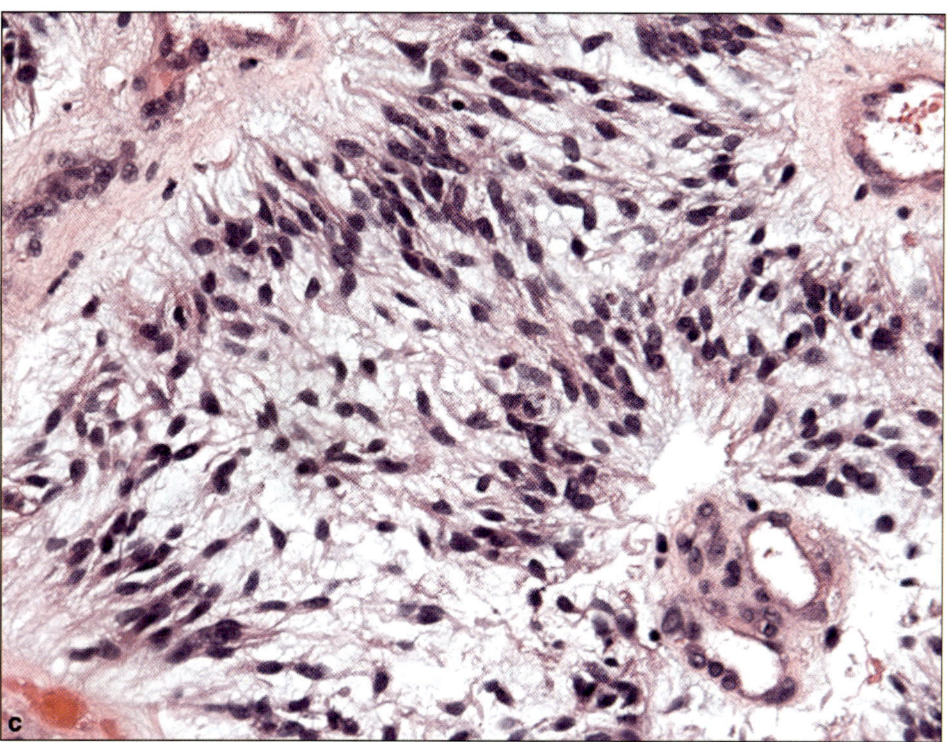

Figure 3.7. *continued* (b) Low-magnification appearance, with spindle cells in a myxoid background, and (c) absence of eosinophilic granular bodies or Rosenthal fibers. Note the prominent microvasculature, identical to that seen in pilocytic astrocytomas.

The tumor cells are characteristically GFAP and S-100 protein positive. Some tumors are positive for synaptophysin. Proliferation measurement such as by the MIB-1 labeling index shows a wide range of reactivity, between 2% and 20%, such that in the lower range between 2% and 4%, this finding could not be used in order to reliably distinguish pilocytic astrocytoma from pilomyxoid astrocytoma.

Figure 3.7. *continued* (d) GFAP immunohistochemistry will highlight perivascular cell processes. Pilomyxoid astrocytomas may also be synaptophysin immunopositive. (e) Proliferative index may be distinctly higher than that of pilocytic astrocytomas.

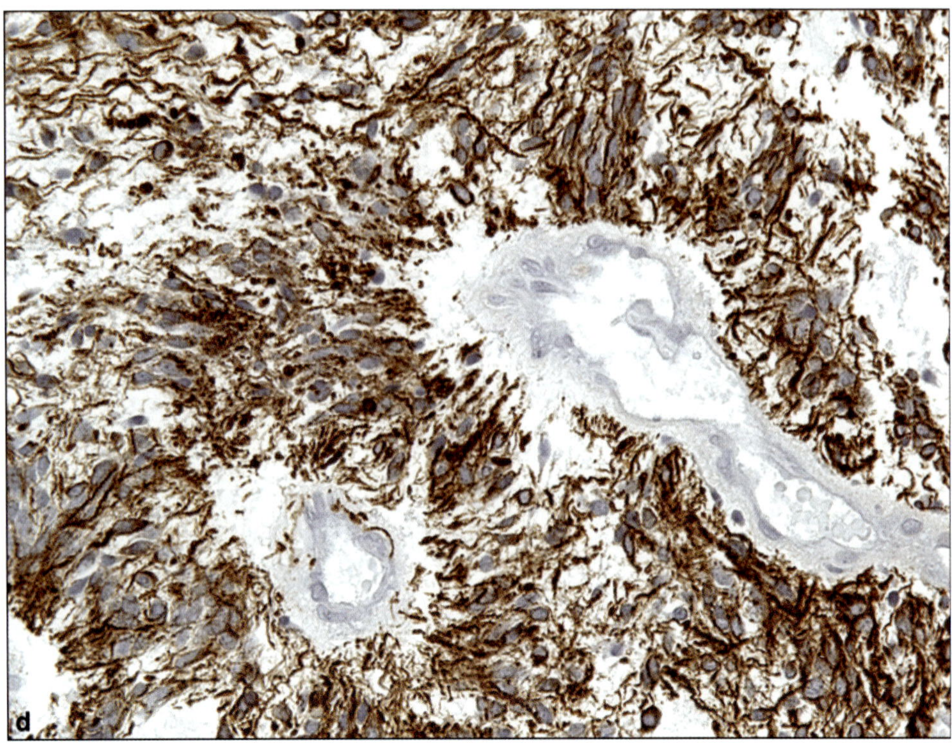

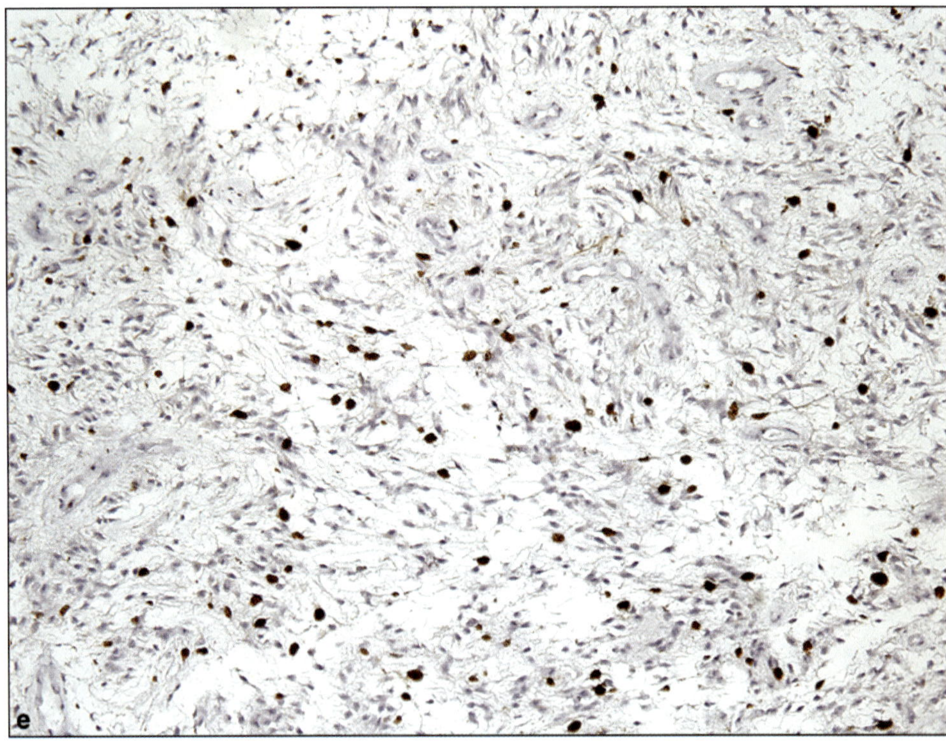

Pleomorphic Xanthoastrocytoma

Clinical and Radiological Features

Pleomorphic xanthoastrocytoma (PXA) is most commonly found as a rather superficial hemispheric, often cystic cortical mass in the temporal or parietal lobes and occurs most often in young adults.

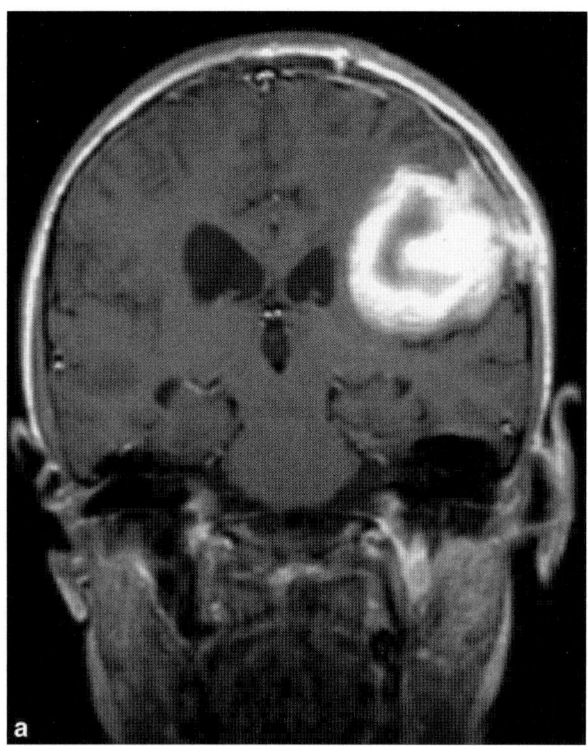

Figure 3.8. Pleomorphic xanthoastrocytoma (PXA), WHO Grade II. (a) Typical radiographic appearance, with bright contrast enhancement of a cystic superficial temporoparietal mass, sometimes discovered in the evaluation of chronic epilepsy.

Radiological features include those of a relatively well-demarcated and rather superficial mass, sometimes with a cyst accompanying the tumor mass, and less peritumoral edema than is typical of higher grade gliomas (Figure 3.8a). They are brightly contrast enhancing. Overlying skull bone may show thinning as with other slow-growing cortical tumors.

Pathology

The pleomorphic xanthoastrocytoma contains fascicles of astrocytic cells with enlarged pleomorphic nuclei (Figure 3.8b–e). A fibrillary background may not be uniformly present, and cell borders are usually quite distinct. Occasional xanthomatous cells may be present but are not required for the diagnosis. A reticulin stain shows characteristic pericellular reticulin deposition, although this is also not a uniform feature of the pleomorphic xanthoastrocytoma. The ultrastructual correlate of this feature is basal lamina around cell membranes, believed to reflect a histogenetic relationship with subpial astrocytes. Mitotic activity and necrosis is rare, and if these are prominent features, a diagnosis of glioblastoma should be considered. Rare examples of anaplastic WHO Grade III pleomorphic xanthoastrocytomas have also been reported.

WHO GRADE III

Anaplastic Astrocytoma

Clinical and Radiological Features

The clinical features are similar to those of space occupying WHO Grade II diffuse astrocytomas although without a prior history, the onset of symptoms

Figure 3.8. *continued*
(b) Marked cytological pleomorphism with a focal abundance of EGBs. (c) Subarachnoid growth of PXA, accompanied by desmoplasia.

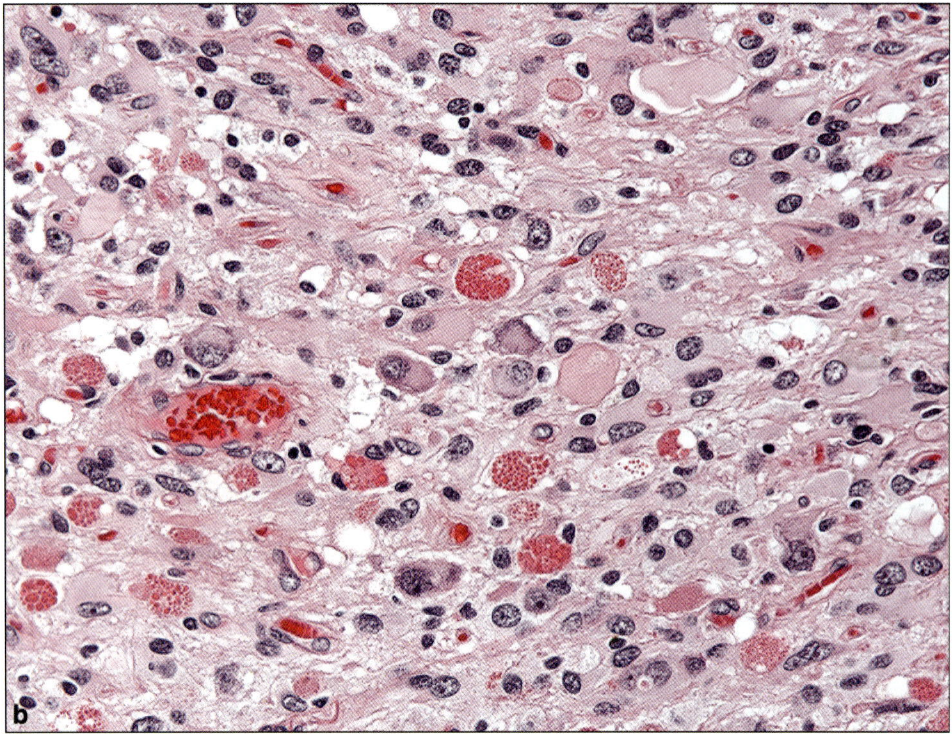

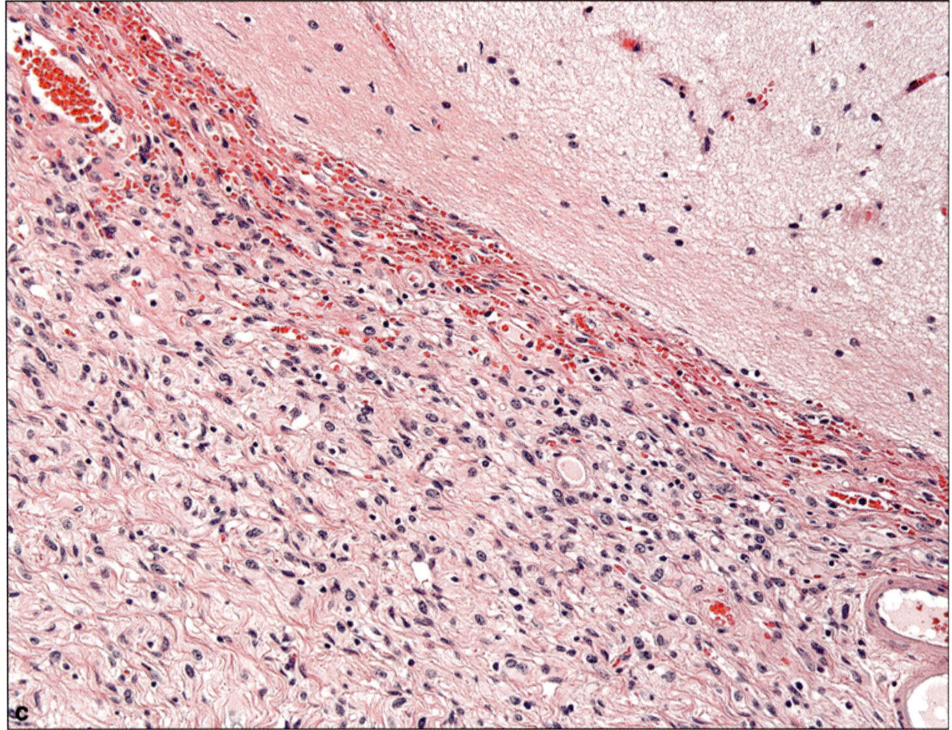

may be more rapid as compared with patients presenting with a WHO Grade II diffuse astrocytoma. They may occur in any location; they, however; are more common in the cerebral hemispheres. MRI imaging shows a range between non focal and focal contrast enhancement.

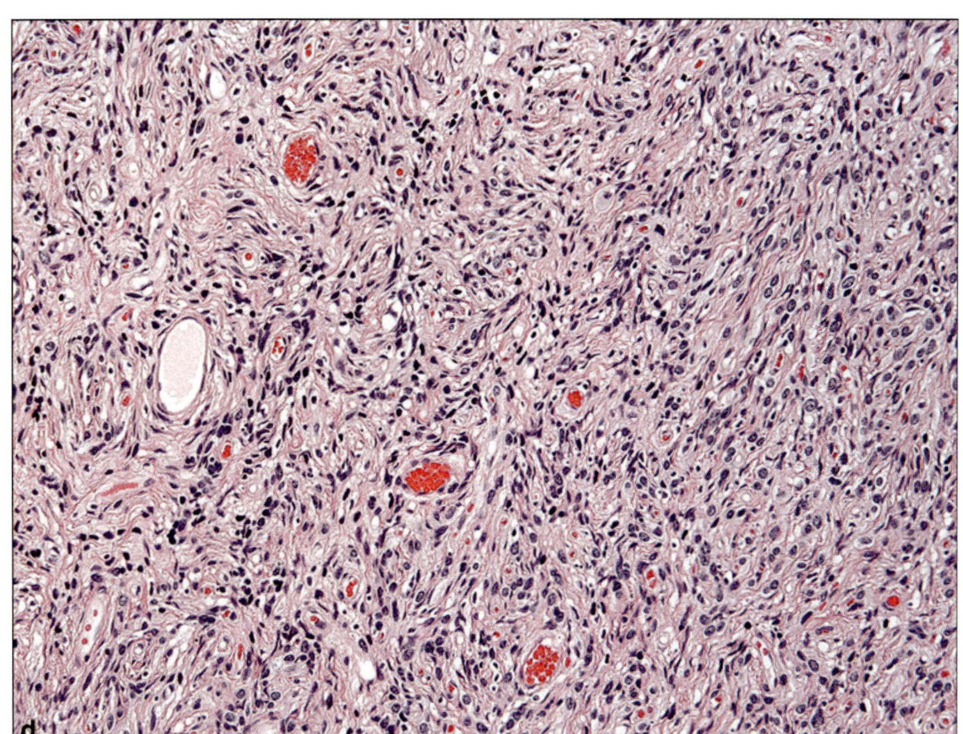

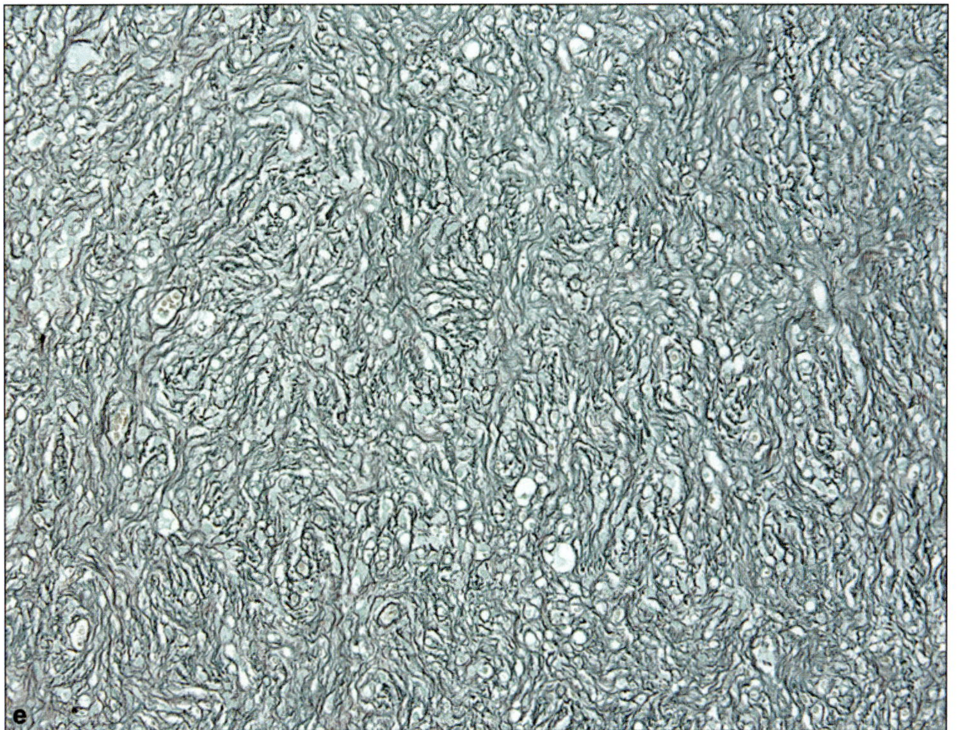

Figure 3.8. *continued*
(d) Desmoplastic region of
PXA, (e) with pericellular
reticulin highlighted by
reticulin stain.

Pathology

The anaplastic astrocytoma displays the features of various WHO grade
II astrocytomas with added mitotic activity and a general increase in
cellularity and cytological atypia (Figure 3.9a,b). Sometimes it is difficult

Figure 3.9. Anaplastic astrocytoma, WHO Grade III. (a) The two essential features are nuclear atypia and mitotic activity without vascular proliferation or necrosis. (b) Large resections stained for proliferating cells may reveal the considerable variation in MIB-1 labeling, which exposes the vulnerability of assigning a grade with very small samples.

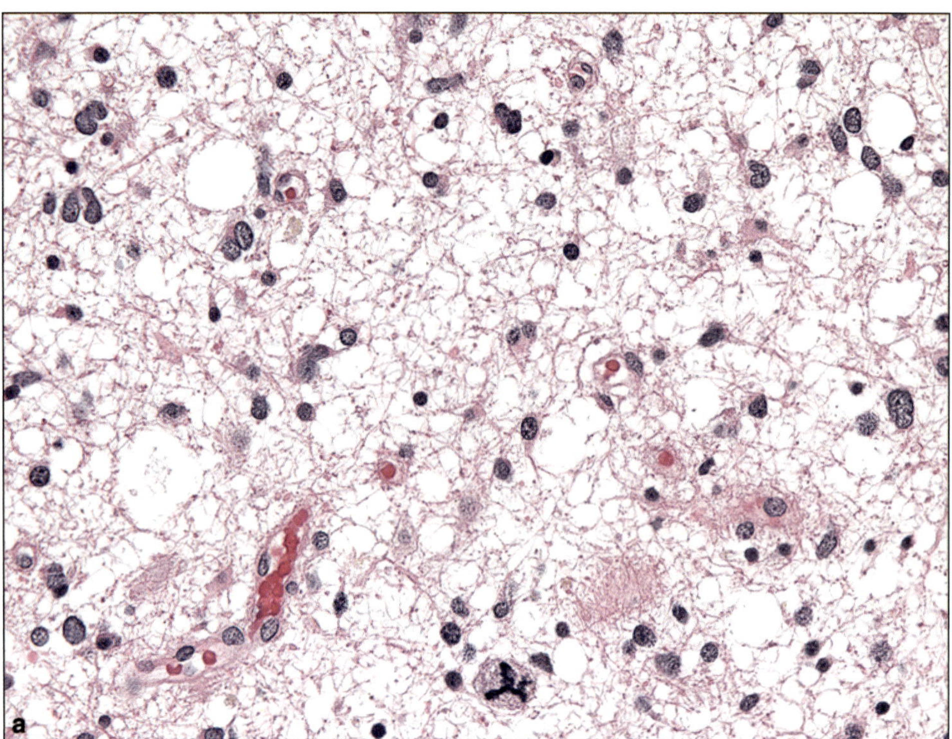

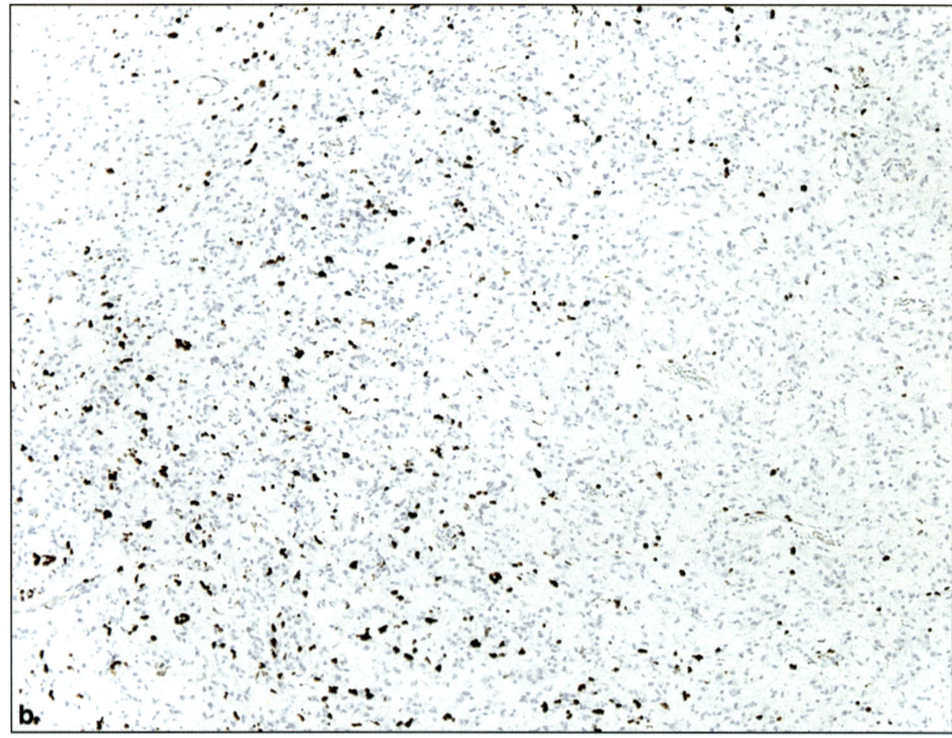

to clearly assign a WHO grade of II or III, and both histological patterns may coexist. Unless WHO grade III features represent a small portion of the sample, a WHO grade of III should be assigned to the lesion since it will most likely determine the most aggressive potential of the

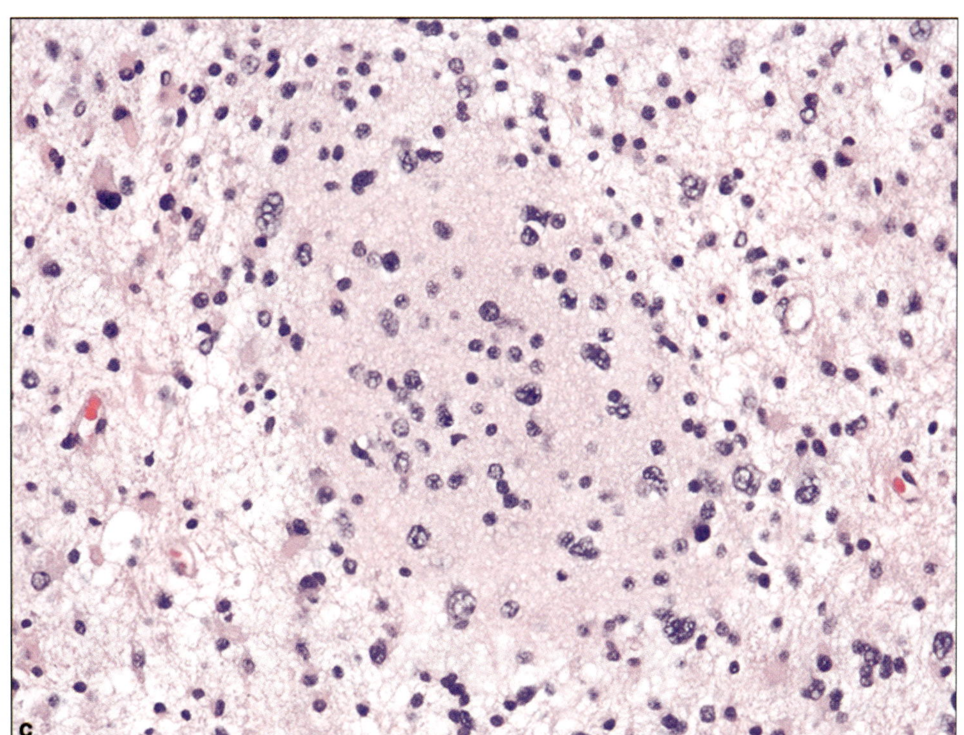

Figure 3.9. *continued* (c) The glioneuronal tumor with neuropil-like islands is a variant of WHO Grade II or III astrocytomas, in which sharply demarcated islands of finely fibrillar neuropil are surrounded by monomorphous small glial cells. Immunohistochemistry for (d) synaptophysin and (e) GFAP will show complimentary staining patterns.

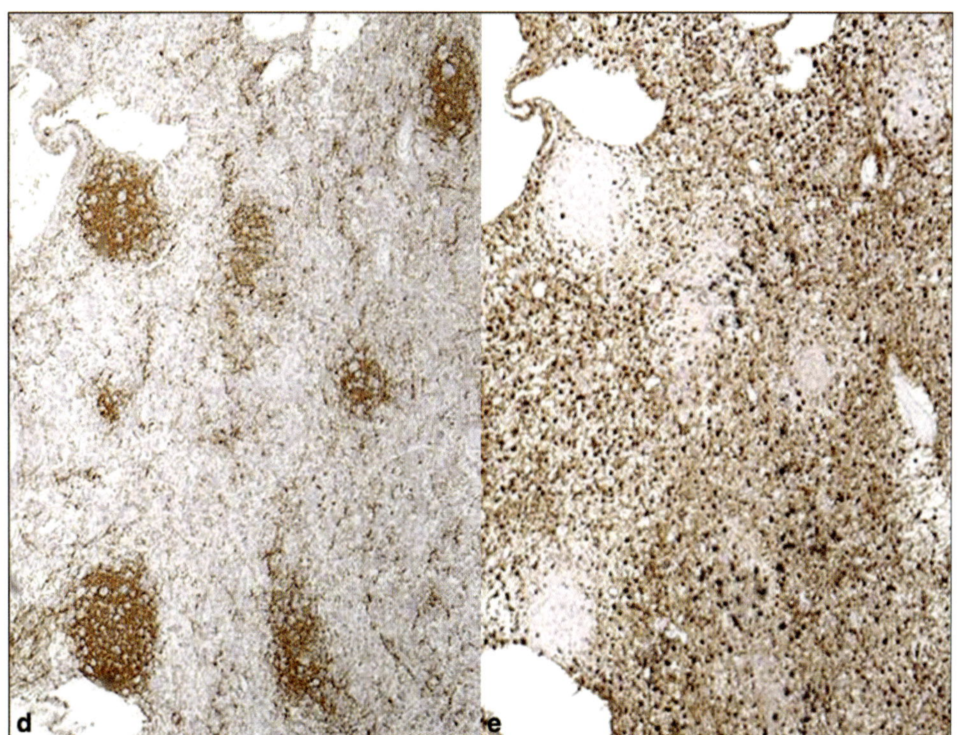

tumor. Vascular proliferation and necrosis are not present, since their presence would indicate a glioblastoma. A variant with neuropil islands has also been described (Figure 3.9c–e). When small stereotactic biopsies indicate features of an anaplastic astrocytoma, it is sometimes impossible to diagnose glioblastoma even though the radiological features are highly suggestive. Microvascular thrombosis has been observed to connote a significantly worse prognosis, drawing the anaplastic astrocytoma one step closer to the diagnostic features of glioblastoma with similar prognostic implications (Tehrani et al., 2008).

WHO GRADE IV

Glioblastoma

Clinical and Radiological Features

Glioblastoma (GBM) is the most common primary glial tumor in adults. It occurs in a bimodal fashion, first affecting the middle-aged adult, typically as a secondary glioblastoma arising in a lower grade astrocytoma, or in older adults as a de novo primary glioblastoma, accounting for the vast majority. Childhood, and even congenital, examples have been reported (Brat et al., 2007b).

The clinical prodrome is on the order of many months in the secondary form, to a more precipitous onset, occurring over days to weeks in the primary form. Symptoms are referable to the region of the CNS that is primarily affected, but are those of a rapidly expanding mass.

Glioblastomas may arise in any region of the CNS, but most commonly in the supratentorial space. By the time they are diagnosed, they have undergone significant microscopic spread, on the order of several centimeters from the radiographically evident lesion (Figure 3.10). This is typically a cystic mass with contrast rim enhancement. The most deceptive form of apparently discrete mass effect is seen in the *giant cell glioblastoma*, and, upon resection, may lead the neurosurgeon to proclaim a gross total resection. Extension along white matter tracts is characteristic, and when the corpus callosum is so involved, the mass can assume a butterfly shape because of the winglike spread across the corpus callosum to involve both hemispheres.

Pathology

Glioblastomas typically show macroscopic areas of necrosis and hemorrhage. There are numerous microscopic patterns seen in glioblastoma, but the two most essential features are *vascular proliferation* and *necrosis* (Figure 3.11). The vascular proliferation has been variously defined as "glomeruloid" or "vascular endothelial proliferation" since simple prominence of endothelial cells does not constitute this diagnostic feature. Vascular proliferation includes all cellular elements of blood vessels: endothelium, pericytes, and fibroblasts. Classic examples contain at least two layers of endothelial cells.

A microscopic hallmark of necrosis in glioblastoma is pseudopalisading necrosis. This phenomenon begins as a small focus of hypoxic tumor

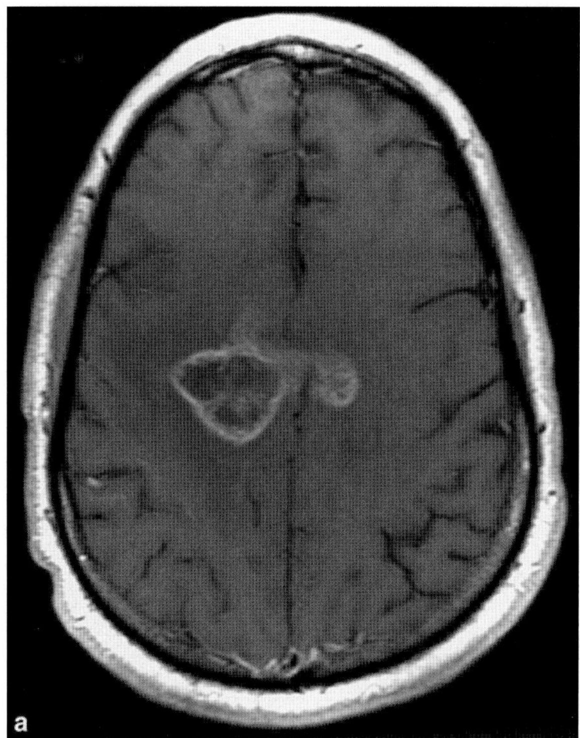

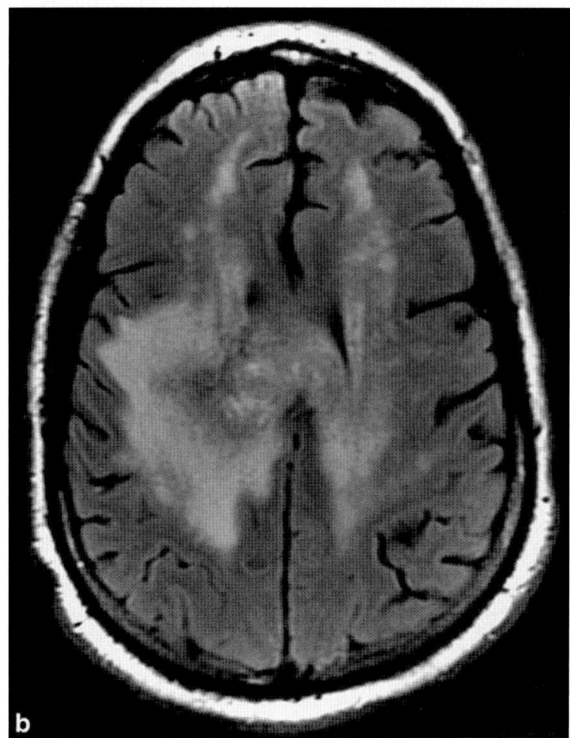

Figure 3.10. Glioblastoma. (a) An axial T1 contrast-enhanced MR image shows a ring-enhancing mass in the right posterior frontal lobe. Centrally within the mass is poor enhancement, probably corresponding to an area of necrosis. (b) An axial FLAIR MR image shows extensive abnormal signal around the areas of enhancement, consistent with vasogenic edema and diffuse tumor infiltration. Glioblastomas, which are highly infiltrative, extend well beyond their areas of enhancement. Biopsies are often targeted at the areas of enhancement. The ring of enhancement is typically thicker and shaggier than that of other ring enhancing cerebral lesions, such as abscesses, hematomas, or demyelinating disease. There is a direct correlation between astrocytoma grade, enhancement, and necrosis.

necrosis attributable to microvascular thrombosis. Surviving tumor cells then migrate away from the growing necrotic focus while at the same time elaborating vasogenic factors (Rong et al., 2006). This leads to two highly characteristic features in the microscopy of glioblastoma: a pseudopalisading of tumor cells

Figure 3.10. *continued*
(c) A cerebral blood volume (CBV) MR map alone and a map, (d) superimposed on top of an axial T2-weighted MR image shows that the nonnecrotic portions of the glioblastoma have high CBV. CBV imaging has been developed over the last decade and is believed to correlate with vascular proliferation or vascular density. There is a direct correlation between CBV and astrocytoma grade. CBV may predict tumor progression independent of tumor grade, and it has been suggested that CBV be used to guide biopsy.

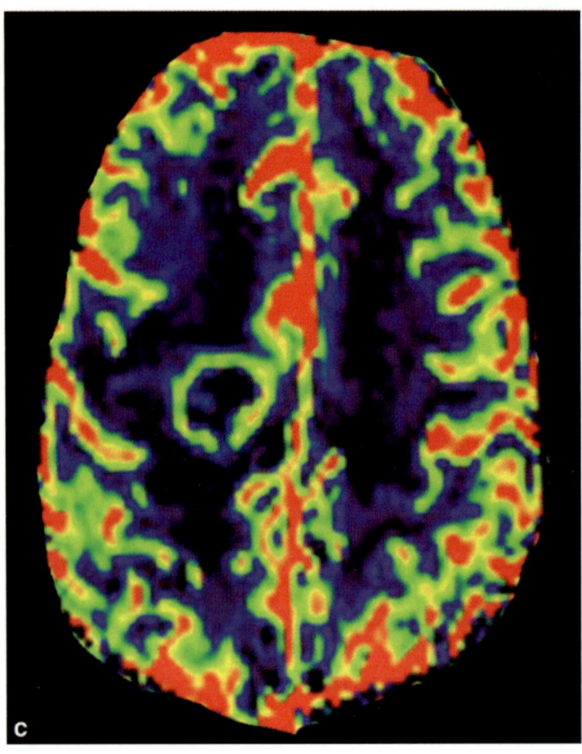

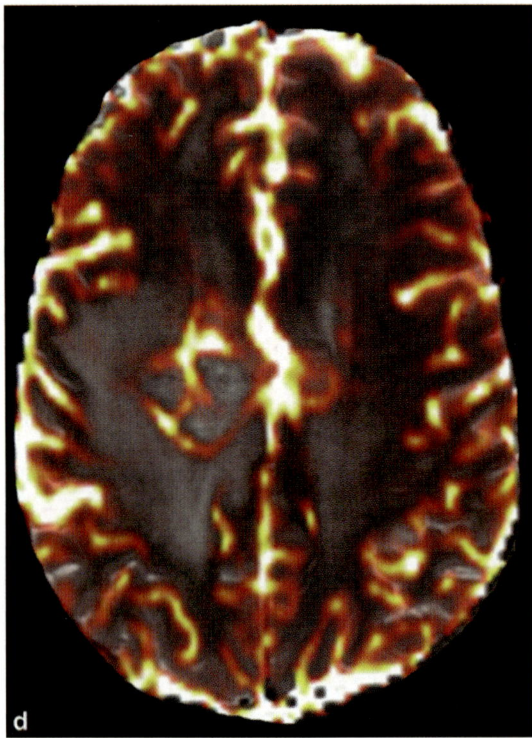

often forming a serpiginous band, and closely adjacent tufts of vascular proliferation.

An interesting variety of microscopic patterns may be seen in glioblastoma. In its quintessential form originally designated multiforme, tumor cells show

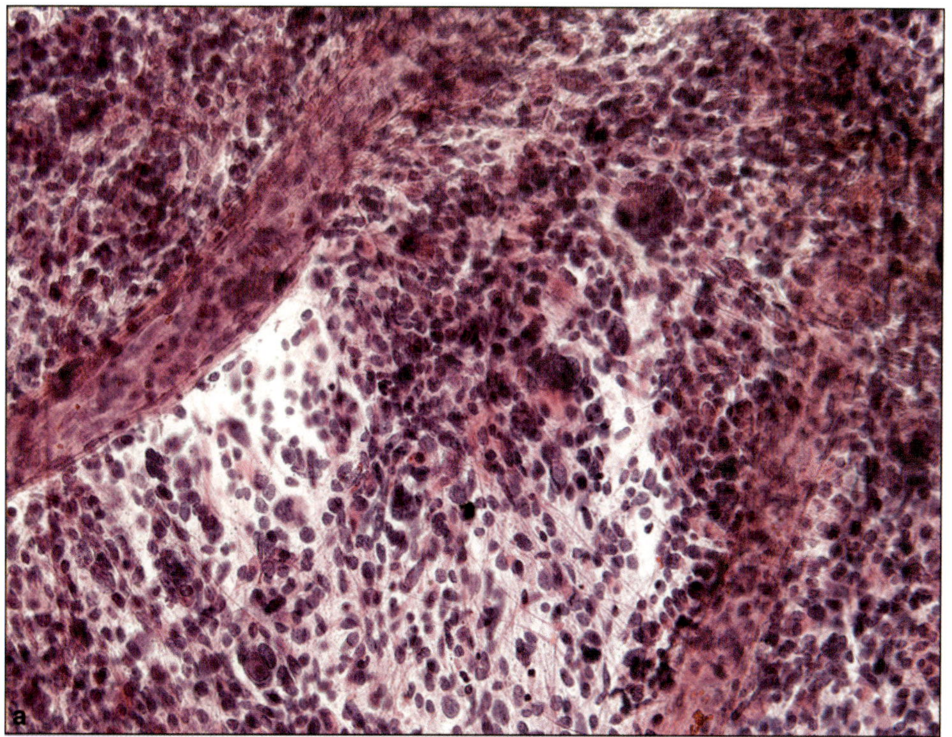

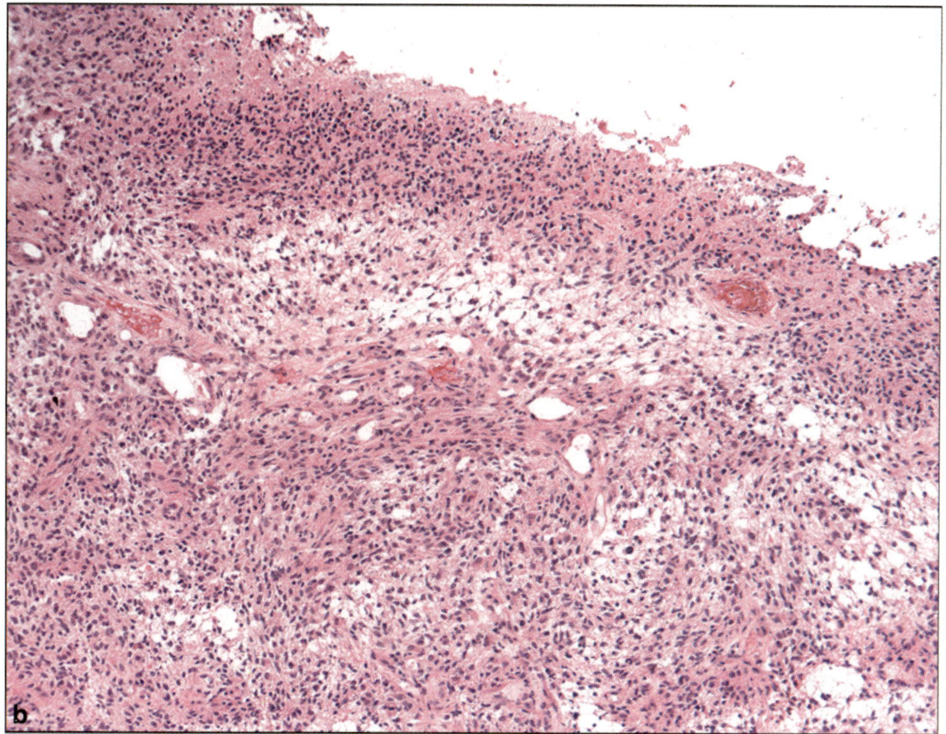

Figure 3.11. Glioblastoma, WHO Grade IV. (a) Squash cytological preparation may have a multiplicity of appearances, but prominent blood vessels a dense cellularity in a fibrillar background may be seen in glioblastoma when relatively pure tumor is sampled. (b) Cryosections and (c) permanent sections may show cleavage of the stereotactice needle biopsy track to include half of a somewhat linear portion of pseudopalisading necrosis, seen at the upper portions of each example, which may be a useful way of detecting necrosis at frozen section that is not centrally located in the specimen. (d) Essential features of glioblastoma are vascular proliferation and necrosis with pseudopalisading seen in this example.

considerable pleomorphism. In its most extreme form, the *giant cell glioblastoma* contains enormous cells with bizarre and wildly pleomorphic nuclei (Figure 3.11g,h) that are immunopositive for nuclear p53. However, a highly monomorphous type composed of closely packed regular and small, nonetheless atypical astrocytic tumor cells, is called *small cell glioblastoma*

Figure 3.11. *continued.*

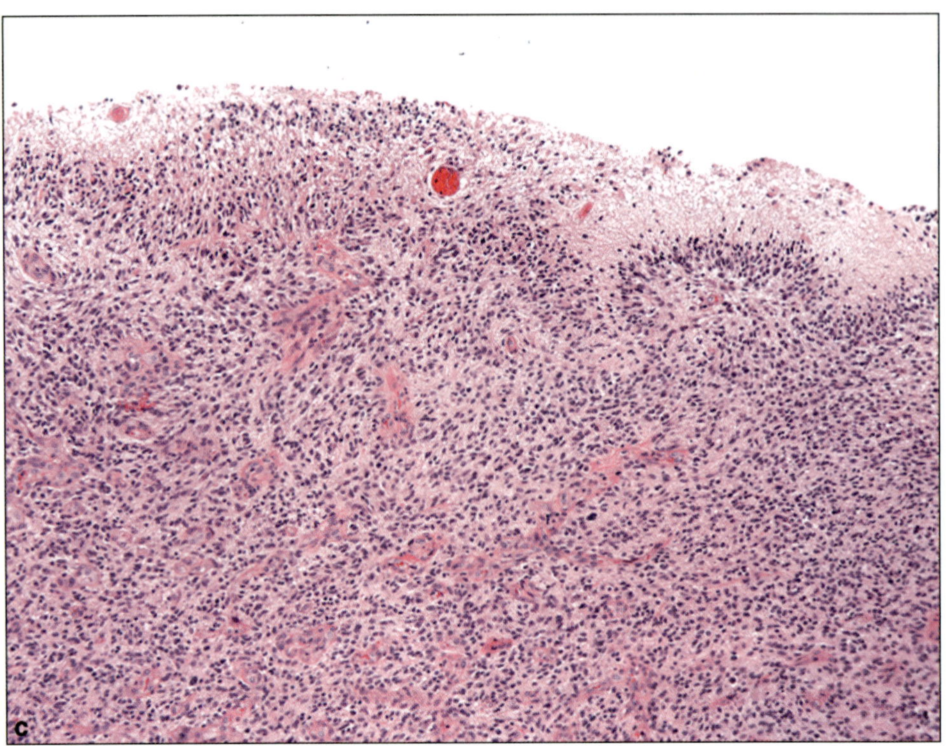

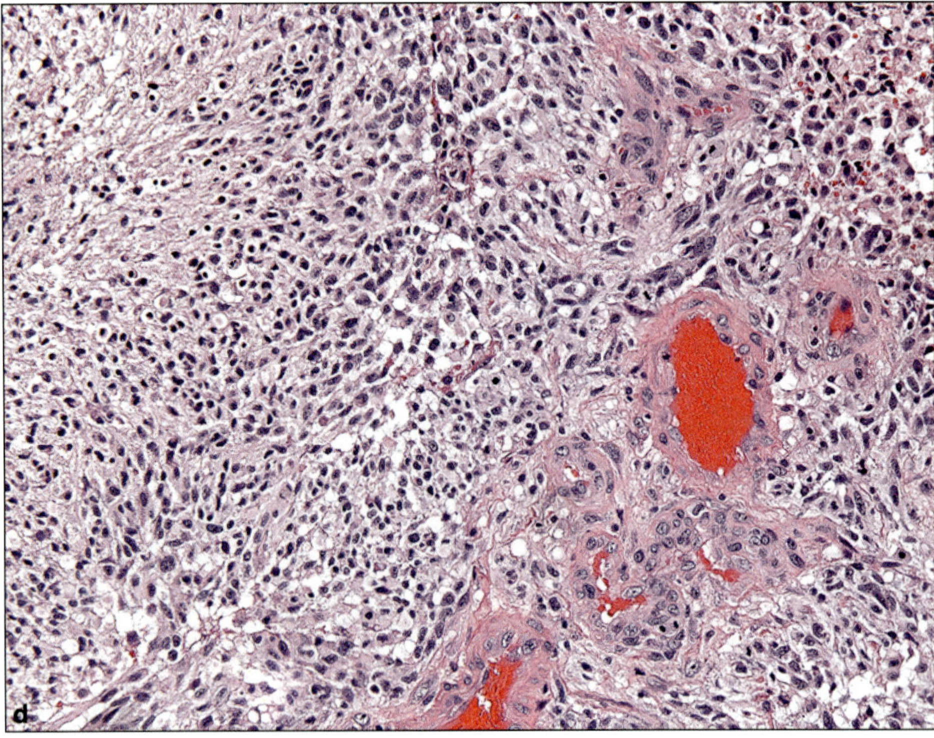

(Figure 3.11i,j). Rarely, glioblastomas may have a prominent myxoid or mucoid background with columnar, epithelioid, or adenomatoid growth patterns (Figure 3.11k,l) (Miyata et al., 2005). Rhabdoid (Figure 3.11m) (Wyatt-Ashmead et al., 2001) and lipidized forms (Queiroz et al., 2005) have

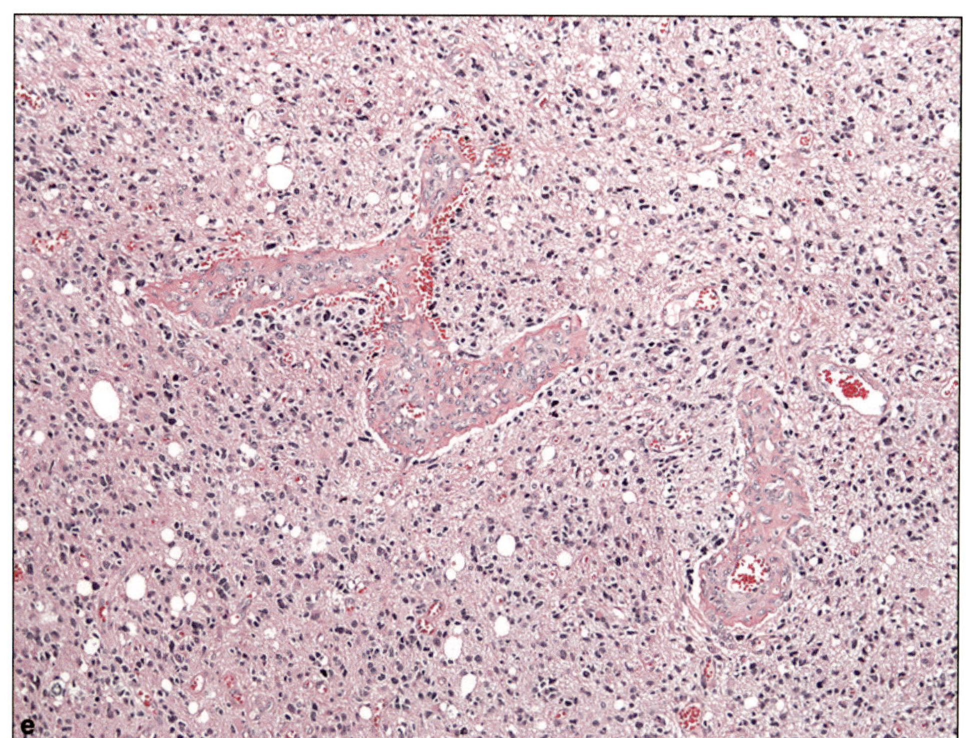

Figure 3.11. *continued* (e) Vascular proliferation alone will suffice to establish the diagnosis of glioblastoma as in this example of a region without necrosis, or (f) in superficial brain cortex showing the potent vasogenic properties of invasive glioblastoma in the overlying subarachnoid space.

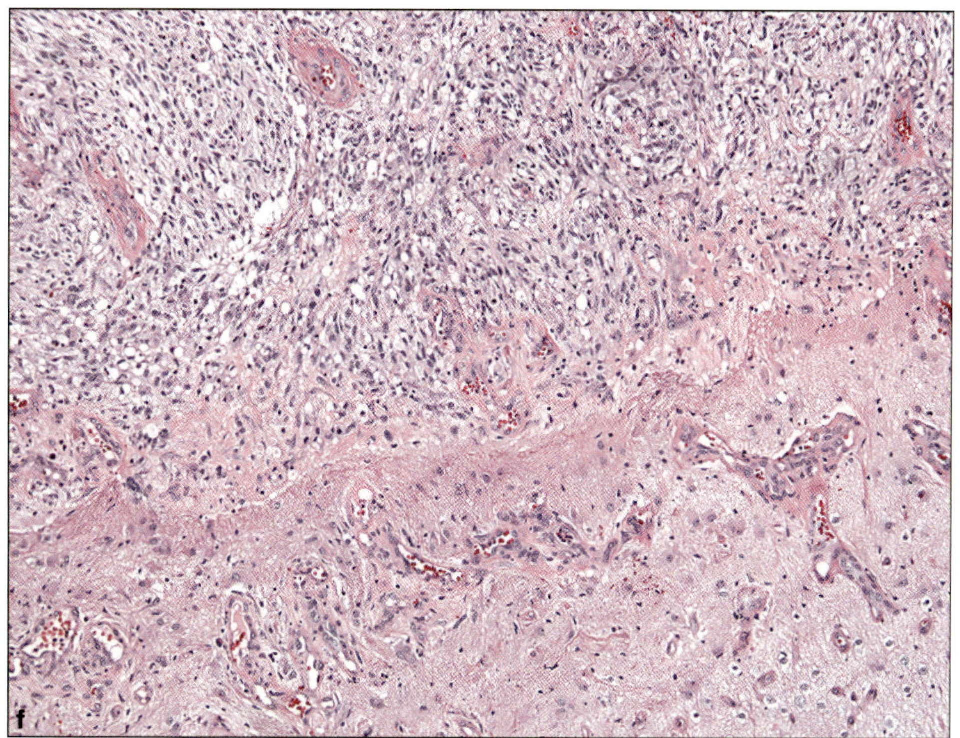

also been reported. When a prominent oligodendroglial component is recognizable in an otherwise astrocytic neoplasm satisfying the criteria for diagnosis of glioblastoma, the term glioblastoma with oligodendroglial features (GBM-O) may be appropriate (Figure 3.11n).

Figure 3.11. *continued*
(g,h) Some glioblastomas
may be composed
predominantly of extremely
pleomorphic cells with
bizarre nuclear features and
when seen in a deceptively
well-circumscribed tumor,
both by neuroimaging and
surgical resection, may
represent a giant cell
glioblastoma.

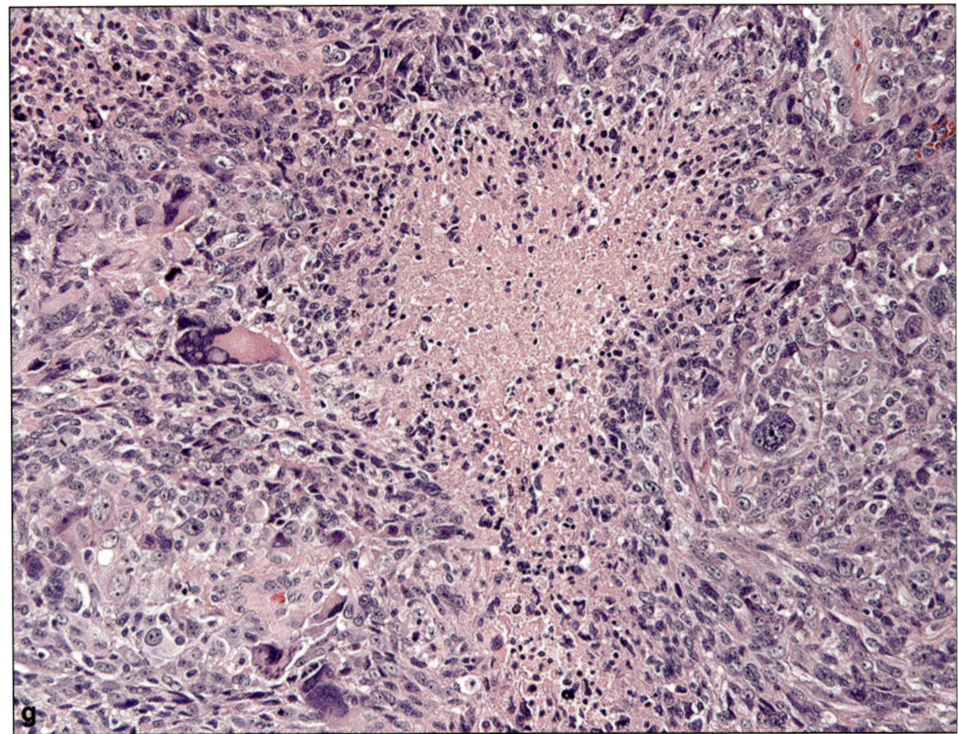

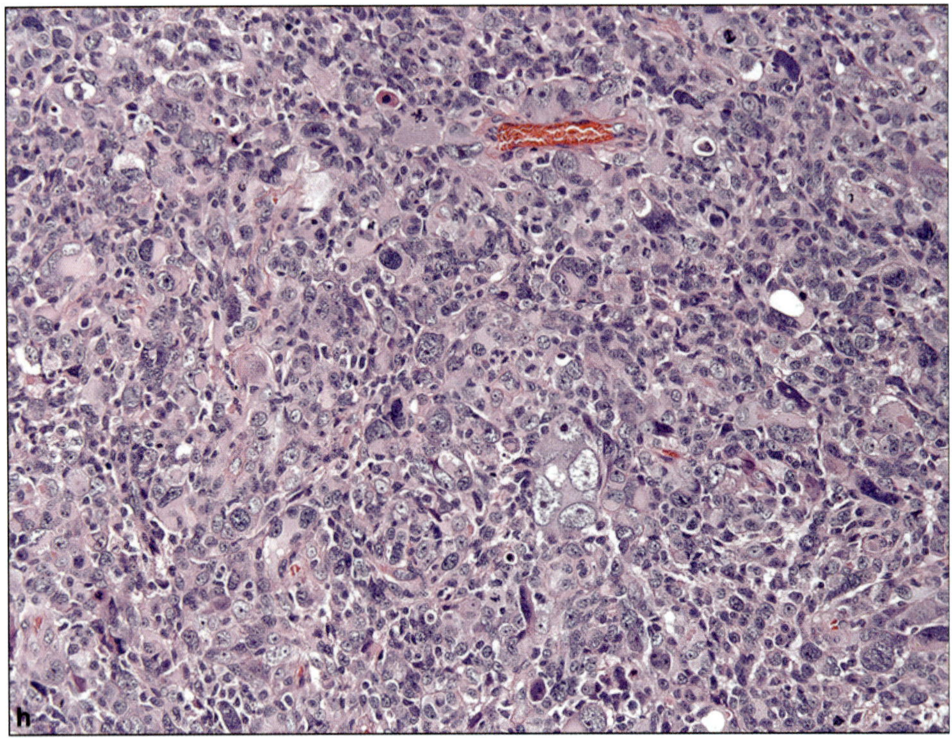

Gliosarcoma

Clinical and Radiological Features

The age distribution of gliosarcoma is similar to that of glioblastoma. They account for 2–8% of all glioblastomas. They are usually located in the cerebral

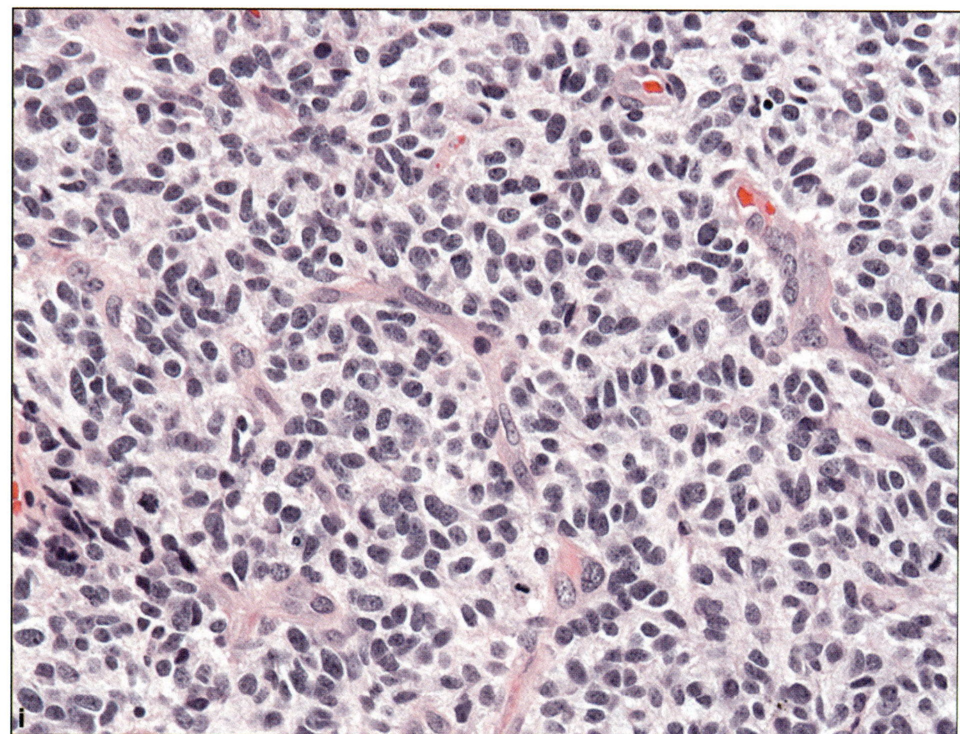

Figure 3.11. *continued*
(i) In contrast, the small cell glioblastoma is a cellular tumor with monotonous nuclei, usually conspicuous mitotic activity, and (j) high proliferative index. Other forms of differentiation in glioblastoma include (k) adenomatoid, and
(l) mucoid, (m) variously termed epithelioid or rhabdoid. (n) Some glioblastomas may contain an easily recognizable oligodendroglial component (GBM-O).

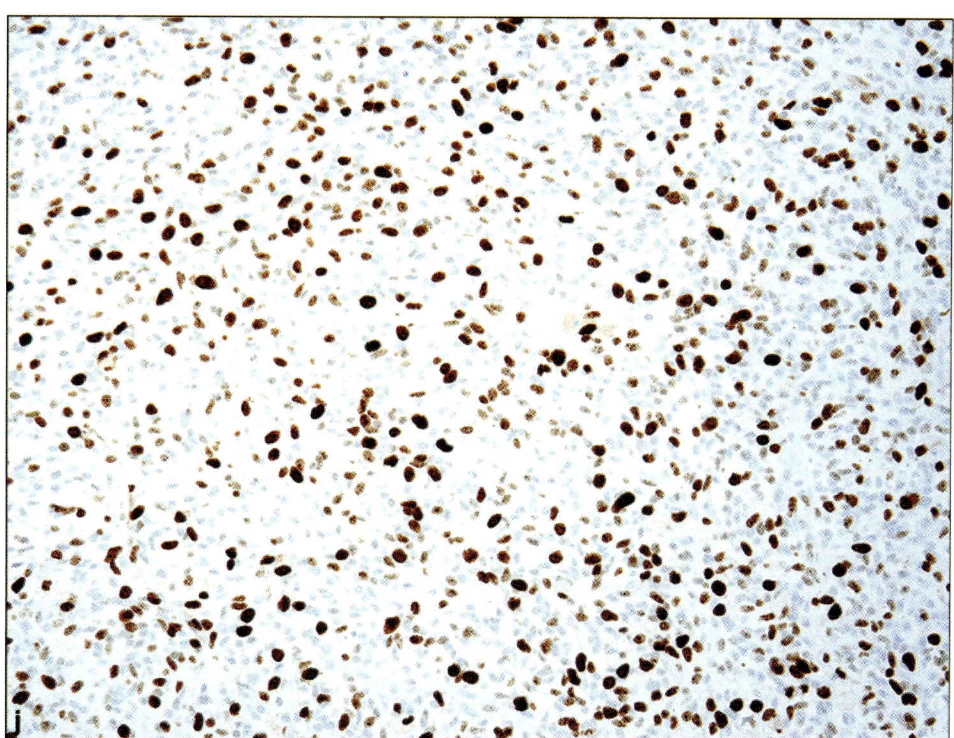

hemispheres, sometimes superficially and are deceptively well circumscribed (Figure 3.12).

Pathology

Glioblastomas may show mesenchymal differentiation, most often akin to fibrosarcoma, but may include regions of osteosarcoma or liposarcoma.

Figure 3.11. *continued.*

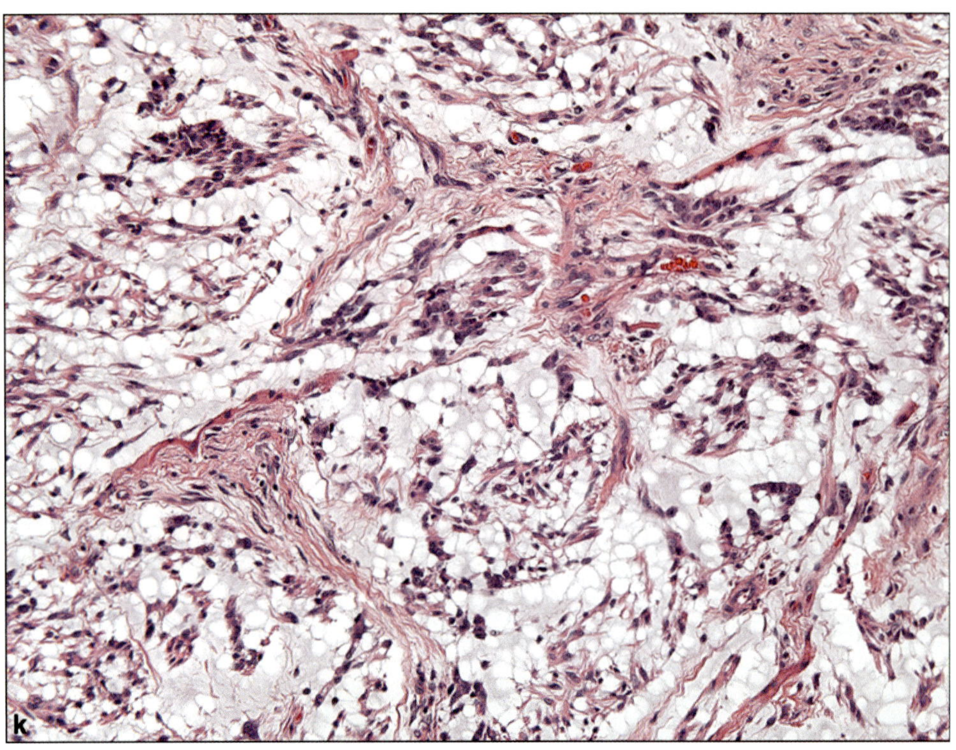

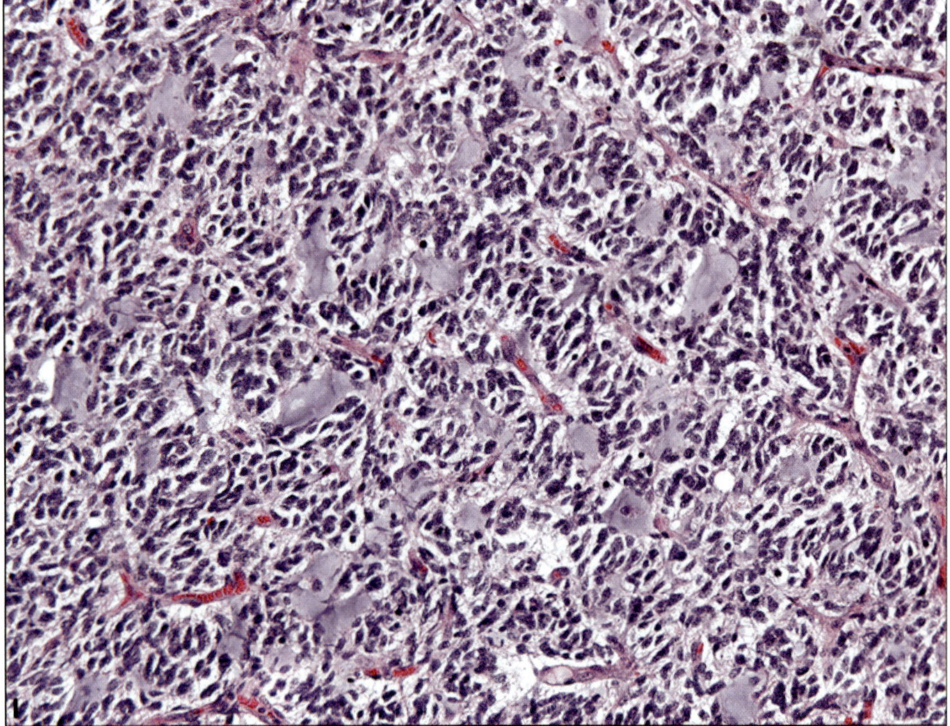

Gliosarcoma is characteristically GFAP immunonegative and reticulin rich, often in sharp contrast to the more straightforward glioblastoma portion of the tumor. This has great importance when either limited sampling or extensive sarcomatous differentiation yields no diagnostic GFAP immunostaining. S-100 expression would be expected to be retained. However, consideration of a metastatic sarcoma under these conditions should also be given.

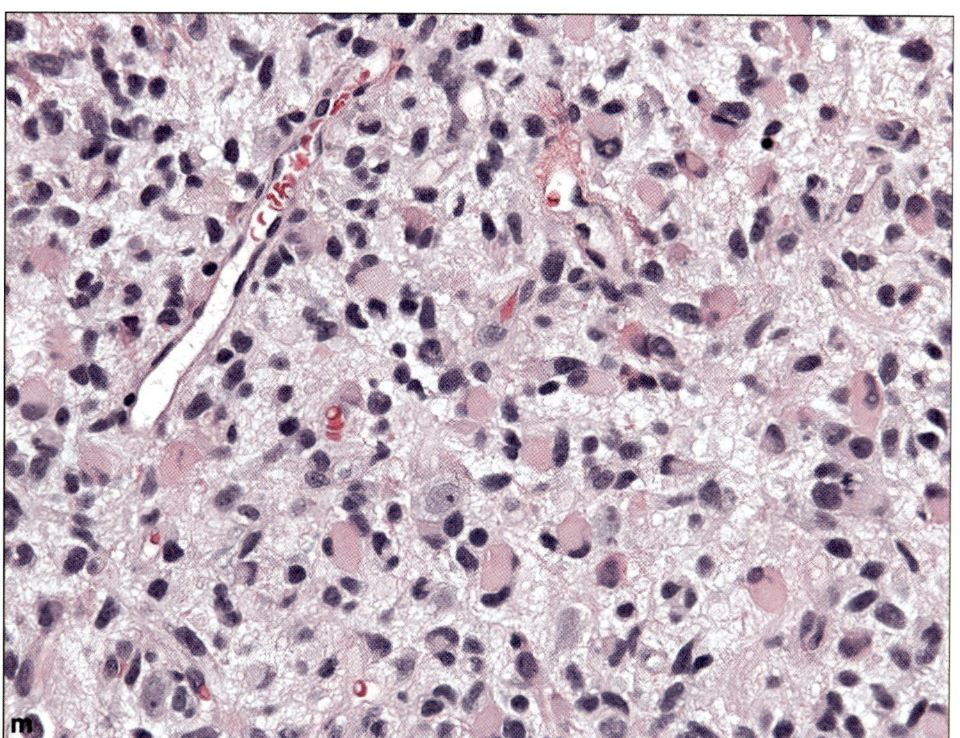

Figure 3.11. *continued.*

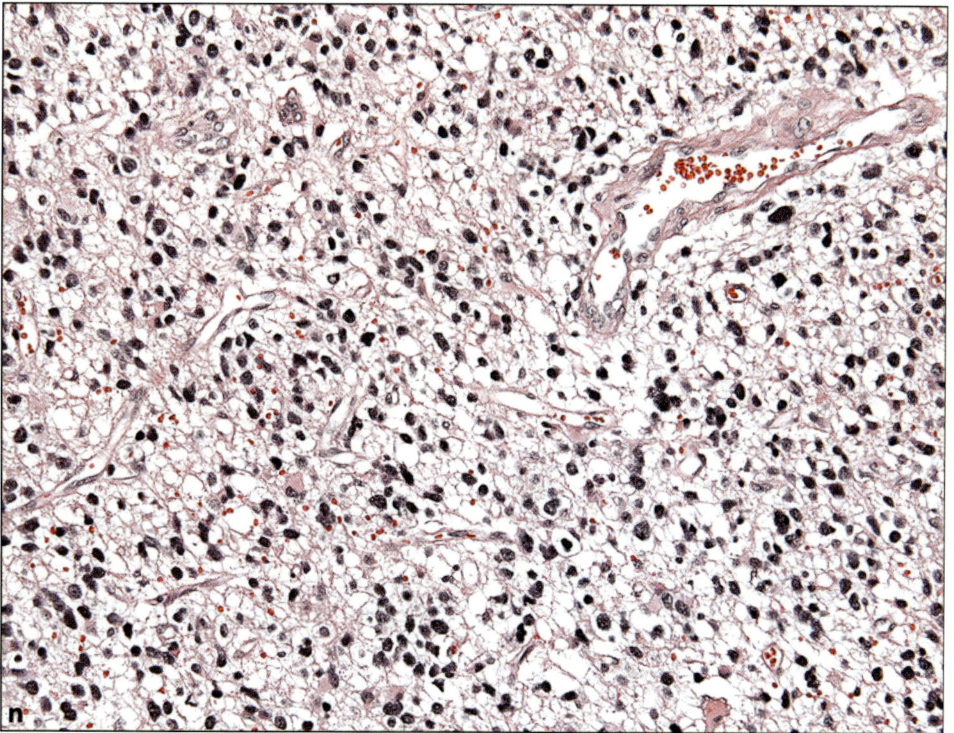

Gliomatosis Cerebri

Clinical and Radiological Features

Gliomatosis cerebri is an unusual and aggressive glial neoplasm, which may occur at any age but is most common in the age range of 40–50 years. Historically,

Figure 3.12. Gliosarcoma, WHO Grade IV. (a) The presence of a spindle cell component in any glioblastoma should suggest the possibility of gliosarcoma, which can be confirmed by the complimentary presence of (b) reticulin deposition in (c) GFAP immunonegative regions. Note that most gliosarcomas have closely intermixed sarcomatous and ordinary glioblastoma elements, but limited sampling of a purely sarcomatous GFAP immunonegative region may not suggest the underlying presence of a primary glial neoplasm.

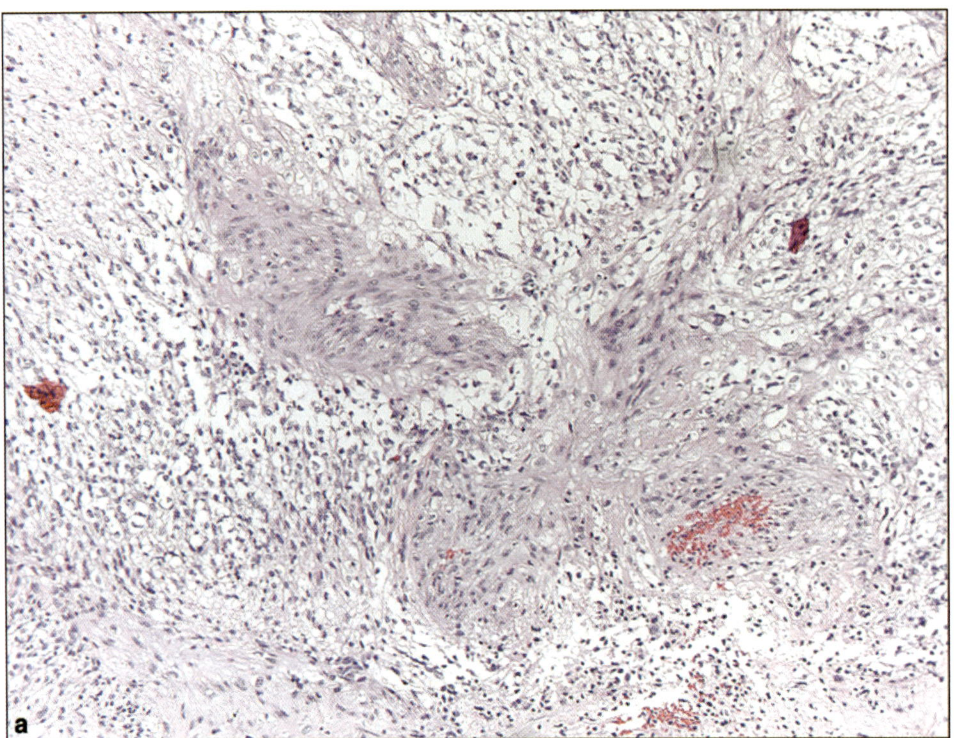

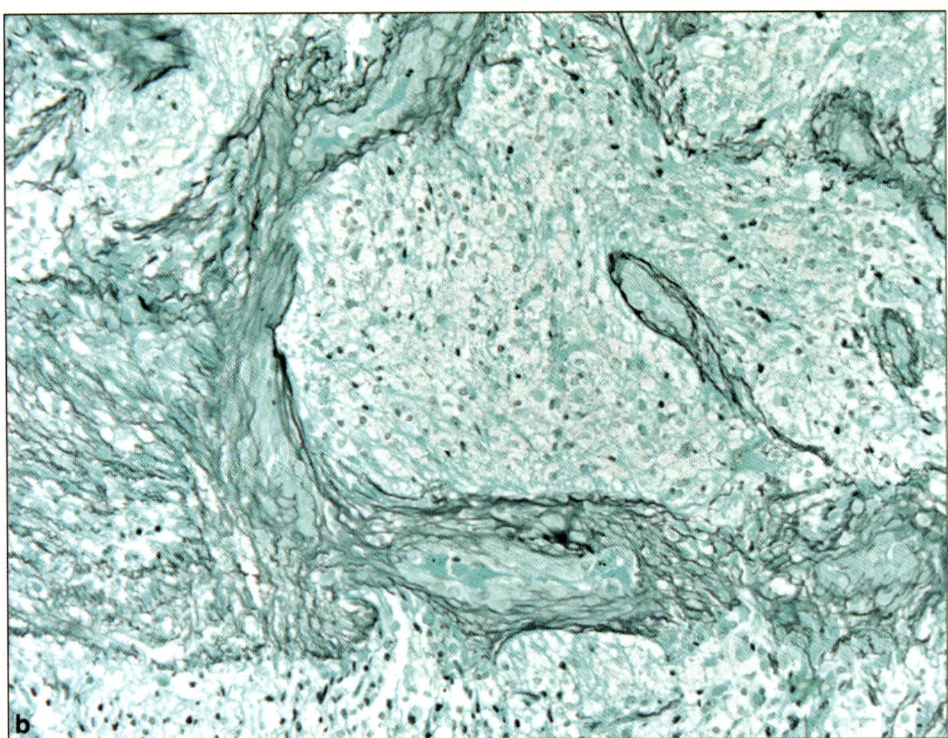

the diagnosis was rarely made in life and produced confusing signs and symptoms, which did not obviously suggest a neoplastic process, such as gradual mental status changes, dementia, lethargy, seizures, headache, or pyramidal symptoms and various other motor and sensory deficits. They are defined as an infiltrative neoplastic

Figure 3.12. *continued.*

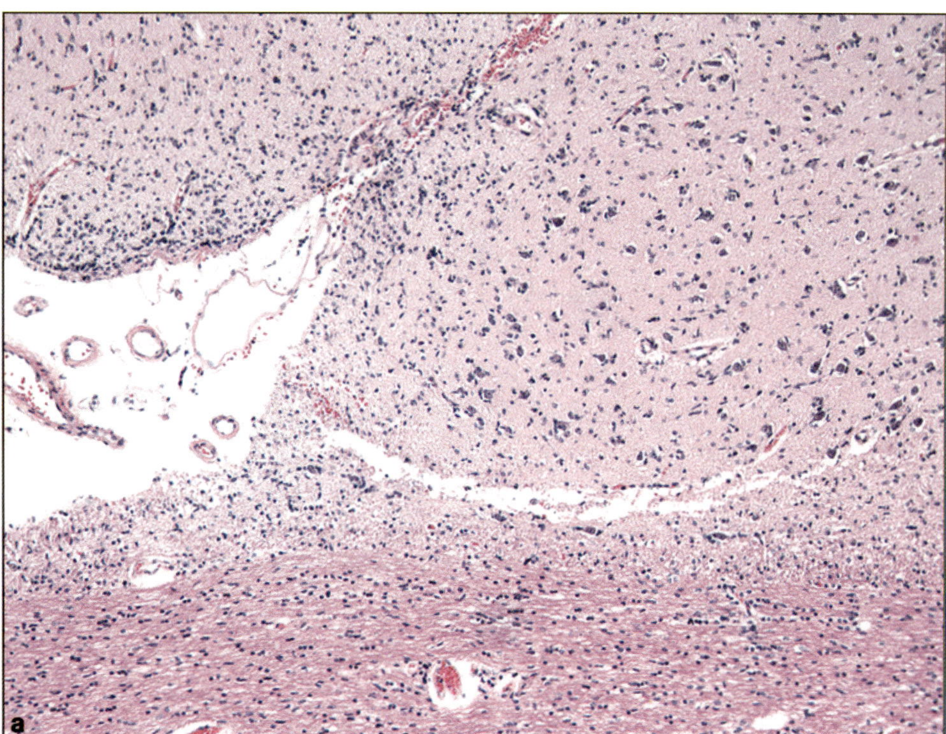

Figure 3.13. Gliomatosis cerebri. (a) Low magnification image shows features of a diffusely infiltrating neoplasm, with characteristic subpial and white matter tract spread and (b) neuronal satellitosis and perivascular spread seen at higher magnification. Infiltrating cells may be quite bland, or possess oligodendroglial features. Lymphomatosis cerebri has also been reported that closely mimics gliomatosis cerebri.

glioma, usually astrocytic, with minimal mass effect but infiltrative involvement of at least three cerebral lobes, usually with bilateral involvement. The process may extend into the brainstem, cerebellum, or spinal cord by the time of diagnosis. MRI imaging studies show conspicuous fluid-attenuated inversion recovery FLAIR sequences with variable contrast enhancement.

Figure 3.13. *continued.*

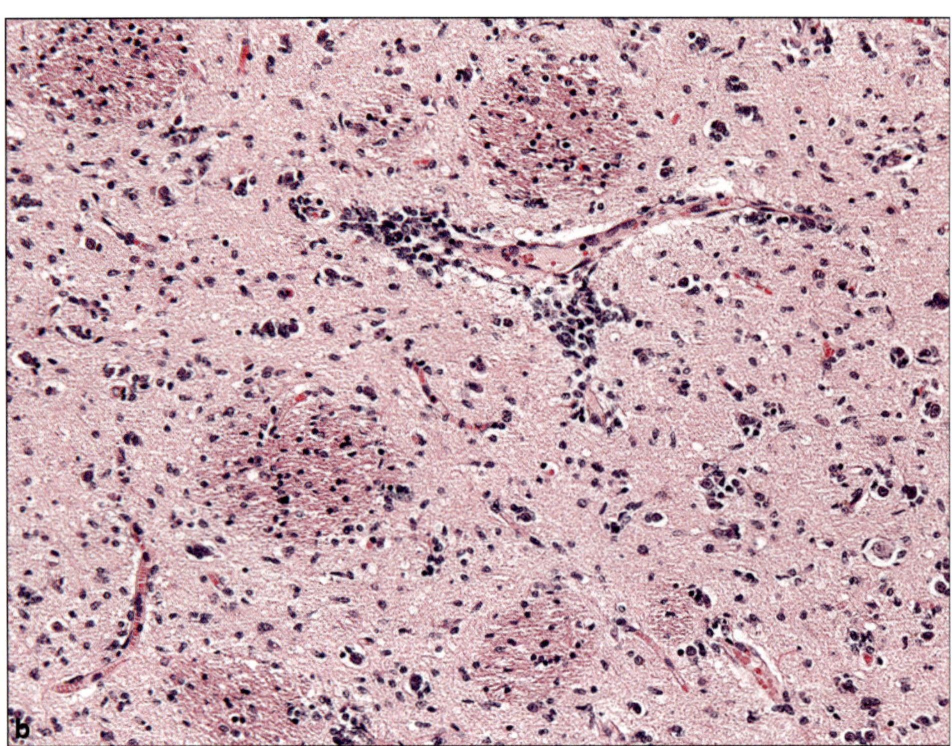

Pathology

Gross inspection of autopsy specimens shows diffuse enlargement of white matter with remarkably little destruction or alteration of anatomy. Microscopic examination indicates a hypercellular process with mildly atypical astrocytic cells, sometimes showing elongated profiles according to their infiltrative behavior (Figure 3.13a,b). Cases have also emerged termed *lymphomatosis cerebri* in which the infiltrating cells closely resemble glial cells but which are in fact lymphocytic as revealed by antilymphocyte immunohistochemistry (Kanai et al., 2008). Oligodendroglial features have also been described in the infiltrating cells. Mitotic figures are infrequent. In classical gliomatosis cerebri, microvascular proliferation and necrosis are absent but may appear in the late stages of the disease. Microglial activation is not a normal feature and its present should raise consideration of a reactive astrocytic process.

Immunohistochemical measurement of proliferative index shows a wide range, between 1 percent and 30 percent. The study may prove especially useful when large and atypical nuclei are seen to be those labeled as proliferative, especially in small biopsies.

REFERENCES

Badie B, Schartner JM. Flow cytometric characterization of tumor-associated macrophages in experimental gliomas. *Neurosurgery* 2000; 46: 957–61; discussion 961–2.
Boesel CP, Paulson GW, Kosnik EJ, Earle KM. Brain hamartomas and tumors associated with tuberous sclerosis. *Neurosurgery* 1979; 4: 410–17.

Brat DJ, Scheithauer BW, Fuller GN, Tihan T. Newly codified glial neoplasms of the 2007 WHO Classification of Tumours of the Central Nervous System: angiocentric glioma, pilomyxoid astrocytoma and pituicytoma. *Brain Pathol* 2007a; 17: 319–24.

Brat DJ, Scheithauer BW, Medina-Flores R, Rosenblum MK, Burger PC. Infiltrative astrocytomas with granular cell features (granular cell astrocytomas): a study of histopathologic features, grading, and outcome. *Am J Surg Pathol* 2002; 26: 750–7.

Brat DJ, Shehata BM, Castellano-Sanchez AA, Hawkins C, Yost RB, Greco C, et al. Congenital glioblastoma: a clinicopathologic and genetic analysis. *Brain Pathol* 2007b; 17: 276–81.

Burger PC. Pathology of brain stem astrocytomas. *Pediatr Neurosurg* 1996; 24: 35–40.

Burger PC. *Tumors of the Central Nervous System*. Washington, D.C.: American Registry of Pathology, 2007.

Ishii N, Sawamura Y, Tada M, Daub DM, Janzer RC, Meagher-Villemure M, et al. Absence of p53 gene mutations in a tumor panel representative of pilocytic astrocytoma diversity using a p53 functional assay. *Int J Cancer* 1998; 76: 797–800.

Jaros E, Perry RH, Adam L, Kelly PJ, Crawford PJ, Kalbag RM, et al. Prognostic implications of p53 protein, epidermal growth factor receptor, and Ki-67 labelling in brain tumours. *Br J Cancer* 1992; 66: 373–85.

Kanai R, Shibuya M, Hata T, Hori M, Hirabayashi K, Terada T, et al. A case of 'lymphomatosis cerebri' diagnosed in an early phase and treated by whole brain radiation: case report and literature review. *J Neurooncol* 2008; 86: 83–8.

Kim SK, Wang KC, Cho BK, Jung HW, Lee YJ, Chung YS, et al. Biological behavior and tumorigenesis of subependymal giant cell astrocytomas. *J Neurooncol* 2001; 52: 217–25.

Louis DN, International Agency for Research on Cancer. *WHO Classification of Tumours of the Central Nervous System*. Lyon: International Agency for Research on Cancer, 2007.

Miyata S, Sugimoto T, Kodama T, Akiyama Y, Nakano S, Wakisaka S, et al. Adenoid glioblastoma arising in a patient with neurofibromatosis type-1. *Pathol Int* 2005; 55: 348–52.

Murayama S, Bouldin TW, Suzuki K. Immunocytochemical and ultrastructural studies of eosinophilic granular bodies in astrocytic tumors. *Acta Neuropathol* 1992; 83: 408–14.

Nakamura Y, Becker LE. Subependymal giant-cell tumor: astrocytic or neuronal? *Acta Neuropathol* 1983; 60: 271–7.

Peiffer J, Kleihues P. Hans-Joachim Scherer(1906–1945), pioneer in glioma research. *Brain Pathol* 1999; 9: 241–5.

Prayson RA, Estes ML. Protoplasmic astrocytoma. A clinicopathologic study of 16 tumors. *Am J Clin Pathol* 1995; 103: 705–9.

Queiroz LS, Faria AV, Zanardi VA, Netto JR. Lipidized giant-cell glioblastoma of cerebellum. *Clin Neuropathol* 2005; 24: 262–6.

Roggendorf W, Strupp S, Paulus W. Distribution and characterization of microglia/macrophages in human brain tumors. *Acta Neuropathol* 1996; 92: 288–93.

Rong Y, Durden DL, Van Meir EG, Brat DJ. 'Pseudopalisading' necrosis in glioblastoma: a familiar morphologic feature that links vascular pathology, hypoxia, and angiogenesis. *J Neuropathol Exp Neurol* 2006; 65: 529–39.

Sasaki A, Yoshida T, Kurihara H, Sasaki T, Nakazato Y. Glioblastoma with large numbers of eosinophilic hyaline droplets in neoplastic astrocytes. *Clin Neuropathol* 2001; 20: 156–62.

Schiffer D, Chio A, Giordana MT, Leone M, Soffietti R. Prognostic value of histologic factors in adult cerebral astrocytoma. *Cancer* 1988; 61: 1386–93.

Selvapandian S, Rajshekhar V, Chandy MJ. Brainstem glioma: comparative study of clinico-radiological presentation, pathology and outcome in children and adults. *Acta Neurochir (Wien)*1999; 141: 721–6; discussion 726–7.

Shepherd CW, Scheithauer BW, Gomez MR, Altermatt HJ, Katzmann JA. Subependymal giant cell astrocytoma: a clinical, pathological, and flow cytometric study. *Neurosurgery* 1991; 28: 864–8.

Sinson G, Sutton LN, Yachnis AT, Duhaime AC, Schut L. Subependymal giant cell astrocytomas in children. *Pediatr Neurosurg* 1994; 20: 233–9.

Tehrani M, Friedman TM, Olson JJ, Brat DJ. Intravascular thrombosis in central nervous system malignancies: a potential role in astrocytoma progression to glioblastoma. *Brain Pathol* 2008; 18: 164–71.

Telfeian AE, Judkins A, Younkin D, Pollock AN, Crino P. Subependymal giant cell astrocytoma with cranial and spinal metastases in a patient with tuberous sclerosis. Case report. *J Neurosurg* 2004; 100: 498–500.

Tihan T, Fisher PG, Kepner JL, Godfraind C, McComb RD, Goldthwaite PT, et al. Pediatric astrocytomas with monomorphous pilomyxoid features and a less favorable outcome. *J Neuropathol Exp Neurol* 1999; 58: 1061–8.

Wyatt-Ashmead J, Kleinschmidt-DeMasters BK, Hill DA, Mierau GW, McGavran L, Thompson SJ, et al. Rhabdoid glioblastoma. *Clin Neuropathol* 2001; 20: 248–55.

Oligodendroglial and Mixed Oligoastrocytic Tumors

Oligodendroglioma

Clinical and Radiological Features

Oligodendrogliomas account for 10%–25% of diffuse gliomas and arise most commonly in the cerebral hemispheres, particularly the frontal lobes. They may rarely occur in the brainstem, spinal cord, or cerebellum. They occur most frequently occur in adulthood with a peak incidence at 40–45 years, and are distinctly rare in childhood (Kreiger et al., 2005). They produce neural deficits such as headache and seizures according to their location, chiefly due to increased intracranial pressure. The pace of the onset of symptoms may predict the grade of tumor, with a more protracted history typical of WHO Grade II tumors.

WHO Grade II lesions are typically nonenhancing with increased T2-weighted signal and FLAIR sequences (Figure 3.14a,b). As anaplasia occurs, contrast enhancement may be seen. Approximately 40% of oligodendrogliomas may show calcification.

Pathology

Oligodendrogliomas show one of the most characteristic microscopic appearances of all neoplasias, roughly recapitulating the appearance of

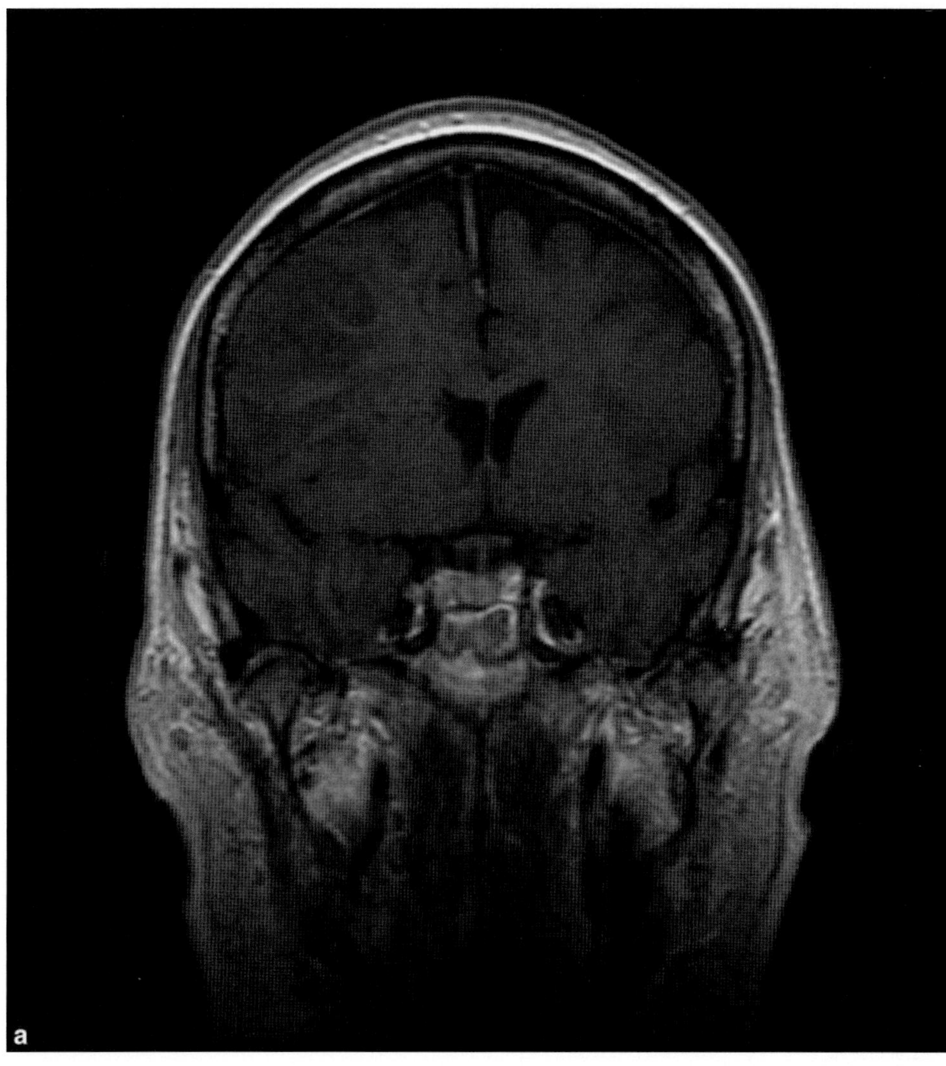

Figure 3.14. (a) WHO Grade II oligodendrogliomas are analogous to astrocytomas of equivalent grade, being typically nonenhancing frontal or temporal lobe lesions, with (b) increased T2-weighted signal and FLAIR sequences. As anaplasia occurs, contrast enhancement may be seen. Approximately 40% of oligodendrogliomas may show calcification. (c) Squash cytological preparations show round nuclei to great advantage. (d) Cryosections or even some rapidly fixed specimens will not show perinuclear halos, an artifact of formalin fixation and paraffin embedding. (e) Typical microscopic appearance, with "fried egg" perinuclear halos and delicate microvasculature, (f) and "ropey myelin", intact myelinated fibers within the infiltrating oligodendroglioma.

nonneoplastic oligodendrocytes (Figure 3.14c–m). Nuclear morphology is a key microscopic feature of all oligodendrogliomas and may be most helpful in distinguishing these from astrocytic tumors. Nuclei are round with sharply defined membranes and inconspicuous chromatin. Formalin fixation yields perinuclear clear halos, yielding the characteristic "fried egg" appearance. Importantly, this is not a feature of cryostat sections and thus would not be a useful diagnostic artifact at the time of frozen section for intraoperative diagnosis.

Another conspicuous feature is the delicate hexagonal array of capillaries, also described as a "chickenwire" pattern. Microcalcifications are also a frequent finding, particularly adjacent to small blood vessels. Mucinous or microcystic areas are occasionally seen but should not be confused with microcystic change in diffuse astrocytomas, or more particularly, low-grade brain tumors with oligodendroglial-like areas and mucinous change such as that seen in the dysembryoplastic neuroepithelial tumor (DNT) or pilocytic astrocytoma.

Figure 3.14. *continued.*

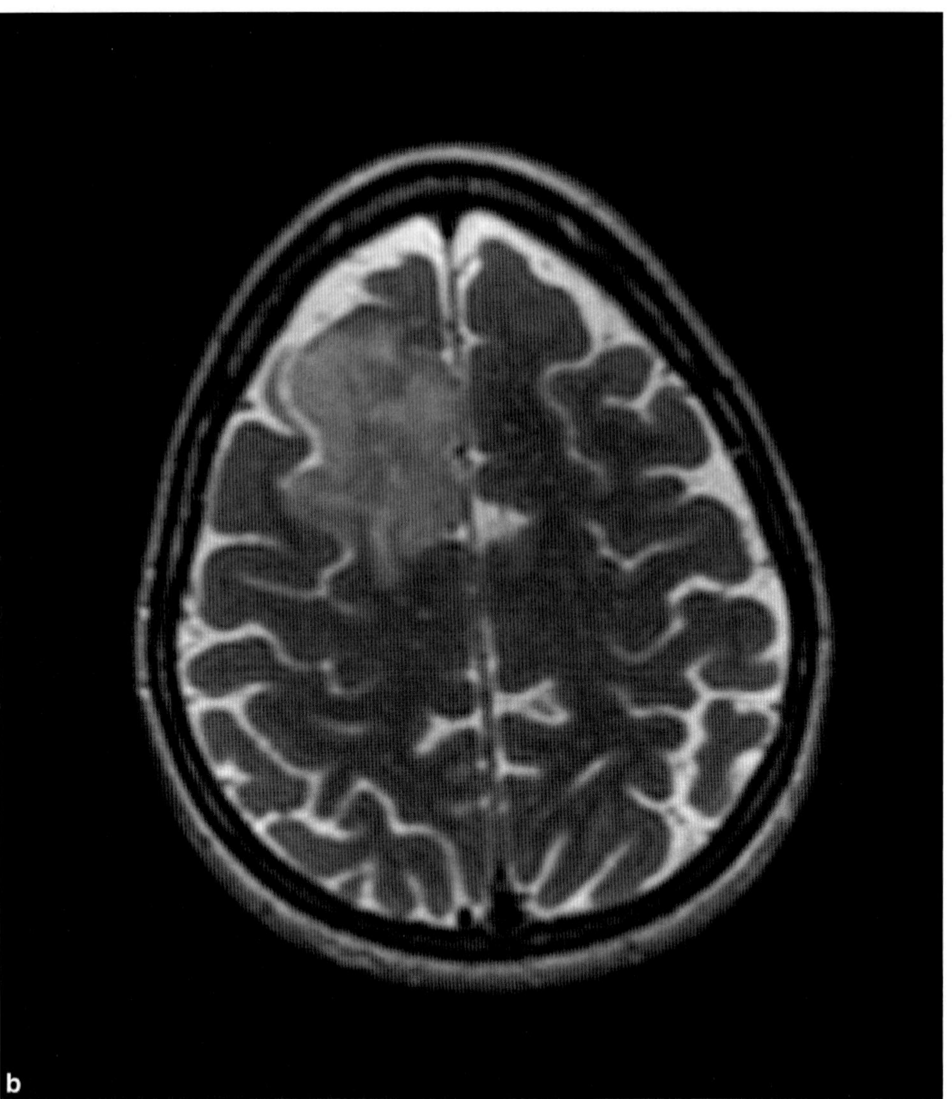

Oligodendrogliomas are also distinctive by their infiltrative behavior, often appearing to arise in subcortical white matter and then diffusely infiltrating the overlying cortex showing perineuronal satellitosis and perivascular spread. This may be a useful microscopic finding when cortex overlying a tumor mass is biopsied. When this microscopic feature is noted, oligodendroglioma should be strongly considered. Neuronal gigantism may be seen as a reactive feature. Within white matter, myelinated fibers may exist as surprisingly intact strands within the oligodendroglioma, known as ropey myelin.

An often-confusing aspect of oligodendrogliomas is the nonetheless relatively frequent presence of cells with distinctly oligodendroglial nuclei but eosinophilic cytoplasm. This is sometimes barely detectable as subtle and eccentrically located paranuclear cytoplasm or may be more conspicuous and conform to the designation of "minigemistocytes." Similar cells with possibly a single detectable cell process are sometimes called glial fibrillary oligodendrocytes because of the perinuclear or circumnuclear GFAP immunopositivity. Such cells may result in difficulty, distinguishing pure oligodendroglioma from mixed oligoastrocytoma or

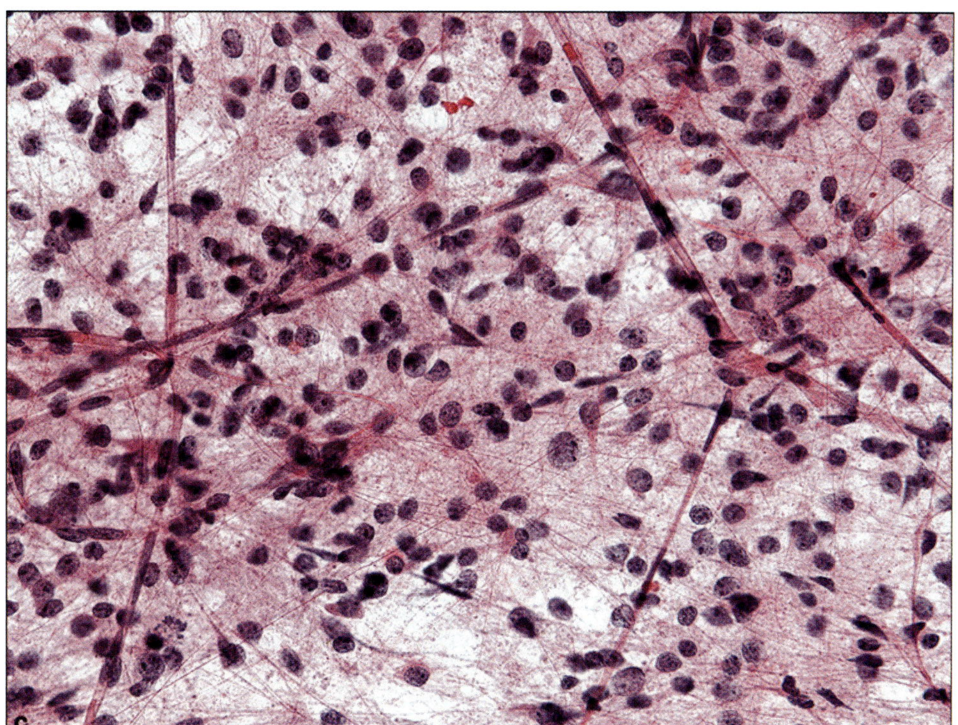

Figure 3.14. *continued.*

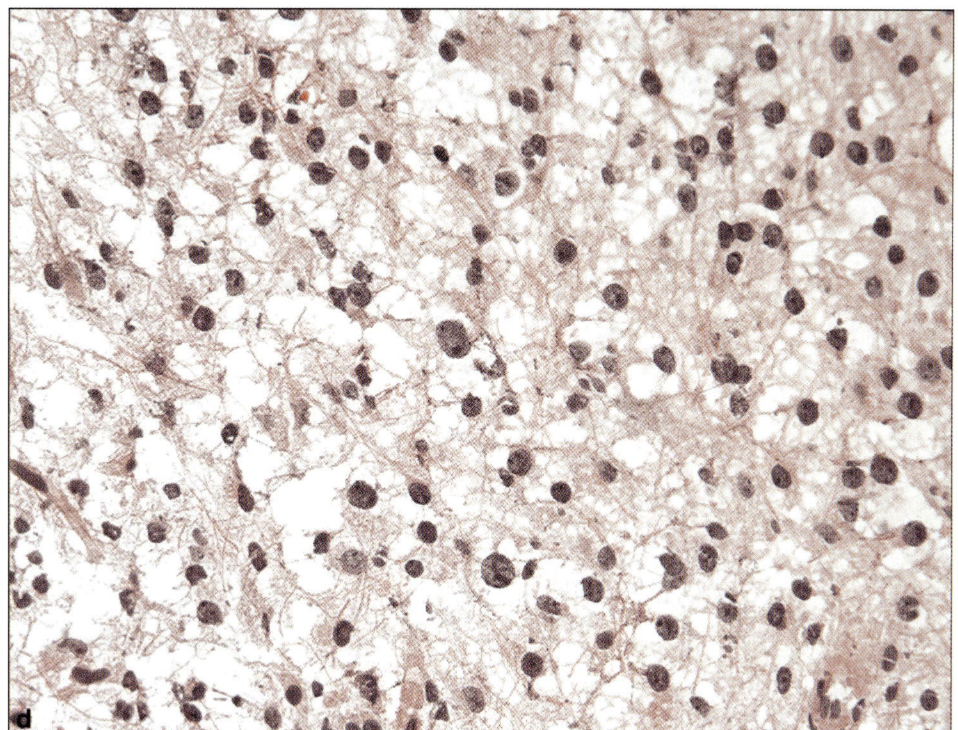

pure astrocytoma; however, oligodendroglial lineage should be favored if the nuclear features are oligodendrocytic.

Immunohistochemical tools for the diagnosis of oligodendroglioma remain quite limited as there is no reliable and specific marker of oligodendrocytes. Immunohistochemistry is most useful in excluding tumors with morphologic

Figure 3.14. *continued.*

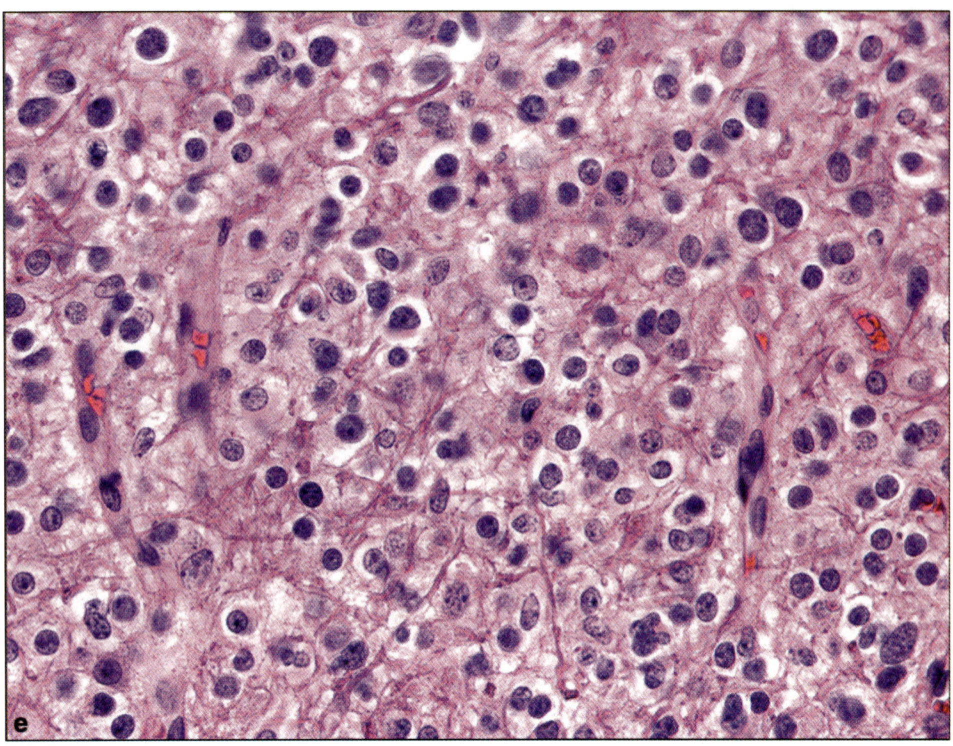

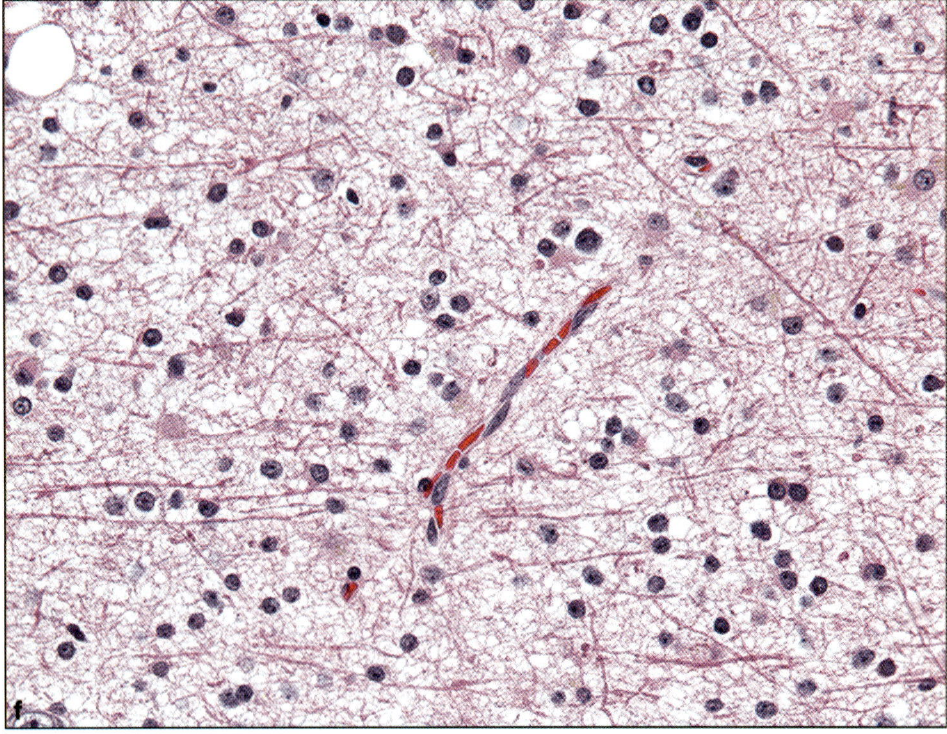

similarities, chiefly clear cell ependymomas, astrocytomas, or oligoastrocytomas. The use of MIB-1 immunostaining may be used to distinguish WHO Grade II examples from more anaplastic forms with average labeling indices of about 1% to 7% or 10% or higher, respectively.

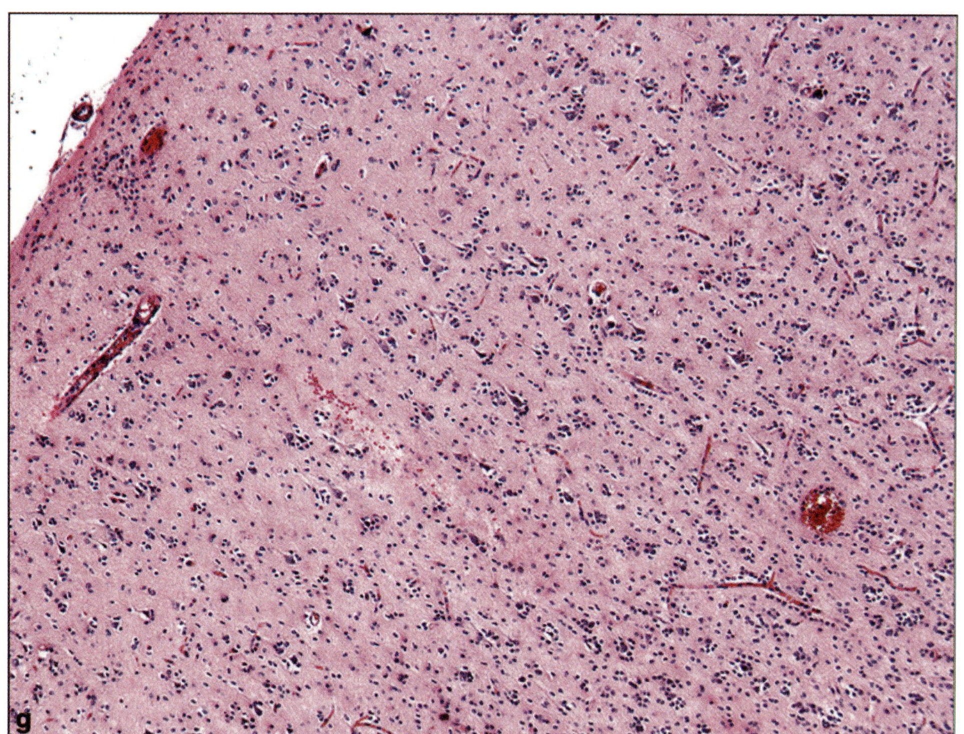

Figure 3.14. *continued*
(g,h) Oligodendrogliomas, irrespective of the favorable 1p/19q codeletion, may show extensive cortical invasion with prominent perinuclear satellitosis, perivascular spread and subpial aggregates.

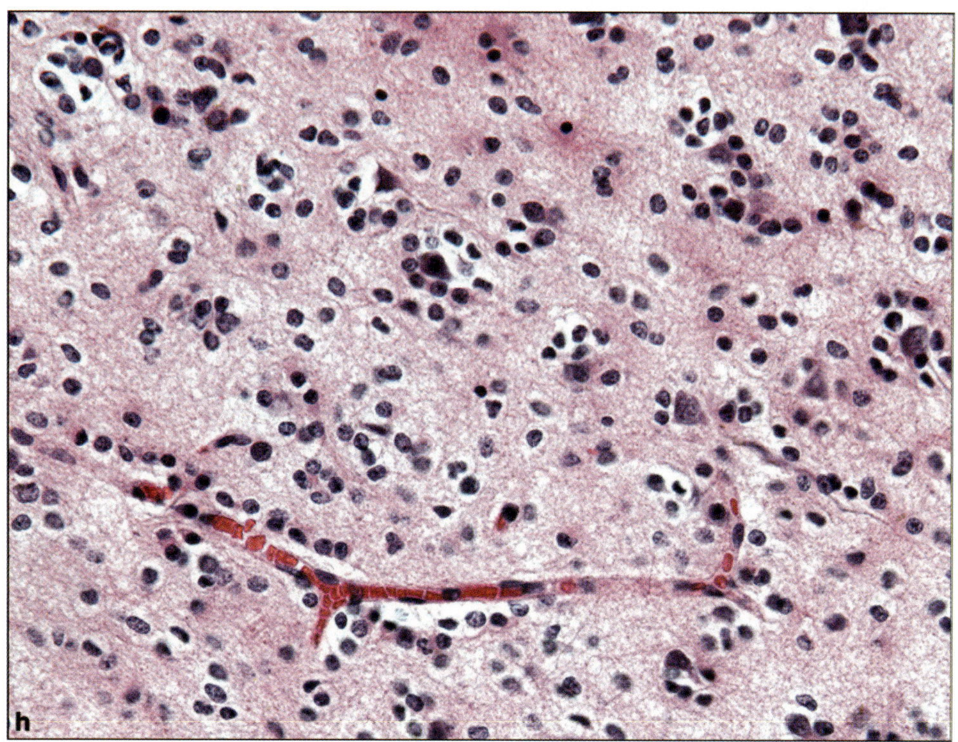

Anaplastic Oligodendroglioma

Clinical and Radiological Features

Anaplastic oligodendrogliomas occur in the same locations as their lower grade counterparts but may feature a shorter prodrome of symptoms. These are also more likely to show focal contrast enhancement.

Figure 3.14. *continued*
(i) Oligodendrogliomas may contain cells such as minigemistocytes with a small amount of eccentric eosinophilic cytoplasm, or gliofibrillary oligodendrocytes, (j) with more extensive perinuclear GFAP immunopositivity, but retaining the round nuclear contour.

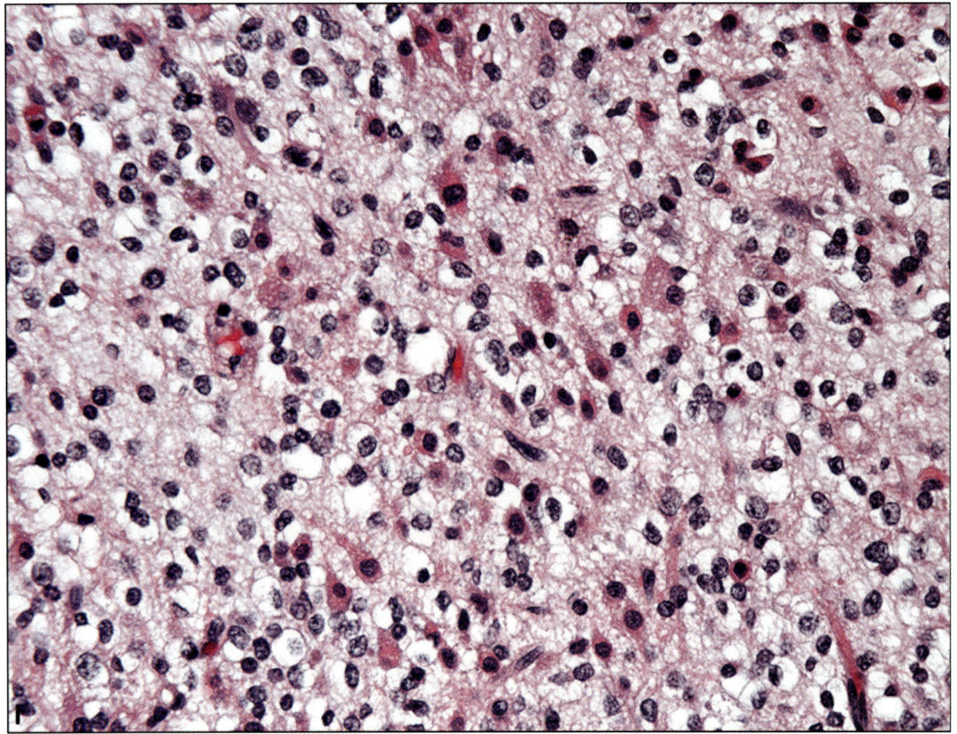

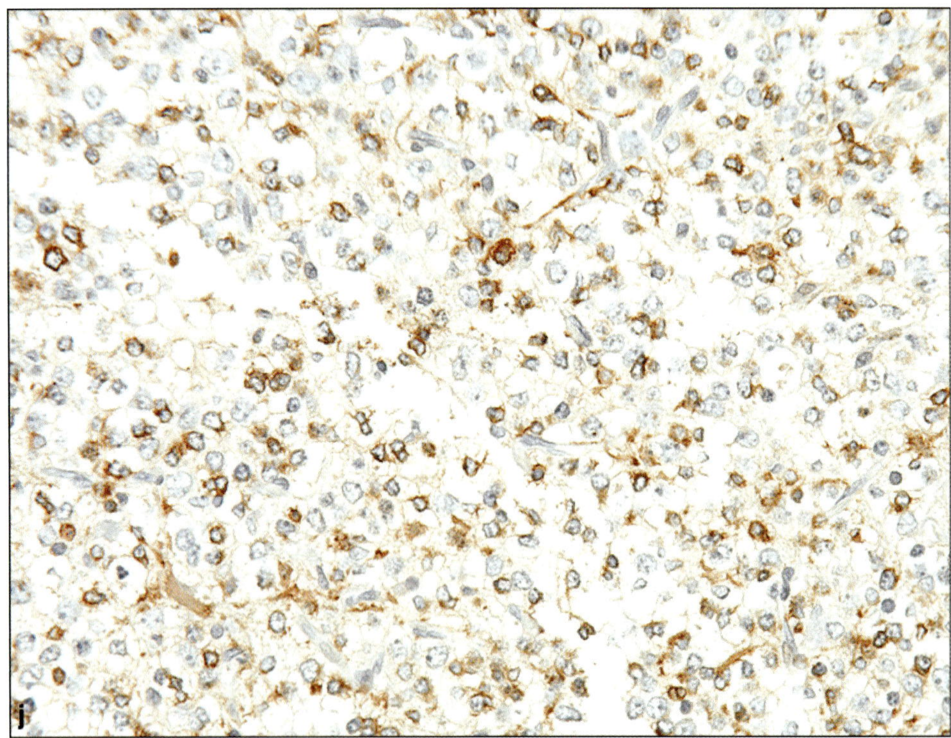

Pathology

The presence of intermediate forms of oligodendroglioma between WHO Grades II and III creates an occasional problem in clearly distinguishing anaplastic oligodendroglioma. Islands of hypercellularity and increased proliferative activity in otherwise uniformly WHO Grade II oligodendrogliomas may

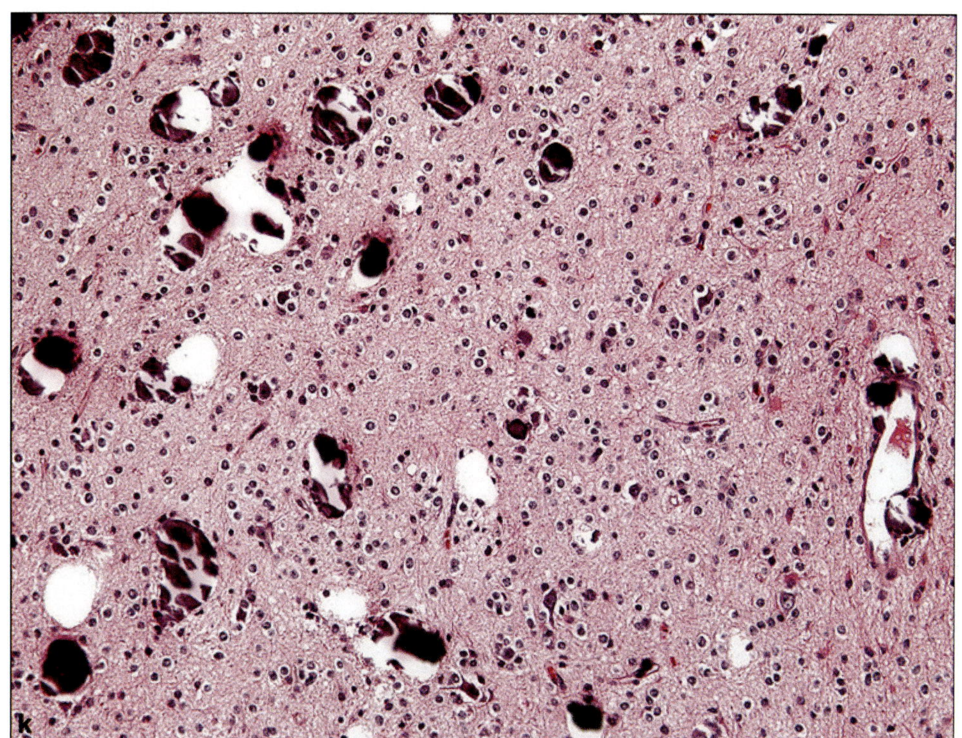

Figure 3.14. *continued*
(k) Microcalcification is especially associated with oligodendrogliomas.
(l) Microcystic change.

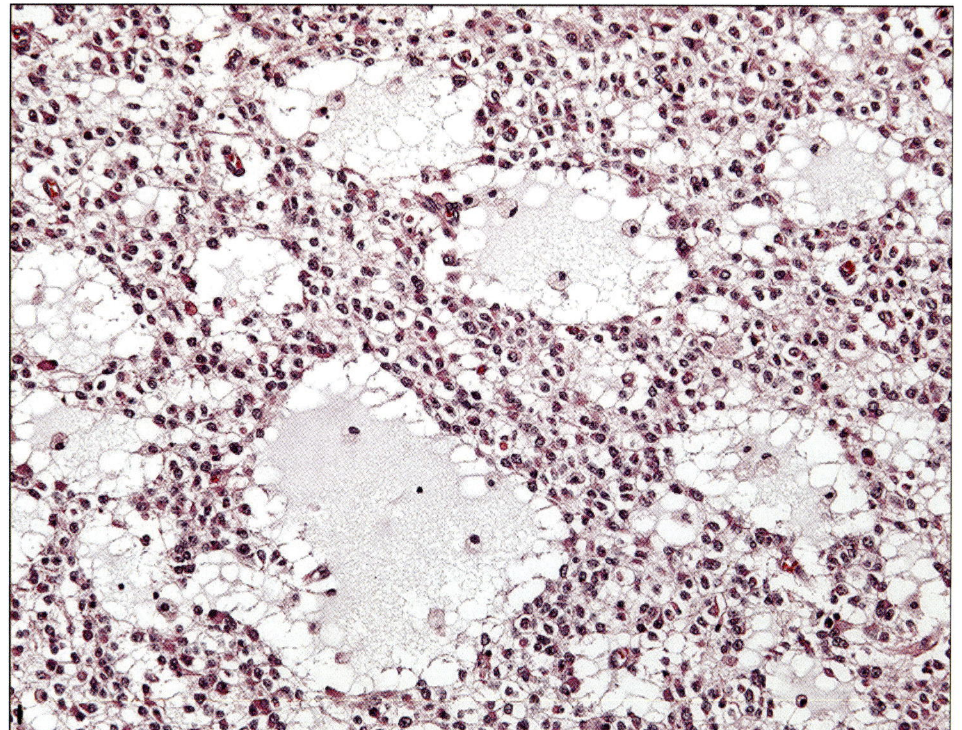

occasionally be seen. An unambiguous anaplastic oligodendroglioma may be diagnosed when high cellularity, nuclear pleomorphism, and vascular proliferation are observed (Figure 3.15). As previously noted, nuclei generally retain their rounded contours in spite of moderate pleomorphism and hyperchromasia. Rows or banks of cells in close parallel alignment may also be present.

Figure 3.14. *continued* (m) Neuronal "gigantism" in infiltrating oligodendroglioma.

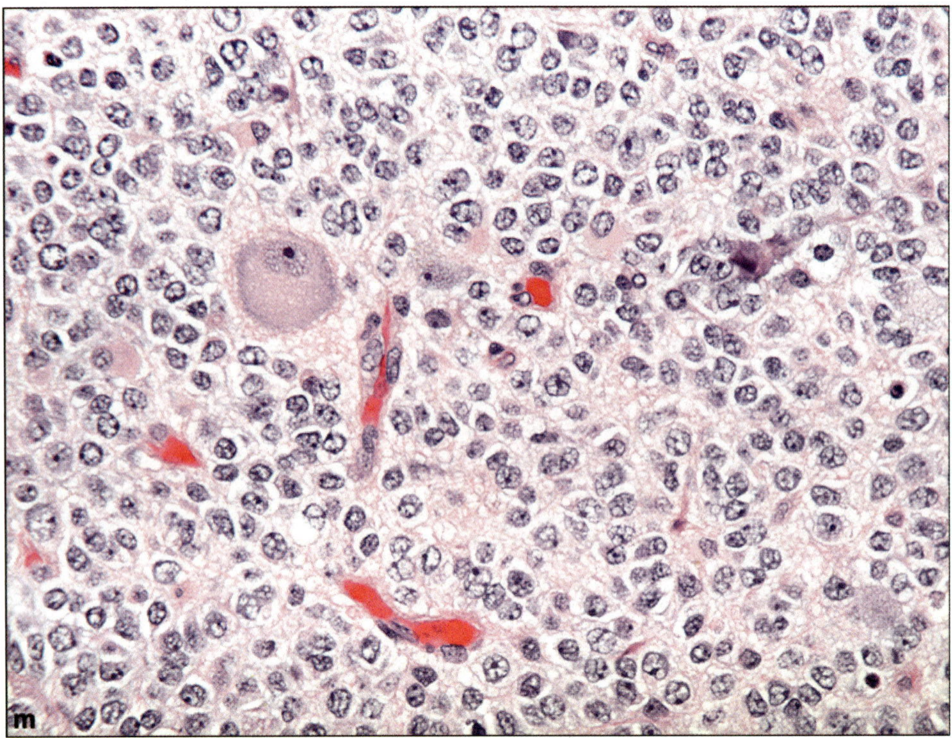

Focal necrosis with pseudopalisading seen in an otherwise oligodendroglial neoplasm, disregard should not prompt a diagnosis of glioblastoma. Variants of anaplastic oligodendroglioma include a spindle-cell type. Occasional neoplastic cells with astrocytic features may be seen. Controversy exists as to the percentage of such cells required to allow for a diagnosis of anaplastic mixed oligoastrocytoma.

Oligoastrocytoma

Clinical and Radiological Features

Oligoastrocytomas of both WHO Grades II and III occur in the same locations as oligodendroglioma neoplasms, proportional to the bulk of lobes of the cerebral hemispheres. Rare examples have been noted in the brainstem. Imaging of oligoastrocytomas shows no distinctive features separable from those of other diffuse gliomas.

Pathology

Oligoastrocytomas were originally conceived as collision tumors between relatively pure oligodendrogliomas and astrocytomas. As the definition evolved, oligoastrocytoma was viewed as a glial neoplasm showing an admixture of oligodendroglioma and astrocytic cells (Figure 3.16). Accordingly, oligoastrocytomas may be divided into biphasic "compact" and intermingled "diffuse"

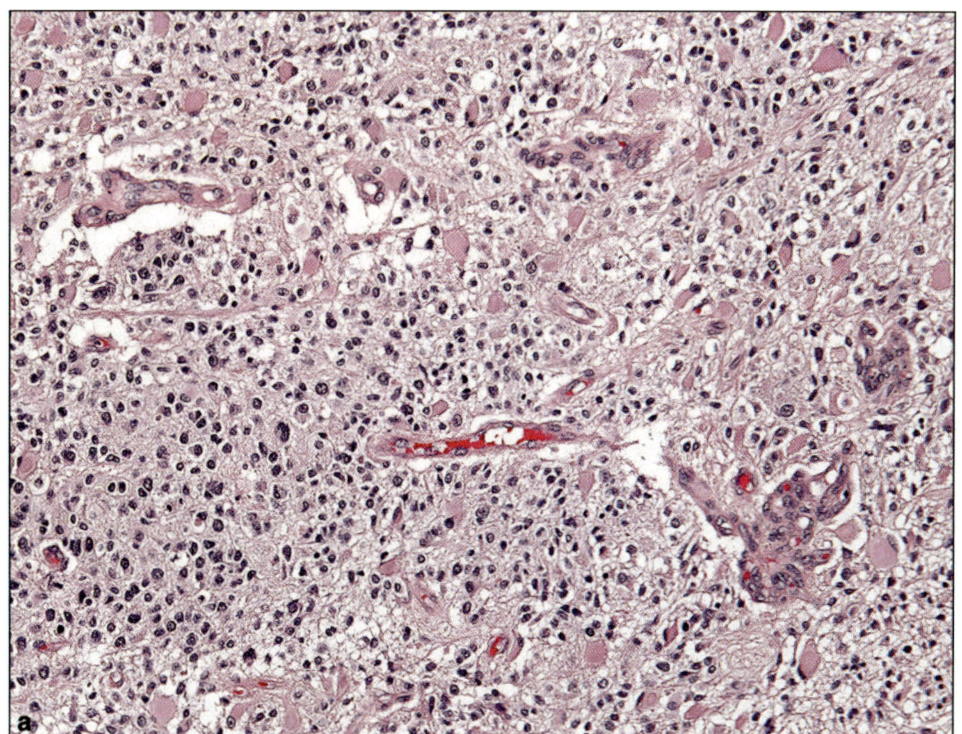

Figure 3.15. Anaplastic oligodendroglioma, WHO Grade III (a) with increased mitotic activity and vascular proliferation but retaining oligodendroglial nuclear morphology. (b) As in astrocytic tumors, oligodendrogliomas have a distinct propensity for regions of increased proliferation, seen here as a nodule of anaplastic oligodendroglioma within a WHO Grade II example.

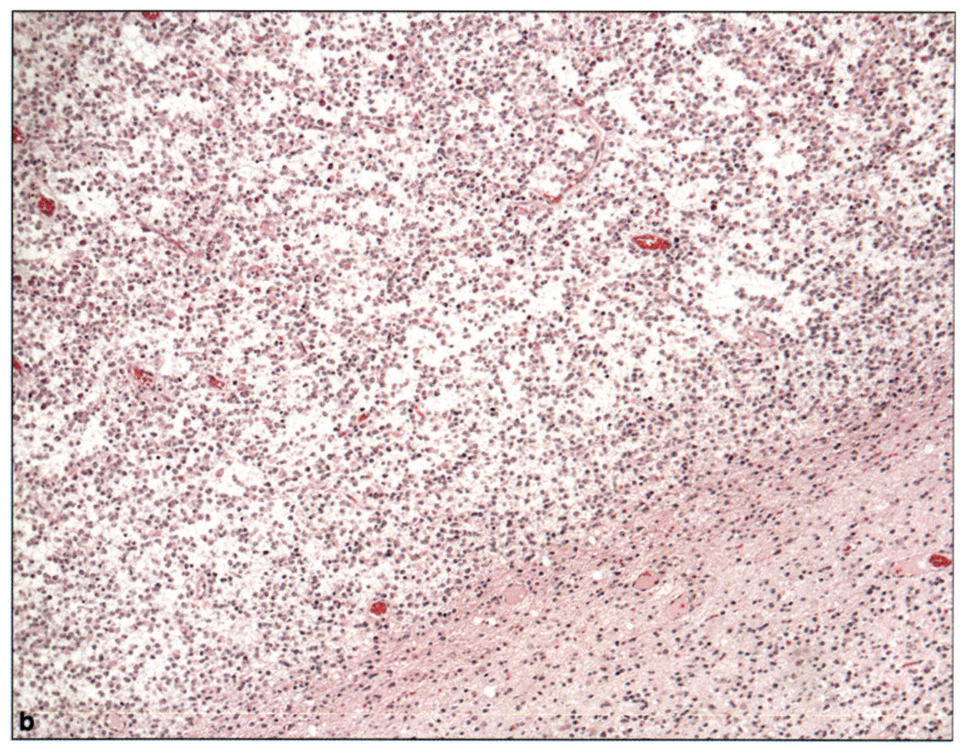

variants (Hart et al., 1974). As noted in the description of oligodendroglioma, the presence of minigemistocytes or gliofibrillary oligodendrocytes should not prompt a diagnosis of oligoastrocytoma. Only the definitive presence of fibrillary, gemistocytic, or protoplasmic elements can be accepted in diagnosing oligoastrocytoma.

Figure 3.15. *continued*
(c) Conspicuous mitotic activity may be seen. (d) An anaplastic oligodendroglioma with granular cell component, associated with either grade.

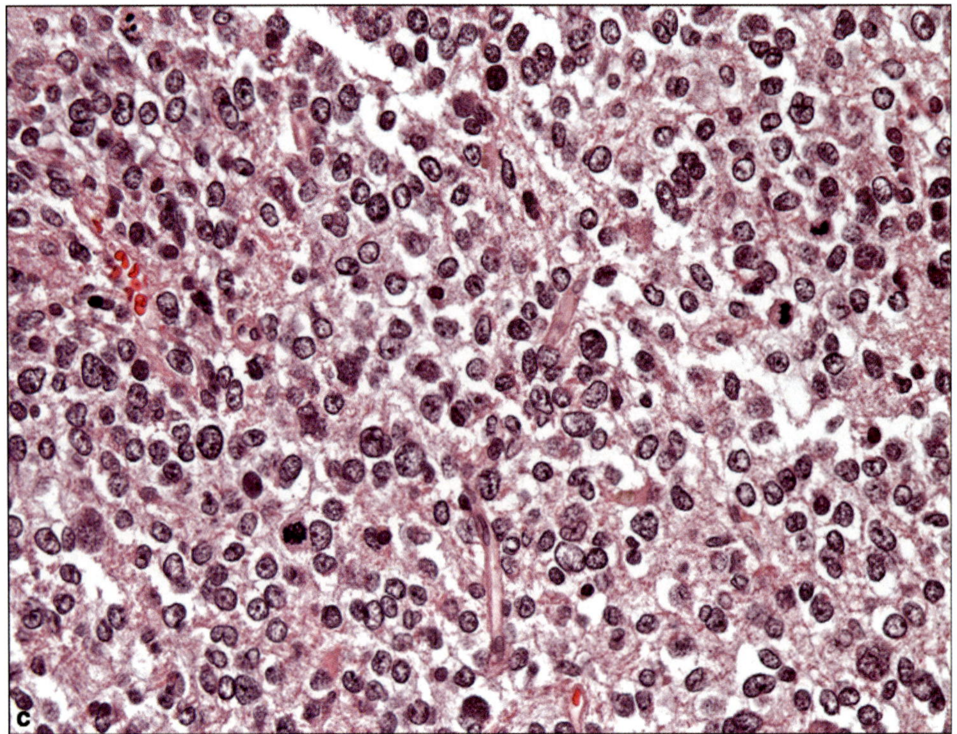

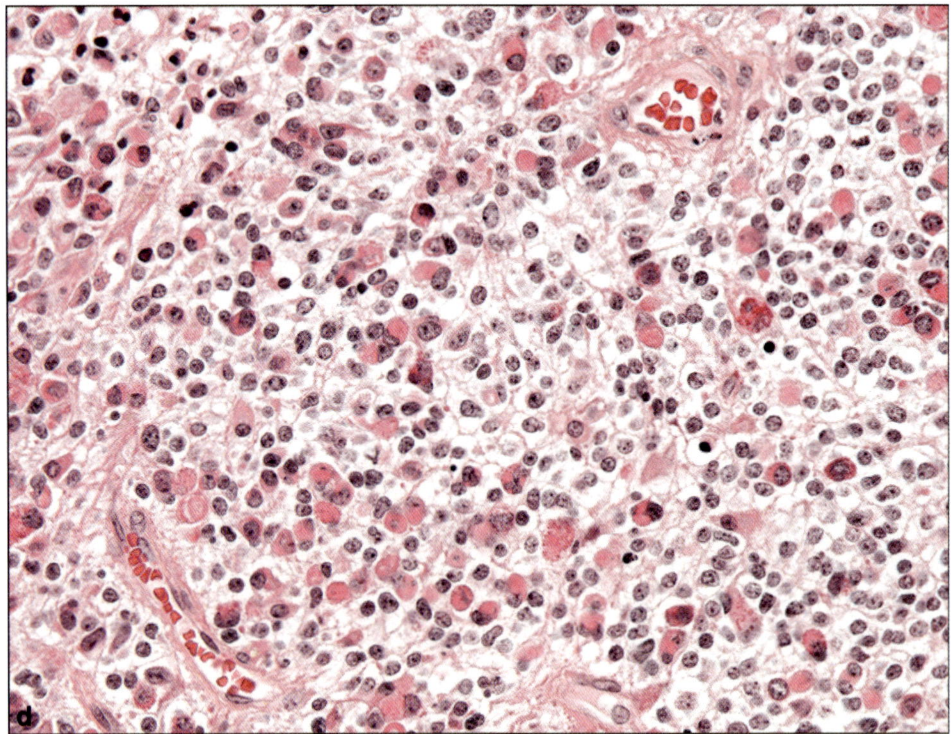

Anaplastic Oligoastrocytoma

Pathology

These tumors are oligoastrocytomas with clear features of anaplasia, including nuclear pleomorphism and atypia, increased cellularity, and high mitotic

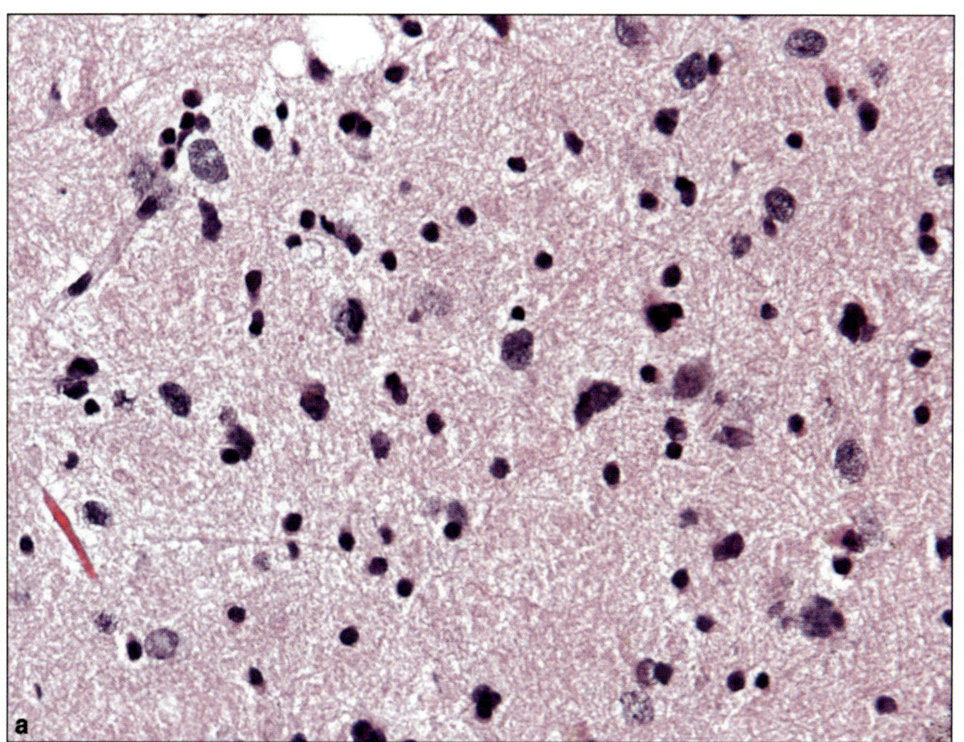

Figure 3.16. (a) Oligoastrocytoma remains a subjective diagnosis involving the recognition of a combination of round oligodendroglial and hyperchromatic angular astrocytic nuclei. (b) Eosinophilic cytoplasm is not necessarily a feature of astrocytic cells; angular nuclear contour and presence of discernable cell processes are more characteristic of astrocytic differentiation, while eosinophilic cytoplasm may be seen in minigemistocytes or gliofibrillary oligodendrocytes.

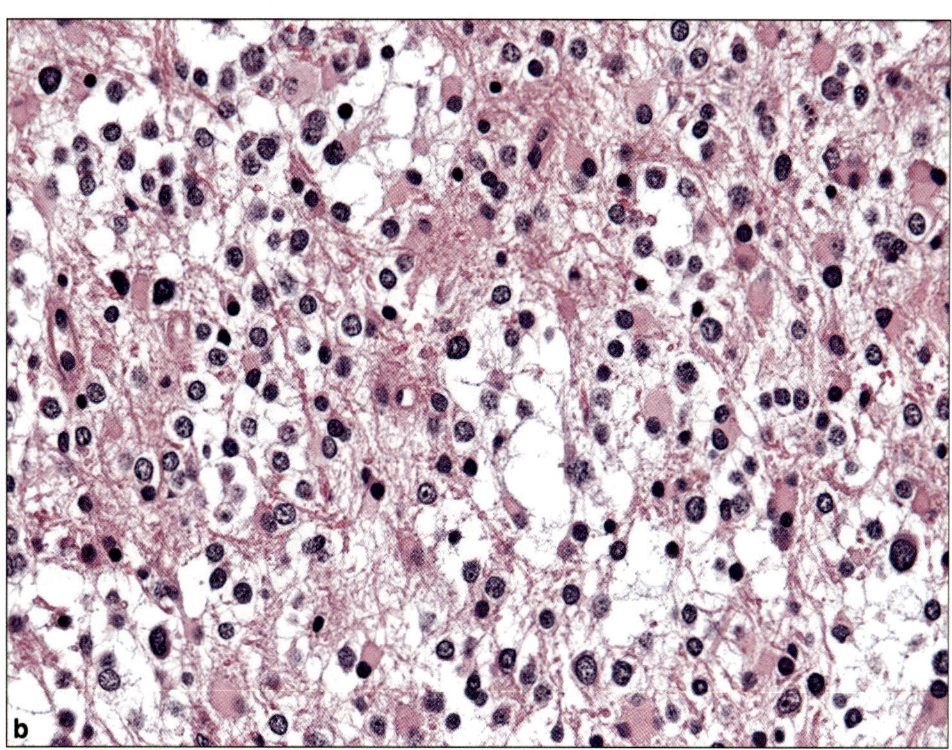

activity. Microvascular proliferation may also be seen (Figure 3.17). However, the presence of necrosis should result in diagnosis of "glioblastoma with oligodendroglial component."

Figure 3.17. Anaplastic oligoastrocytoma WHO Grade III. (a) Oligoastrocytomas with clear features of anaplasia, including nuclear pleomorphism and atypia, increased cellularity, and high mitotic activity. Microvascular proliferation may also be seen. (b) Strong nuclear immunopositivity for p53 is present in some oligoastrocytomas.

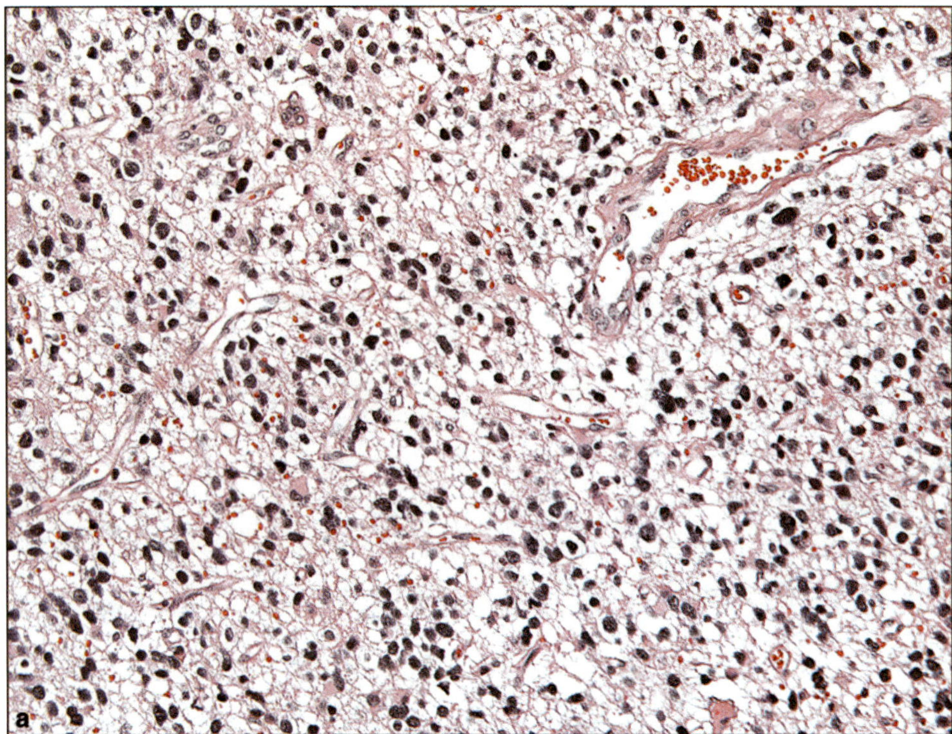

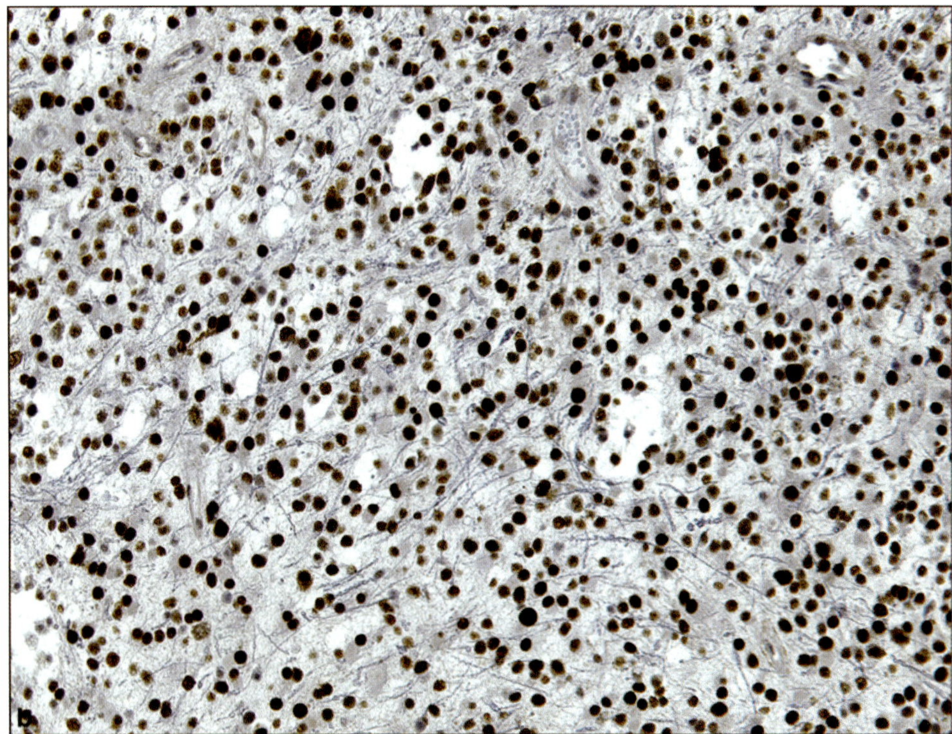

MOLECULAR TESTING IN OLIGODENDROGLIAL TUMORS

Given that the presence of codeleted 1p/19q or 1p deletion alone confers a significant survival advantage and prediction of favorable response to chemotherapy (Fallon et al., 2004), it is now commonplace to test for these

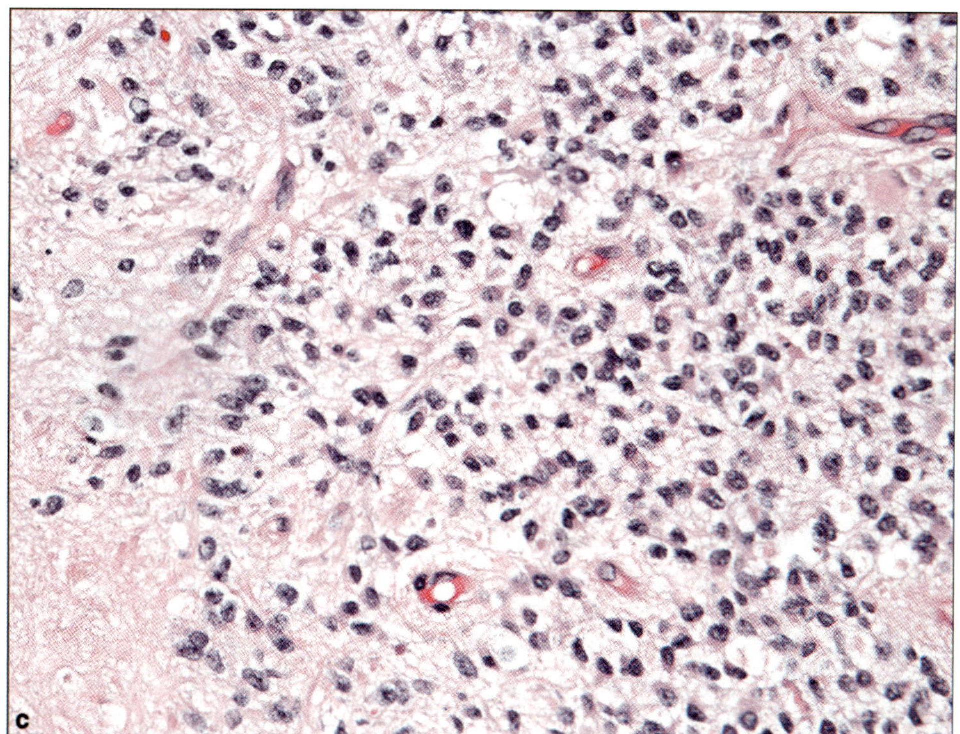

Figure 3.17. *continued*
(c) However, the presence of necrosis should result in diagnosis of "glioblastoma with oligodendroglial component."

abnormalities, most commonly by fluorescence in situ hybridization (FISH), polymerase chain reaction (PCR)-based strategies for the detection of loss of heterozygosity (Kelley et al., 2005) or by comparative genomic hybridization (CGH). FISH offers the advantage of the use of representative paraffin sections or touch cytological preparations from fresh tumor samples, however, skill in recognizing neoplastic cells is required in interpreting the results. Laboratories vary in their threshold for diagnosing gene deletion; however, a typical percentage is approximately 30% or above to constitute deletion, again making this determination by FISH in infiltrated tissue a distinct challenge.

Current observations from published clinicopathological research include the following:

1. Deletions of the entire 1p and 19q arms are associated with the favorable connotation of this finding, apparently related to an unbalanced 1p/19q translocation (Griffin et al., 2006; Jenkins et al., 2006).
2. Between 10% and 20% of oligodendrogliomas of classic histology do not have the 1p/19q codeletion, therefore histology is not completely predictive.
3. Testing for 1p deletion with a FISH probe to 1p36, as is currently commercially available, will not distinguish between the 1p microdeletion that is found in gliomas and other highly diverse human neoplasms, however, in combination with highly characteristic oligodendroglioma morphology (Aldape et al., 2007), most likely reflects loss of the entire 1p arm. Otherwise, FISH probes to a combination of other loci outside 1p36 may be superior.

4. CGH can reveal the status of 1p and 19q deletion but requires non-neoplastic genomic tissue to perform the assay. This may be isolated from blood leukocytes.

5. Conventional cytogenetics is not a reliable tool in this regard because the 1p/19q translocation is not detected by this technique. About half of oligoastrocytomas may have the 1p/19q codeletion; however, there is no conclusive data regarding its prognostic value in such cases.

6. 1p/19q codeletion is not a feature of pediatric oligodendrogliomas.

REFERENCES

Aldape K, Burger PC, Perry A. Clinicopathologic aspects of 1p/19q loss and the diagnosis of oligodendroglioma. *Arch Pathol Lab Med* 2007; 131: 242–51.

Fallon KB, Palmer CA, Roth KA, Nabors LB, Wang W, Carpenter M, et al. Prognostic value of 1p, 19q, 9p, 10q, and EGFR-FISH analyses in recurrent oligodendrogliomas. *J Neuropathol Exp Neurol* 2004; 63: 314–22.

Griffin CA, Burger P, Morsberger L, Yonescu R, Swierczynski S, Weingart JD, et al. Identification of der(1;19)(q10;p10) in five oligodendrogliomas suggests mechanism of concurrent 1p and 19q loss. *J Neuropathol Exp Neurol* 2006; 65: 988–94.

Hart MN, Petito CK, Earle KM. Mixed gliomas. *Cancer* 1974; 33: 134–40.

Jenkins RB, Blair H, Ballman KV, Giannini C, Arusell RM, Law M, et al. A t(1;19)(q10;p10) mediates the combined deletions of 1p and 19q and predicts a better prognosis of patients with oligodendroglioma. *Cancer Res* 2006; 66: 9852–61.

Kelley TW, Tubbs RR, Prayson RA. Molecular diagnostic techniques for the clinical evaluation of gliomas. *Diagn Mol Pathol* 2005; 14: 1–8.

Kreiger PA, Okada Y, Simon S, Rorke LB, Louis DN, Golden JA. Losses of chromosomes 1p and 19q are rare in pediatric oligodendrogliomas. *Acta Neuropathol* 2005; 109: 387–92.

Neuronal and Mixed Neuronal–Glial Tumors

The presence of neuronal differentiation in primary brain tumors has always represented an interpretive challenge. The largest number of newly recognized tumors of neuroepithelial derivation is among the neural and mixed neuronal and glial tumors. Neuronal differentiation varies from relatively undifferentiated neurocytes, most closely resembling granular neurons, to large ganglionic cells, which should display at least some dysplastic feature in order to be distinguished from entrapped cortical or other gray matter neurons. Small neurocytic aggregates may also be mimicked by lymphocytic perivascular aggregates, which may actually be part of a mixed glial and neuronal tumor just as they may be seen in pure astrocytic tumors. The problem is complicated by the lack of specificity of antineuronal antibodies, which may not enable the diagnostician to clearly distinguish between neoplastic ganglion cells and nonneoplastic neurons or entrapped neuronal processes. Immunohistochemistry for dendritic processes such as microtubular associated protein 2 (MAP 2) may highlight an organized or laminar architectural arrangement of neurons, thus favoring invaded gray matter, whereas clusters or irregular aggregates of ganglionic cells favor neoplastic growth. The detection of binucleate neuronal cells is invaluable in diagnosing mixed glial and neuronal tumors as clear evidence of dysplasia or neoplasia.

WHO GRADE I

Desmoplastic Infantile Astrocytoma and Ganglioglioma

Clinical and Radiological Features

Desmoplastic infantile astrocytomas/gangliogliomas (DIA/G) essentially always occur before the age of 12 months. They are distinctly rare tumors although their presentation is stereotypical. They occur as large cystic tumors involving the leptomeninges, often with a dural attachment and the superficial cerebral cortex involving more than one lobe, most commonly the frontal and the parietal (Figure 3.18a). Clinical signs include increased head circumference, bulging fontanelles, lethargy, and the orbital setting sun sign (downward deviation of an infant's or a young child's eyes as a result of pressure on cranial nerves III, IV, and VI, a late and ominous sign of increased intracranial pressure). Perhaps because of the superficial location, there is a generally good prognosis after surgical resection with the possibility of long-term survival, and thus these are classified as WHO Grade I.

Pathology

The solid portions are usually superficial and extracerebral, denoting lepto-meningeal involvement and the dural attachment. The cysts are large and multi-loculated. Both gross and microscopic necrosis and significant mitotic activity are absent. These neoplasms, as indicated by their name, display a prominent desmo-plastic stroma in which tumor cells are arranged in streaming fascicles (Figure 3.18b–g). The reticulin stain shows pericellular deposition. Astrocytic cells range from gemistocytic to elongated forms. When gangliocytic differentiation occurs, it ranges between cells with obvious gangliocytic differentiation to less differentiated small neurocytes, all of which, however, typically express neuronal antigens by immunohistochemistry such as that for synaptophysin or neurofilament. The poorly differentiated areas may also costain for GFAP and neuronal markers (Paulus et al., 1992; Rushing et al., 1993; VandenBerg, 1993). Foci of poorly differentiated epithelial cells may be seen representing an immature component. The proliferative index is generally less than 5% although examples may be seen with significantly higher values.

Dysembryoplastic Neuroepithelial Tumor

Clinical and Radiological Features

Most DNTs occur in the first three decades of life and almost always in patients younger than 50 years of age. They occur most frequently in the supratentorial cortex and are discovered after the diagnosis of long-standing intractable partial seizures (Daumas-Duport, 1993). There are believed to account for 18% of tumors

Figure 3.18. DIA/G.
(a) Radiographic images
displaying a superficial cystic
mass with dural association,
with contrast enhancement in
the T1-weighted image
(arrow). (b) Interface of
superifical cortical and
subarachnoid extension of
DIA/G demonstrating the
acquisition of desmoplastic
morphology in the
subarachnoid portion,
(c) highlighted by the
reticulin stain on the same
area. Cytomorphology may
vary significantly between (d)
spindled, (e) astrocytic with
gemistocytes, and (f)–(g)
poorly differentiated
neuronal differentiation.
Figures (d)–(g) are
generously provided by Dr.
Gregory Fuller, M.D.
Anderson Cancer Center,
Houston, TX.

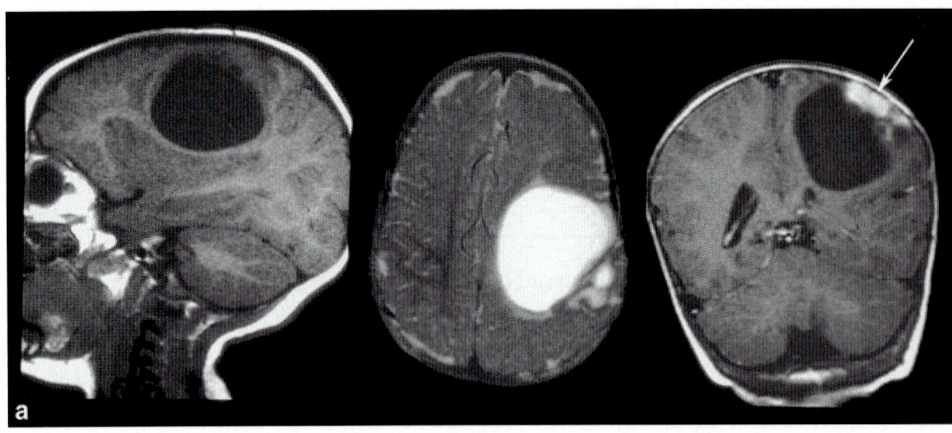

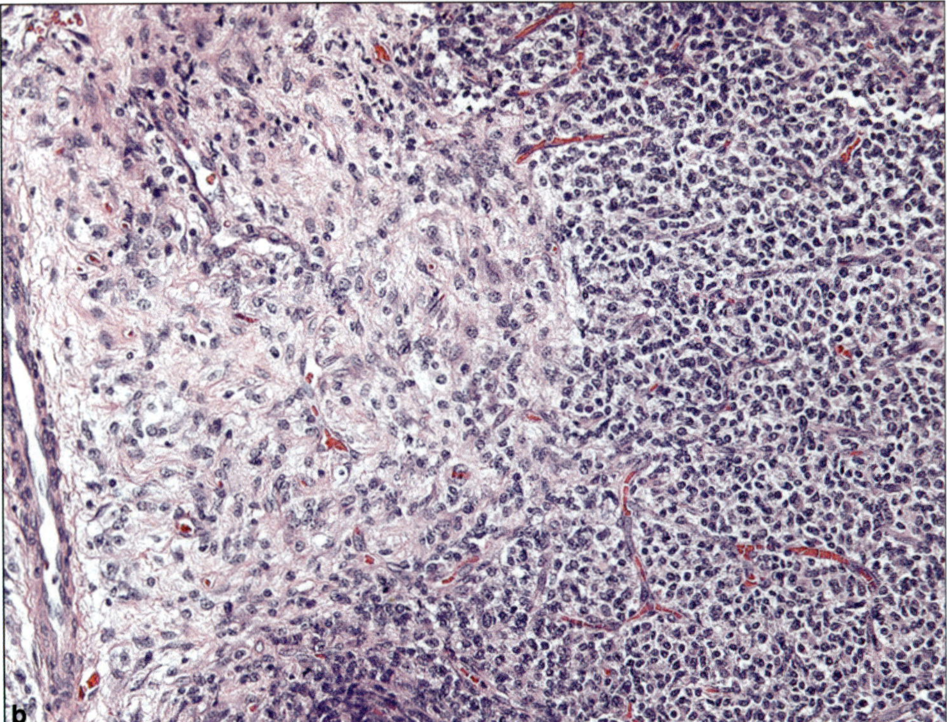

causing temporal lobe epilepsy (TLE). Infratentorial examples as well as a DNT-like tumor of the septum pellucidum have been reported (Baisden et al., 2001).

Radiological findings typically reveal a mass encompassing the thickness of the cortex with focal white matter extension (Figure 3.19a). In a minority of cases, they are hyper intense or isointense on T1-weighted images and may show a multicystic appearance. Deformation of the overlying calvarium may be an indicator of chronicity. Calcification is frequent on CT scans. Contrast enhancement may be focal. More complex forms include the presence of cortical dysplasia in the contiguous adjacent cortex. They occur most commonly in the temporal lobe, particularly the medial portions.

Pathology

The most characteristic microscopic appearance of a DNT is represented by loose columns of monotonous neurocytic cells arranged around vascular cores

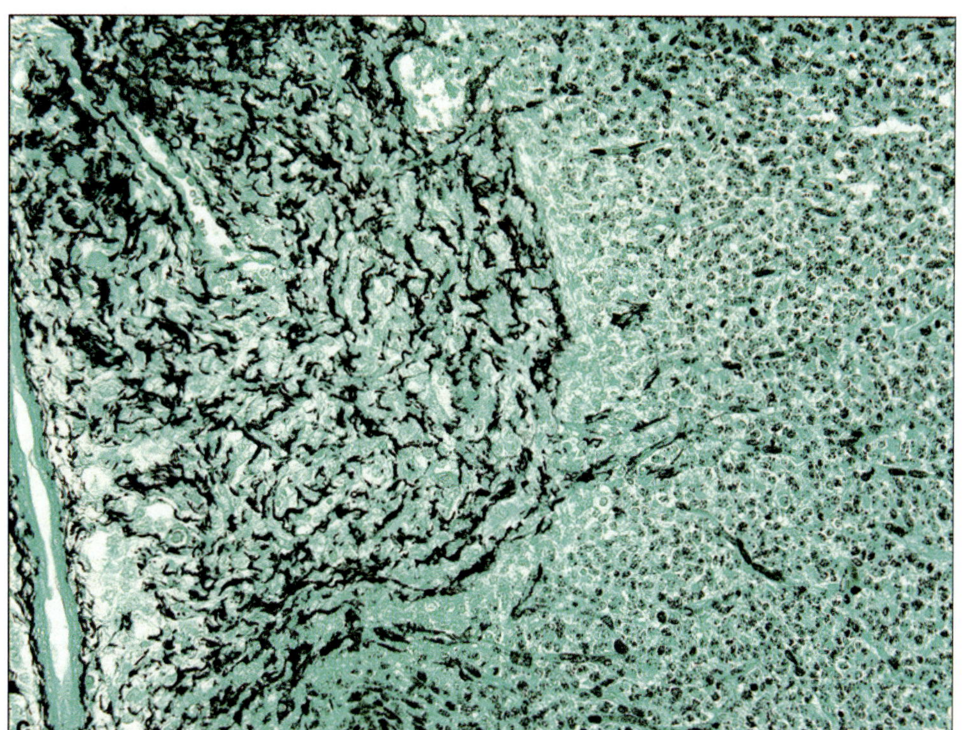

Figure 3.18. *continued.*

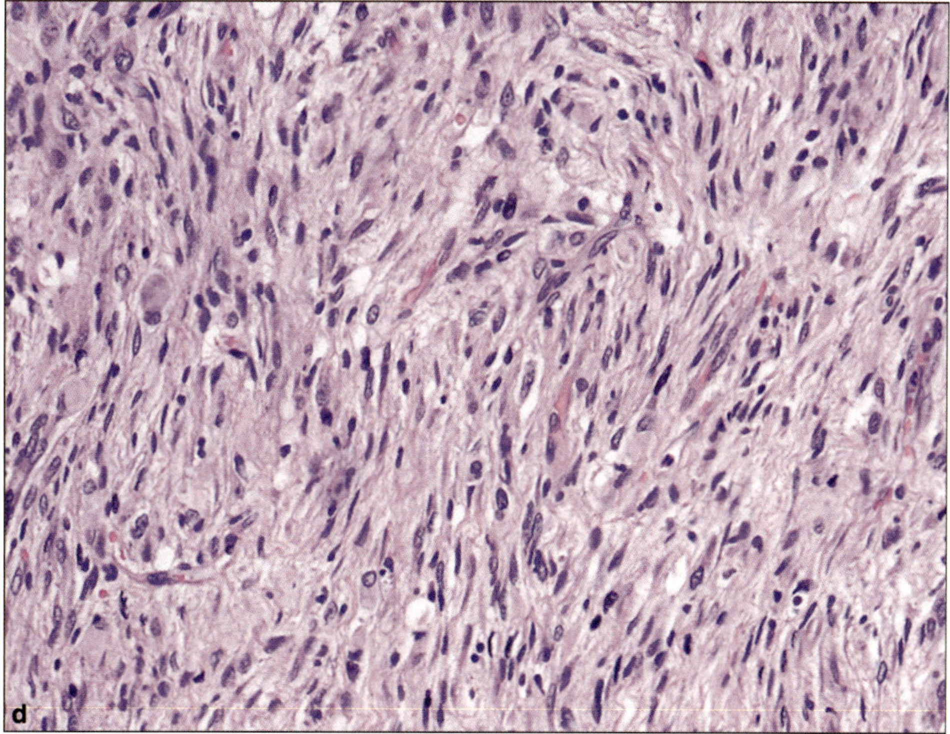

with intervening microcystic spaces (Figure 3.19b–e). Immunohistochemistry will highlight neuronal cell processes in parallel arrays with antisynaptophysin antibodies. Neuronal markers may also highlight floating neurons within microcystic spaces. Large areas of tumor may show clear cell or oligodendroglioma-like areas. These are typically GFAP immunonegative but positive for S-100 protein. The proliferative index is generally quite low.

Figure 3.18. *continued.*

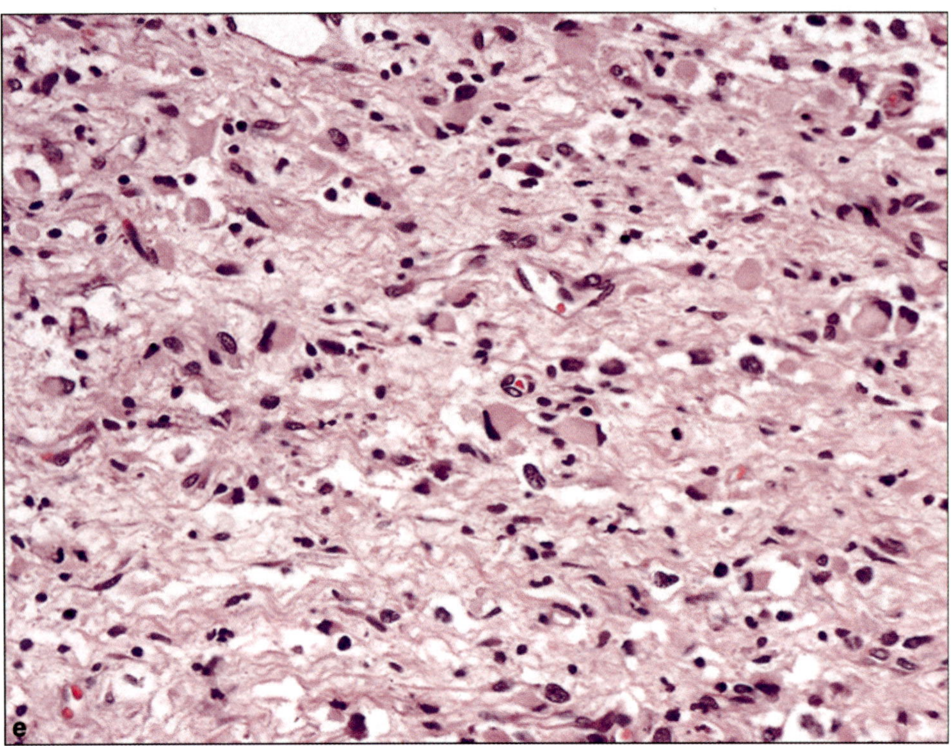

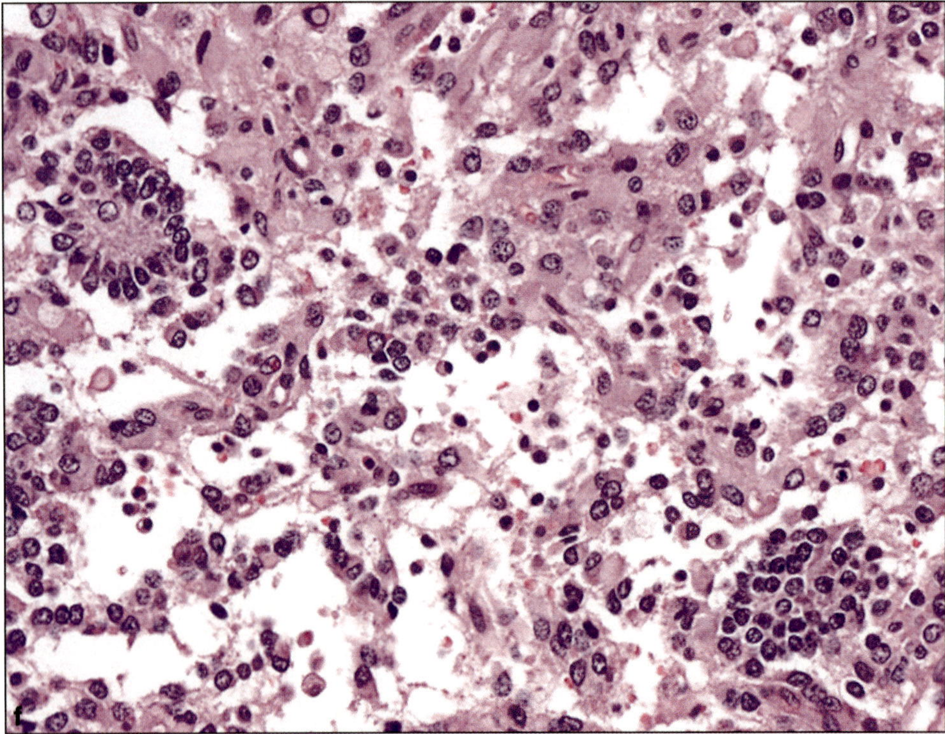

The DNT poses a particular problem in differential diagnosis, as it may be incorrectly diagnosed as a higher grade lesion. Care must be exercised to avoid the diagnosis of oligodendroglioma or other diffuse astrocytomas or glioneuronal tumors. When oligodendroglioma is suspected, molecular genetic analysis for 1p and 19q deletions may aid in the diagnosis by being present in some oligodendrogliomas.

Figure 3.18. *continued.*

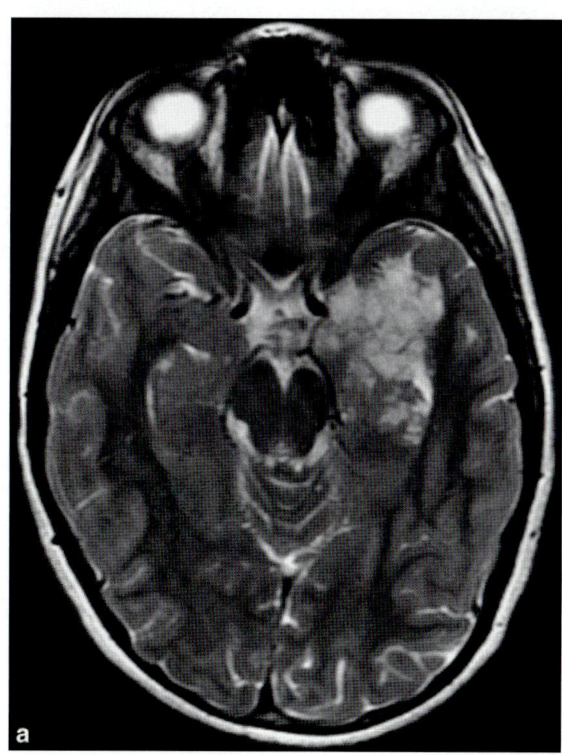

Figure 3.19.
DNT. (a) An axial T2-weighted MR image shows a bubbly, very high signal mass in the left mesiotemporal lobe with minimal enhancement. The mass involves the entire cortical thickness and is not surrounded by vasogenic edema. There may also be benign remodeling of the adjacent calvarium and no enhancement.

Ganglioglioma and Gangliocytoma

Clinical and Radiological Features

The peak incidence is from childhood to mid-adulthood. These neoplasms account for approximately 1% of all brain tumors but for 40% of tumors causing TLE. They may occur anywhere within the neuroaxis, but most commonly occur

Figure 3.19. *continued*
(b) Low-magnification view shows the typical multicentricity also seen radiographically in DNT.
(c) Parallel strands of oligodendrioglia-like cells may be seen in certain panes of section, which would be highlighted by synaptophysin immunohistochemistry.

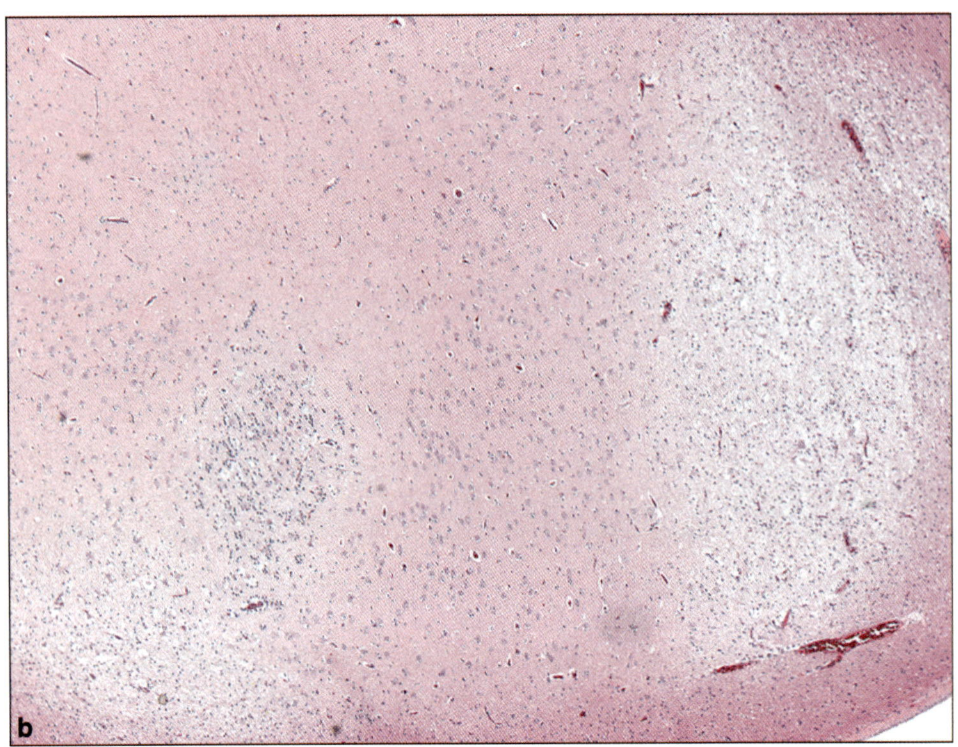

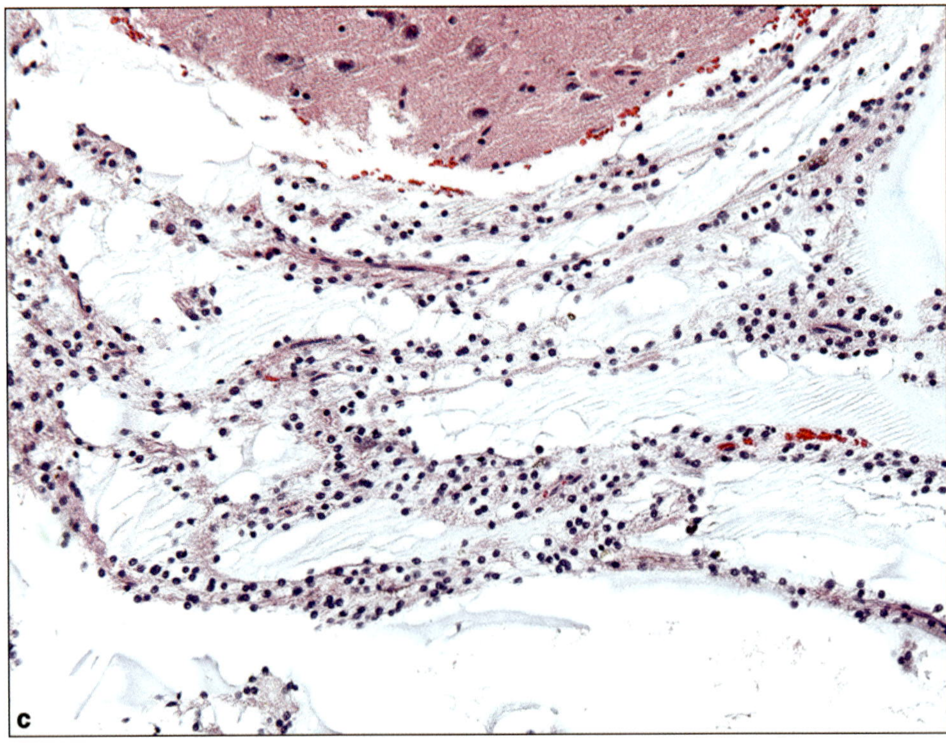

in the temporal lobe. Radiographically, these may be solid or cystic and WHO Grade I examples typically show contrast enhancement (Figure 3.20a).

Pathology

Gangliocytomas consist exclusively of ganglionic cells, but the more common occurrence in ganglion cell tumors is of mixed glial and neuronal cell populations

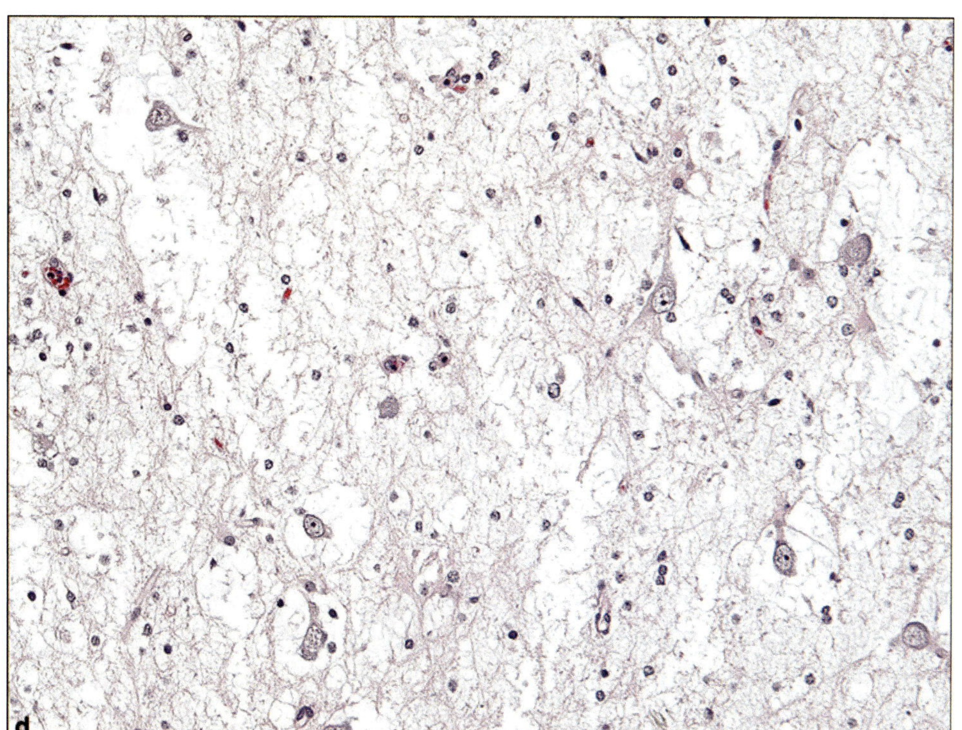

Figure 3.19. *continued* (d) "Floating neurons" in myxoid spaces. (e) Example of DNT of the septum pellucidum.

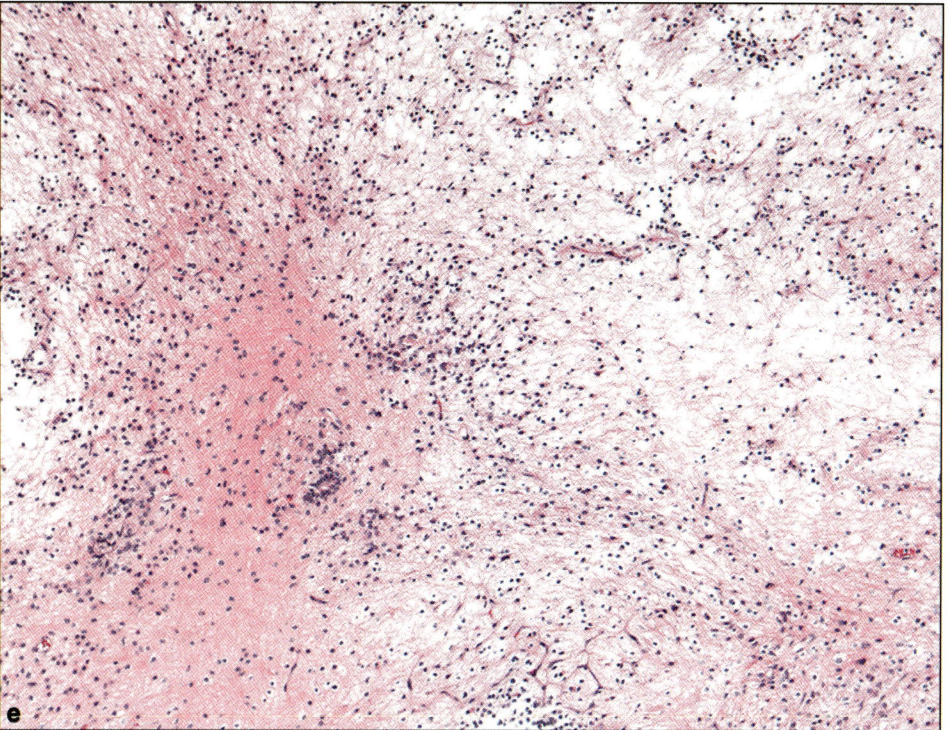

(Figure 3.20b–g). The identification of gangliocytic dysplasia is of paramount importance since otherwise pure astrocytomas may invade the cortex to the extent that cortical neuronal cytoarchitecture is unapparent, and neuronal gigantism or other reactions may occur to alter the appearance of nonneoplastic ganglion cells. Binucleated forms, marginated Nissl substance, and highly irregular cytoarchitectural arrangements and orientations, as defined by a haphazard

Figure 3.20. Ganglion cell tumors. (a) MRI showing the typical appearance of a temporal lobe ganglioglioma, with contrast enhancement of the solid protein of a cystic tumor, often discovered for the evaluation of epilepsy. (b) The simplest form of ganglion cell tumor is the gangliocytoma, with atypical and haphazardly arranged ganglion cells and no obvious glial component. (c) Higher magnification shows an EGB, and neurofibrillary change (arrow), (d) highlighted by silver impregnation (arrow). (e) Gangliogliomas may have a very loose glial background somewhat reminiscent of pilocytic astrocytoma, in this example with numerous EGBs.

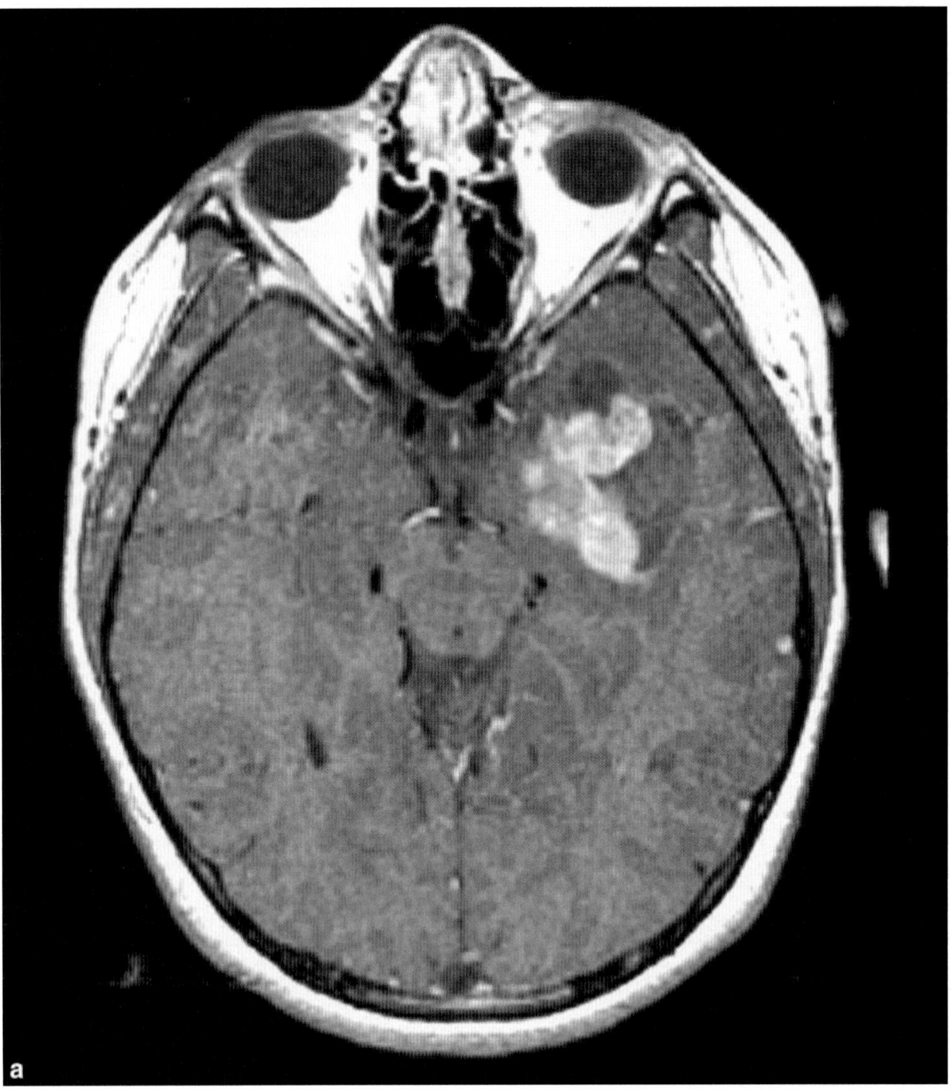

array of cell processes, are reliable findings. These may be accentuated by anti-neuronal antibody immunostaining, particularly for MAP 2. Small areas of less differentiated neurocytes may be present, which in turn may be imitated by perivascular lymphocytic infiltrates, also not an uncommon finding in gangliogliomas.

The astrocytic portion of the tumor is often highly reminiscent of pilocytic astrocytoma, estimated to occur in approximately two-thirds of gangliogliomas: a biphasic pattern of perivascular compact and looser microcystic areas may be observed, along with the presence of Rosenthal fibers and eosinophilic granular bodies. In lesions with strong contrast enhancement, prominent vasculature as is seen in pilocytic astrocytomas may also be found.

Subarachnoid spread is quite common in superficially located tumors, which does not necessarily portend a higher grade. Necrosis and mitotic activity are distinctly rare unless the astrocytic component warrants a worsening in grade, and according to current criteria, WHO Grade II lesions are not formally recognized. Anaplastic examples warrant WHO Grade III or anaplastic ganglioglioma. The existence of WHO Grade II "intermediate" examples has been suggested, but the criteria have not been validated or independently confirmed (Luyken et al., 2004).

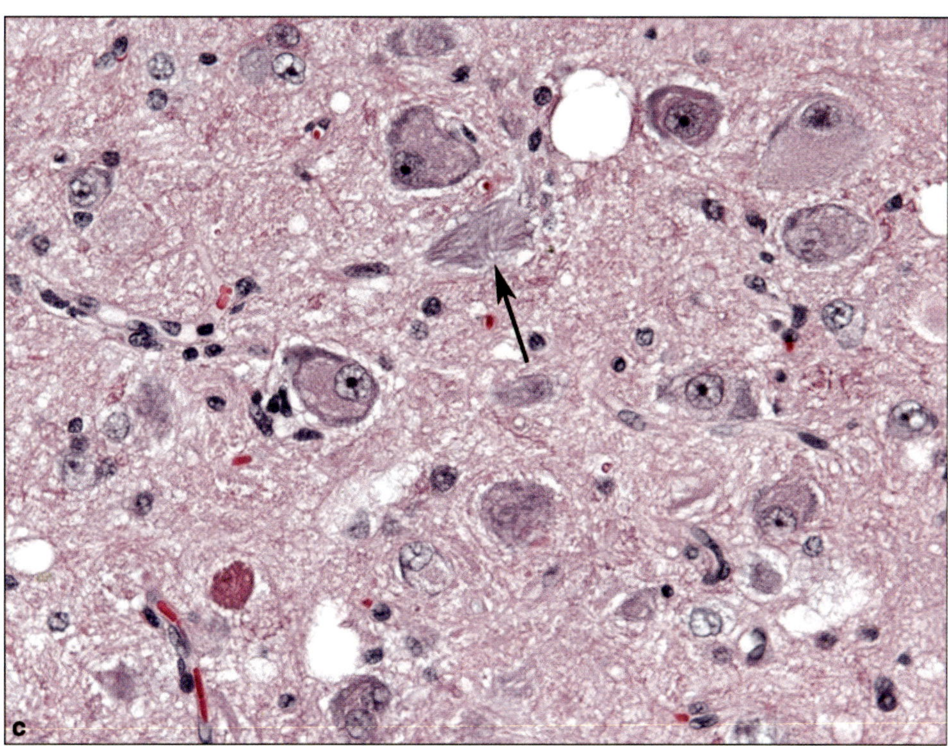

Figure 3.20. *continued.*

Dysplastic Gangliocytoma of the Cerebellum (Lhermitte – Duclos Disease)

Clinical and Radiological Features

This lesion is usually associated with the autosomal dominant disorder due to loss of activity mutations in the PTEN gene, resulting in Cowden disease.

Figure 3.20. *continued.*

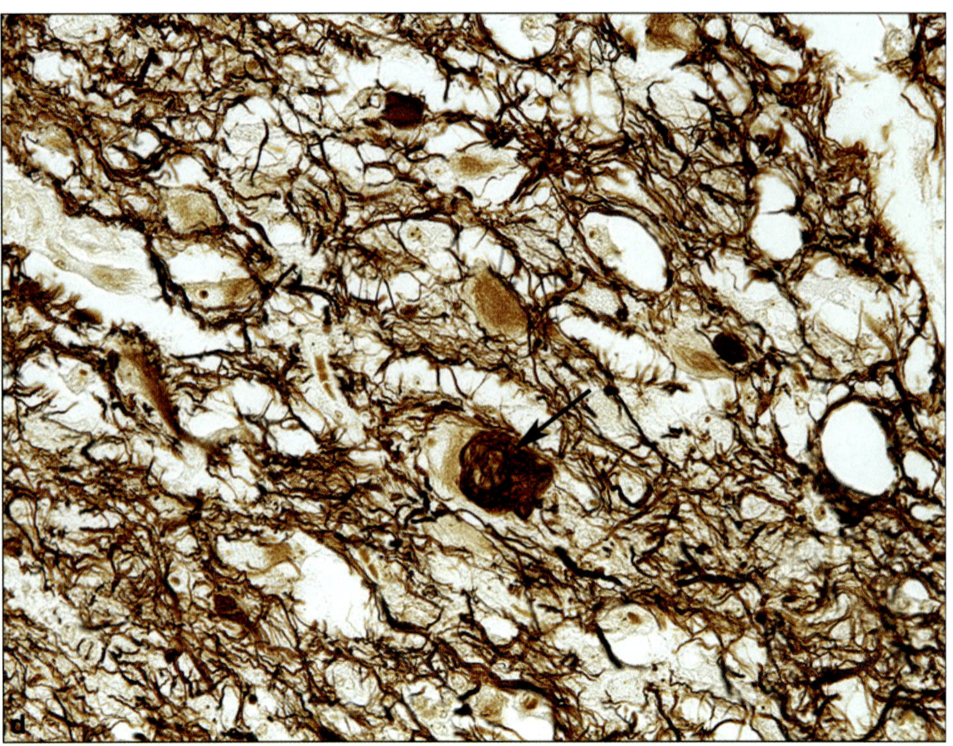

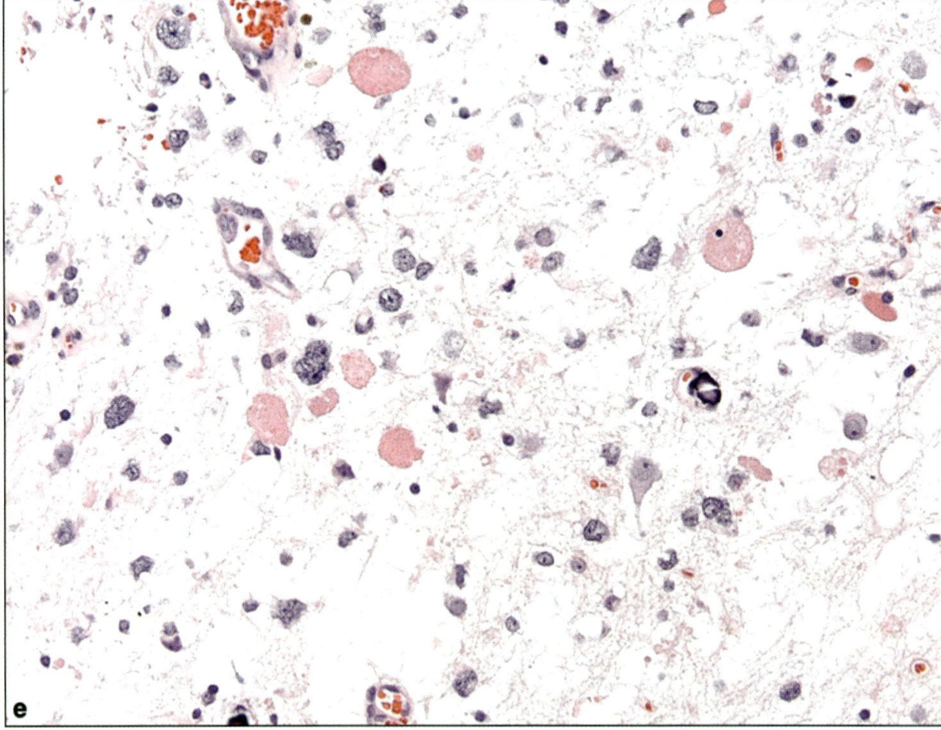

Other associated neoplasms include breast, nonmedullary thyroid, and endometrial cancers as well as hamartomas, including trichilemmoma. These occur rarely, generally between the second and seventh decade with the peak incidence in mid-adulthood. Childhood-onset cases are not associated with PTEN mutations (Zhou et al., 2003).

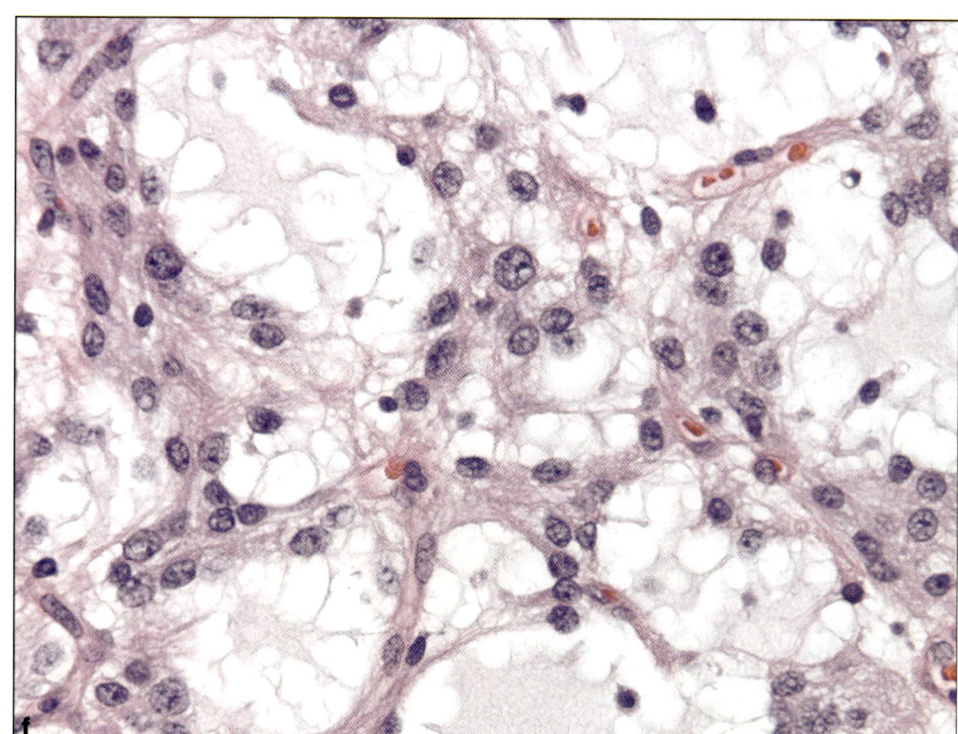

Figure 3.20. *continued*
(f) Some ganglion cell tumors do not show obvious ganglionic cell morphology, but cells with prominent round nuclei should otherwise prompt consideration of a neuronal cell type, (g) confirmed with MAP 2 immunohistochemistry.

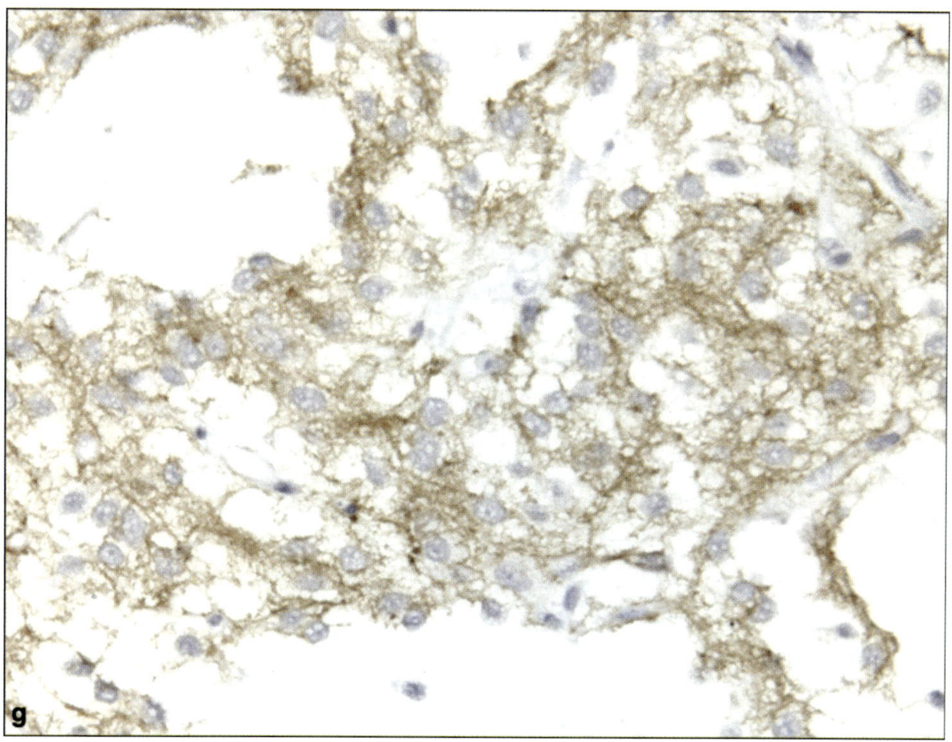

The most common clinical presentation is due to abnormalities in cerebellar function including dysmetria and other manifestations of mass effect including macrocephaly and seizures. The appearance of dysplastic gangliocytoma of the cerebellum may precede other manifestations of Cowden disease. Thus, comprehensive clinical evaluation of the patient would include screening for other associated malignancies, particularly breast carcinoma in females.

Figure 3.20. *continued*
(h) Gangliogliomas have a distinct predisposition, also like pilocytic astrocytomas, to locally invade the subarachnoid space. The parenchymal lesion in this cortical gyrus is accompanied by a mound of subpial spread, (i) seen at higher magnification.

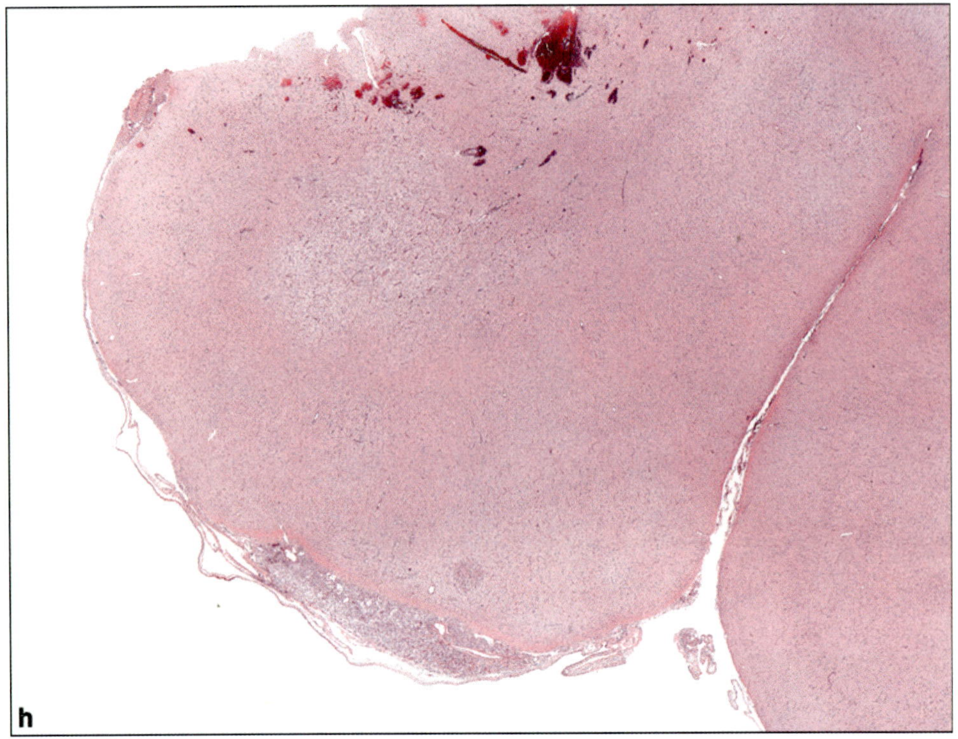

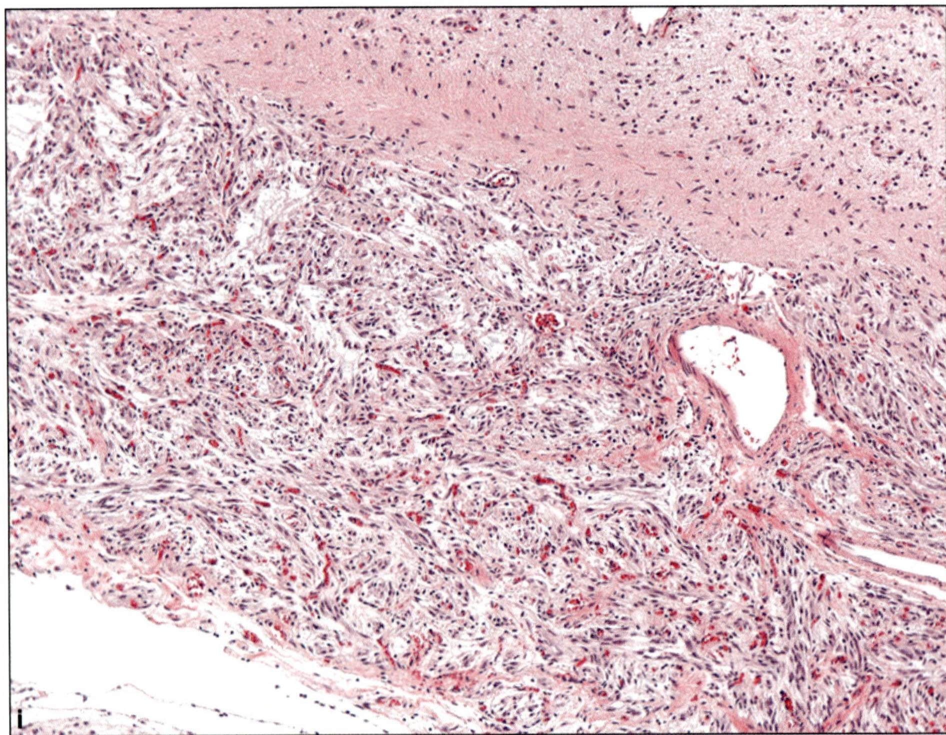

Neuroimaging studies will demonstrate the abnormal architecture of the otherwise enlarged cerebellar hemisphere (Figure 3.21a), sometimes accompanied by cystic changes (Milbouw et al., 1988). The tumor is usually unilateral but may be multifocal. Debate persists whether this is hamartomatous or neoplastic; however, in the context of neoplasia, the grade is WHO Grade I.

Pathology

The gross appearance of this lesion reflects the radiologic impression of enlarged folia. The microscopic diagnosis is most esthetically achieved with sections that demonstrate the altered folial architecture whereby the molecular and internal granular layers are architecturally intact but diffusely enlarged and filled by ganglionic cells of varying sizes (Figure 3.21b). The outer molecular layer may be covered by a layer of myelinated fibers, sometimes yielding the impression of an inverted cerebellar cortex. Small aggregates of misplaced granule cells may be present in the molecular layer or in subpial locations. Purkinje cells are either diminished or absent. Calcification and vascular ectasia may also be present.

Paraganglioma

Clinical and Radiological Features

Paragangliomas of the CNS are most commonly located in the filum terminale cauda equina region with an obvious association with the filum terminale or nerve roots. These tumors most commonly occur in adults, with the peak incidence in the fourth through sixth decades. They most commonly present with a chronic history of low back pain and a surprising lack of motor or sensory deficits. Paragangliomas in the head and neck region typically arise from the glomus jugulare or the carotid bodies, with a similar recurrence in mid-adulthood and a Caucasian predilection (Jackson, 2001). Intracranial examples are exceedingly rare and usually result from extension by jugulotympanic lesions. By neuroimaging, paragangliomas typically appear as isodense, homogeneously enhancing, sharply circumscribed, and occasionally partially cystic masses.

Tumor location is the most important prognostic feature. Glomus jugulare tumors may recur locally in almost half of cases (Lack et al., 1979). Most cauda equina paragangliomas are curable by complete resection.

Pathology

These tumors are frequently accompanied by notable hemorrhage upon resection. Their microscopic appearance is similar to normal paraganglia and otherwise shows typical neuroendocrine features, with monotonous cells arranged in nests or lobules bordered by a delicate fibrovascular capillary network (Figure 3.22). Degenerative nuclear pleomorphism may be seen. Some paragangliomas contain mature ganglionic elements, analogous to the visceral "gangliocytic paragangliomas." Others might contain prominent spindle-cell or melanocytic components.

Immunohistochemistry will confirm neuroendocrine differentiation, with synaptophysin and chromogranin usually being immunopositive. Sustentacular cells may be detected by anti-S-100 immunohistochemistry. Paranuclear cytokeratin immunopositivity is prominent in cauda equina lesions (Chetty, 1999).

Figure 3.21. Dysplastic gangliocytoma of the cerebellum (Lhermitte–Duclos disease).
(a) Radiographic imaging may show preservation of the overall structure of the cerebellum but with peculiar accentuation through mass effect. (b) Expansion of the granule neuron cell layer by the dysplastic gangliocytic element of the tumor, with the distinctive overlying parallel layers of myelinated fibers in the more superficial molecular layer creating the illusion of inverted cerebellar folial architecture.

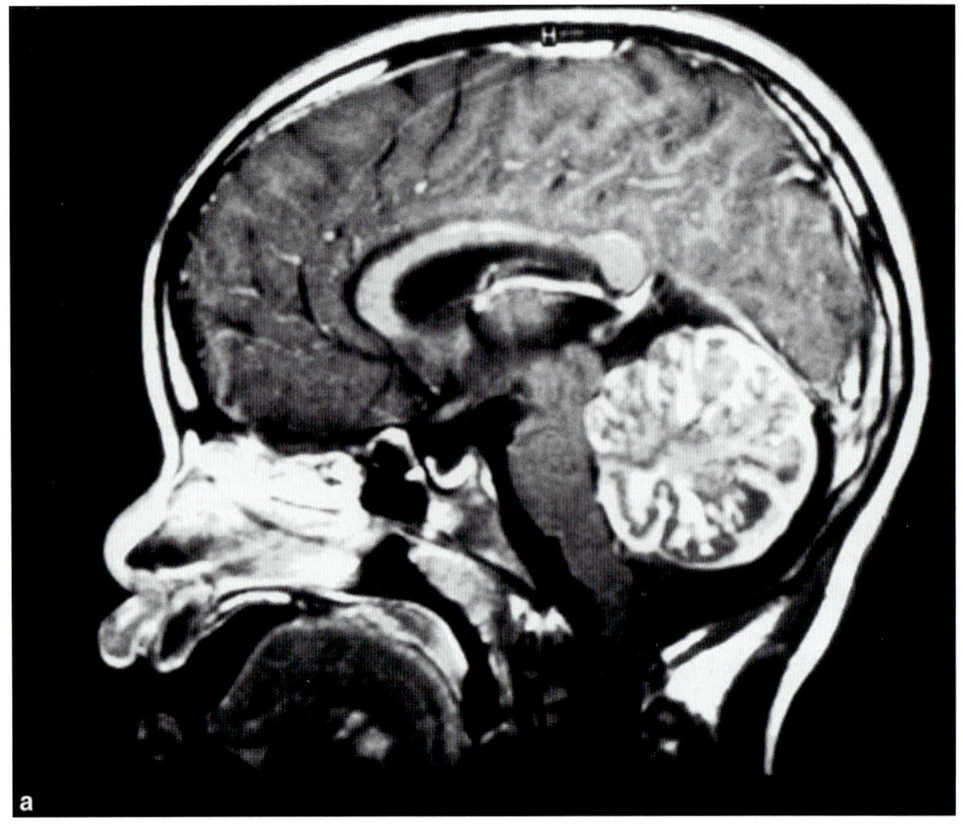

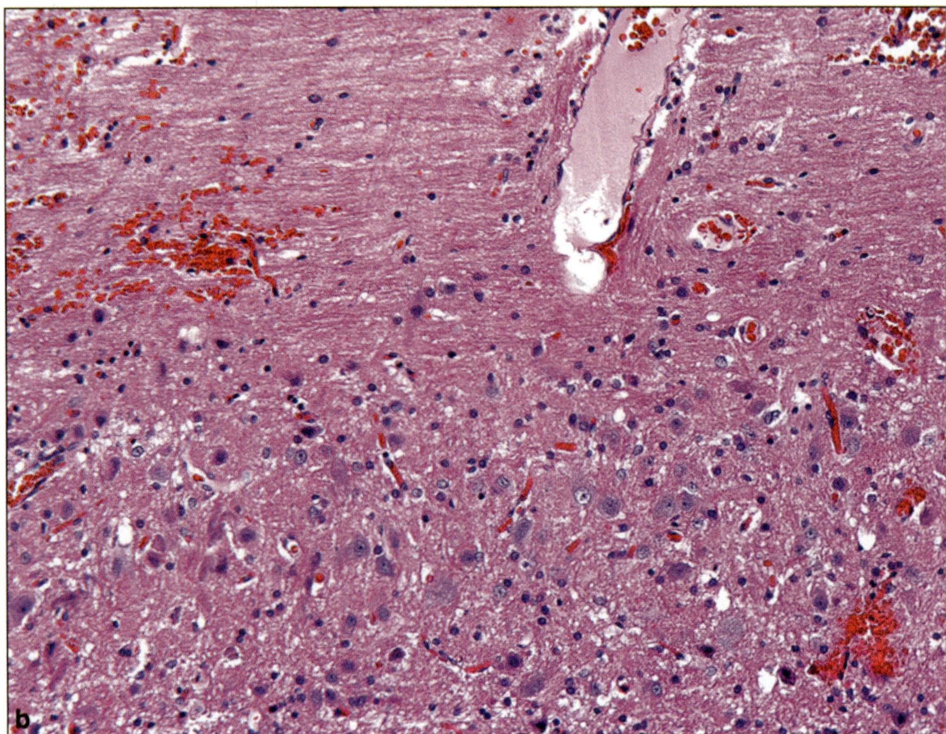

Papillary Glioneuronal Tumor

Clinical and Radiological Features

This recently recognized tumor was originally conceived as a variant of ganglio-glioma. Only a small number have been reported; therefore, there is no age predilection

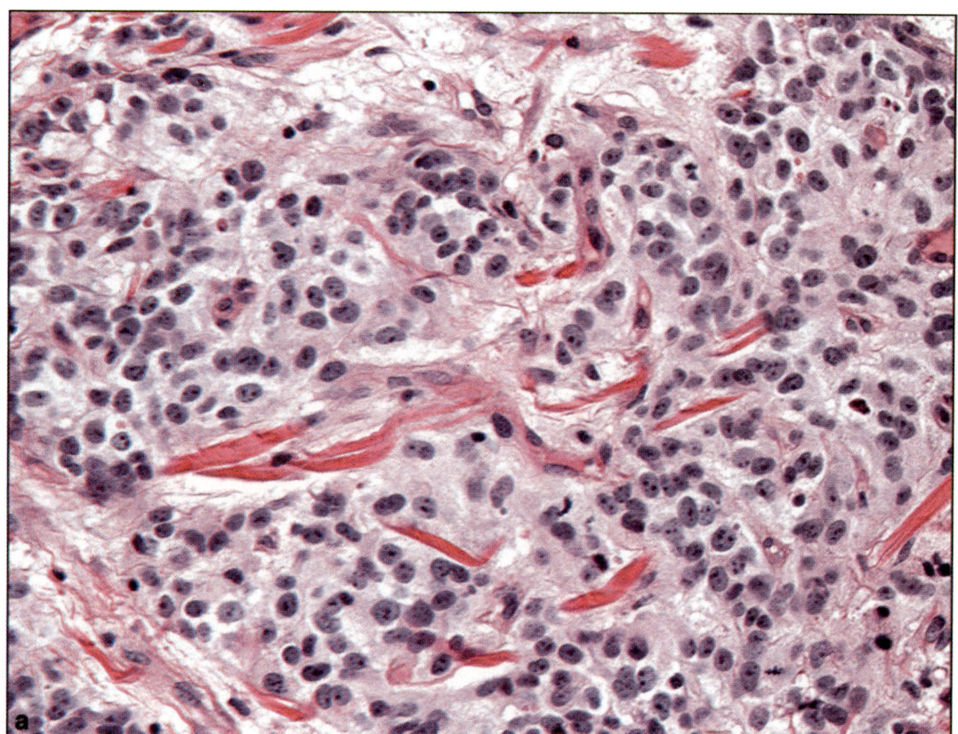

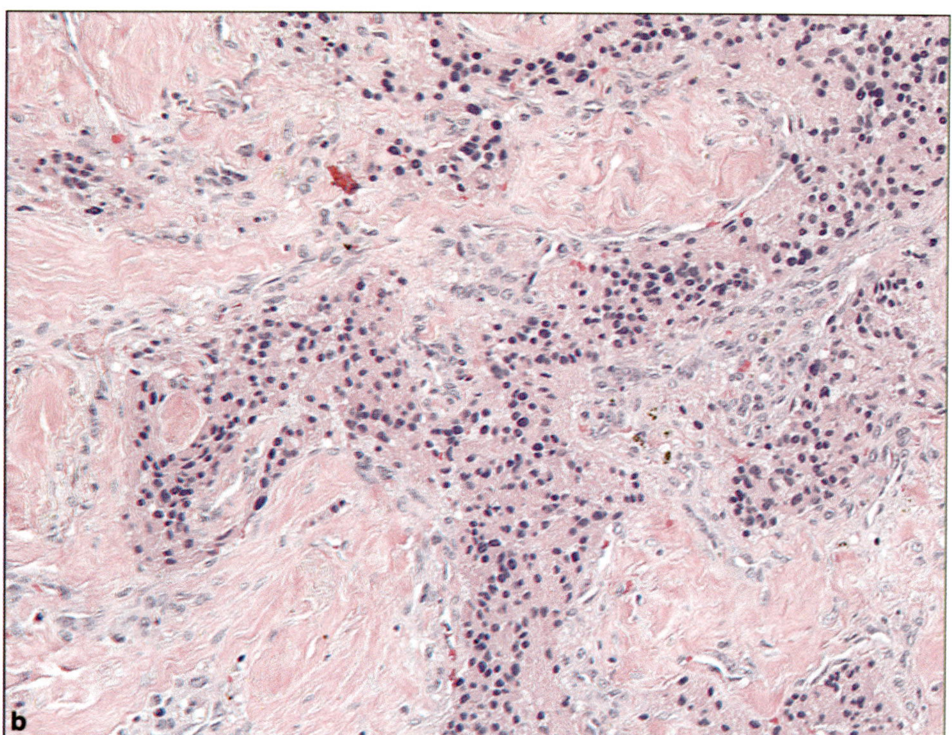

Figure 3.22. (a) Paragangliomas usually show histological features of a monomorphous neuroendocrine neoplasm with a tendency for nesting. (b) Some examples result in regional sclerosis, with tumor cells accentuated by (c) synaptophysin immunostaining, and (d) identification of sustentacular cells by S-100 immunolabeling.

noted thus far; they have been described from childhood to late adulthood. They generally occur in cerebral hemispheres, although spinal pediatric examples have been reported (Harris and Horoupian, 2000). Gross total resection usually requires no additional treatment and is predictive of recurrence-free long-term survival.

The clinical presentation is similar to that of other hemispheric mixed glial and neuronal tumors by causing seizures or other focal neurologic deficits.

Figure 3.22. *continued.*

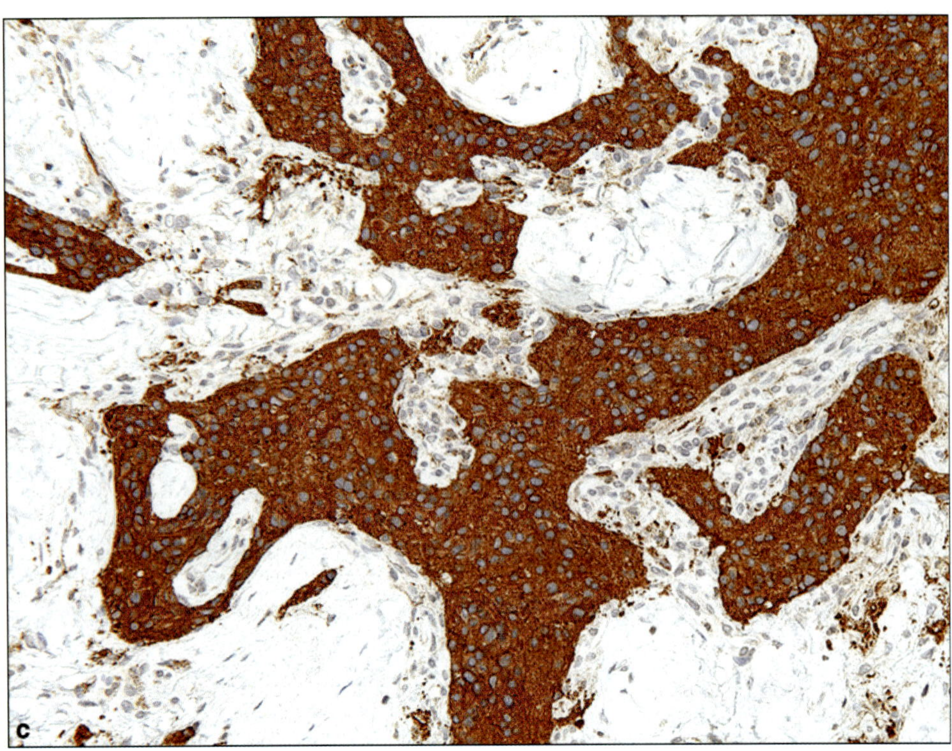

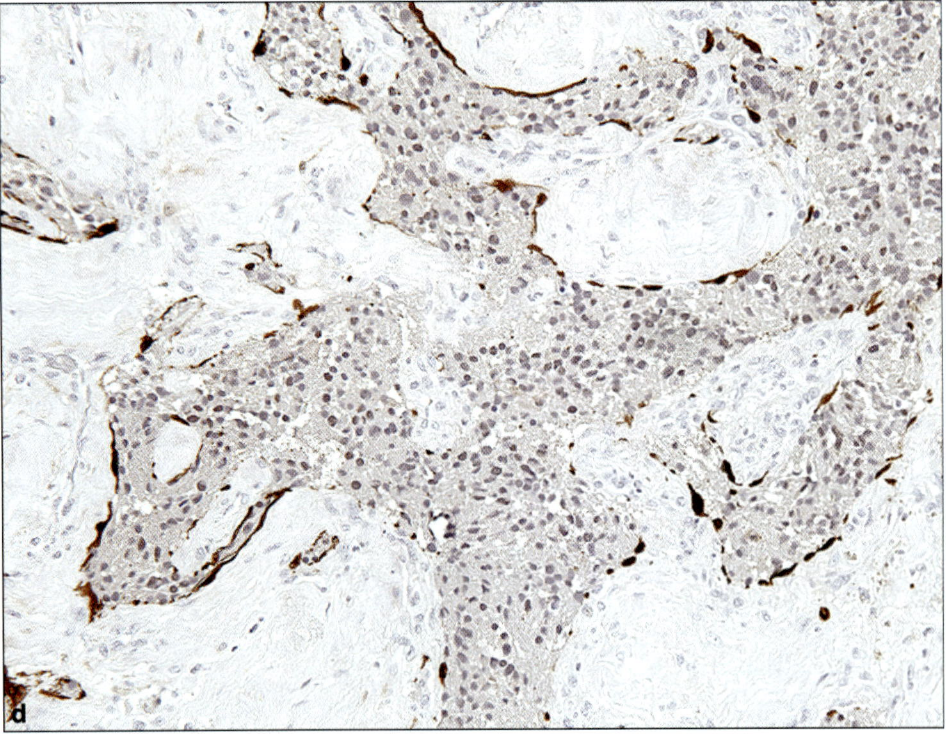

Radiographically, they may demonstrate a cystic component with contrast enhancement of the solid portion.

Pathology

As the name implies, the tumor is composed of delicate papillary structures in which thin fibrovascular septae are lined by a slightly crowded arrangement of

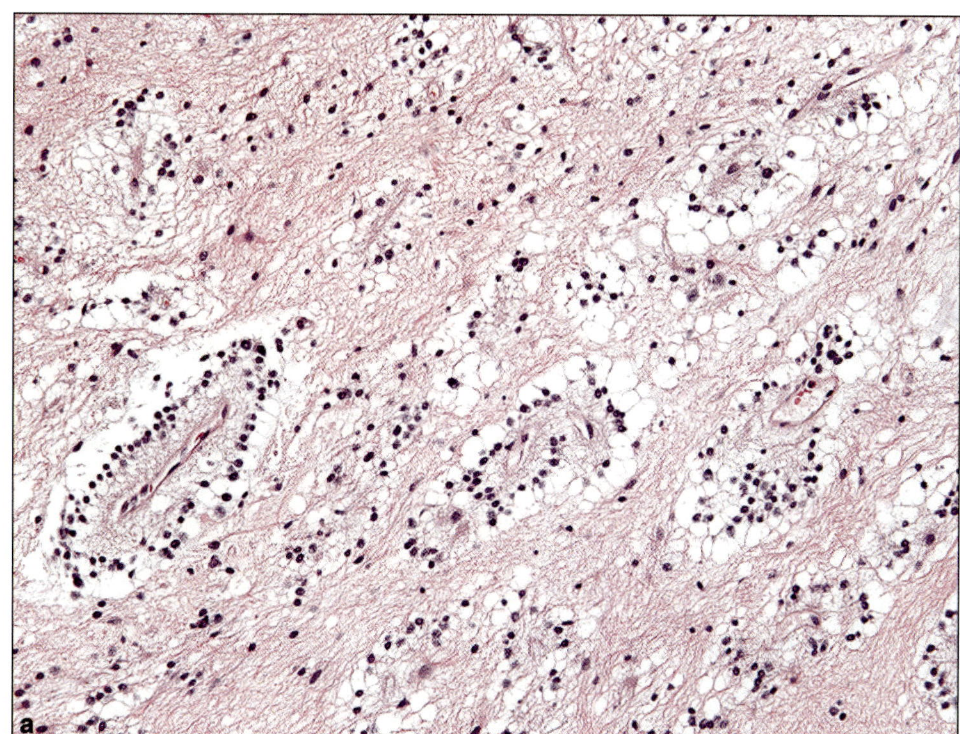

Figure 3.23. (a) Papillary glioneuronal tumor, with small neurocytic cells forming fibrovascular papillae, (b) highlighted by synaptophysin immunostaining, and (c) demonstrating relative lack of GFAP immunopositivity as compared with surrounding neuropil.

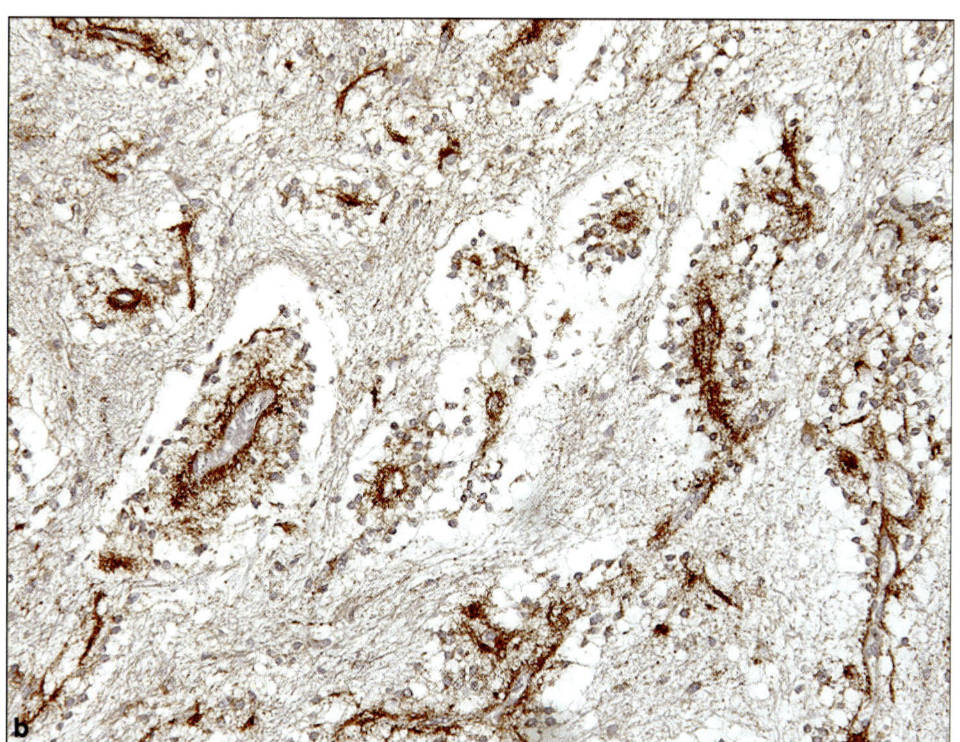

monotonous small round cells conforming to neurocytes (Figure 3.23). The papillary blood vessels may show hyalinization. Frankly ganglionic elements may be noted (Komori et al., 1998). Mitotic activity and necrosis are not observed. Immunohistochemically, the tumor characteristically coexpresses GFAP as well as neuronal markers including synaptophysin, class III beta tubulin, and CD56.

Figure 3.23. *continued.*

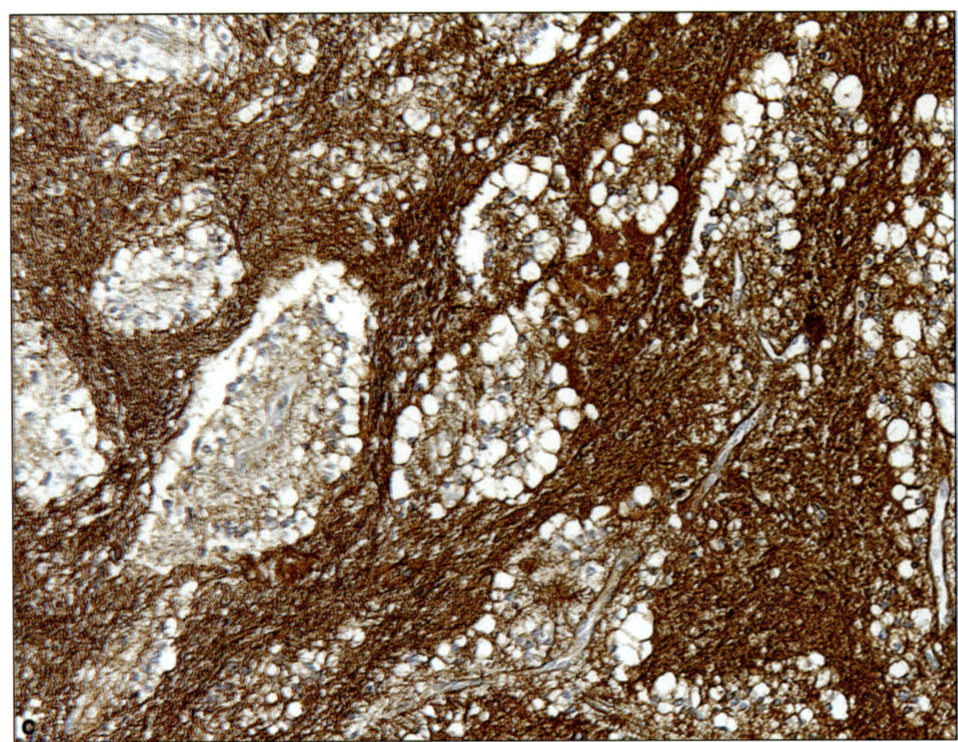

Figure 3.24. (a) Rosette-forming glioneuronal tumor of the fourth ventricle, showing microcytic change with mixed astrocytic and neurocytic elements.

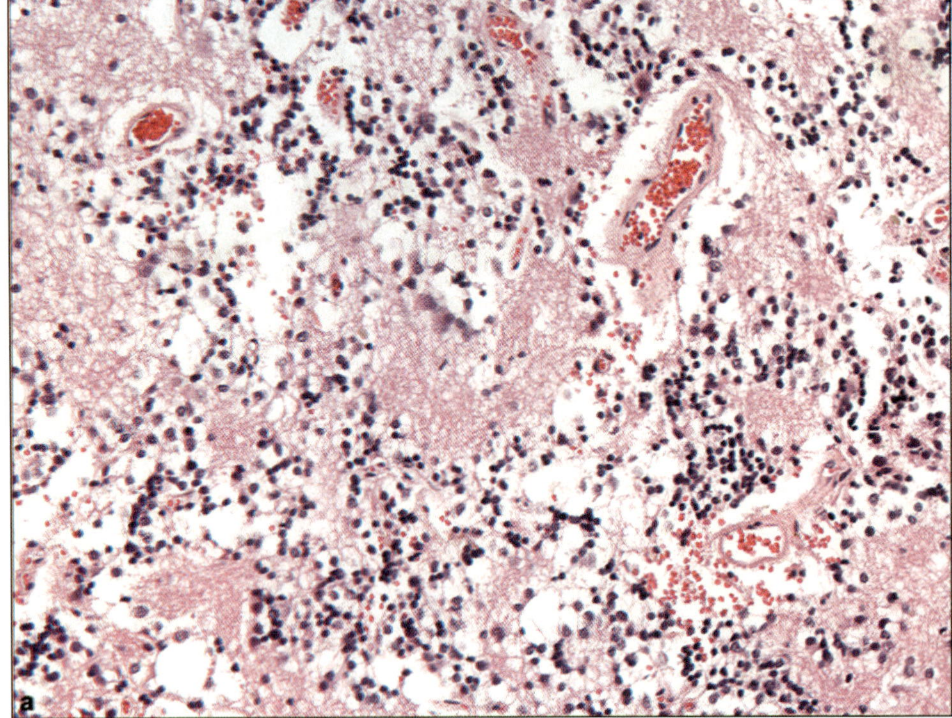

Rosette-Forming Glioneuronal Tumor of the Fourth Ventricle

Clinical and Radiological Features

This is an extremely rare and newly described tumor of young adults. Its distinct status is warranted by a highly characteristic histological appearance. Because of the location, symptoms are usually attributable to obstruction of

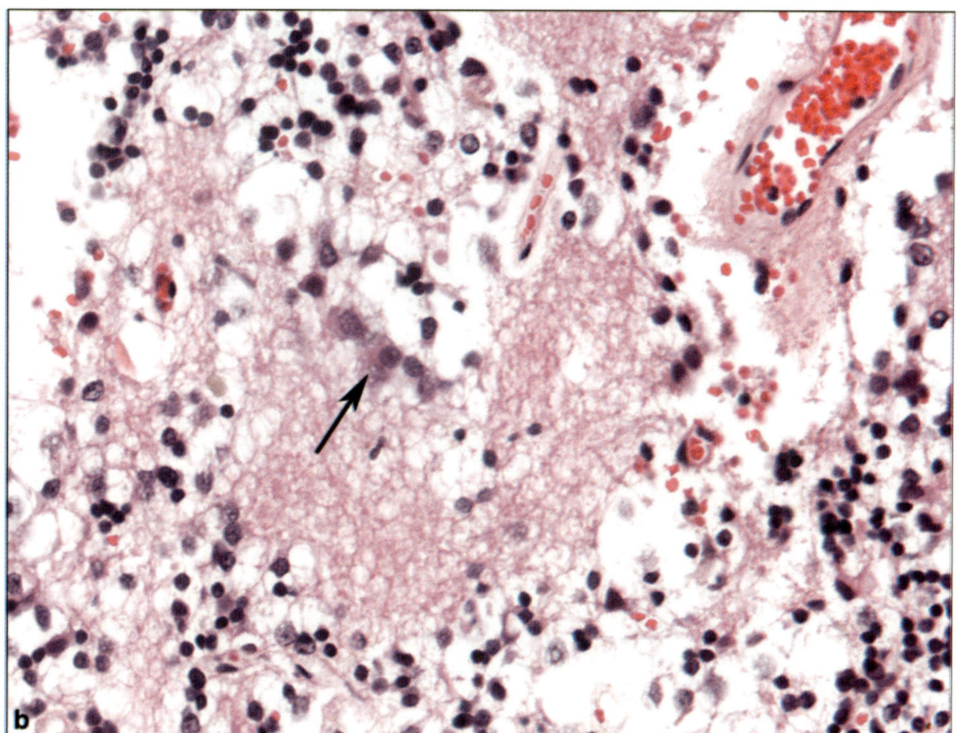

Figure 3.24. *continued*
(b) Higher magnification
shows frank gangliocytic
differentiation (arrow).

cerebrospinal fluid (CSF) flow and consequent hydrocephalus. Histological examples are particularly unusual because such lesions may be managed with CSF shunting and radiological monitoring without biopsy. Because of the difficulty of surgical resection, the morbidity carried by this lesion is most often related to surgical intervention.

Pathology

The histopathology of the small number of reported cases indicates a biphasic tumor composed of neurocytic and glial components (Figure 3.24). The neurocytic component includes monotonous neurocyte-forming rosettes or perivascular pseudorosettes. Microcystic or mucinous regions may be noted. The astrocytic component is reported to most closely resemble pilocytic astrocytoma including oligodendroglioma-like areas and Rosenthal fibers, eosinophilic granular bodies, microcalcification, and prominent microvasculature. As in the other mixed glioneuronal tumors, immunoreactivity for neuronal markers such as synaptophysin and MAP 2 may be noted in the neuronal component and GFAP and S-100 in the glial component, generally absent in the neurocytic rosettes.

WHO GRADE II

Central Neurocytoma and Extraventricular Neurocytoma

Clinical and Radiological Features

Central neurocytomas account for less than 1% of brain tumors. They are generally tumors of young adults but may occur up to the seventh decade. They most often occur around the midline between the lateral and third ventricles in

Figure 3.25. Central neurocytoma. (a) Axial T1-weighted contrast-enhanced image shows a heterogeneous, enhancing, well-demarcated, partially cystic mass intimately associated with the septum pellucidum in this young adult. About half of central neurocytomas have calcifications visible on CT; this mass does not display any obvious calcification on MR. (b) Squash preparation shows monomorphous cells with round nuclei and finely punctate nuclear chromatin.

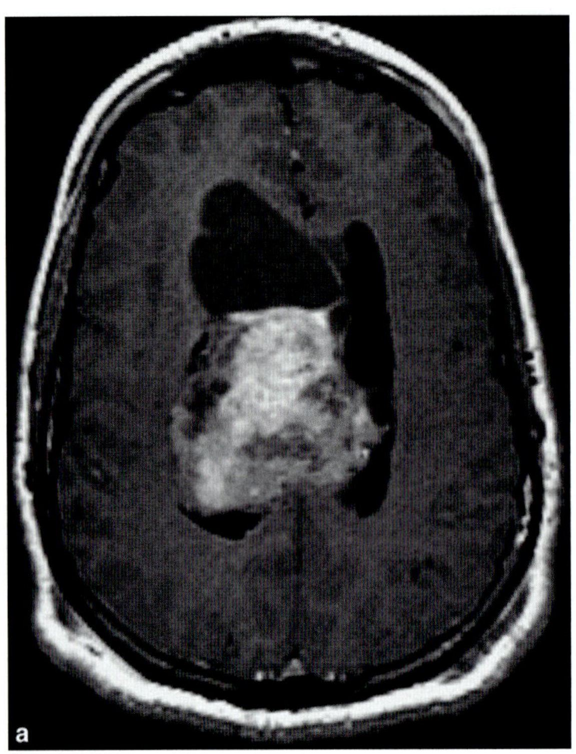

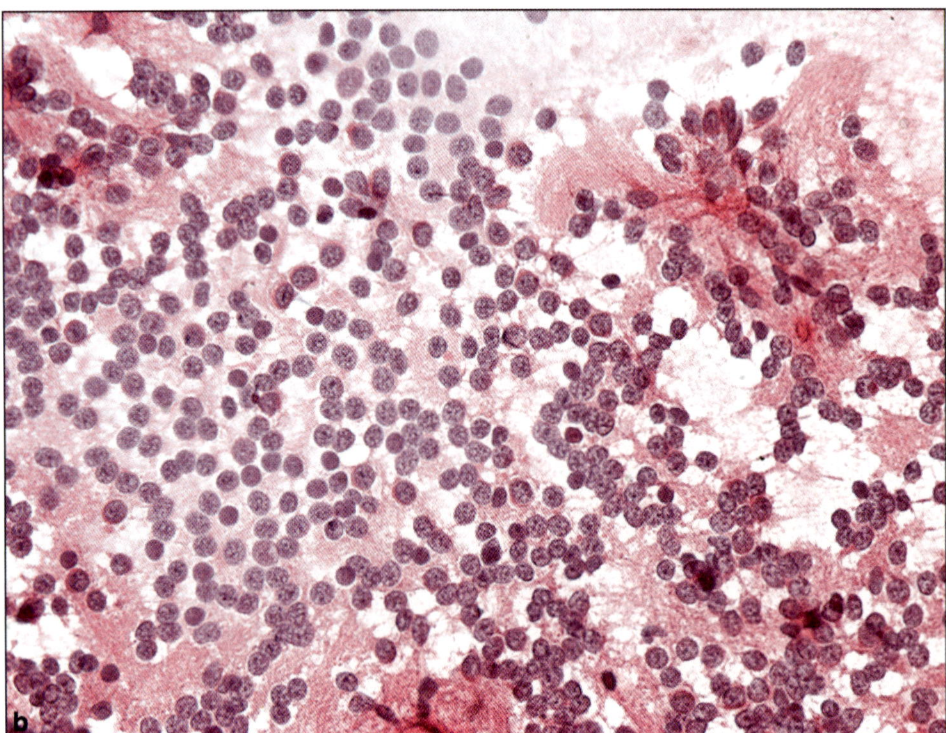

the region of the foramen of Munro. Extraventricular neurocytomas are now well documented. Intraventricular examples usually present with symptoms of obstructive hydrocephalus or more acutely due to hemorrhage. Extraventricular examples usually result in focal symptoms.

Radiographic imaging will indicate a contrast-enhancing lesion with heterogeneous hyperintensity on T1-weighted and hyperintensity on T2-weighted

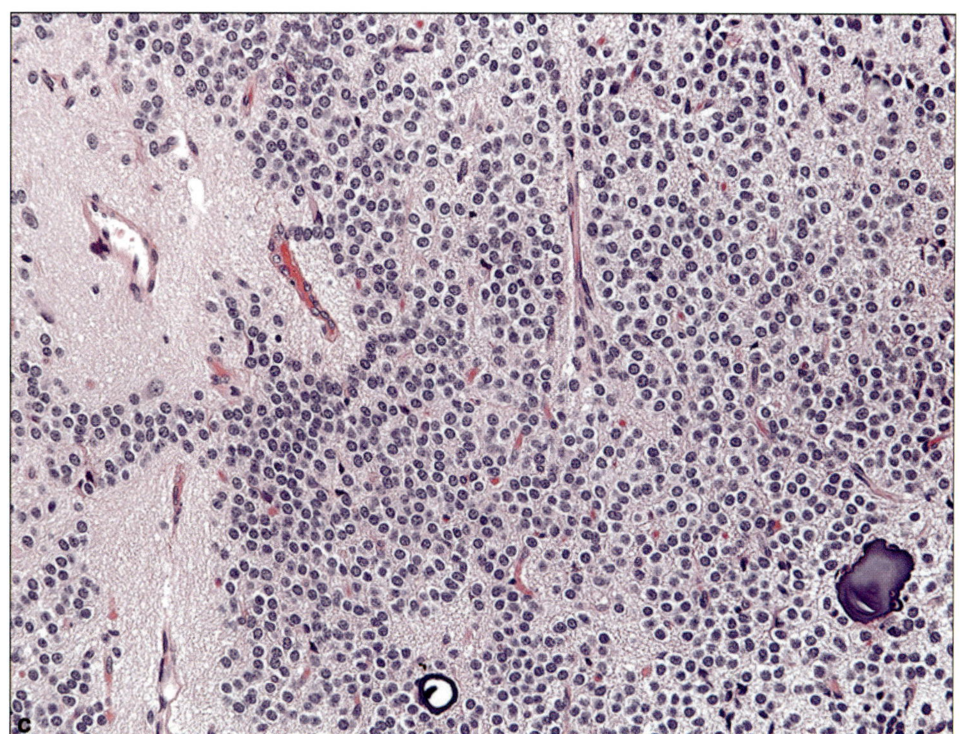

Figure 3.25. *continued* (c) Typical appearance of neurocytomas, with focal calcification and anuclear areas of neuropil. (d) Strong and diffuse synaptophysin immunopositivity.

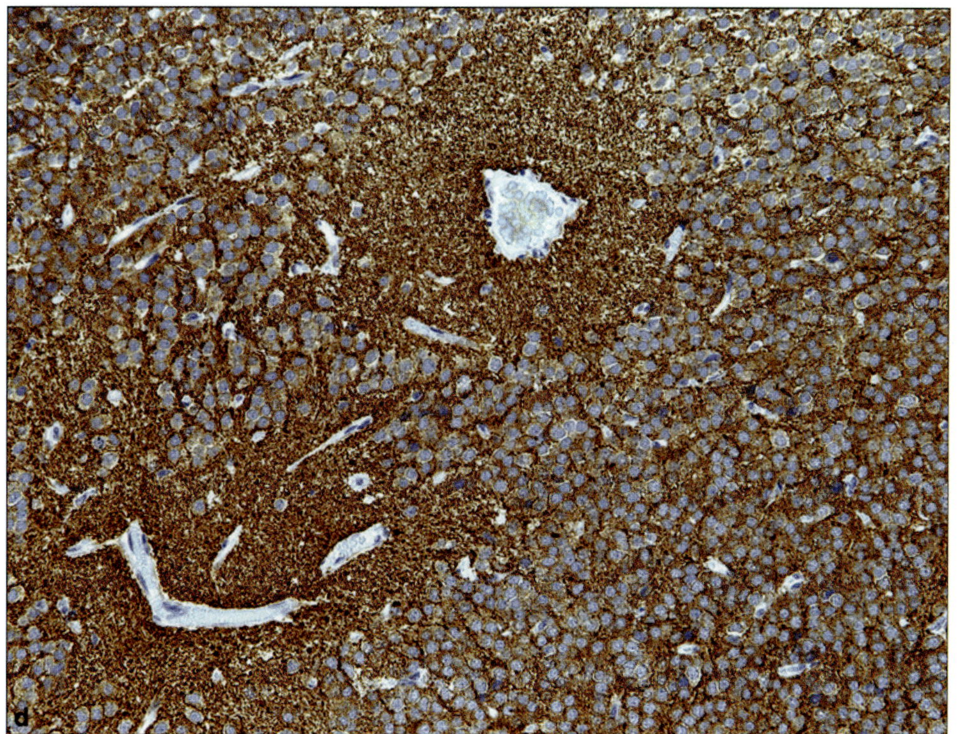

images. Calcification or cystic change may be noted. In spite of the low-grade histology, these tumors may achieve significant size and thus prevent total resection, leading to local recurrence.

Pathology

The histologic appearance of this tumor is perhaps best introduced by indicating that before its recognition as a distinct entity, it was considered to be an intraventricular oligodendroglioma or clear cell ependymoma. The tumor is thereby composed of monotonous sheets of round cells, sometimes even with perinuclear halos. Careful examination will demonstrate neuropil-like anuclear fibrillary areas (Figure 3.25). Calcifications are present in half of the cases. Rarely, anaplastic features may be noticed, including an increased mitotic rate, microvascular proliferation, and necrosis, all of which are of no definite significance in worsening the prognosis. Immunohistochemistry shows diffuse strong synaptophysin positivity with GFAP immunopositivity limited to entrapped or reactive astrocytes.

Cerebellar Liponeurocytoma

Clinical and Radiological Features

This rare lesion occurs in adults with a steady increase in incidence according to age. The tumor was originally considered WHO Grade I; however, examples of recurrence have resulted in reclassification as WHO Grade II. Clinical symptoms are usually attributable to increased pressure within the posterior fossa or obstructive hydrocephalus. The tumors occur most commonly in cerebellar hemispheres and less commonly in the vermis or cerebellopontine angle.

Neuroimaging may show a heterogeneously enhancing lesion on T1-weighted MRI studies with heterogeneous contrast enhancement. Certain irregularities may reflect the presence of lipidized components. The prognosis is generally favorable, although recurrence has been noted in almost two-thirds of patients (Aker et al., 2005).

Figure 3.26. Cerebellar liponeurocytoma.

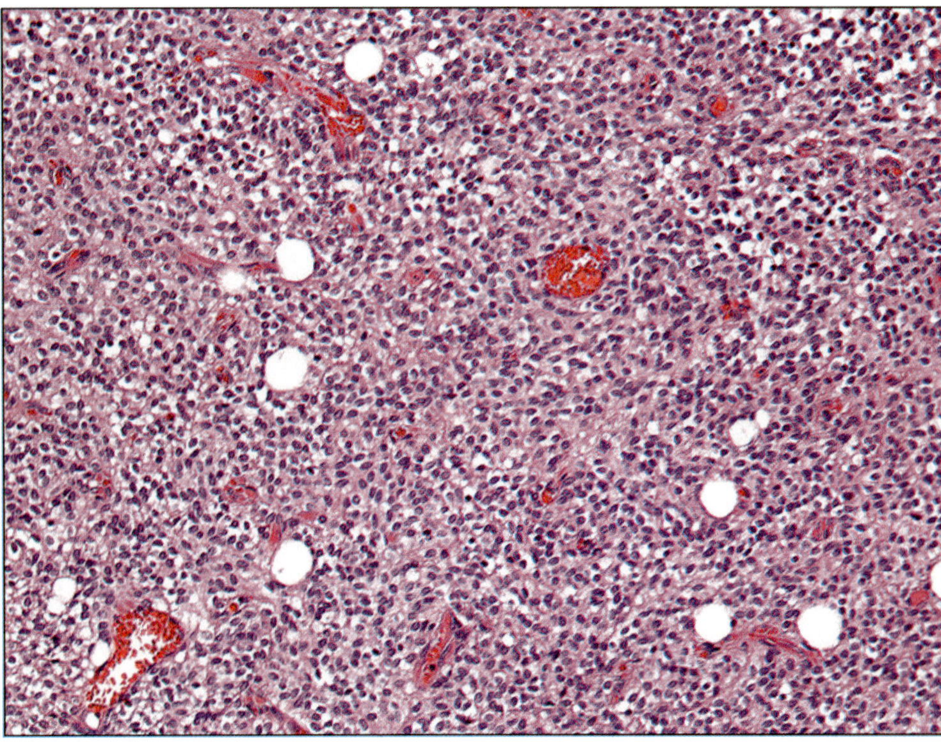

Pathology

The name largely describes the histopathology of this lesion, which is composed of sheets or small clusters of adipocytes in a background of monomorphous neurocytic cells, often yielding a biphasic appearance (Figure 3.26). The cytomorphology may suggest oligodendroglioma or clear cell ependymoma. Careful interpretation of immunohistochemical stains will reveal that both neurocytic and lipidized portions express neuronal markers such as synaptophysin and MAP 2. This signifies metaplastic differentiation of tumor cells rather than entrapment of fat cells or, more importantly, the occasional presence of lipid-laden macrophages in ordinary medulloblastomas. GFAP may be focally expressed (Soylemezoglu et al., 1996).

REFERENCES

Aker FV, Ozkara S, Eren P, Peker O, Armagan S, Hakan T. Cerebellar liponeurocytoma/ lipidized medulloblastoma. *J Neurooncol* 2005; 71: 53–9.

Baisden BL, Brat DJ, Melhem ER, Rosenblum MK, King AP, Burger PC. Dysembryoplastic neuroepithelial tumor-like neoplasm of the septum pellucidum: a lesion often misdiagnosed as glioma: report of 10 cases. *Am J Surg Pathol* 2001; 25: 494–9.

Chetty R. Cytokeratin expression in cauda equina paragangliomas. *Am J Surg Pathol* 1999; 23: 491.

Daumas-Duport C. Dysembryoplastic neuroepithelial tumours. *Brain Pathol* 1993; 3: 283–95.

Harris BT, Horoupian DS. Spinal cord glioneuronal tumor with "rosetted" neuropil islands and meningeal dissemination: a case report. *Acta Neuropathol* 2000; 100: 575–9.

Jackson CG. Glomus tympanicum and glomus jugulare tumors. *Otolaryngol Clin North Am* 2001; 34: 941–70, vii.

Komori T, Scheithauer BW, Anthony DC, Rosenblum MK, McLendon RE, Scott RM, et al. Papillary glioneuronal tumor: a new variant of mixed neuronal-glial neoplasm. *Am J Surg Pathol* 1998; 22: 1171–83.

Lack EE, Cubilla AL, Woodruff JM. Paragangliomas of the head and neck region. A pathologic study of tumors from 71 patients. *Hum Pathol* 1979; 10: 191–218.

Luyken C, Blumcke I, Fimmers R, Urbach H, Wiestler OD, Schramm J. Supratentorial gangliogliomas: histopathologic grading and tumor recurrence in 184 patients with a median follow-up of 8 years. *Cancer* 2004; 101: 146–55.

Milbouw G, Born JD, Martin D, Collignon J, Hans P, Reznik M, et al. Clinical and radiological aspects of dysplastic gangliocytoma (Lhermitte-Duclos disease): a report of two cases with review of the literature. *Neurosurgery* 1988; 22: 124–8.

Paulus W, Schlote W, Perentes E, Jacobi G, Warmuth-Metz M, Roggendorf W. Desmoplastic supratentorial neuroepithelial tumours of infancy. *Histopathology* 1992; 21: 43–9.

Rushing EJ, Rorke LB, Sutton L. Problems in the nosology of desmoplastic tumors of childhood. *Pediatr Neurosurg* 1993; 19: 57–62.

Soylemezoglu F, Soffer D, Onol B, Schwechheimer K, Kleihues P. Lipomatous medulloblastoma in adults. A distinct clinicopathological entity. *Am J Surg Pathol* 1996; 20: 413–8.

VandenBerg SR. Desmoplastic infantile ganglioglioma and desmoplastic cerebral astrocytoma of infancy. *Brain Pathol* 1993; 3: 275–81.

Zhou XP, Marsh DJ, Morrison CD, Chaudhury AR, Maxwell M, Reifenberger G, et al. Germline inactivation of PTEN and dysregulation of the phosphoinositol-3-kinase/ Akt pathway cause human Lhermitte–Duclos disease in adults. *Am J Hum Genet* 2003; 73: 1191–8.

Astroblastoma

Clinical and Radiological Features

This unusual neoplasm occurs predominantly in childhood through early adulthood. Based upon the limited number of reported cases, there may be a female predominance. They occur most frequently in the cerebral hemispheres (Figure 3.27a,b) and cause focal neurological deficits. Because of limited clinical experience with this entity, no WHO grade assignment has been made (Aldape and Rosenblum, 2007).

Pathology

Astroblastomas most closely resemble ependymomas such that they demonstrate perivascular pseudorosettes of cells with a variably nuclear free zone around blood vessels (Figure 3.28a,b). The conspicuous difference with the ependymal perivascular pseudorosettes is that in astroblastoma, the perivascular processes are thickened and stubby as they approach the vascular wall. Other regular features in this entity include thick hyalinized blood vessels, a papillary growth pattern, and signet ring differentiation. Like ependymomas, the tumor border is relatively well demarcated or pushing. Anaplastic examples have been reported, evidenced by conspicuous mitotic activity and cytological atypia (Navarro et al., 2005).

WHO GRADE I

Angiocentric Glioma

Clinical and Radiological Features

This recently recognized entity is typically a superficial hemispheric cortical tumor causing epilepsy (Wang et al., 2005). The most frequent tumor locations reflect the general volume of the brain lobes with frontoparietal compartment being most common followed by temporal lobes. The prognosis is favorable after surgical excision without adjunctive therapy. Radiographic imaging typically shows a well-demarcated, solid nonenhancing cortical mass with extension into subcortical white matter, sometimes extending to the ventricular surface.

Pathology

The angiocentric glioma is composed of elongated glial cells and careful inspection of the lesion will show focal areas with perivascular perpendicularly arranged tumor cells (Figure 3.29a–c). They are typically strongly GFAP positive and also show distinctive dot like epithelial membrane antigen (EMA) positivity, reminiscent of ependymomas.

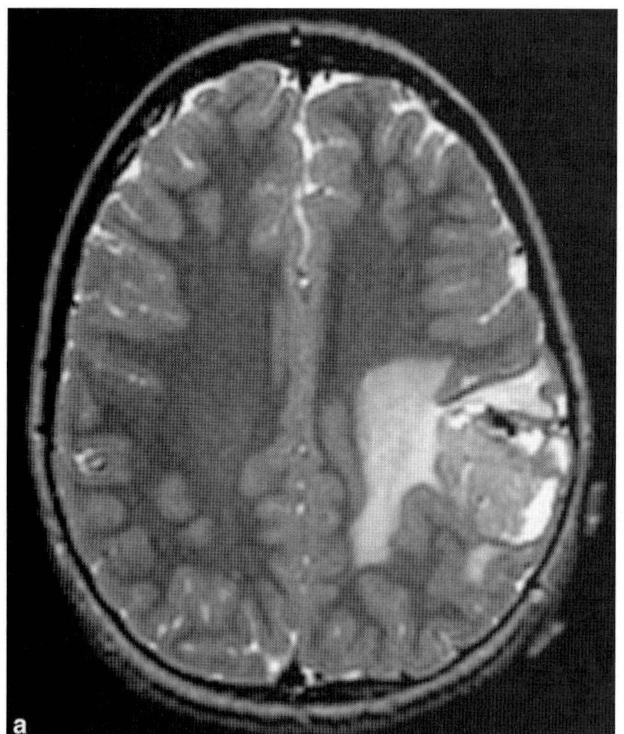

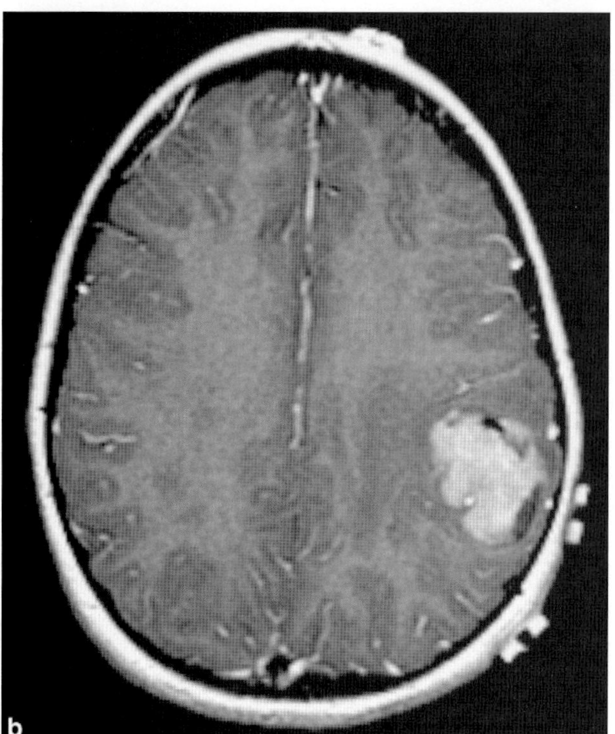

Figure 3.27. (a) An axial T2-weighted image shows cystic areas within the mass and surrounding vasogenic edema. The hypointensity in the anterior aspect of the mass is probably a calcification. Astroblastomas often have a multicystic appearance and most reported cases describe calcifications, which are visible on CT (Bell et al., 2007). (b) An axial T1-weighted contrast enhance image shows a circumscribed enhancing mass centered within the parietal lobe and displacing the central sulcus anteriorly.

WHO GRADE II

Chordoid Glioma of the Third Ventricle

Clinical Features

This extremely rare entity occurs only in the third ventricle and typically causes obstructive hydrocephalus with headache, nausea, and ataxia (Brat et al.,

Figure 3.28. (a) Perivascular processes in astroblastoma, with thick processes as distinguished from the thin tapering processes of a perivascular pseudorosette in ependymomas. Nuclear features are closely reminiscent of those in ependymomas. b) Thick perivascular processes are highlighted by GFAP immunohistochemistry.

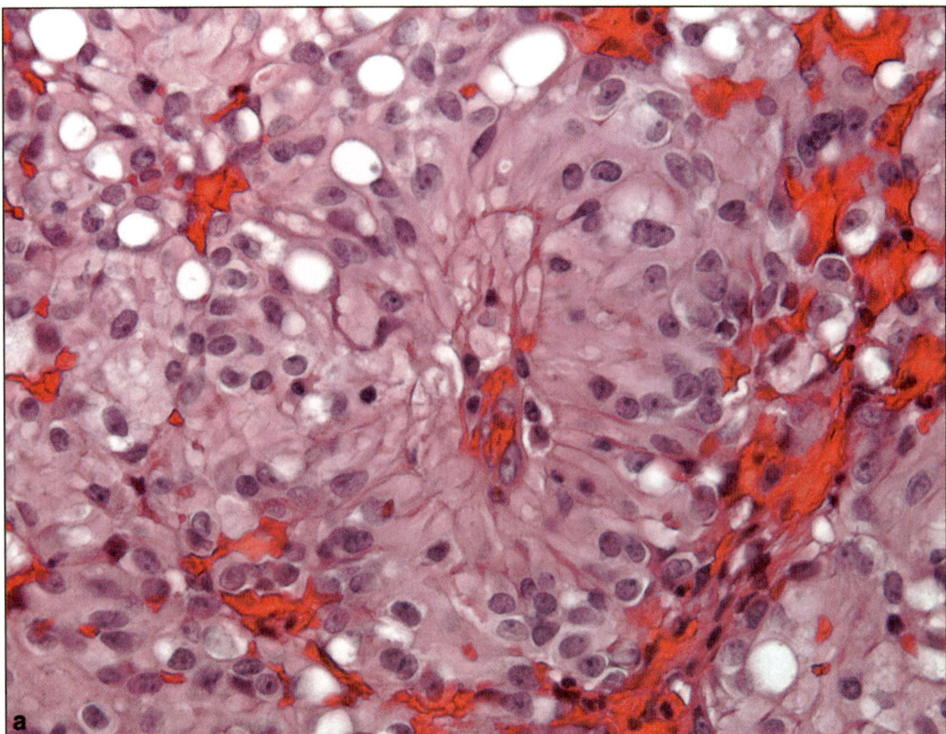

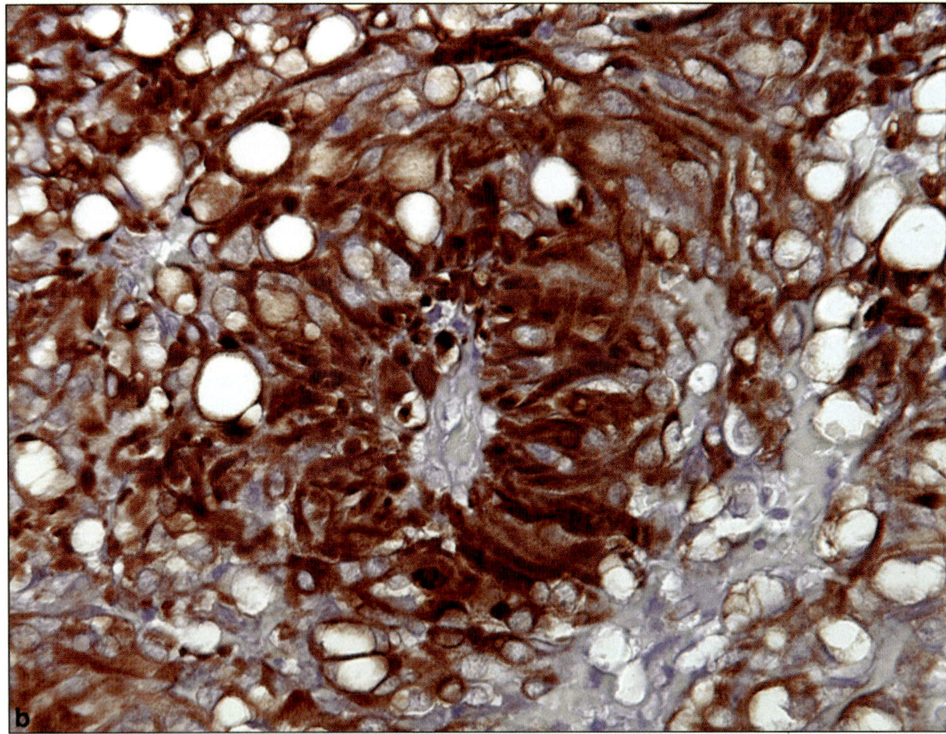

1998). Endocrine, visual, and psychiatric disturbances have also been reported because of compression of local structures. They generally occur in adults between the ages of 30 and 60 years.

Pathology

As indicated by the name, these tumors are composed of cords or clusters of epithelioid cells surrounded by a mucinous matrix, highly reminiscent of

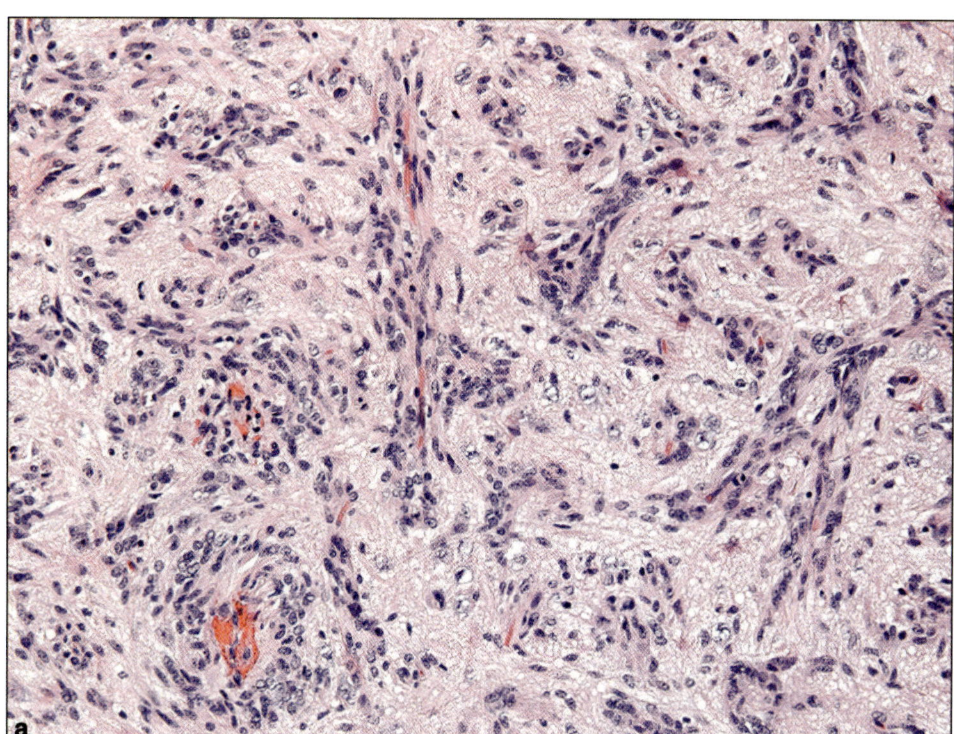

Figure 3.29. (a) Typical perivascular aggregates of glial tumor cells, which (b) extends into surrounding brain tissue in angiocentric glioma.

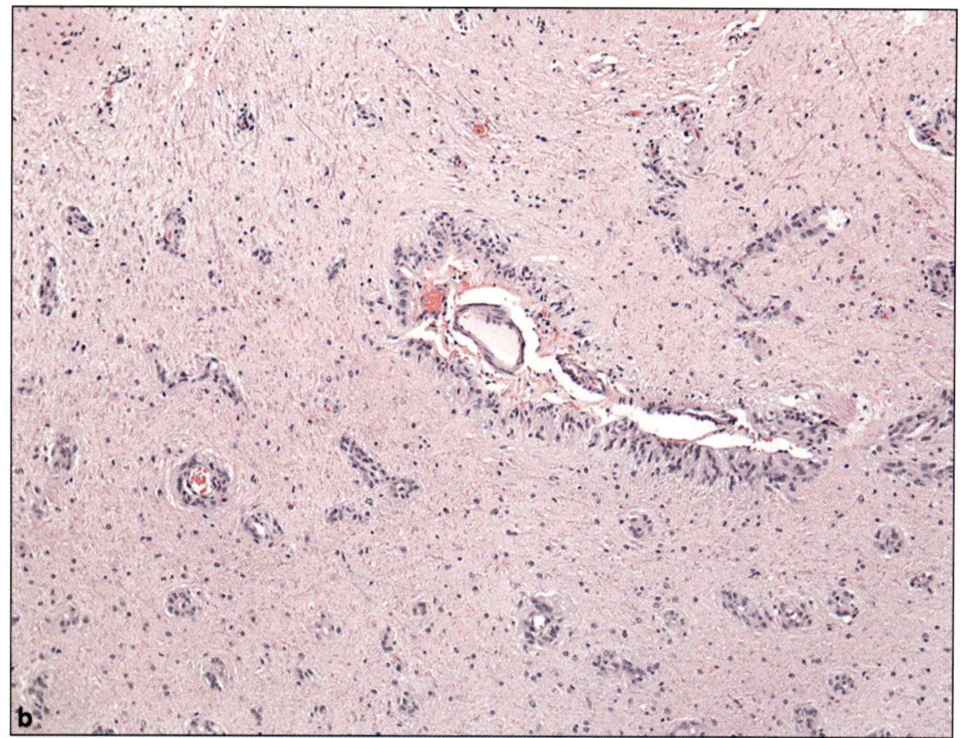

and sometimes virtually indistinguishable from chordoma (Figure 3.30a–c). Cells tend to lack the prominent vacuolation of chordoma cells. Despite their rarity, a regular feature is a lymphoplasmacytic infiltrate. Cytological atypicality, mitotic activity, and necrosis are not present.

Figure 3.29. *continued*
(c) EMA reactivity is seen as punctate cytoplasmic dots.

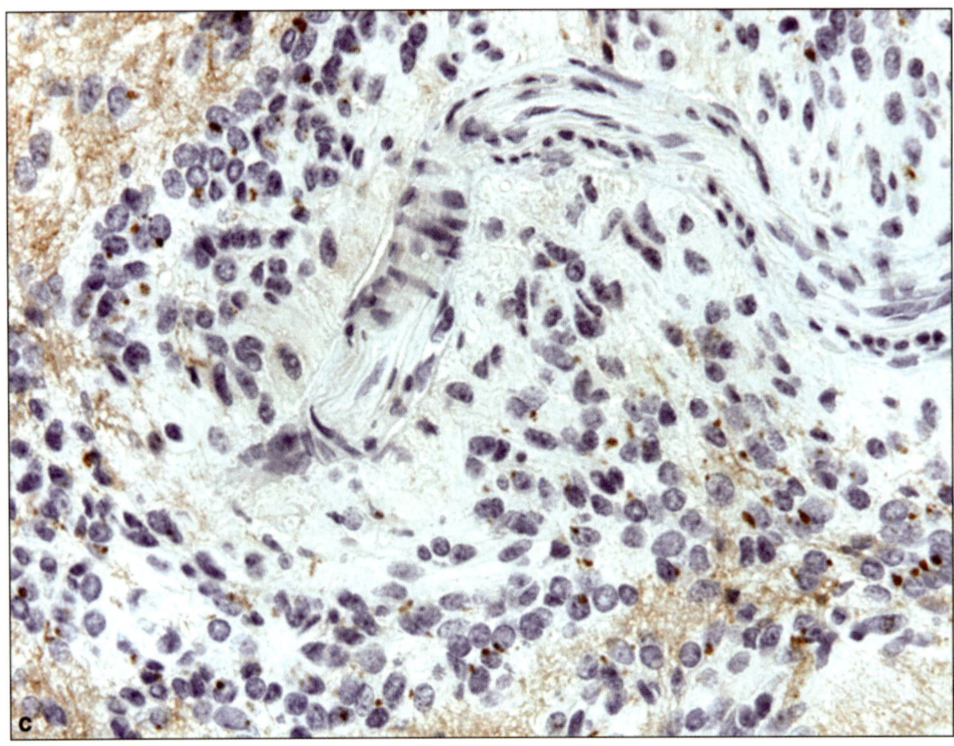

Figure 3.30. (a) The chordoid glioma bears remarkable microscopic similarity with chordomas, including a myxoid background, (b) however, closer inspection will reveal the absence of the vacuolation in tumor cell cytoplasm. (c) Chordoid gliomas are strongly immunopositive for GFAP. Photomicrographs are generously provided by D. Brat, Emory University School of Medicine, Atlanta, GA.

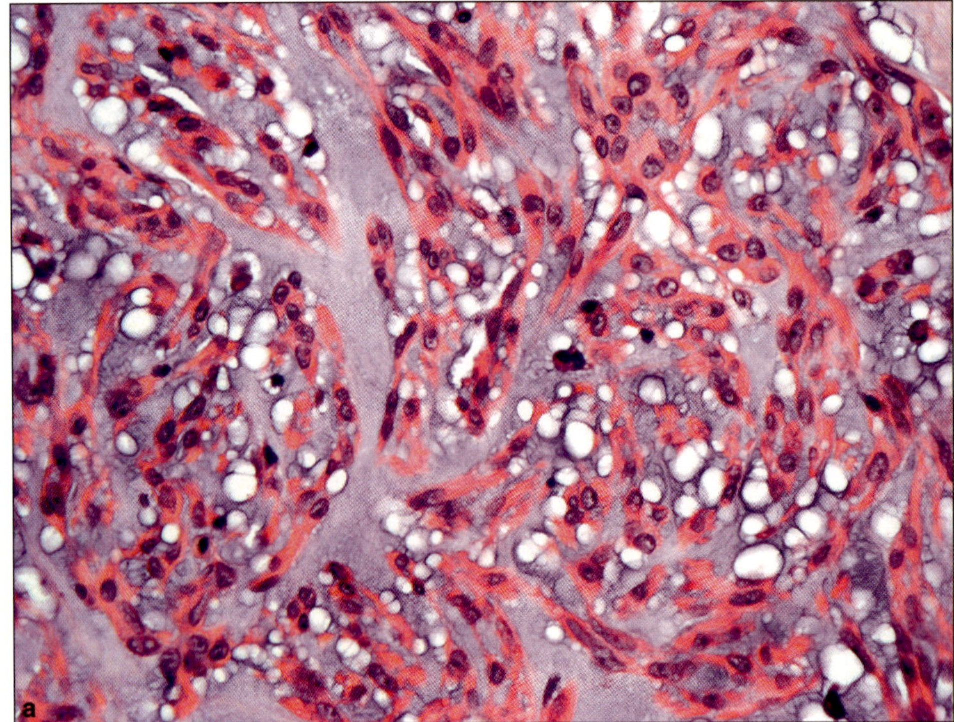

Immunohistochemistry provides the diagnostic distinction as these tumors are strongly GFAP positive but do not show the characteristic cytokeratin positivity of chordomas, although S-100 immunopositivity may be focally present.

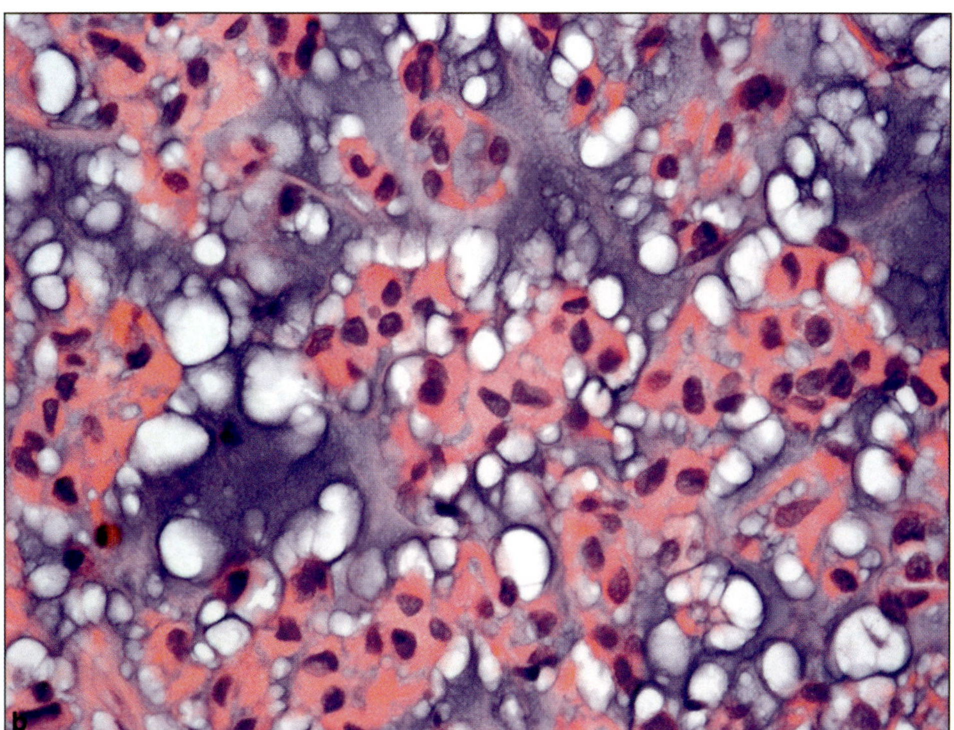

Figure 3.30. *continued.*

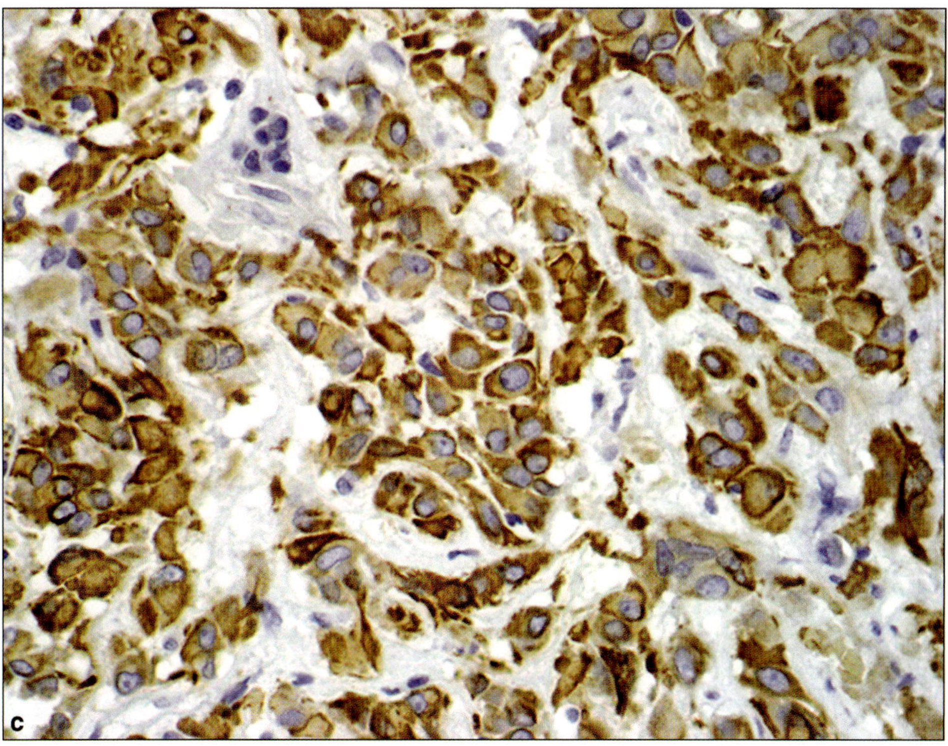

REFERENCES

Aldape KD, Rosenblum MK. Astroblastoma. In: *WHO Classification of Tumours of the Central Nervous System. Louis DN, editor.* Lyon: International Agency for Research on Cancer, 2007. 88–9.

Brat DJ, Scheithauer BW, Staugaitis SM, Cortez SC, Brecher K, Burger PC. Third ventricular chordoid glioma: a distinct clinicopathologic entity. *J Neuropathol Exp Neurol* 1998; 57: 283–90.

Navarro R, Reitman AJ, de Leon GA, Goldman S, Marymont M, Tomita T. Astroblastoma in childhood: pathological and clinical analysis. *Childs Nerv Syst* 2005; 21: 211–20.

Wang M, Tihan T, Rojiani AM, Bodhireddy SR, Prayson RA, Iacuone JJ, et al. Monomorphous angiocentric glioma: a distinctive epileptogenic neoplasm with features of infiltrating astrocytoma and ependymoma. *J Neuropathol Exp Neurol* 2005; 64: 875–81.

Ependymal Tumors

WHO GRADE I

Subependymoma

Clinical and Radiological Features

These are indolent, benign gliomas, which occur in middle to late adulthood with a male to female incidence of greater than two to one (Rushing et al., 2007). It is not unusual for subependymomas to be found incidentally at autopsy (Ernestus and Schroder, 1993). They typically appear as a pedunculated intraventricular mass most commonly in the fourth ventricle and 50–60% of cases, followed by the lateral ventricles in 30–40% of cases. Rarely, subependymomas occur in the cervical or thoracic spinal cord as an intramedullary lesion and rarely as an extramedullary mass (Jallo et al., 1996). Subependymomas can be cured by surgical excision but may recur if incompletely resected.

Subependymomas produced symptoms largely through the obstruction of CSF flow and resultant raised intracranial pressure. They may undergo extensive intratumoral or subarachnoid hemorrhage to the extent that the underlying tumor may be obscured by the accumulated blood (Lindboe et al., 1992; Marra et al., 1991). The radiological appearance is highly suggestive in the appropriate clinical context (Figure 3.31).

Pathology

Subependymomas are firm well-demarcated tumors often protruding as a pedunculated mass from the wall of a ventricle. The histologic features are quite characteristic, consisting of loose clusters of bland, rather monomorphous cells with nuclear features of ependymal differentiation in a rich fibrillary background (Figure 3.32). Microcystic degeneration as well as microcalcification are common. These tumors are GFAP immunopositive. As with other neoplasms associated with ependymal differentiation, cilia or microvilli may be seen ultrastructurally. It is important to recognize that gliomas with mixed ependymal and subependymal morphologies constitute a distinct entity with the prognosis determined by the grade of the ependymal portion.

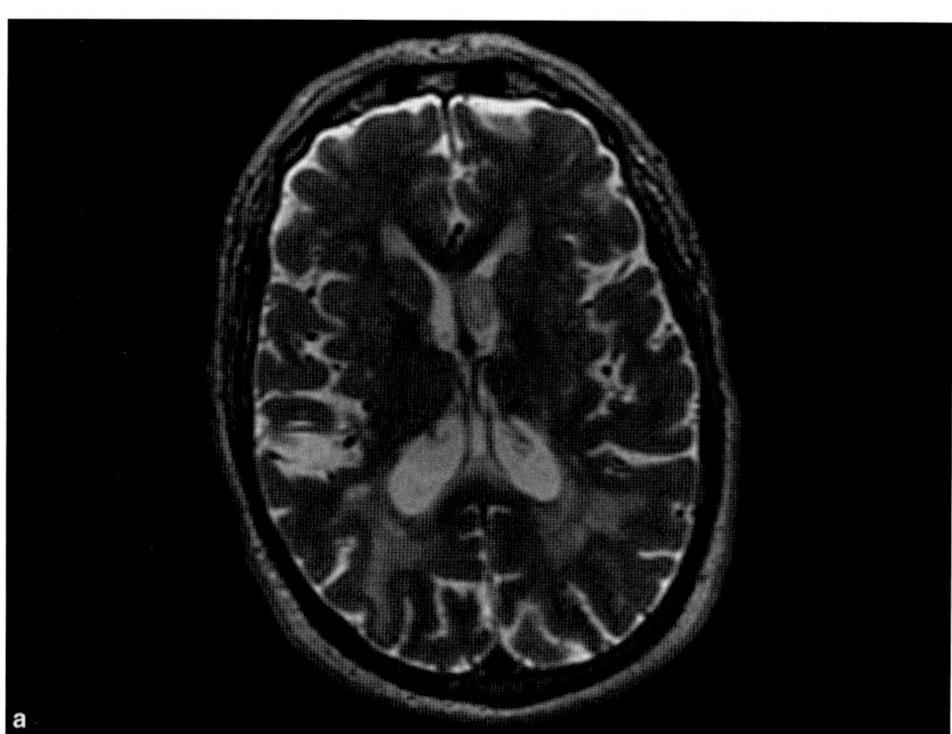

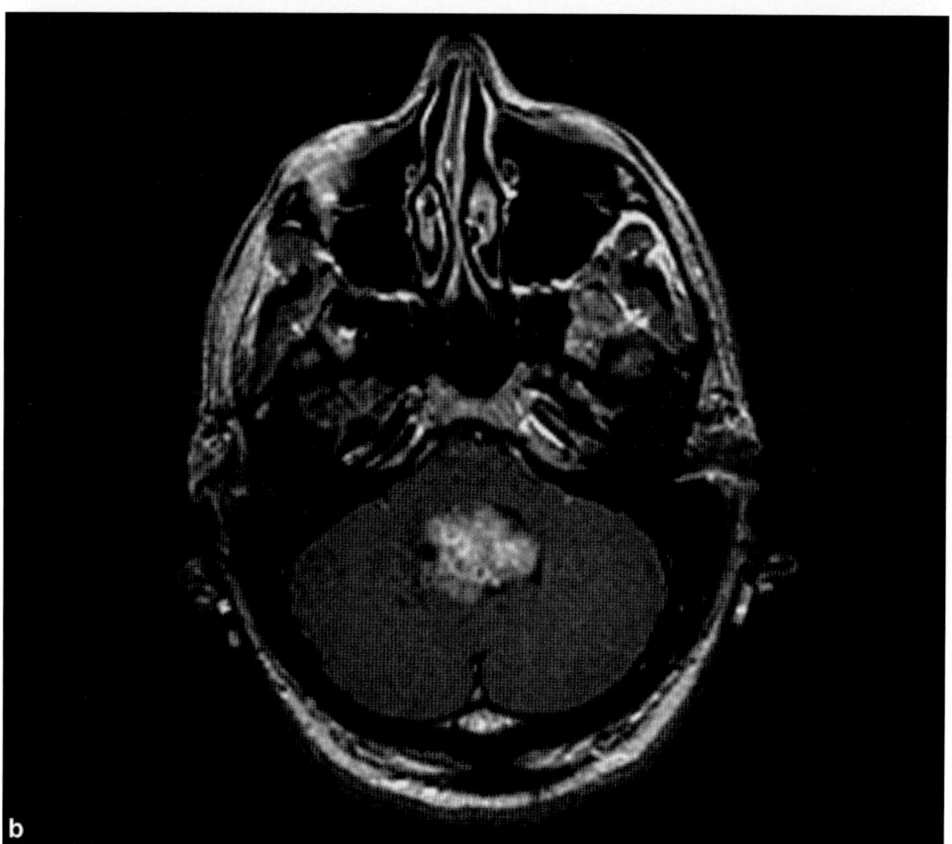

Figure 3.31. Just as they appear grossly, subependymomas by neuroimaging show a sharply circumscribed nodular mass, which is typically noncontrast-enhancing (Chiechi et al., 1995) in (a) the lateral ventricle or (b) the fourth ventricle. Calcification and hemorrhage may be seen.

Figure 3.32. (a) Subependymomas are often an incidental finding at autopsy, as was this small example in the floor of the fourth ventricle. (b) The-low power appearance of subependymomas reveals its hypocellularity and loose clusters of cells in a fibrillary background.

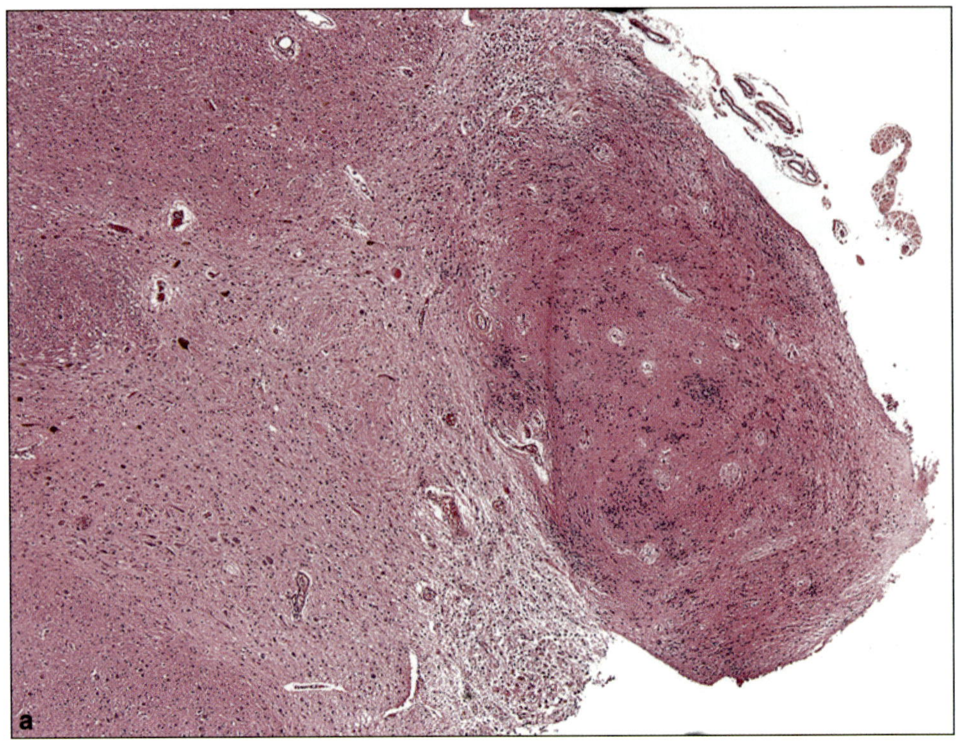

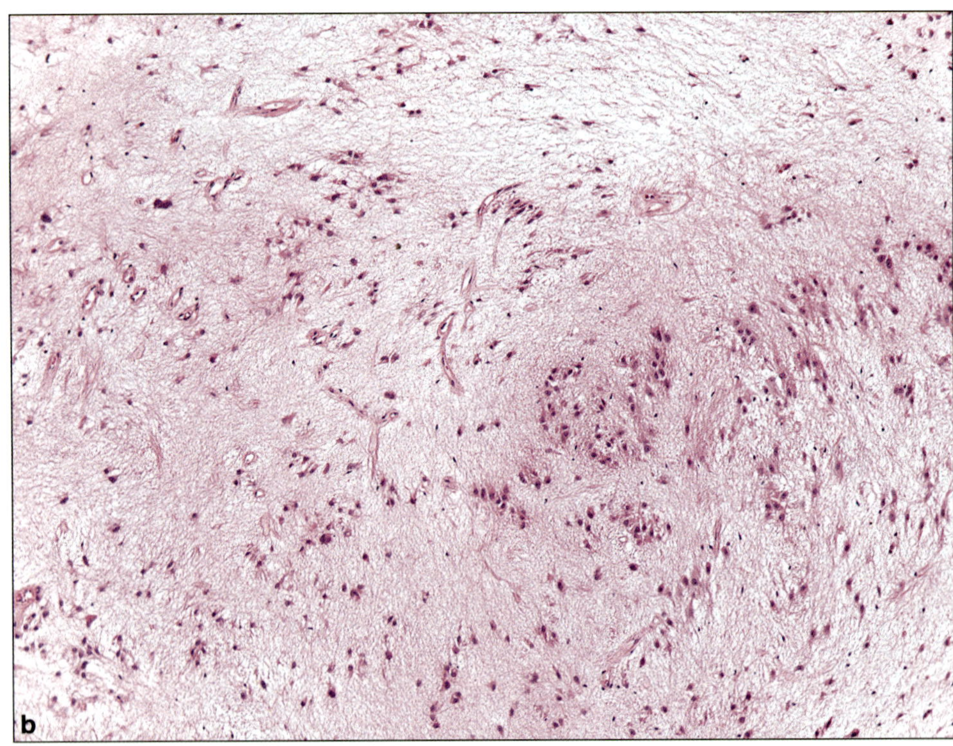

Myxopapillary Ependymoma

Clinical and Radiological Features

The myxopapillary ependymoma occurs within the broad age range but most commonly in young adults in the third and fourth decades with a greater

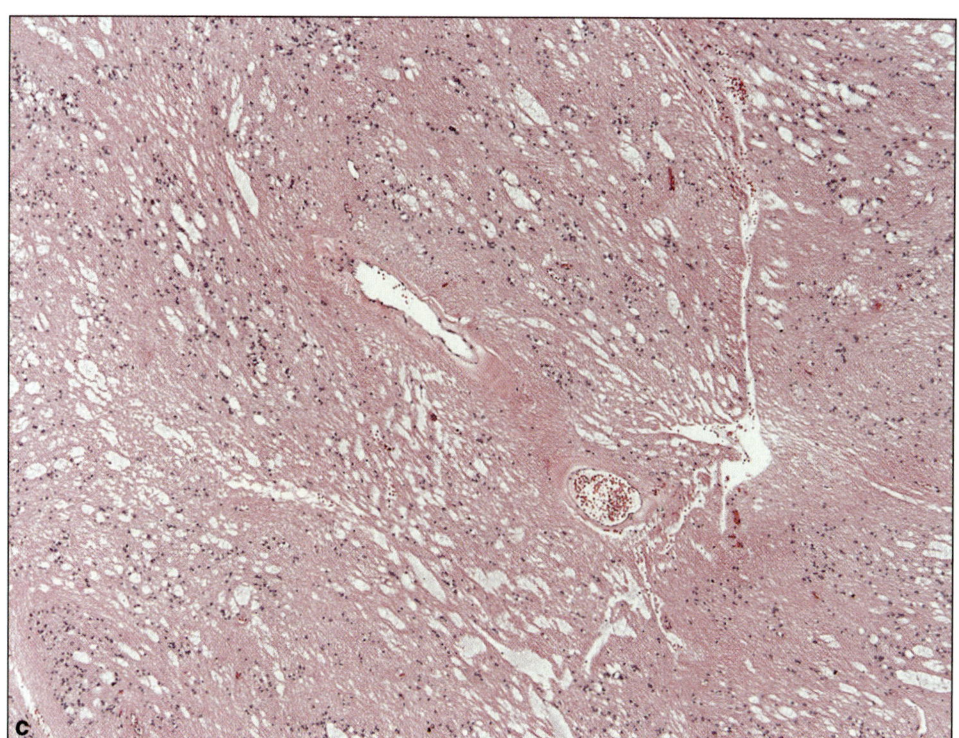

Figure 3.32. *continued* (c) Microcystic degeneration is a regular feature of subependymomas. (d) Closer inspection of nuclei reveals the ovoid shapes reminiscent of an ependymal lineage.

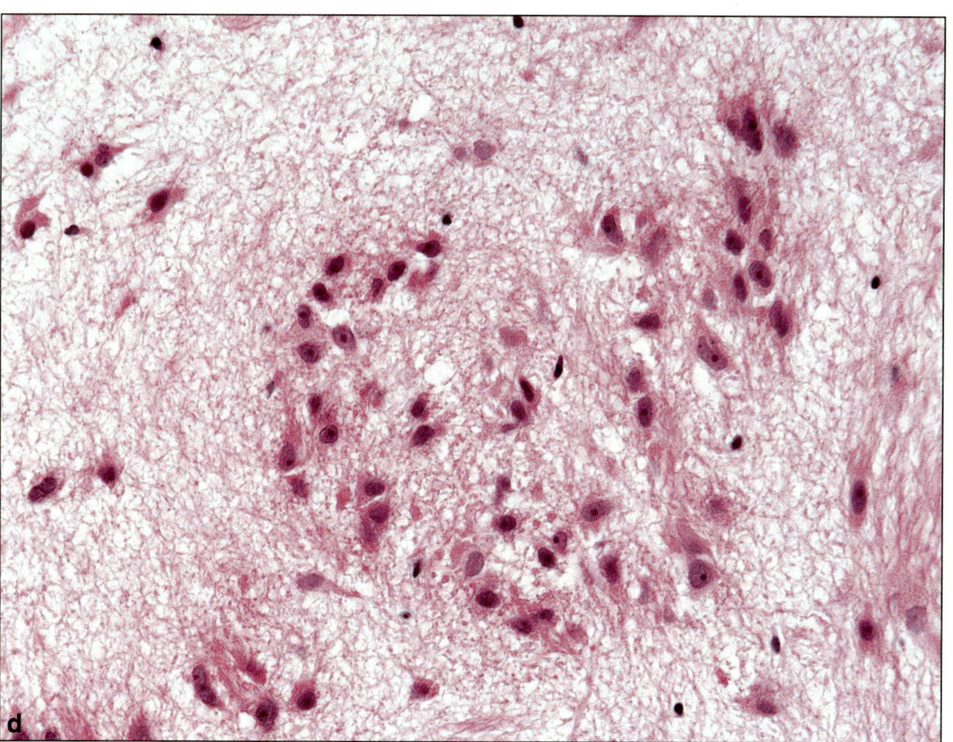

than 2:1 incidence in males as compared with females (Kurt et al., 2006). They are the most common intramedullary neoplasm of the spinal cauda equina and are essentially only found in this location (Figure 3.33). Sacrococcygeal subcutaneous examples have been reported and may be associated with a higher rate of regrowth or even distant metastases (Helwig and Stern, 1984; Ilhan et al., 1998). The quite favorable prognosis after total or sometimes even partial

Figure 3.33. This mid-sagittal MRI shows the sausage shape of the myxopapillary ependymoma in the region of the cauda equina, with inhomogeneous contrast enhancement.

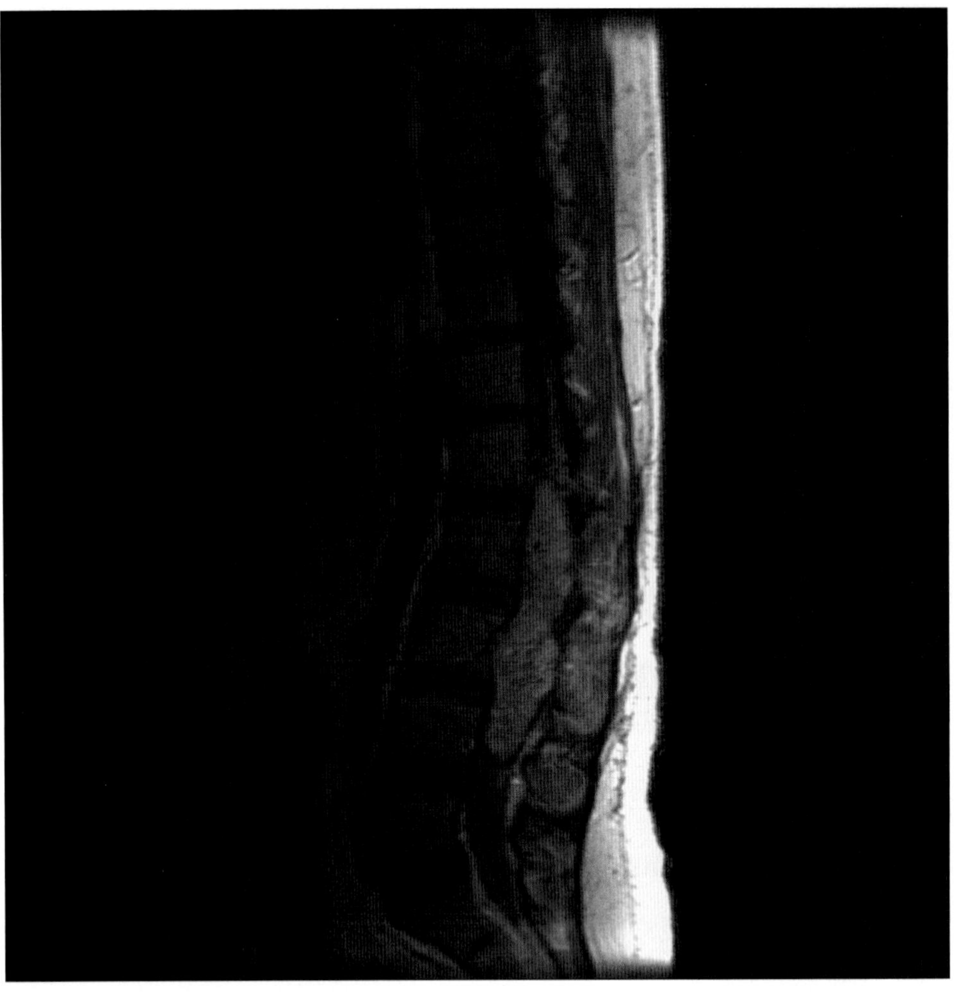

resection is reflective of the WHO Grade I classification. If tumor spillage occurs in resection, there may be a local and inexorable infiltrative recurrence. CNS metastases may also occur (Fassett et al., 2005).

Pathology

When operative conditions permit, the gross resection specimen will be an elongated and encapsulated mass, thus indicating a successful en bloc resection. The cut surface is soft and gray with a lobulated texture. Microscopically, myxopapillary ependymomas are composed of sometimes only vaguely recognizable papillary structures rimmed by glial cells with nuclear features of ependymal derivation, namely ovoid nuclei with finely stippled chromatin (Figure 3.34). Sometimes the cells are noticeably elongated and may show perivascular delicate processes. The myxoid component of these tumors may also be difficult to discern but special stains such as Alcian blue or periodic acid–Schiff (PAS) may highlight small amounts of myxoid matrix. While there may be mild nuclear pleomorphism, proliferative activity is minimal. Tumor cells are GFAP and S-100 immunopositive, and negative for cytokeratin staining, which may be helpful in distinguishing this tumor from metastatic papillary epithelial neoplasms.

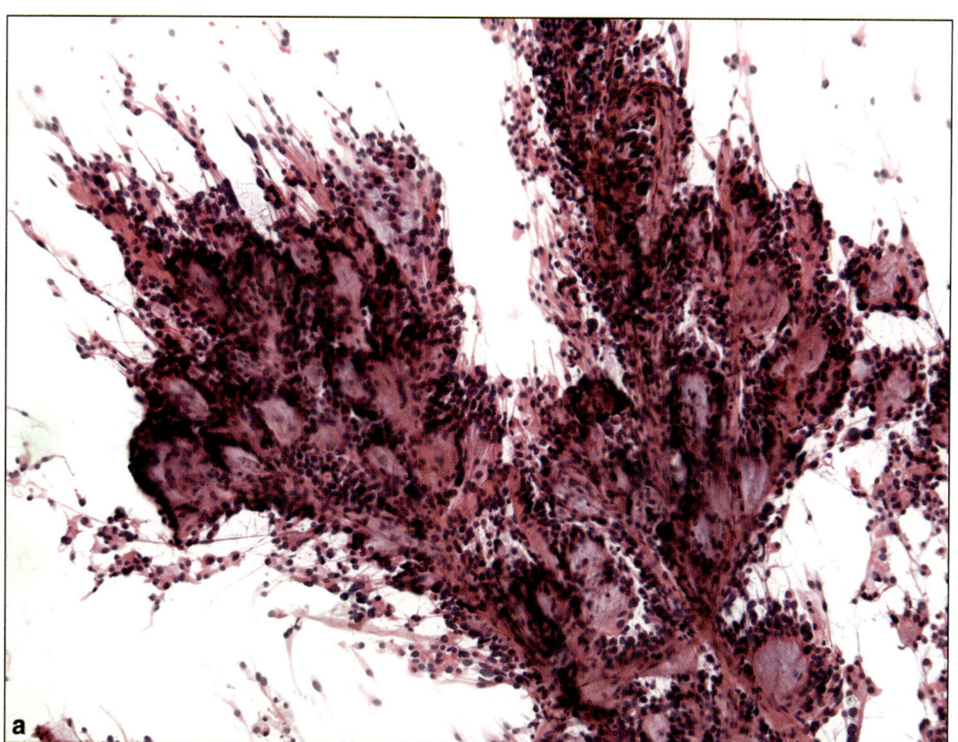

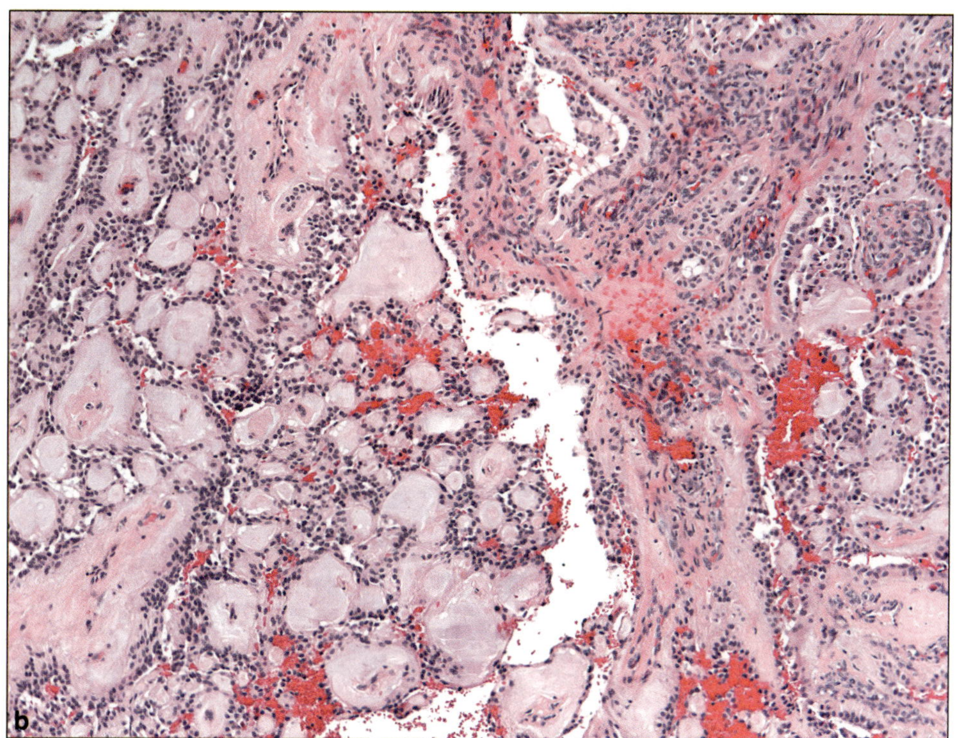

Figure 3.34. (a) Squash preparation of a myxopapillary ependymoma showing preservation of its distinctive papillary architecture. (b) Papillary growth is not always obvious, as seen in the upper right corner.

WHO GRADE II

Ependymoma

Clinical and Radiological Features

Ependymomas are most common in the pediatric population; however, they may occur well into late adulthood (Reni et al., 2007). There are distinct

Figure 3.34. *continued*
(c) Nuclear morphology is ependymal, with ovoid shapes and small but distinct nucleoli. (d) The Alcian blue stain highlights the myxoid component, which may be quite focal and much less extensive than in this example.

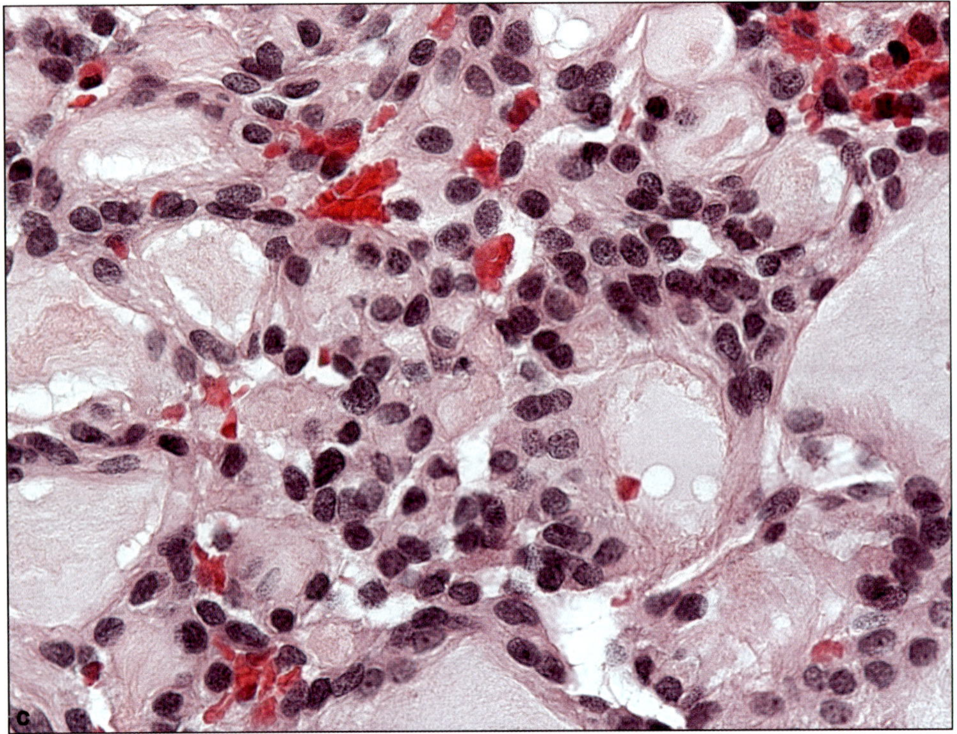

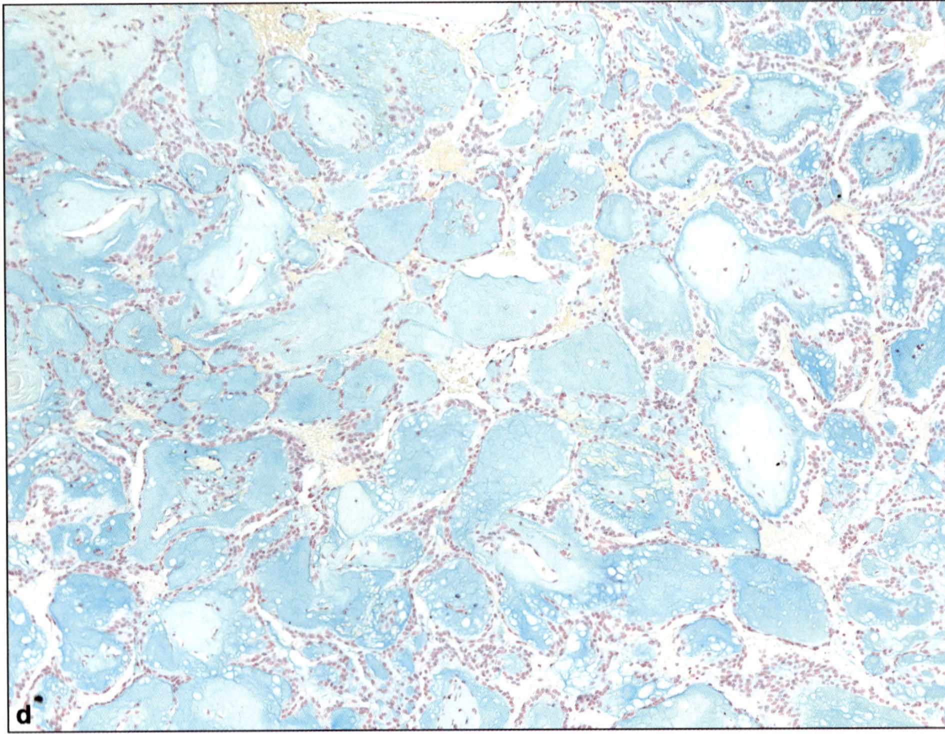

predilections for location according to the age of the patient. Posterior fossa examples predominate in childhood and typically arise within the fourth ventricle at a lateral recess. They tend to grow through the foramina of Luschka and may extend into the subarachnoid space of the ventral pons and encase the basilar

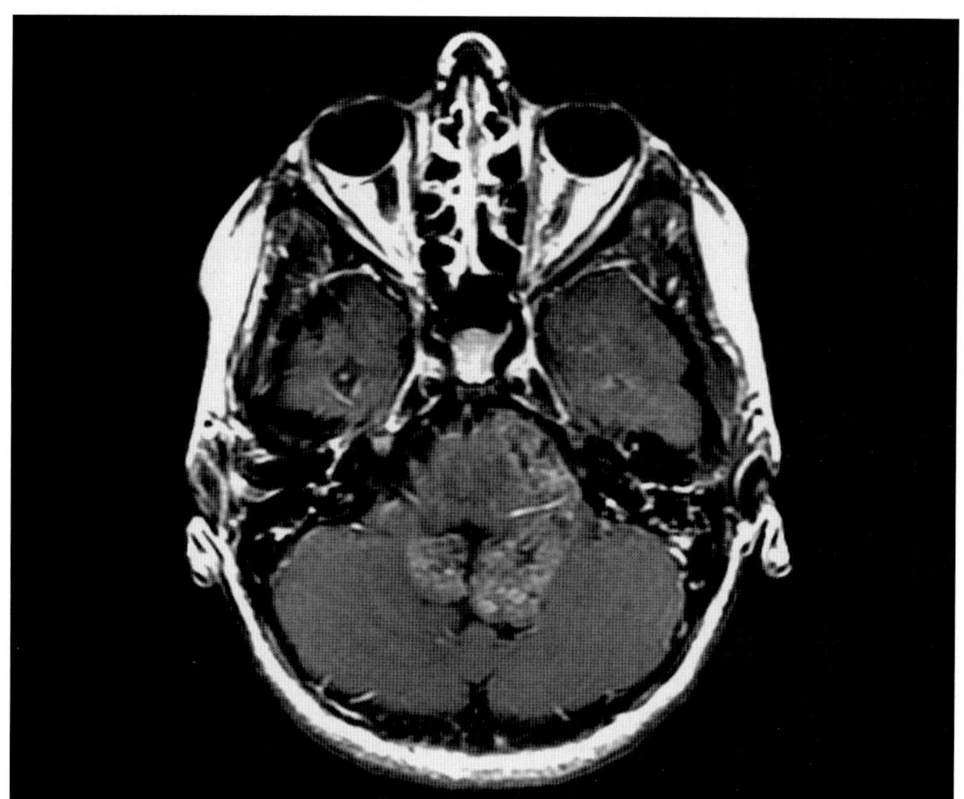

Figure 3.35. Ependymomas are typically well demarcated by neuroimaging and show variable contrast enhancement. Extensive calcification may sometimes be seen. This example shows the characteristic tendency of ependymomas to extend from the fourth ventricle into the prepontine space, sometimes encasing the basilar artery.

artery (Figure 3.35). Spinal ependymomas are more common in adults. Rare examples exist for pelvic (Duggan et al., 1989; Hofman et al., 2001) and ovarian ependymomas (Garcia-Barriola et al., 2000). Supratentorial ependymomas occur in both age groups.

The symptoms of ependymomas depend on the location. Posterior fossa tumors tend to produce obstructive hydrocephalus. Supratentorial examples produce effects referable to space-occupying lesion and increased intracranial pressure, such as headache, dizziness, nausea, and vomiting. Spinal ependymomas produce motor and sensory deficits.

The prognosis for ependymomas depends heavily upon the extent of surgical resection, as chemotherapy and radiation therapy are of limited effectiveness with this tumor. The clear cell ependymoma may be associated with a more aggressive course (Fouladi et al., 2003). A study of posterior fossa childhood ependymomas suggests that the extent of resection and age above 3 years are the most important positive prognostic predictors, and grading does not carry equally significant prognostic importance (Tihan et al., 2008).

Ependymomas are distinctive among most glial tumors in that the borders are comparatively better demarcated, without the tendency seen in astrocytomas for extensive single cell infiltration far into adjacent brain or spinal cord tissue. This has important implications for intraoperative consultations since a neurosurgeon may successfully achieve total resection of an ependymoma and thus ensure the likelihood of long-term survival (McGirt et al., 2008), whereas the infiltrative nature of an astrocytoma would argue against an attempt at complete resection.

Figure 3.36. Classic ependymoma. (a) Squash preparations of ependymomas may allow for preservation of the perivascular pseudorosettes. (b) Classic low-power appearance of ependymoma in cryosection in which perivascular pseudorosettes may be seen in spite of suboptimal histological representation of the sample, and should always prompt consideration of ependymoma even when present in vague forms.

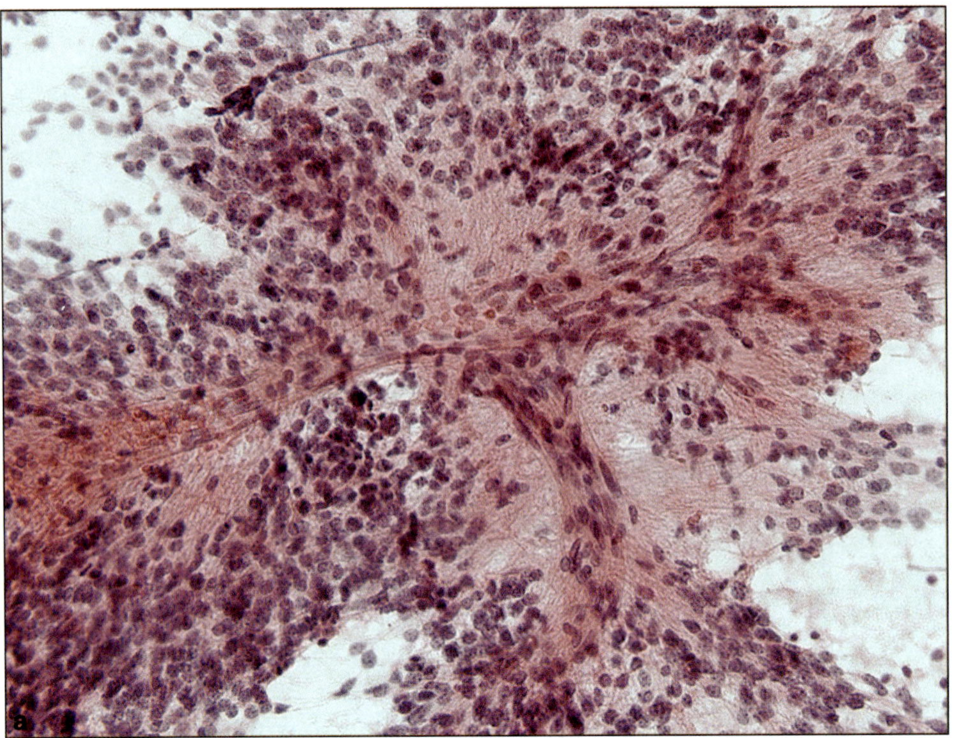

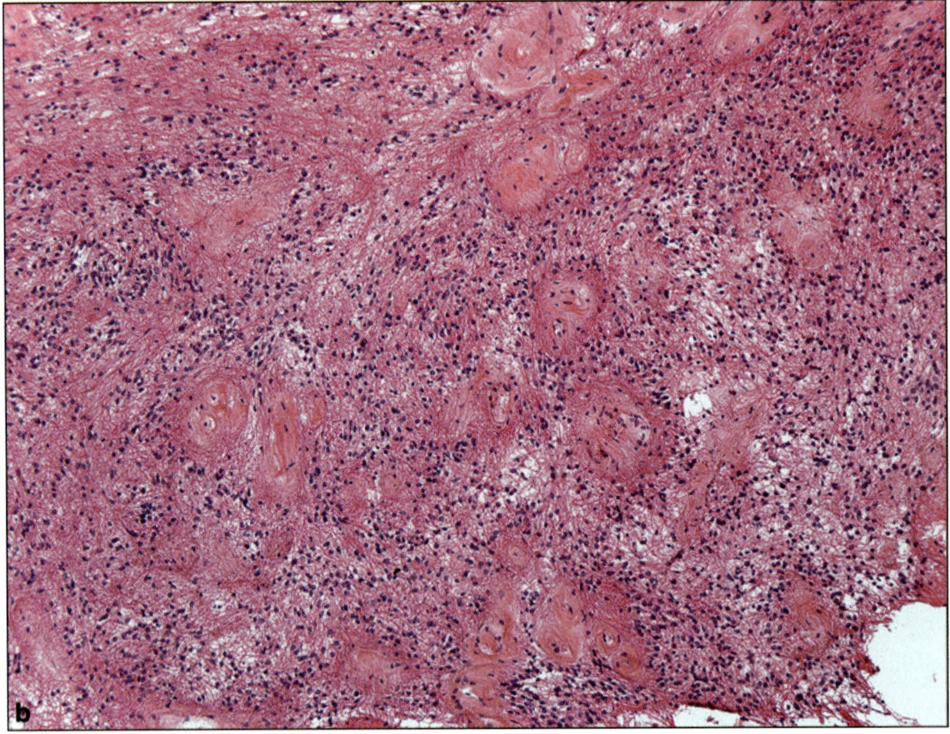

Pathology

Ependymomas are divided into classic forms and variants as listed, also classified as WHO Grade II tumors. They tend to share a distinctive nuclear morphology consisting of monomorphous ovoid nuclei with finely punctate

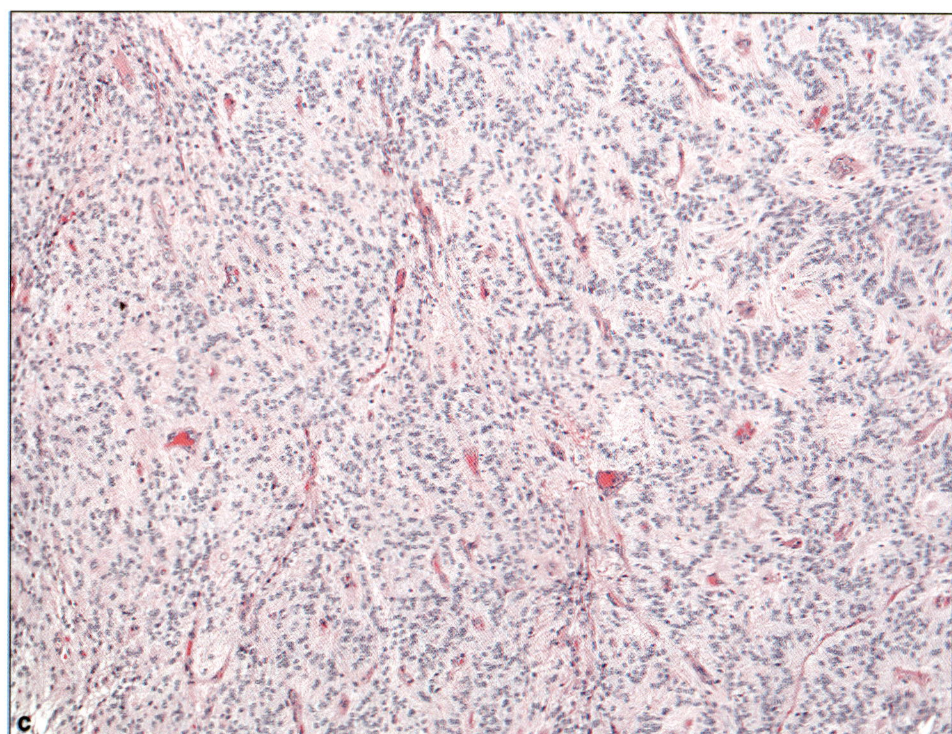

Figure 3.36. *continued* (c) Typical appearance of ependymoma, with frequent perivascular pseudorosettes in the right field of the figure, while the portion in the left illustrates the variable extent of this finding. (d) True ependymal rosettes are usually much rarer than perivascular pseudorosettes and (e) are highlighted by EMA immunohistochemistry in addition to characteristic dotlike cytoplasmic positivity of ependymomas.

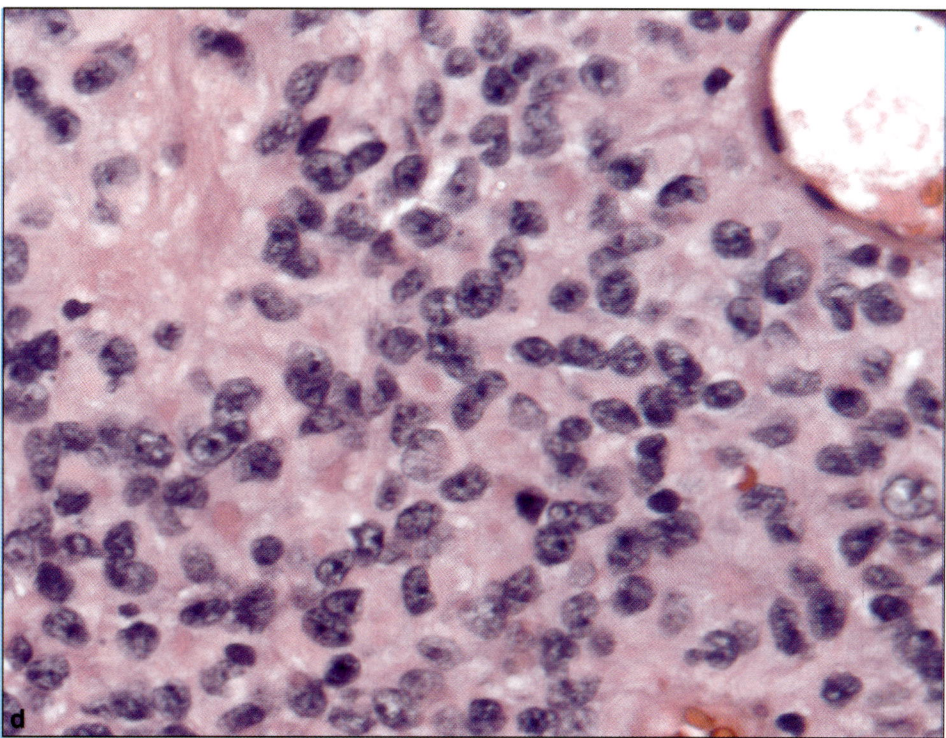

chromatin and a small but distinct nucleolus. The glial nature of ependymomas can be vividly seen in cytological squash preparations through the rich fibrillary background, which may also highlight perivascular cell processes (Figure 3.36).

The most useful diagnostic histological feature in ependymomas is the perivascular pseudorosette; when encountered in either frozen or permanent

Figure 3.36. *continued.*

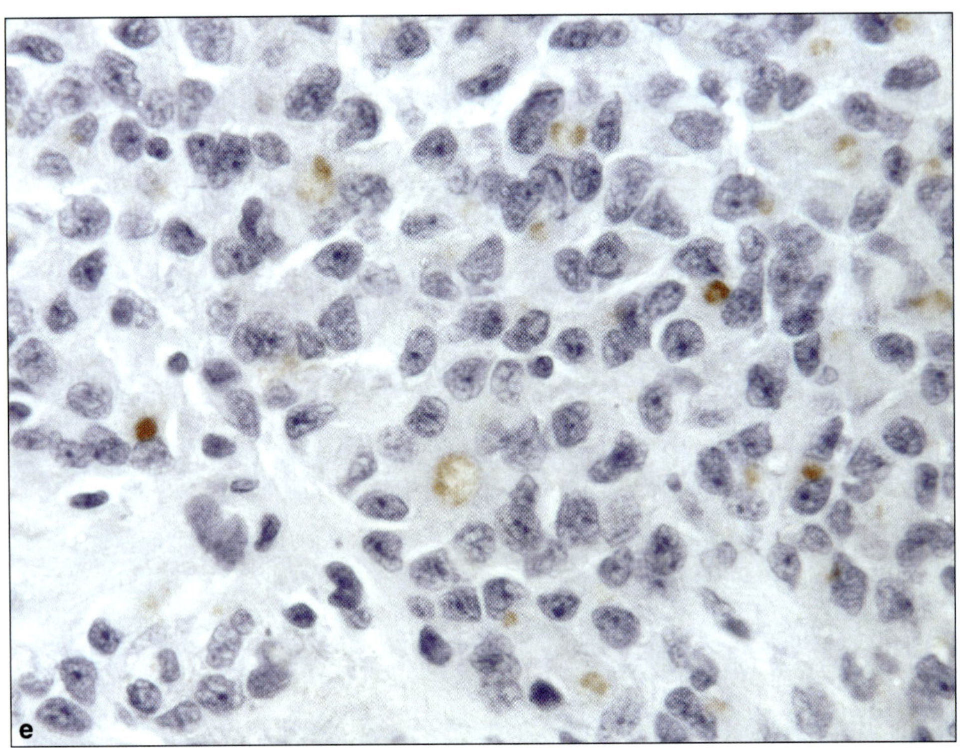

sections, the diagnosis of ependymoma can be made with relative ease. This is usually apparent as an anuclear perivascular zone of varying width. The hematoxylin and eosin (H&E) stain may not reveal the perpendicular and tapering glial processes of which the perivascular pseudorosette is composed. However, portions of the tissue demonstrating a pulling artifact or a GFAP immunostain would serve to highlight the perivascular pseudorosette cell processes. This is an approach that may be applied to all forms of ependymoma, particularly those with vague perivascular pseudorosettes.

Less commonly, true ependymal rosettes may be found, in which cells are arranged in a small circle around a lumen lined by cilia or more commonly, basal bodies or blepharoplasts along the apical surfaces of the tumor cells. Such lumina would be highlighted along the periphery by EMA immunostaining. Another immunohistochemical feature in several types of ependymoma, which may be of key diagnostic value, is the presence of EMA-positive dotlike cytoplasmic inclusions, representing microlumina in tumor cells (Takei et al., 2007).

Blood vessels are relatively inconspicuous in WHO Grade II ependymomas. Necrosis should prompt consideration of an anaplastic ependymoma; however, necrosis may be found in otherwise WHO Grade II ependymomas of the posterior fossa and should not result in a designation of WHO Grade III.

Metaplastic change in the form of cartilage or bone formation may be seen. Some supratentorial or extraventricular ependymomas may show such extensive and dense calcification as to obscure the ependymal nature of the tumor. Myxoid degeneration and tumor hemorrhage may also be seen. Other forms of differentiation include lipomatous (Onaya et al., 2005; Sharma et al., 2000), giant cell

(Brown et al., 1998; Fourney et al., 2004; Pimentel et al., 2001; Zec et al., 1996), extensive vacuolation or signet ring cell differentiation (Hirato et al., 1997; Mizuno et al., 2005; Vajtai et al., 1999), and melanotic pigment (Chan et al., 2003).

Most ependymomas are GFAP immunopositive with S-100 and vimentin coexpressions. The aforementioned EMA immunopositivity may be diffuse in rare cases in contrast to the usual dotlike cytoplasmic positivity. Cytokeratin positivity may be seen in unusual cases, complicating the process of distinguishing them from metastatic tumors (Mannoji and Becker, 1988). Ependymomas of the third ventricle have been shown to express thyroid transcription factor 1 (TTF1) (Zamecnik et al., 2004). Neuronal antigens of unknown clinical significance may be present (Rodriguez et al., 2007), although interestingly, neuN immunoreactivity has been noted in ependymomas, particularly in the anaplastic examples (Parker et al., 2001).

Cellular Ependymoma

These are associated with supratentorial extraventricular origins (Shuangshoti et al., 2005), and are distinguished from classic ependymomas by increased nuclear density without an increase in mitotic activity (Figure 3.37). Accordingly, pseudorosettes may be less apparent.

Papillary Ependymoma

Papillary growth within ependymomas may often appear as the focal consequence of the artifactual pulling apart of tissue. However, when fingerlike projections forming genuine papillae are present, the term papillary ependymoma may be used. These may be particularly difficult to distinguish from other papillary tumors such as choroid plexus papillomas (Park et al., 1996) or metastatic carcinomas. The papillary ependymoma would demonstrate extensive GFAP immunopositivity in contrast to a relative or complete lack of GFAP expression in choroid plexus papillomas or metastatic carcinomas.

Clear Cell Ependymoma

The clear cell ependymoma is stated to be more common in supratentorial locations of young children and is associated with a poorer prognosis (Fouladi et al., 2003). They are dominated by monomorphous cells with clear cytoplasm yet retaining nuclear features of an ependymoma (Figure 3.38). These may nonetheless be difficult to distinguish from other clear cell gliomas, particularly oligodendroglioma or regions of other gliomas such as pilocytic astrocytoma, ganglioglioma, or the DNT with oligodendrocyte-like components. Immunohistochemistry for GFAP may be especially useful in highlighting perivascular pseudorosettes and for EMA by revealing cytoplasmic dotlike immunoreactivity.

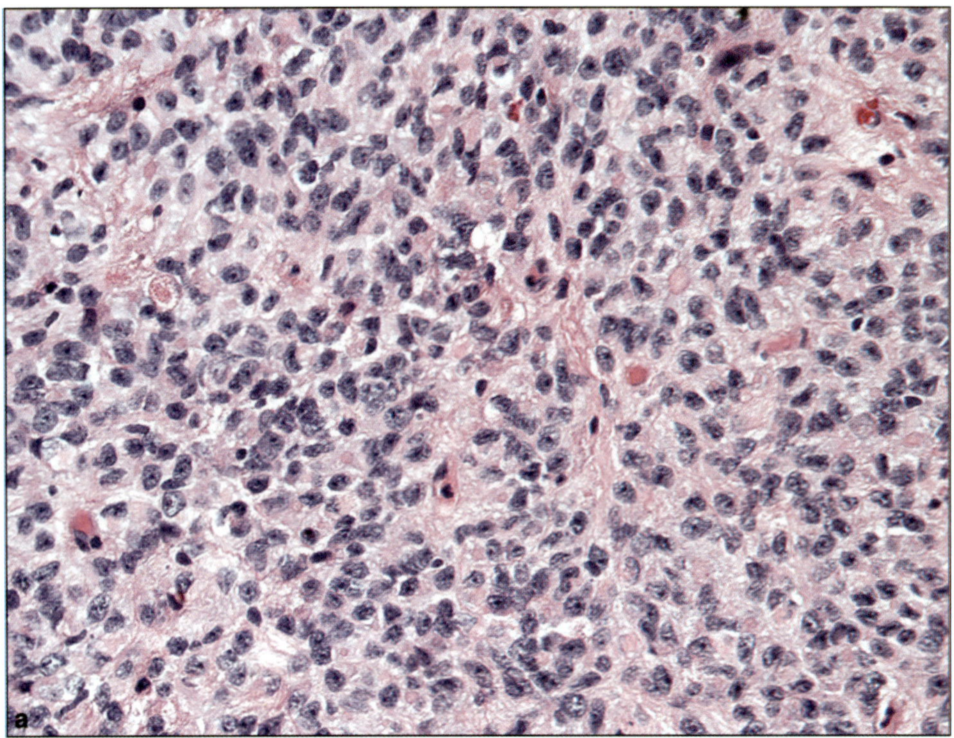

Figure 3.37. (a) Cellular ependymomas are characterized by increased cellularity without anaplasia, which may obscure the presence of usual perivascular pseudorosettes. (b) As in all ependymomas, GFAP immunohistochemistry may reveal the slender perivascular tumor processes that are not appreciable in H&E-stained sections.

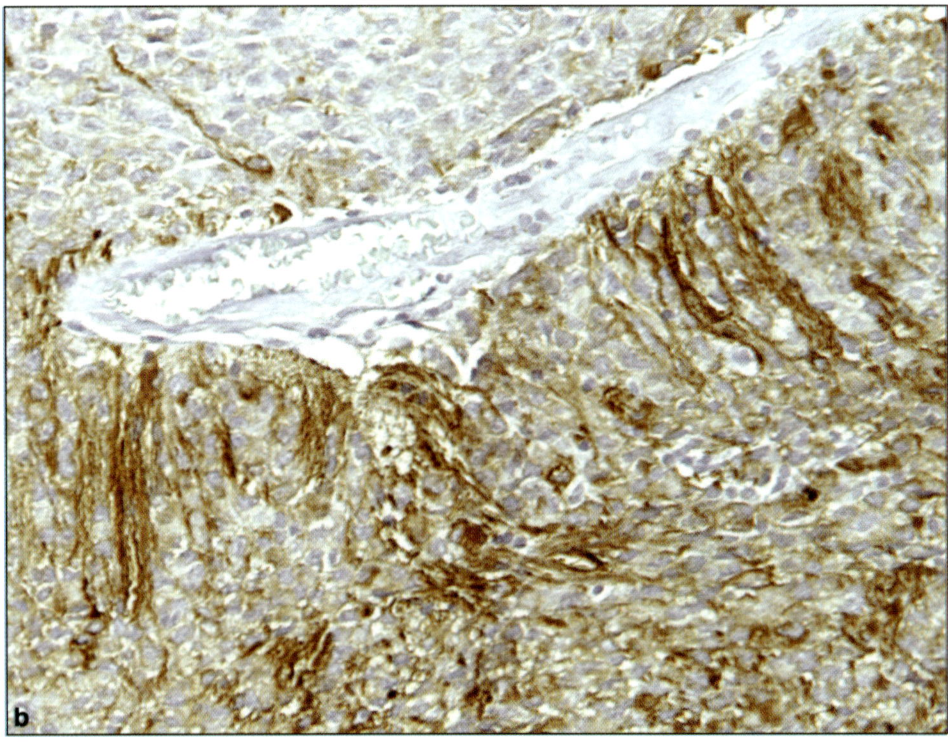

Tanycytic Ependymoma

The name derives from tanycytes, which are periventricular spindle cells with perpendicular cytoplasmic processes. This rare form of ependymoma is

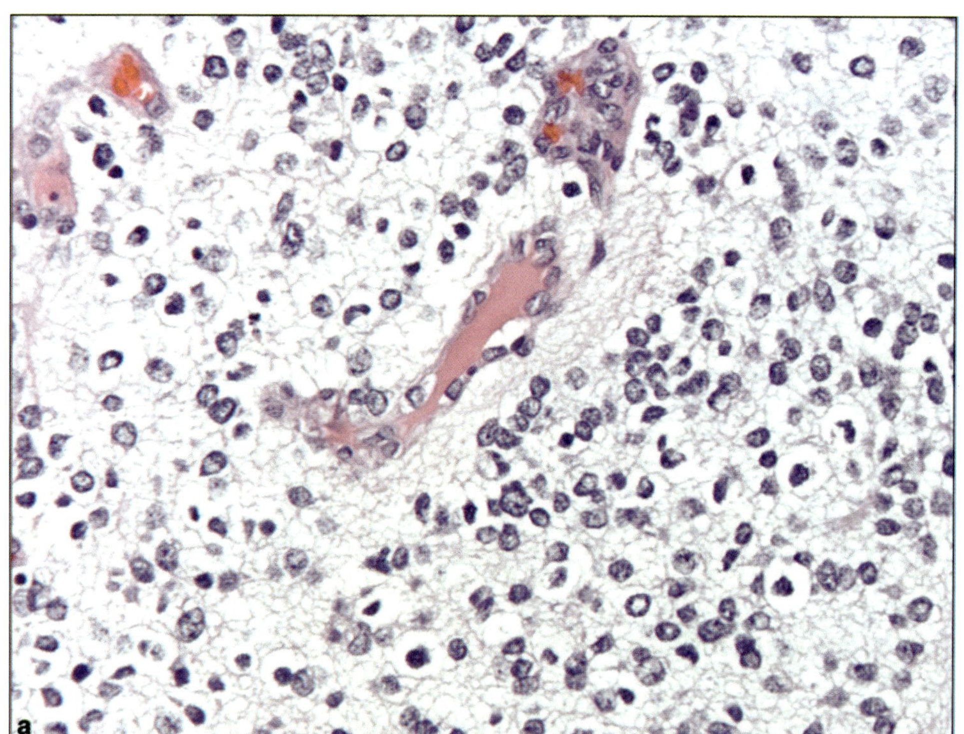

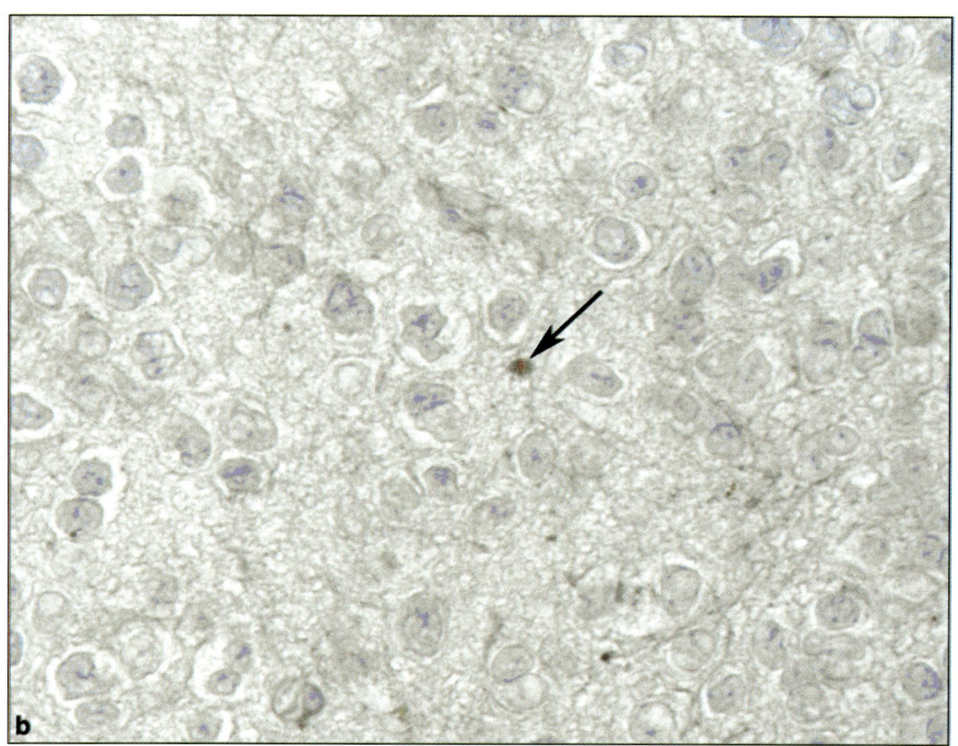

Figure 3.38. (a) Clear cell ependymomas raise the differential diagnosis between other CNS clear cell tumors, chiefly oligodendrogliomas and clear cell meningiomas. (b) Immunohistochemistry for EMA will show cytoplasmic dotlike positivity in some cells (arrow).

especially associated with spinal locations (Kobata et al., 2001; Sato et al., 2005) but is also found in the supratentorial compartment (Daneyemez et al., 1999; Ragel et al., 2005; Richards et al., 2004). An association with NF2 has been reported (Kobata et al., 2001; Ueki et al., 2001).

Figure 3.39. (a) Tanycytic ependymomas shows features more reminiscent of spindle cell neoplasms such as schwannomas or some meningiomas. b) Close inspection shows vague perivascular pseudorosettes and characteristic ependymal nuclear morphology.

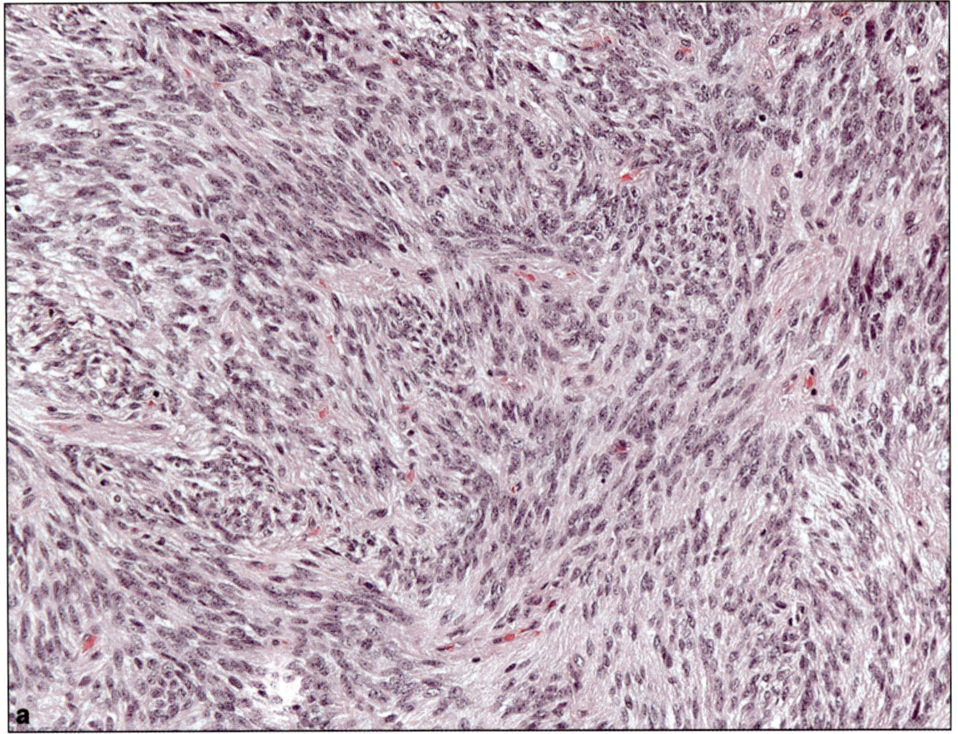

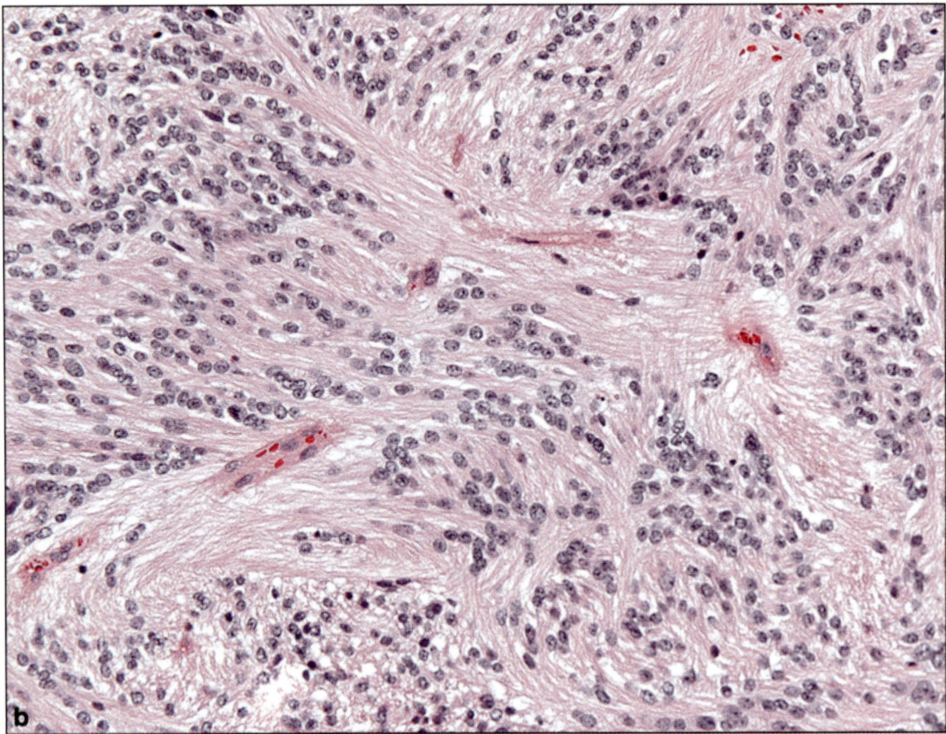

It is dominated by fascicles of spindle cells; pseudorosettes may be especially difficult to recognize (Figure 3.39). Again, nuclear features are ependymal in nature, which may be important in distinguishing this from fibrous meningiomas or other spindle-cell neoplasms.

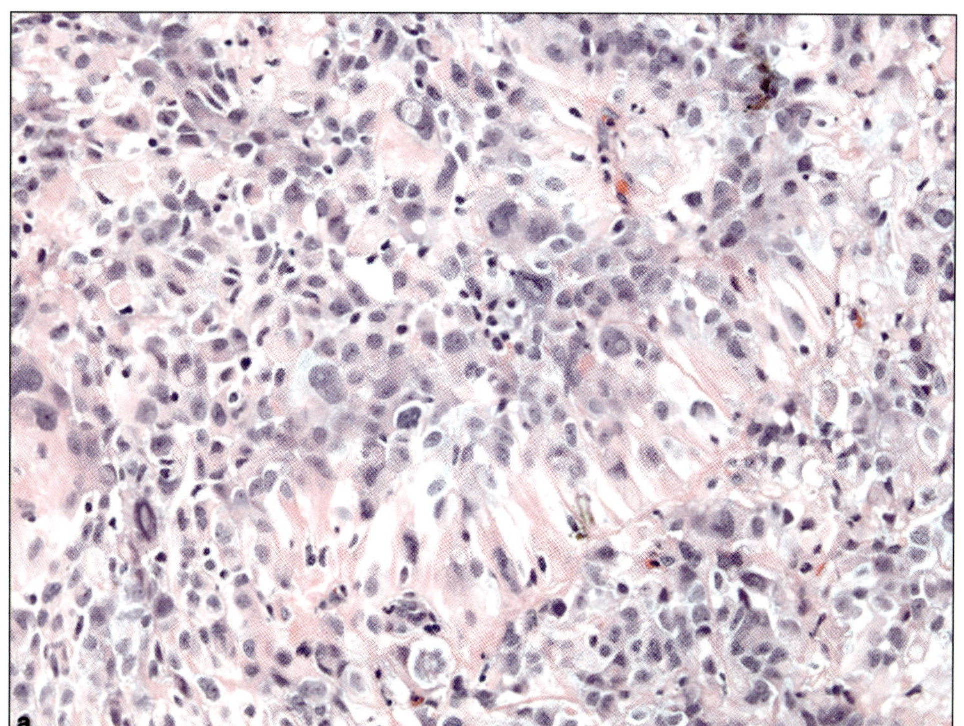

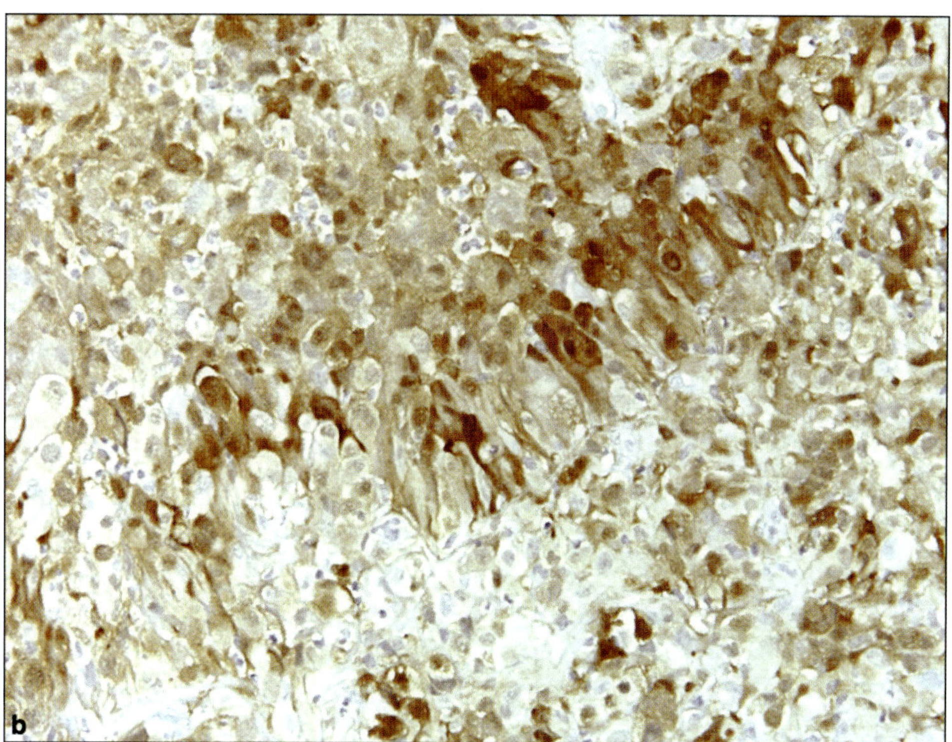

Figure 3.40. (a) Giant cell ependymoma may be unrecognizable as an ependymoma, although focal areas of typical differentiation may occur. Immunohistochemical profile is characteristic of most ependymomas, including positivity for (b) S-100, (c) GFAP, and (d) CD99.

Giant Cell Ependymoma

This type of ependymoma has been recognized by the most recent WHO classification as a variant pattern; however, several reports indicate the possible distinctiveness of this entity. It has been reported to predominantly occur in adolescents, originally in the filum terminale but later in posterior fossa and supratentorial locations (Adamek et al., 2008; Brown et al., 1998; Fourney et al., 2004; Pimentel et al., 2001).

Figure 3.40. *continued.*

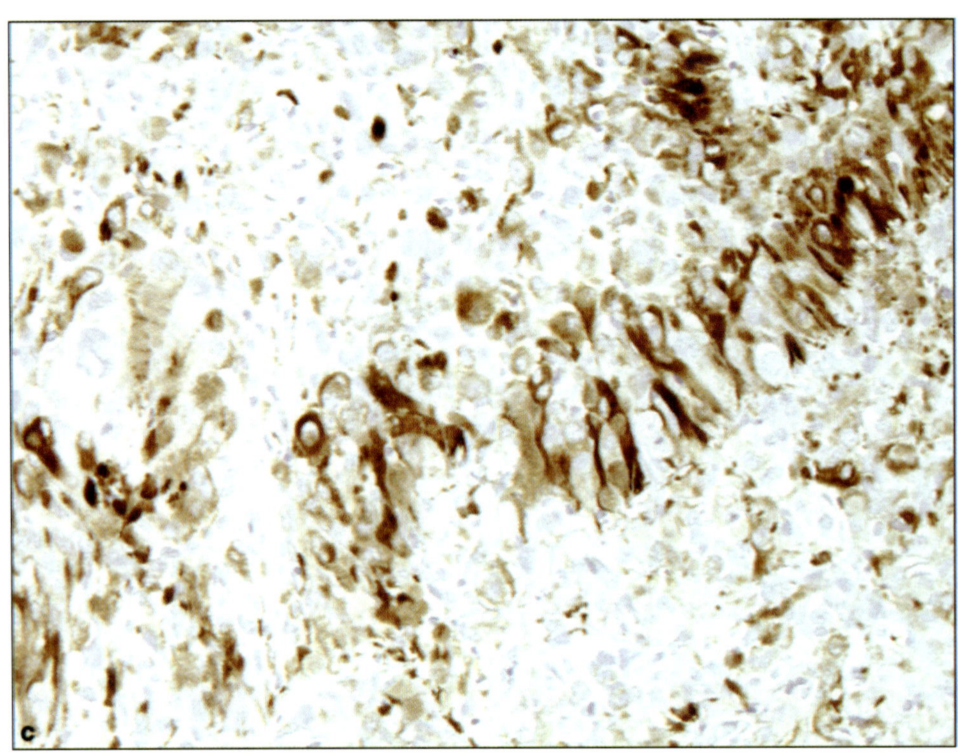

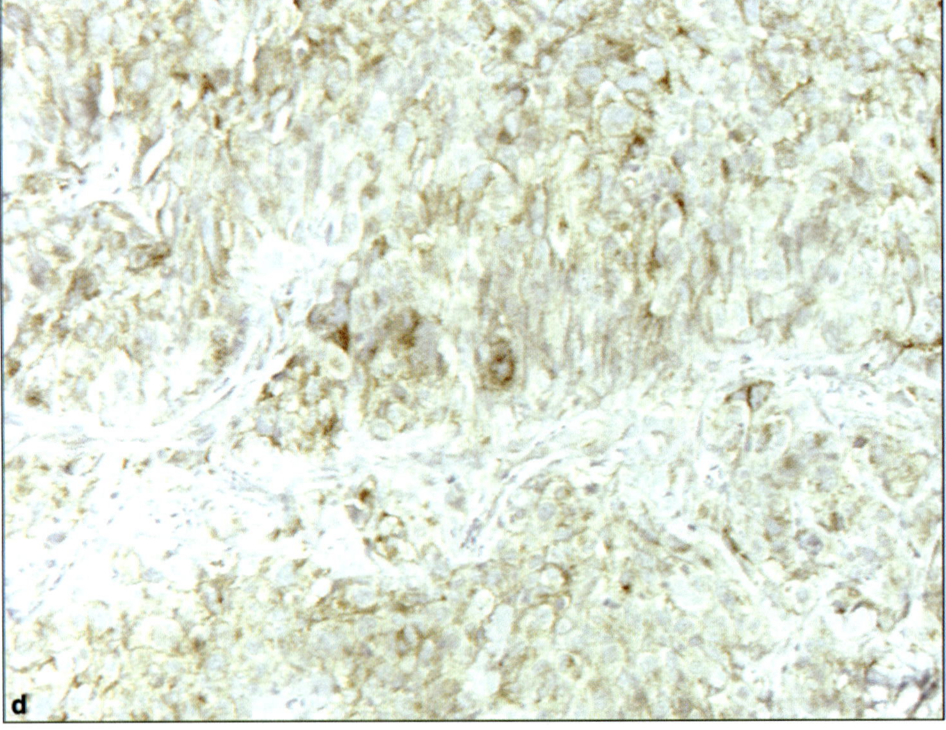

Microscopically, these tumors are barely recognizable as ependymomas (Figure 3.40); however, the focal presence of perivascular pseudorosettes, GFAP immunopositivity, and characteristic ultrastructural findings of junctional complexes and cytoplasmic lumina with microvillous projections support the diagnosis of giant cell ependymoma.

WHO GRADE III

Anaplastic Ependymoma

Clinical and Radiological Features

Anaplastic ependymomas may occur in any location in which WHO Grade II ependymomas occur but are particularly associated with childhood and the

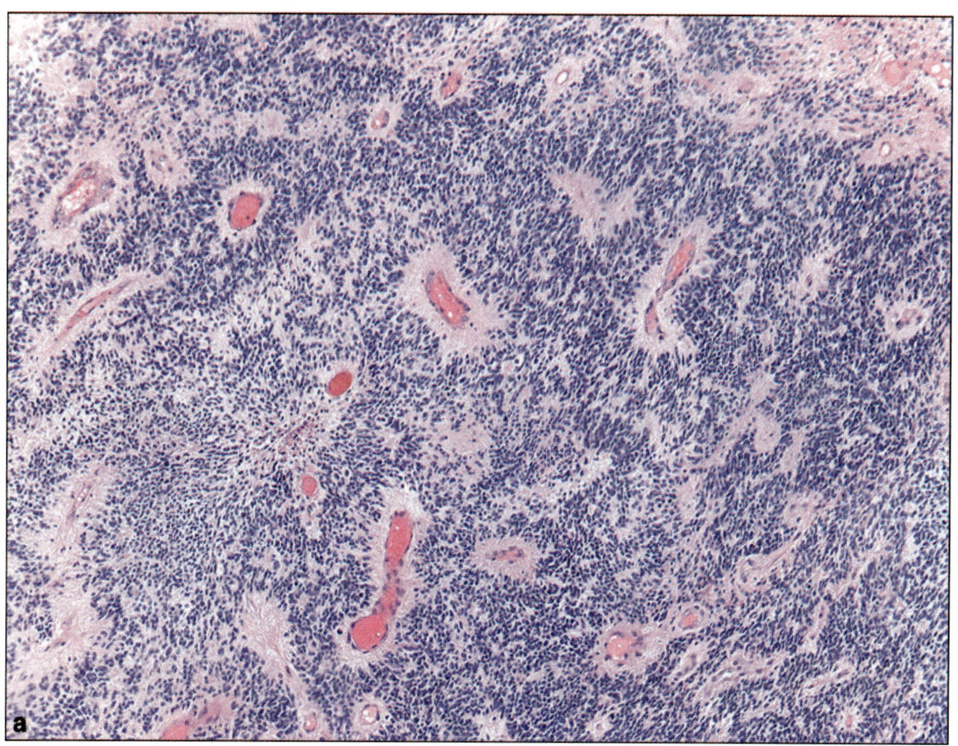

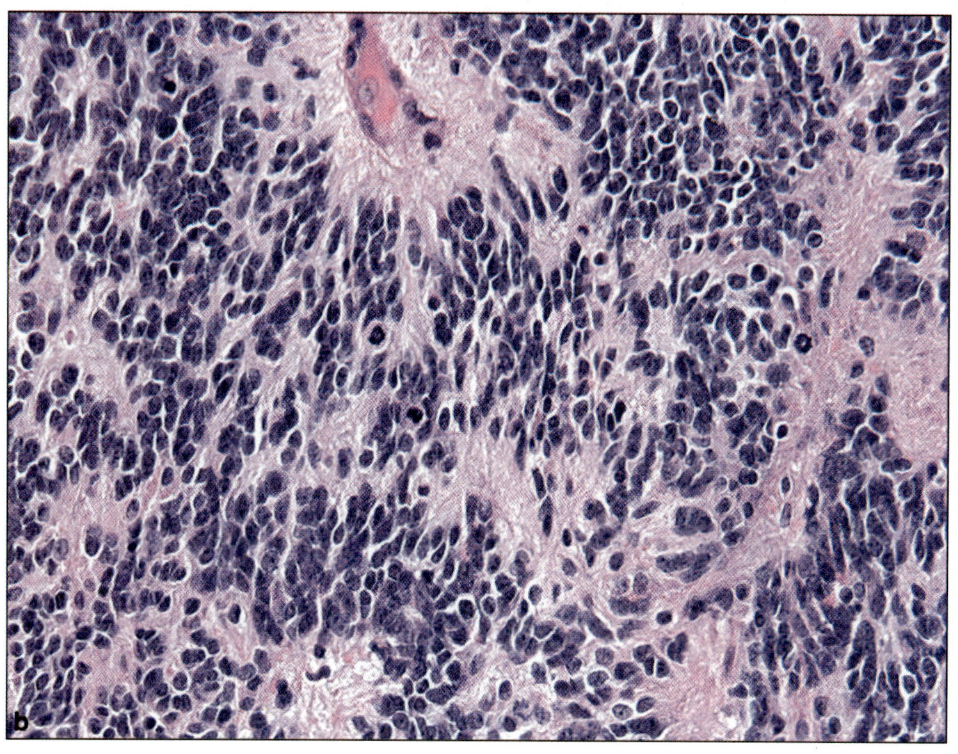

Figure 3.41. (a) Anaplastic ependymoma, WHO Grade III, is marked by a significant increase in cellularity resulting in sheets of crowded cells. (b) Readily identifiable mitotic figures are another hallmark of anaplastic ependymomas.

Figure 3.41. *continued*
(c) Pseudopalisading necrosis
and microvascular
proliferation may be features
of anaplastic ependymoma,
thus raising the importance of
distinguishing them from
WHO Grade IV
glioblastomas.

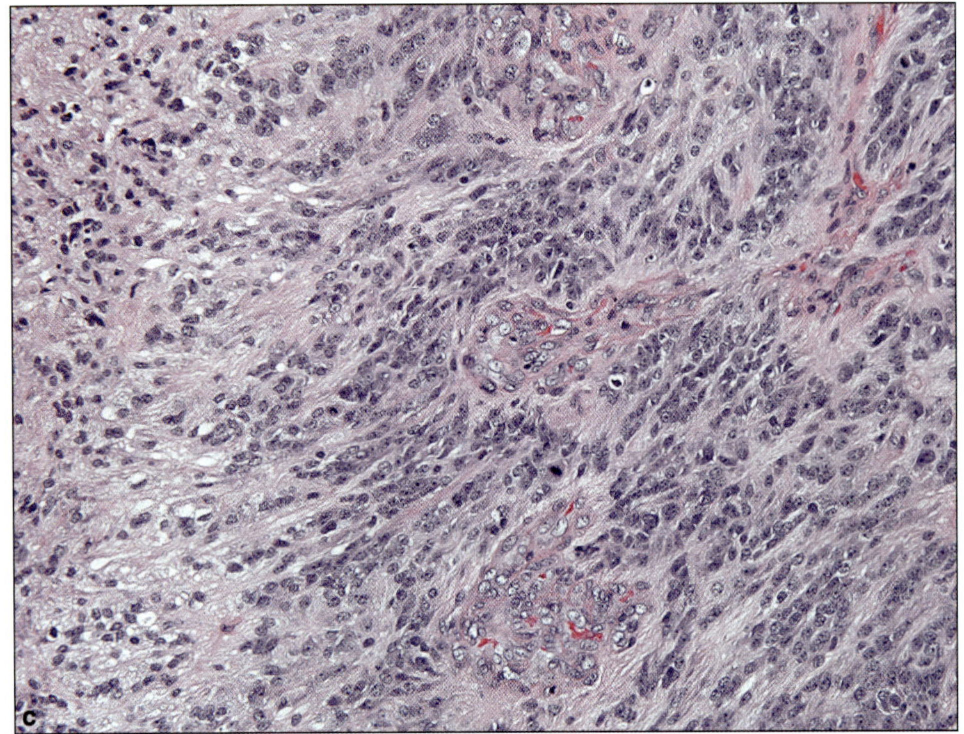

posterior fossa. They are associated with aggressive behavior and poor response to therapy. Neuroimaging typically shows contrast enhancement.

Pathology

The parameters for the distinction of anaplastic ependymoma from WHO Grade II ependymoma are not clear in borderline situations. However, an ependymoma with sheets of densely packed cells, increased mitotic activity (Schiffer et al., 1991), vascular proliferation, and necrosis should be considered anaplastic (Figure 3.41). Cartilaginous and osseous metaplasia has also been reported (Mridha et al., 2007). Perivascular pseudorosettes may be inconspicuous and true ependymal rosettes are essentially nonexistent. As stated, isolated necrosis in an otherwise WHO Grade II ependymoma of the posterior fossa should not be considered evidence of anaplasia (Tihan et al., 2008). Anaplastic ependymomas usually retain GFAP immunopositivity although sometimes to a lesser extent than in WHO Grade II examples.

REFERENCES

Adamek D, Dec M, Sobol G, Urbanowicz B, Jaworski M. Giant cell ependymoma: A case report. *Clin Neurol Neurosurg* 2008; 110: 176–81.

Brown DF, Chason DP, Schwartz LF, Coimbra CP, Rushing EJ. Supratentorial giant cell ependymoma: a case report. *Mod Pathol* 1998; 11: 398–403.

Chan AC, Ho LC, Yip WW, Cheung FC. Pigmented ependymoma with lipofuscin and neuromelanin production. *Arch Pathol Lab Med* 2003; 127: 872–5.

Daneyemez M, Can C, Izci Y, Beduk A, Timuckaynak E. The tanycytic ependymoma of the lateral ventricle: case report. *Minim Invasive Neurosurg* 1999; 42: 201–3.

Duggan MA, Hugh J, Nation JG, Robertson DI, Stuart GC. Ependymoma of the uterosacral ligament. *Cancer* 1989; 64: 2565–71.

Ernestus RI, Schroder R. [Clinical aspects and pathology of intracranial subependymoma – 18 personal cases and review of the literature]. *Neurochirurgia (Stuttg)* 1993; 36: 194–202.

Fassett DR, Pingree J, Kestle JR. The high incidence of tumor dissemination in myxopapillary ependymoma in pediatric patients. Report of five cases and review of the literature. *J Neurosurg* 2005; 102: 59–64.

Fouladi M, Helton K, Dalton J, Gilger E, Gajjar A, Merchant T, et al. Clear cell ependymoma: a clinicopathologic and radiographic analysis of 10 patients. *Cancer* 2003; 98: 2232–44.

Fourney DR, Siadati A, Bruner JM, Gokaslan ZL, Rhines LD. Giant cell ependymoma of the spinal cord. Case report and review of the literature. *J Neurosurg* 2004; 100: 75–9.

Garcia-Barriola V, De Gomez MN, Suarez JA, Lara C, Gonzalez JE, Garcia-Tamayo J. Ovarian ependymoma. A case report. *Pathol Res Pract* 2000; 196: 595–9.

Helwig EB, Stern JB. Subcutaneous sacrococcygeal myxopapillary ependymoma. A clinicopathologic study of 32 cases. *Am J Clin Pathol* 1984; 81: 156–61.

Hirato J, Nakazato Y, Iijima M, Yokoo H, Sasaki A, Yokota M, et al. An unusual variant of ependymoma with extensive tumor cell vacuolization. *Acta Neuropathol* 1997; 93: 310–16.

Hofman V, Isnard V, Chevallier A, Motamedi JP, Michiels JF, Hassoun J, et al. Pelvic ependymoma arising from the small bowel. *Pathology* 2001; 33: 26–9.

Ilhan I, Berberoglu S, Kutluay L, Maden HA. Subcutaneous sacrococcygeal myxopapillary ependymoma. *Med Pediatr Oncol* 1998; 30: 81–4.

Jallo GI, Zagzag D, Epstein F. Intramedullary subependymoma of the spinal cord. *Neurosurgery* 1996; 38: 251–7.

Kobata H, Kuroiwa T, Isono N, Nagasawa S, Ohta T, Tsutsumi A. Tanycytic ependymoma in association with neurofibromatosis type 2. *Clin Neuropathol* 2001; 20: 93–100.

Kurt E, Zheng PP, Hop WC, van der Weiden M, Bol M, van den Bent MJ, et al. Identification of relevant prognostic histopathologic features in 69 intracranial ependymomas, excluding myxopapillary ependymomas and subependymomas. *Cancer* 2006; 106: 388–95.

Lindboe CF, Stolt-Nielsen A, Dale LG. Hemorrhage in a highly vascularized subependymoma of the septum pellucidum: case report. *Neurosurgery* 1992; 31: 741–5.

Mannoji H, Becker LE. Ependymal and choroid plexus tumors. Cytokeratin and GFAP expression. *Cancer* 1988; 61: 1377–85.

Marra A, Dario A, Scamoni C, Cerati M, Crivelli G, Dorizzi A. Intraventricular subependymoma presenting as subarachnoid hemorrhage. Case report. *J Neurosurg Sci* 1991; 35: 213–15.

McGirt MJ, Chaichana KL, Atiba A, Attenello F, Woodworth GF, Jallo GI. Neurological outcome after resection of intramedullary spinal cord tumors in children. *Childs Nerv Syst* 2008; 24: 93–7.

Mizuno J, Nakagawa H, Inoue T, Kondo S, Hara K, Hashizume Y. Signet-ring cell ependymoma with intratumoral hemorrhage in the medulla oblongata. *J Clin Neurosci* 2005; 12: 711–14.

Mridha AR, Sharma MC, Sarkar C, Garg A, Singh MM, Suri V. Anaplastic ependymoma with cartilaginous and osseous metaplasia: report of a rare case and review of literature. *J Neurooncol* 2007; 82: 75–80.

Onaya M, Kujas M, Tominaga I, Arthuis F, Marsault C, Poirier J. [Intramedullary lipomatous ependymoma: case report]. *Ann Pathol* 2005; 25: 240–3.

Park SH, Park HR, Chi JG. Papillary ependymoma: its differential diagnosis from choroid plexus papilloma. *J Korean Med Sci* 1996; 11: 415–21.

Parker JR, Armstrong DL, Strother D, Rudman DM, Dauser RC, Laurent JP, et al. Antineuronal nuclei immunohistochemical staining patterns in childhood ependymomas. *J Child Neurol* 2001; 16: 548–52.

Pimentel J, Kepes JJ, Moura Nunes JF, Bentes C, Miguens J, Antunes JL. Supratentorial giant cell ependymoma. *Clin Neuropathol* 2001; 20: 31–7.

Ragel BT, Townsend JJ, Arthur AS, Couldwell WT. Intraventricular tanycytic ependymoma: case report and review of the literature. *J Neurooncol* 2005; 71: 189–93.

Reni M, Gatta G, Mazza E, Vecht C. Ependymoma. *Crit Rev Oncol Hematol* 2007; 63: 81–9.

Richards AL, Rosenfeld JV, Gonzales MF, Ashley D, Mc Lean C. Supratentorial tanycytic ependymoma. *J Clin Neurosci* 2004; 11: 928–30.

Rodriguez FJ, Scheithauer BW, Robbins PD, Burger PC, Hessler RB, Perry A, et al. Ependymomas with neuronal differentiation: a morphologic and immunohistochemical spectrum. *Acta Neuropathol* 2007; 113: 313–24.

Rushing EJ, Cooper PB, Quezado M, Begnami M, Crespo A, Smirniotopoulos JG, et al. Subependymoma revisited: clinicopathological evaluation of 83 cases. *J Neurooncol* 2007; 85: 297–305.

Sato K, Kubota T, Ishida M, Handa Y. Spinal tanycytic ependymoma with hematomyelia – case report. *Neurol Med Chir (Tokyo)* 2005; 45: 168–71.

Schiffer D, Chio A, Giordana MT, Migheli A, Palma L, Pollo B, et al. Histologic prognostic factors in ependymoma. *Childs Nerv Syst* 1991; 7: 177–82.

Sharma MC, Arora R, Lakhtakia R, Mahapatra AK, Sarkar C. Ependymoma with extensive lipidization mimicking adipose tissue: a report of five cases. *Pathol Oncol Res* 2000; 6: 136–40.

Shuangshoti S, Rushing EJ, Mena H, Olsen C, Sandberg GD. Supratentorial extraventricular ependymal neoplasms: a clinicopathologic study of 32 patients. *Cancer* 2005; 103: 2598–605.

Takei H, Bhattacharjee MB, Rivera A, Dancer Y, Powell SZ. New immunohistochemical markers in the evaluation of central nervous system tumors: a review of 7 selected adult and pediatric brain tumors. *Arch Pathol Lab Med* 2007; 131: 234–41.

Tihan T, Zhou T, Holmes E, Burger PC, Ozuysal S, Rushing EJ. The prognostic value of histological grading of posterior fossa ependymomas in children: a Children's Oncology Group study and a review of prognostic factors. *Mod Pathol* 2008; 21: 165–77.

Ueki K, Sasaki T, Ishida T, Kirino T. Spinal tanycytic ependymoma associated with neurofibromatosis type 2 – case report. *Neurol Med Chir (Tokyo)* 2001; 41: 513–16.

Vajtai I, Mucsi Z, Varga Z, Bodi I. Signet-ring cell ependymoma: case report with implications for pathogenesis and differential diagnosis. *Pathol Res Pract* 1999; 195: 853–8.

Zamecnik J, Chanova M, Kodet R. Expression of thyroid transcription factor 1 in primary brain tumours. *J Clin Pathol* 2004; 57: 1111–13.

Zec N, De Girolami U, Schofield DE, Scott RM, Anthony DC. Giant cell ependymoma of the filum terminale. A report of two cases. *Am J Surg Pathol* 1996; 20: 1091–101.

Choroid Plexus Tumors

Clinical and Radiological Features

Choroid plexus tumors occur in intraventricular locations where native choroid plexus epithelium normally exists. Eighty percent of tumors occur in patients younger than 20 years of age, particularly those of the lateral ventricle (Janisch and Staneczek, 1989; Rickert and Paulus, 2001). Pediatric choroid plexus tumors are especially common in the first year of life, even occurring

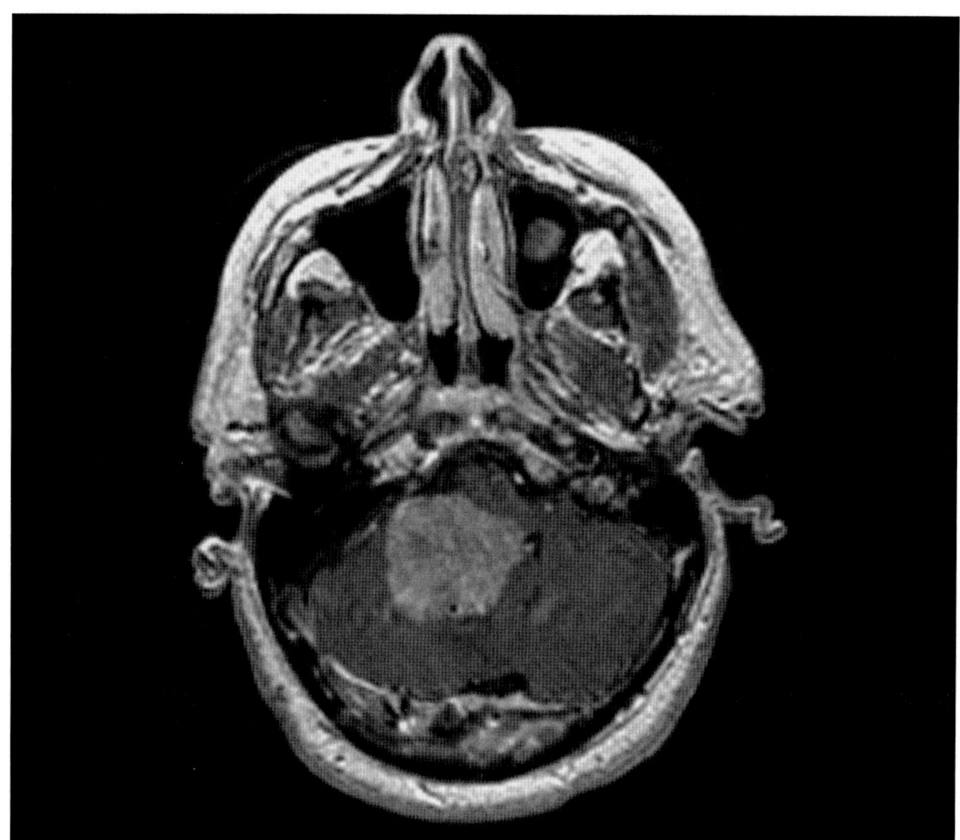

Figure 3.42. Posterior fossa choroid plexus papilloma originating at the cerebellopontine angle, showing diffuse contrast enhancement.

as fetal or congenital examples, accounting for 10–20% of brain tumors in this age category. However, choroid plexus tumors of the fourth ventricle occur at all ages without a predilection for childhood. Five percent of choroid plexus tumors may occur in the third ventricle and may very rarely occur in extra-ventricular locations (Beskonakli et al., 1998).

They tend to produce symptoms by blocking the flow of CSF and thus causing obstructive hydrocephalus, with increased head circumference in infants and increased intracranial pressure in older patients. Choroid plexus papillomas are also believed to cause hydrocephalus through the over production of CSF (Fujimura et al., 2004).

CT or MRI typically shows a well-demarcated irregularly contrast-enhancing mass that is T1 - isodense and T2 - hyperdense, which may be unusually large by the time of diagnosis. Some tumors are irregular in outline or disseminated (Figures 3.42 and 3.43).

WHO GRADE I

Choroid Plexus Papilloma

Pathology

These are well-circumscribed lobular and papilliform masses that may compress or adhere to adjacent ventricular walls but are not invasive. Cyst formation and hemorrhage may occur.

Figure 3.43. Choroid plexus carcinoma in the lateral ventricle with marked local mass effect and markedly enlarged ventricles due to obstruction and possibly also related to overproduction of CSF.

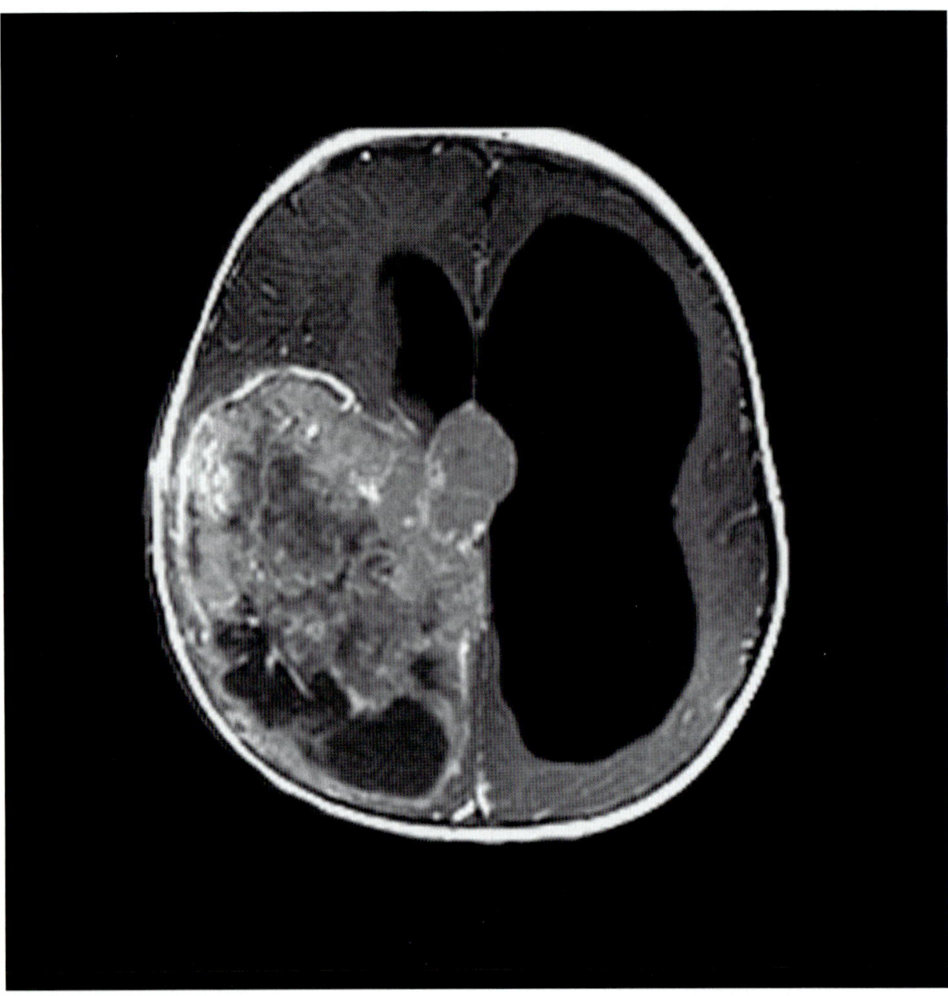

Figure 3.44. (a) Choroid plexus papillomas show fibrovascular papillae lined by crowded epithelium with heaped up nuclei in contrast to the orderly single array of benign choroid plexus epithelium seen for comparison in the upper left portion of the field.

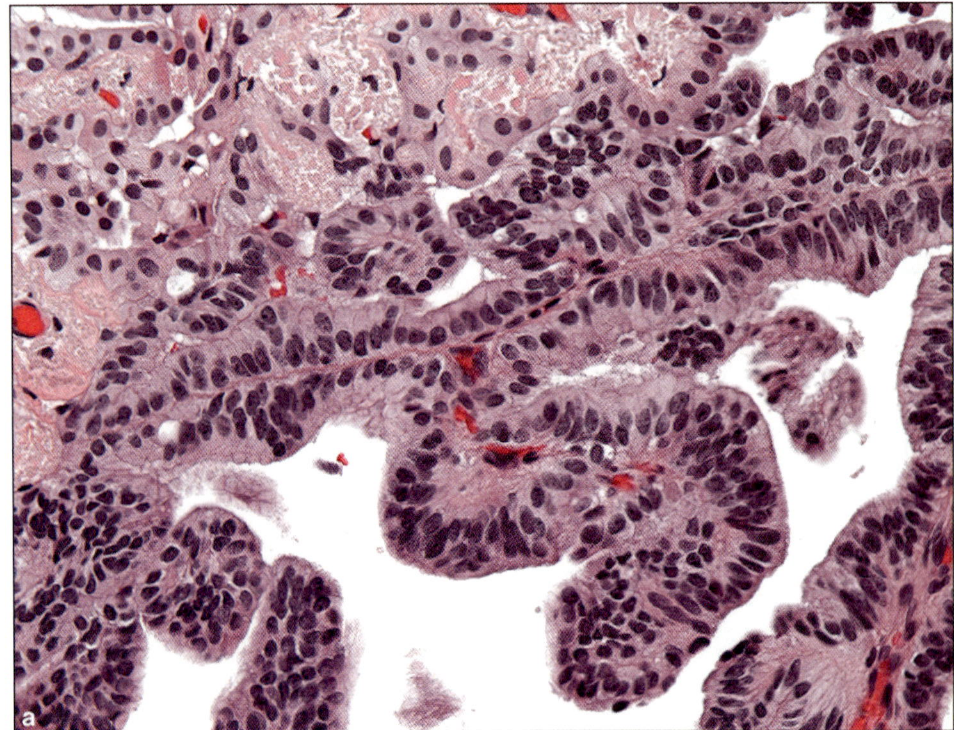

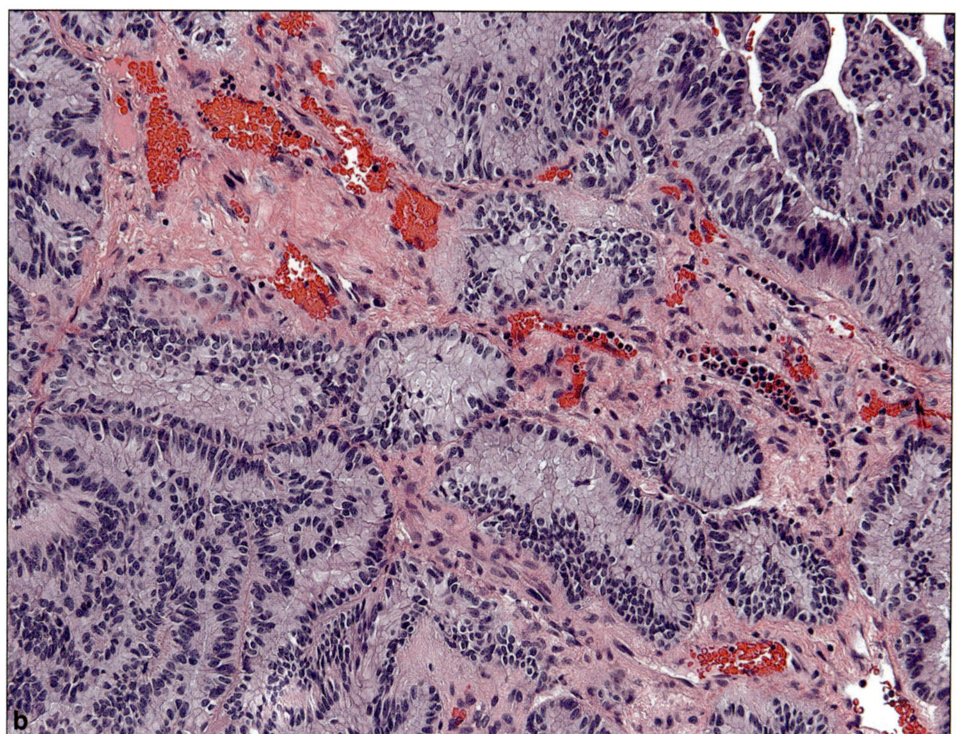

Figure 3.44. *continued*
(b) Care must be exercised in avoiding the interpretation of tangentially cut invaginations at the base of stalks as evidence of invasive growth.

Microscopically, WHO Grade I choroid plexus papillomas show a delicate papillary architecture. They are distinguishable from native choroid plexus epithelium by the crowded and more irregular alignment of tall columnar, stratified nuclei along the fibrovascular cores, in contrast to the even and low cuboidal choroid plexus epithelium (Figure 3.44a,b).

Choroid plexus papillomas have only minimal cytological atypia and mitotic activity. A variety of histological alterations may also exist such as oncocytic (Diengdoh and Shaw, 1993; Stefanko and Vuzevski, 1985), mucinous, or melanotic change (Vajtai et al., 1995), tubular architecture, and metaplastic chondroid or bone formation (Corcoran et al., 2001; Kocaeli et al., 2007; Yap et al., 1997). Choroid plexus papillomas have now been added to the list of gliomas that may contain neuropil-like islands (Hasselblatt et al., 2008).

The immunohistochemistry of choroid plexus papillomas reflects their neuroepithelial derivation and are thus S-100 and at least focally GFAP positive (Figure 3.45). They are also transthyretin (prealbumin) (Figure 3.46), CD99, keratin, and vimentin positive. An intriguing incidental finding was immunopositivity of both native choroid plexus epithelium and papillomas and even choroid plexus carcinomas for synaptophysin (Kepes and Collins, 1999) (Figure 3.51), which may be useful in differentiating these from metastatic papillary carcinomas. Immunostaining for inward rectifier potassium channel Kir7.1 (Figure 3.48) has been reported as a marker of both native choroid plexus epithelium and its tumors and is an example of an immunoprobe derived from a microarray based search for diagnostic antibodies (Hasselblatt et al., 2006).

Figure 3.45. GFAP immunohistochemistry in choroid plexus papilloma.

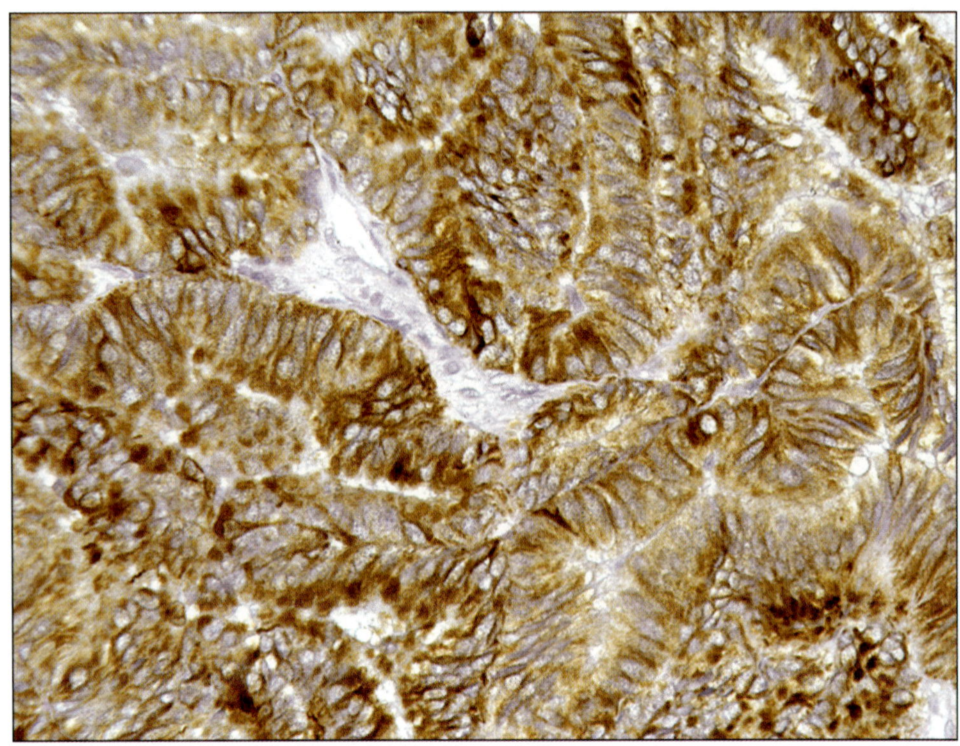

Figure 3.46. Transthyretin immunohistochemistry in choroid plexus papilloma.

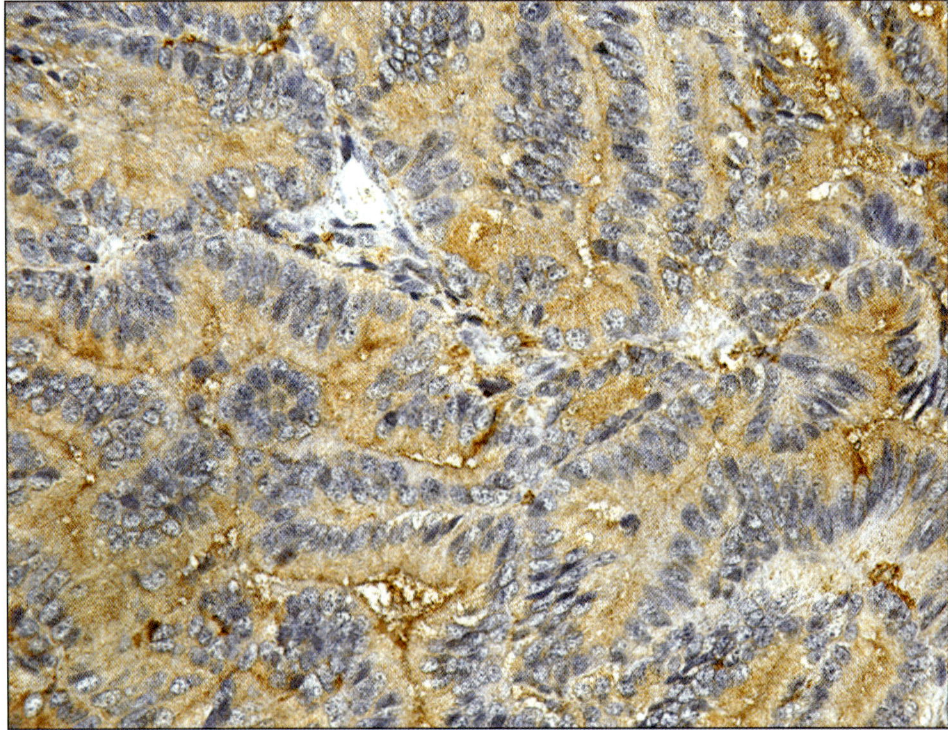

WHO GRADE II

Atypical Choroid Plexus Papilloma

Pathology

This entity arose from the recognition of choroid plexus tumors, which are more akin to WHO Grade I choroid plexus papillomas in gross characteristics

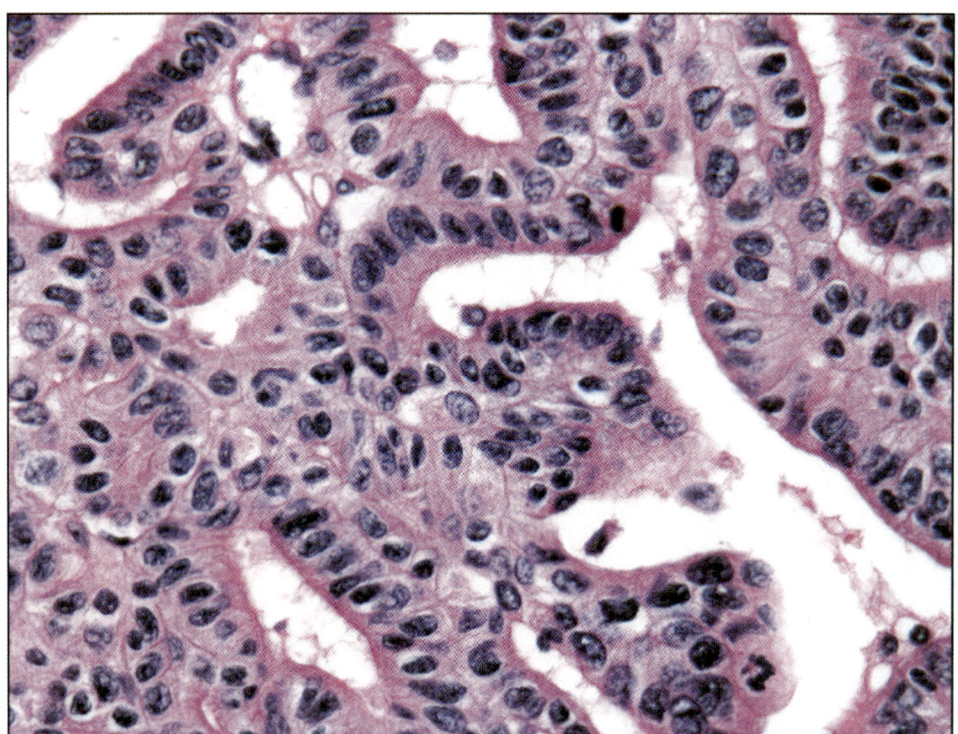

Figure 3.47. Atypical choroid plexus papilloma, showing increased mitotic activity without significant pleomorphism or other frankly carcinomatous features.

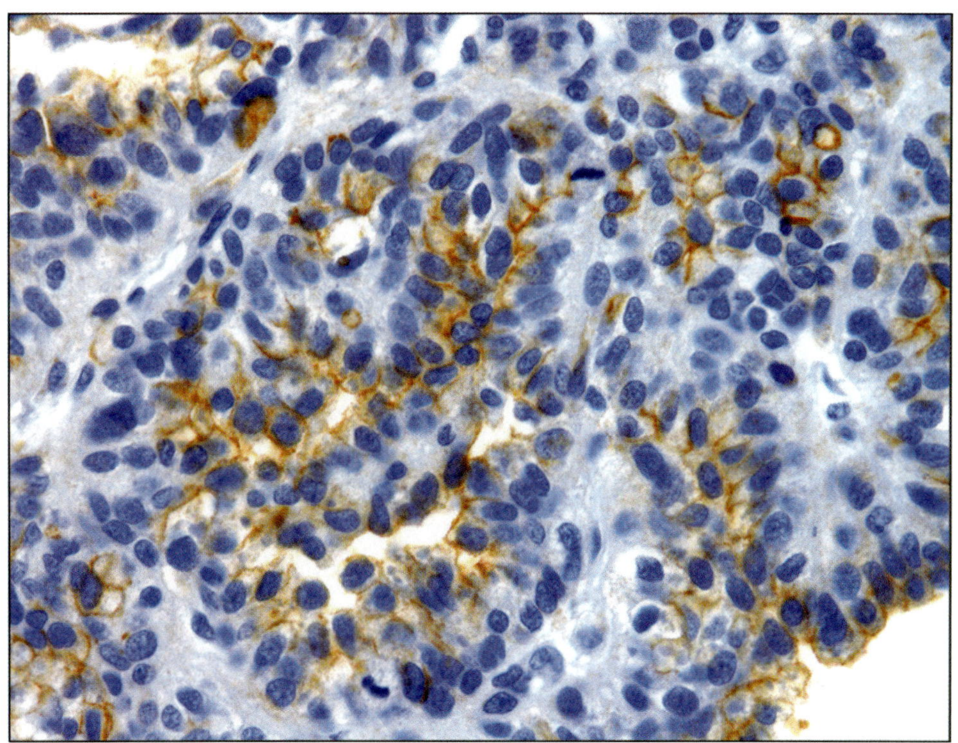

Figure 3.48. Kir7.1 immunostaining of an atypical choroid plexus papilloma. (Image generously provided by Prof. Werner Paulus, Muenster, Germany.)

and histological appearance but with increased mitotic activity of greater than or equal to two mitoses per ten high-power fields and thus an increased likelihood of local recurrence (Jeibmann et al., 2006) or spinal metastasis (Uff et al., 2007). As WHO Grade II neoplasms, they are somewhat analogous to

Figure 3.49. Choroid plexus carcinoma with marked anaplasia with mixed papillary and solid growth.

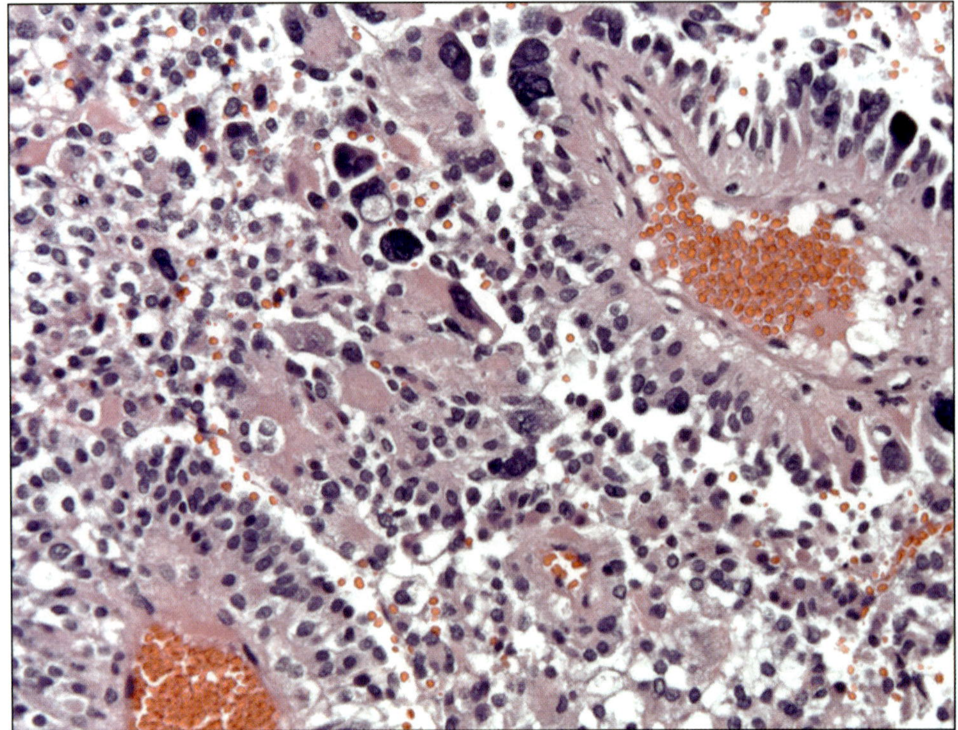

Figure 3.50. GFAP in choroid plexus carcinoma, with diminished staining in comparison with choroid plexus papillomas.

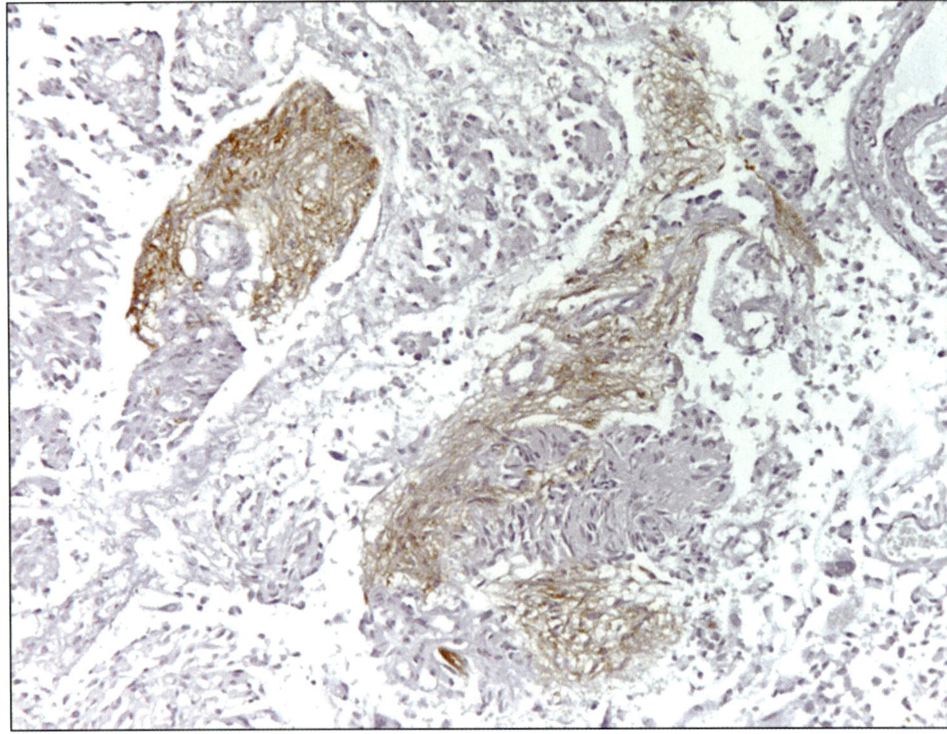

atypical meningiomas, showing an increase in mitotic activity without other obviously atypical features (Figure 3.47). There should be no features of frank malignancy such as poorly differentiated morphology or necrosis.

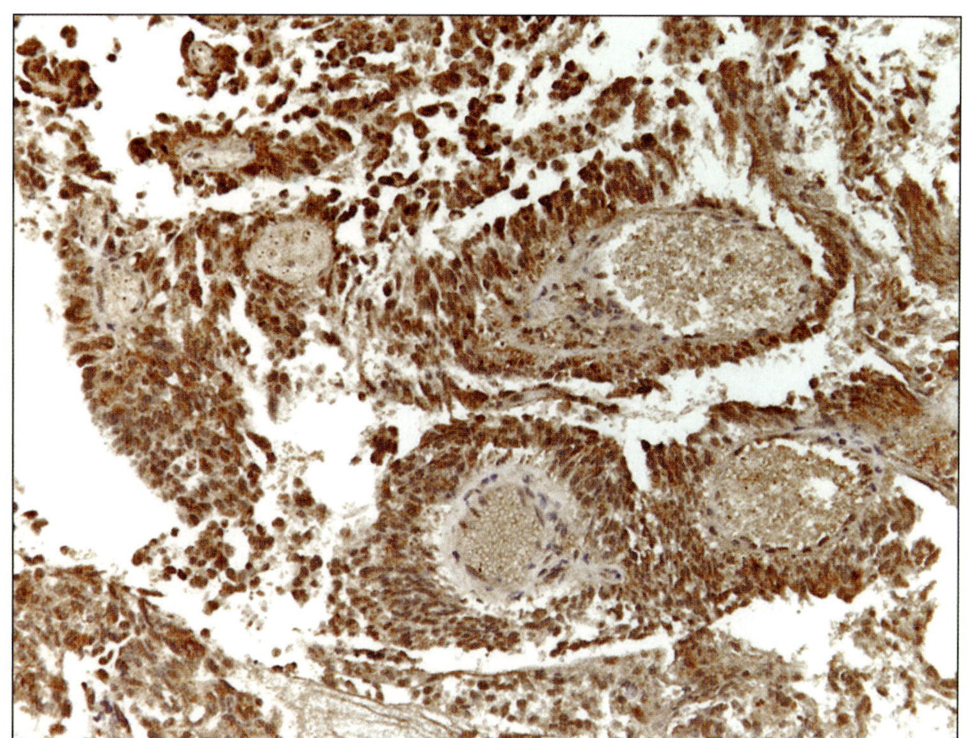

Figure 3.51. Synaptophysin immunopositivity is a feature of choroid plexus papillomas and is retained in this choroid plexus carcinoma.

WHO GRADE III

Choroid Plexus Carcinoma

Pathology

Grossly, these are large infiltrative masses with hemorrhage and necrosis. Microscopically, choroid plexus carcinomas are sometimes barely recognizable as a papillary neoplasm, demonstrating significant nuclear pleomorphism, increased cellularity, and mitotic activity, with solid growth (Figure 3.49). Immunohistochemical markers such as transthyretin and GFAP (Figures 3.50, 3.51) may show diminished positivity with increasing degrees of dedifferentiation.

REFERENCES

Beskonakli E, Cayli S, Bostanci U, Kulacoglu S, Yalcinlar Y. Choroid plexus papillomas of the posterior fossa: extraventricular extension, intraventricular and primary extraventricular location. Report of four cases. *J Neurosurg Sci* 1998; 42: 37–40.

Corcoran GM, Frazier SR, Prayson RA. Choroid plexus papilloma with osseous and adipose metaplasia. *Ann Diagn Pathol* 2001; 5: 43–7.

Diengdoh JV, Shaw MD. Oncocytic variant of choroid plexus papilloma. Evolution from benign to malignant "oncocytoma". *Cancer* 1993; 71: 855–8.

Fujimura M, Onuma T, Kameyama M, Motohashi O, Kon H, Yamamoto K, et al. Hydrocephalus due to cerebrospinal fluid overproduction by bilateral choroid plexus papillomas. *Childs Nerv Syst* 2004; 20: 485–8.

Hasselblatt M, Bohm C, Tatenhorst L, Dinh V, Newrzella D, Keyvani K, et al. Identification of novel diagnostic markers for choroid plexus tumors: a microarray-based approach. *Am J Surg Pathol* 2006; 30: 66–74.

Hasselblatt M, Jeibmann A, Guerry M, Senner V, Paulus W, McLendon RE. Choroid plexus papilloma with neuropil-like islands. *Am J Surg Pathol* 2008; 32: 162–6.

Janisch W, Staneczek W. [Primary tumors of the choroid plexus. Frequency, localization and age]. *Zentralbl Allg Pathol* 1989; 135: 235–40.

Jeibmann A, Hasselblatt M, Gerss J, Wrede B, Egensperger R, Beschorner R, et al. Prognostic implications of atypical histologic features in choroid plexus papilloma. *J Neuropathol Exp Neurol* 2006; 65: 1069–73.

Kepes JJ, Collins J. Choroid plexus epithelium (normal and neoplastic) expresses synaptophysin. A potentially useful aid in differentiating carcinoma of the choroid plexus from metastatic papillary carcinomas. *J Neuropathol Exp Neurol* 1999; 58: 398–401.

Kocaeli H, Yilmazlar S, Abas F, Aksoy K. Total ossification of choroid plexus papilloma mimicking calcified petrous bone pathology. *Pediatr Neurosurg* 2007; 43: 67–71.

Rickert CH, Paulus W. Tumors of the choroid plexus. *Microsc Res Tech* 2001; 52: 104–11.

Stefanko SZ, Vuzevski VD. Oncocytic variant of choroid plexus papilloma. *Acta Neuropathol* 1985; 66: 160–2.

Uff CE, Galloway M, Bradford R. Metastatic atypical choroid plexus papilloma: a case report. *J Neurooncol* 2007; 82: 69–74.

Vajtai I, Varga Z, Bodosi M, Voros E. Melanotic papilloma of the choroid plexus: report of a case with implications for pathogenesis. *Noshuyo Byori* 1995; 12: 151–4.

Yap WM, Chuah KL, Tan PH. Choroid plexus papilloma with chondroid metaplasia. *Histopathology* 1997; 31: 386–7.

Pineal Parenchymal Tumors

Pineal tumors are rare, accounting for less than 1% of all intracranial neoplasms, with pineal parenchymal tumors accounting for 14–27% of tumors in this location (Konovalov and Pitskhelauri, 2003; Regis et al., 1996). They produce symptoms by compressing local structures including the cerebral aqueduct and, brainstem, and may extend into the third ventricle. Parinaud syndrome occurs when the mass lesion causes compression on the superior colliculi, resulting in paralysis of upward gaze.

Any basic awareness of the difficulty in surgically approaching the pineal gland and its tumors along with increasing preference of stereotactic biopsy over invasive techniques predicts biopsies of sizes barely adequate for permanent sections, not to mention for frozen section diagnosis. Under these circumstances, cytological preparations can be of distinct diagnostic utility (Parwani et al., 2005).

WHO GRADE I

Pineocytoma

Clinical and Radiological Features

Pineocytomas occur evenly between the second and seventh decades, roughly equally between males and females. Pineocytomas behave

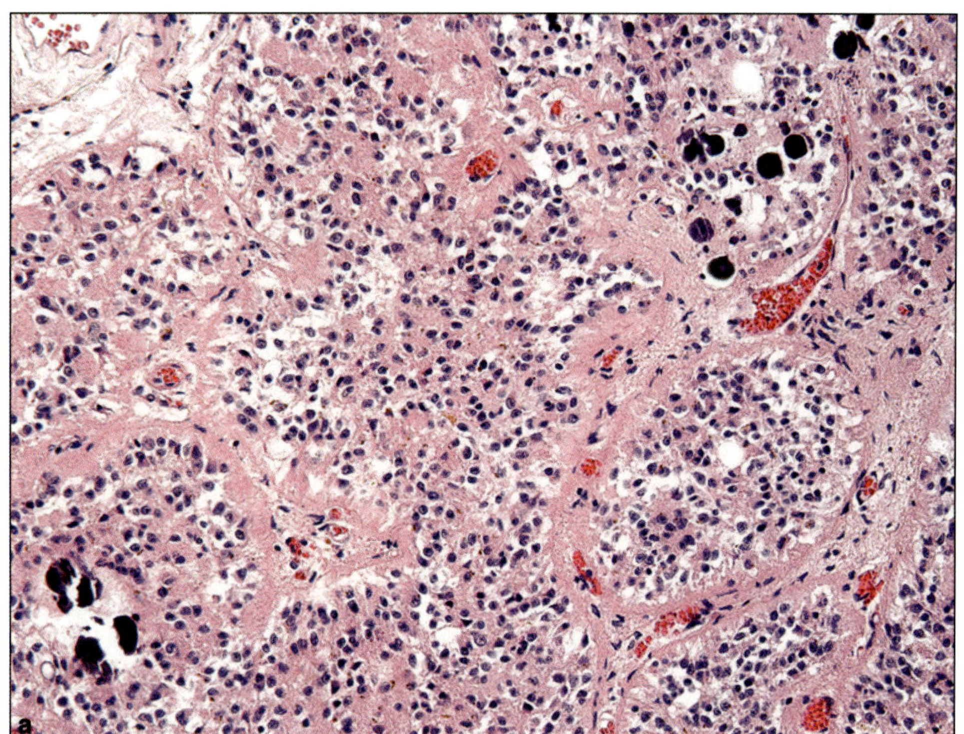

Figure 3.52. (a) Normal pineal gland (autopsy specimen). Failure to appreciate normal histology can result in misdiagnosis of pineal gland as pineocytoma. (b) Slightly more crowded yet well-differentiated cell proliferation of pineocytoma. Note the circular aggregates of cells forming pineocytomatous rosettes.

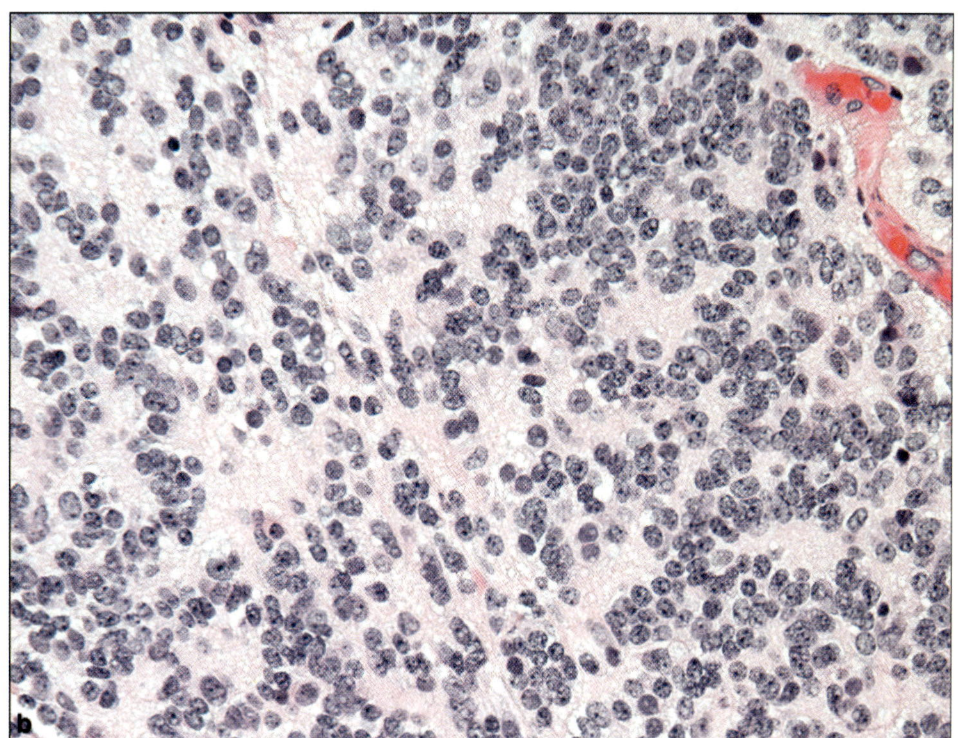

in an indolent fashion without a propensity for metastasis or subarachnoid spread.

Radiographic imaging indicates a well circumscribed mass generally less than 3 cm in diameter, sometimes showing peripheral calcification or cystic

Figure 3.52. *continued*
(c) Strong and diffuse
synaptophysin positivity.

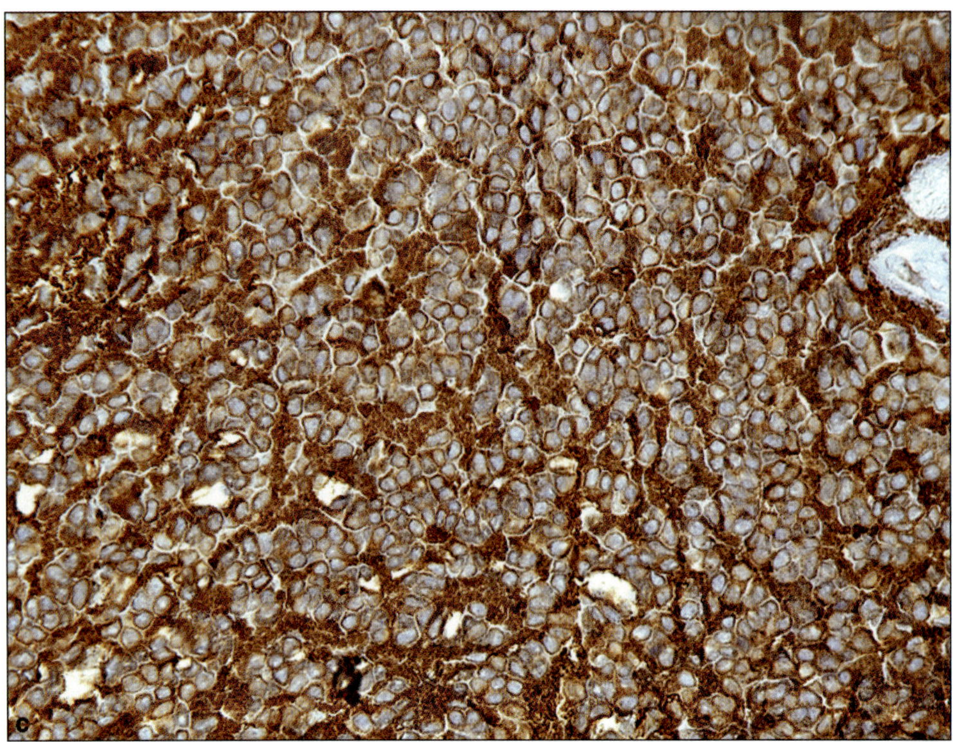

changes (Chiechi et al., 1995; Schild et al., 1993). These tumors generally show strong homogeneous contrast enhancement.

Pathology

The histopathology of pineocytomas is fraught with difficulty in distinguishing them from the nonneoplastic pineal gland. Diagnosticians should familiarize themselves with the normal histologic appearance of the pineal gland (Figure 3.52a) in order to avoid this pitfall. The situation is further complicated by the receipt of a biopsy barely visible to the naked eye owing to the precarious territory for stereotactic biopsy: the pineal gland is bordered by several deep cerebral veins.

Pineocytomas show an increased cellularity, moderate in degree; however, the cytological features closely resemble those of normal pineocytes (Figure 3.52b). Biopsies or sufficient size may show the architectural presence of pineocytomatous rosettes, which are neurocytic cells arranged in a wide arc around a neuropil-like central area composed of delicate cell processes.

Cytological pleomorphism with ganglion cells (Mena et al., 1995) or multinucleated cells may be seen, which does not appear to have prognostic significance. Mitotic activity and necrosis are essentially absent.

Immunohistochemical studies show neuronal reactivity with antibodies to synaptophysin (Figure 3.52c), with neurofilament highlighting cytoplasmic processes. The retinal S-antigen may be demonstrable.

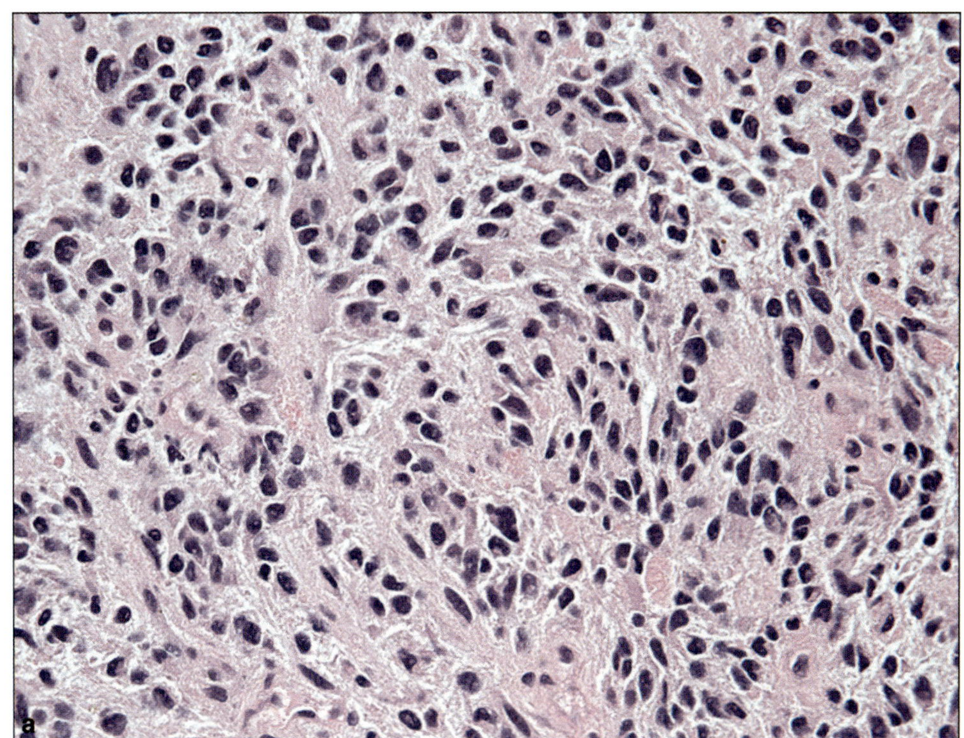

Figure 3.53. Pineal parenchymal tumor of intermediate differentiation. (a)–(c) Spectrum of varied histological features, with distinctly greater cellularity, absence of pineocytomatous rosettes, but without the overt features of an embryonal tumor as seen in pineoblastoma. (d) Spindle cell component retains synaptophysin immunopositivity.

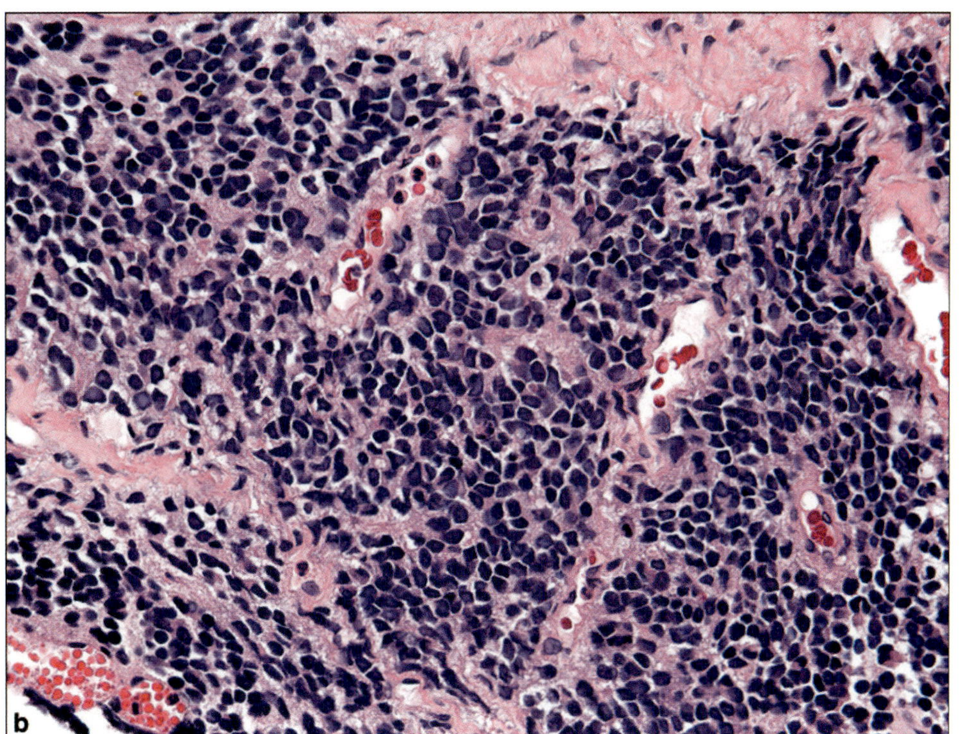

Figure 3.53. *continued.*

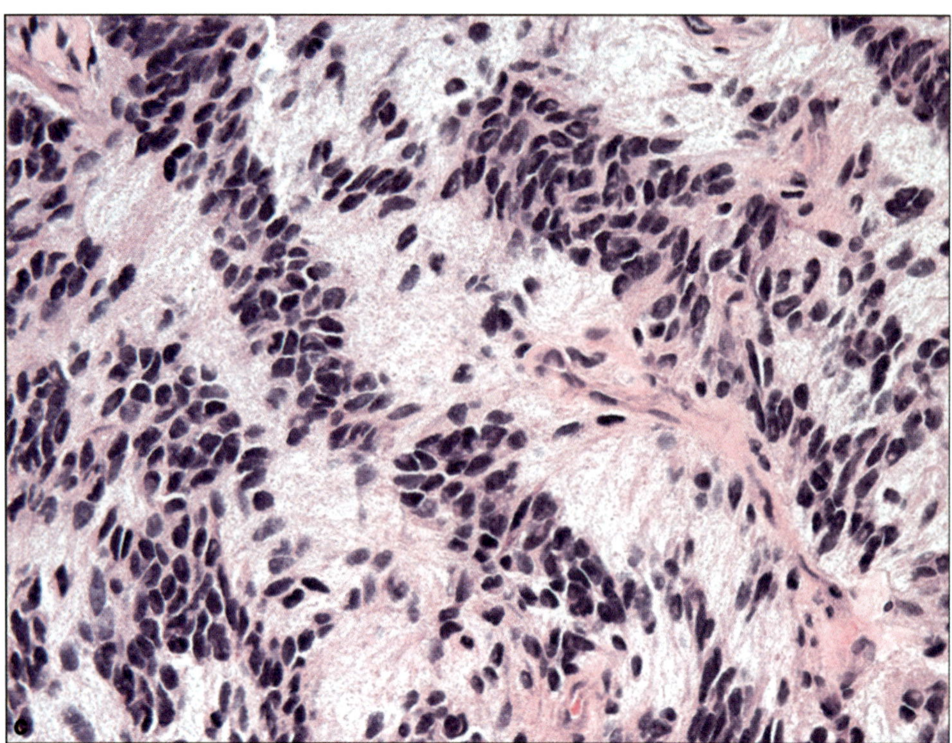

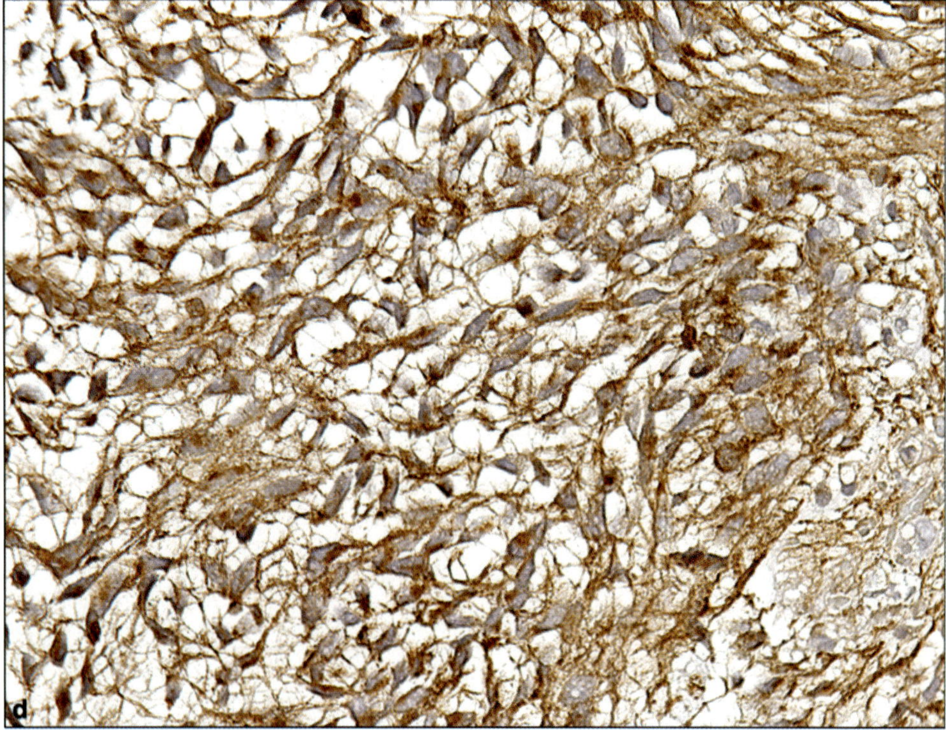

WHO GRADE II OR III

Pineal Parenchymal Tumor of Intermediate Differentiation

Clinical and Radiological Features

The concept of this tumor was developed in order to accommodate pineocytomas with atypical features or pineoblastomas with an unusual degree of differentiation (Schild et al., 1993). Some authors consider this entity to more closely approximate true pineoblastomas because of their distinctly poorer prognosis. They occur in an age distribution similar to that of pineocytomas, with a slight female preponderance. The clinical presentation is quite similar to that of pineocytoma namely due to compression of local structures and increased intracranial pressure.

Pathology

This designation is not meant to include tumors with coexistent pineocytoma and pineoblastoma but rather represents a true intermediate histology (Schild et al., 1993). This tumor shows either diffuse or lobular growth, and there is a distinctly higher cellularity than that seen in pineocytoma (Figure 3.53). There may be mild-to-moderate nuclear atypia, or even distinct cytological pleomorphism (Sasaki et al., 2006), and mitotic activity, which should be used to ultimately distinguish between WHO Grades II and III. The proposal has been made that the diagnosis of pineal parenchymal tumor of intermediate differentiation with a more favorable prognosis may be made when there are fewer than six mitoses and positive neurofilament immunolabeling (Jouvet et al., 2000). Homer Wright rosettes may be seen, but pineocytomatous rosettes are not.

Papillary Tumor of the Pineal Region

Clinical and Radiological Features

This recently described rare entity occurs at any age but more frequently in adults (Fevre-Montange et al., 2006; Jouvet et al., 2003; Roncaroli and Scheithauer, 2007). Time will tell whether this unique cytoarchitecture and immunophenotype may occur in other locations in the central nervous system (CNS). The symptoms are referable to local mass effect, with obstructive hydrocephalus, headache, and other nonspecific symptoms. Radiographic imaging shows contrast enhancement. They may reach relatively large sizes of up to 4 cm.

Pathology

This neoplasm is dominated by epithelial appearance with papillary growth (Figure 3.54a). Intervening cellular areas most closely invoke a similarity with ependymomas. Indeed, some authors have attributed the histogenesis of this tumor with the specialized ependymal cells of the subcommisural organ. Mitotic activity is generally low but may number between 0 and 10 per high-power field. Necrosis may be present.

The diagnosis rests upon the typical histochemical profile whereby these tumors are reactive for both cytokeratin antibodies (Figure 3.54c), including

Figure 3.54. Papillary tumor of the pineal region. (a) Papillary growth with crowded but relatively monomorphous tumor cells. Immunostaining may show (b) focal GFAP, (c) mixed cytokeratin, and (d) synaptophysin positivity.

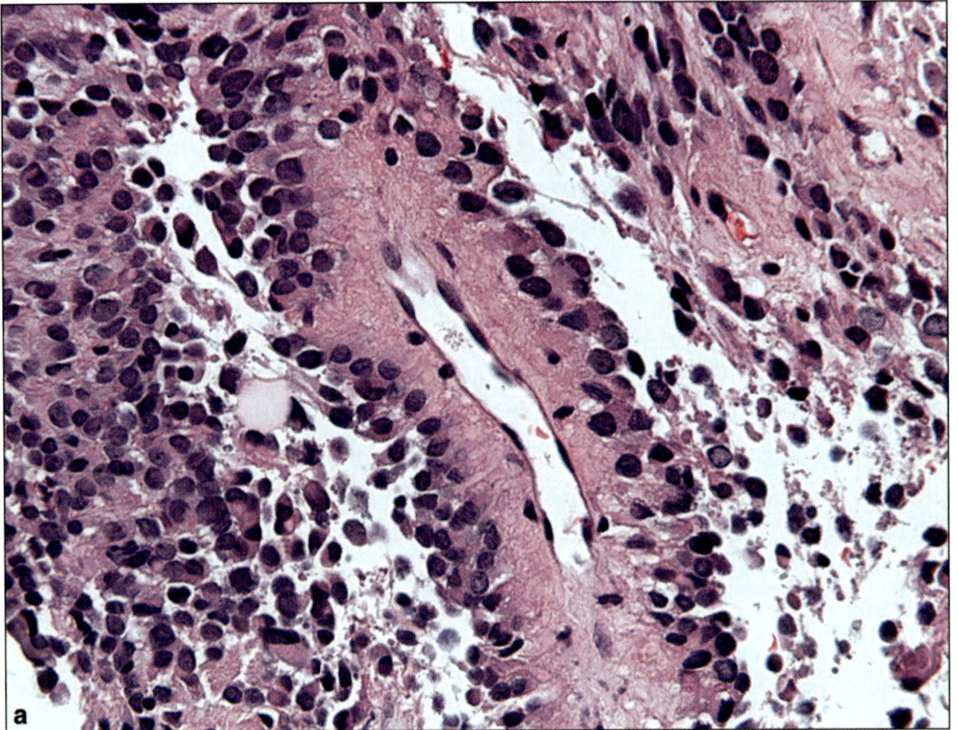

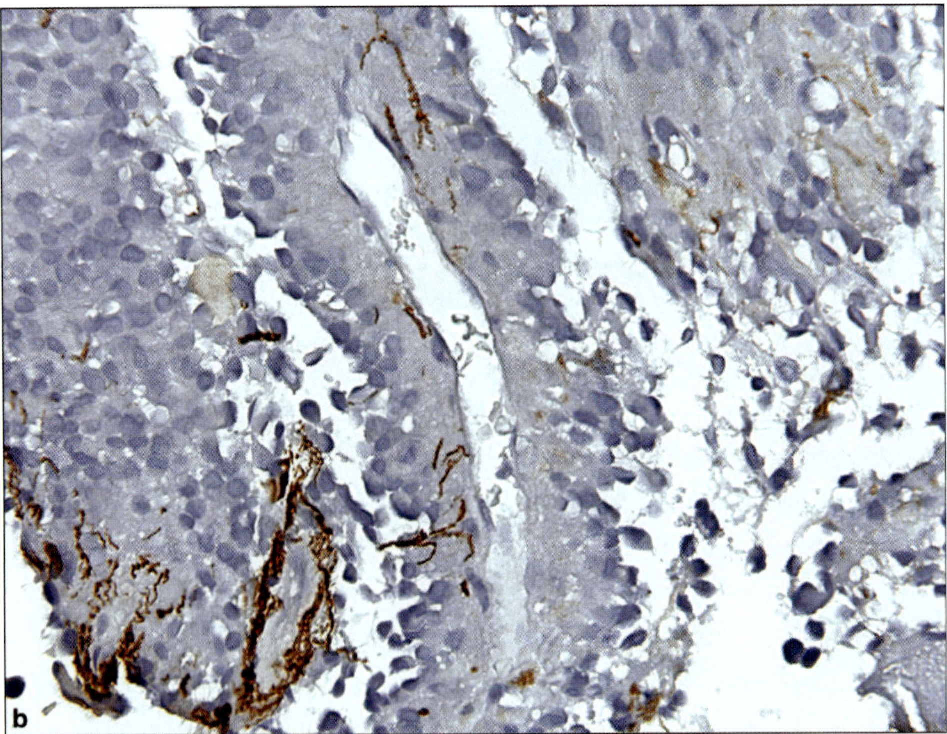

anti-AE1/AE3, CAM 5.2, and CK18. This is combined with limited GFAP expression (Figure 3.54b), which should help distinguish them from ependymomas. However like ependymomas, the papillary tumor of the pineal region may show dotlike cytoplasmic or focal membrane staining for epithelial

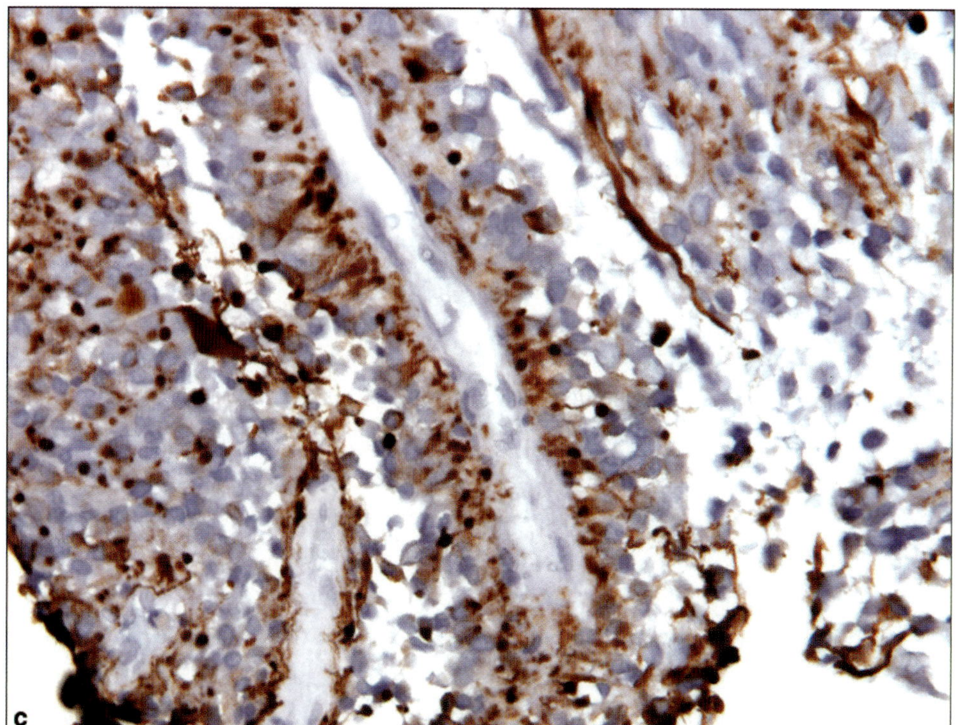

Figure 3.54. *continued.*

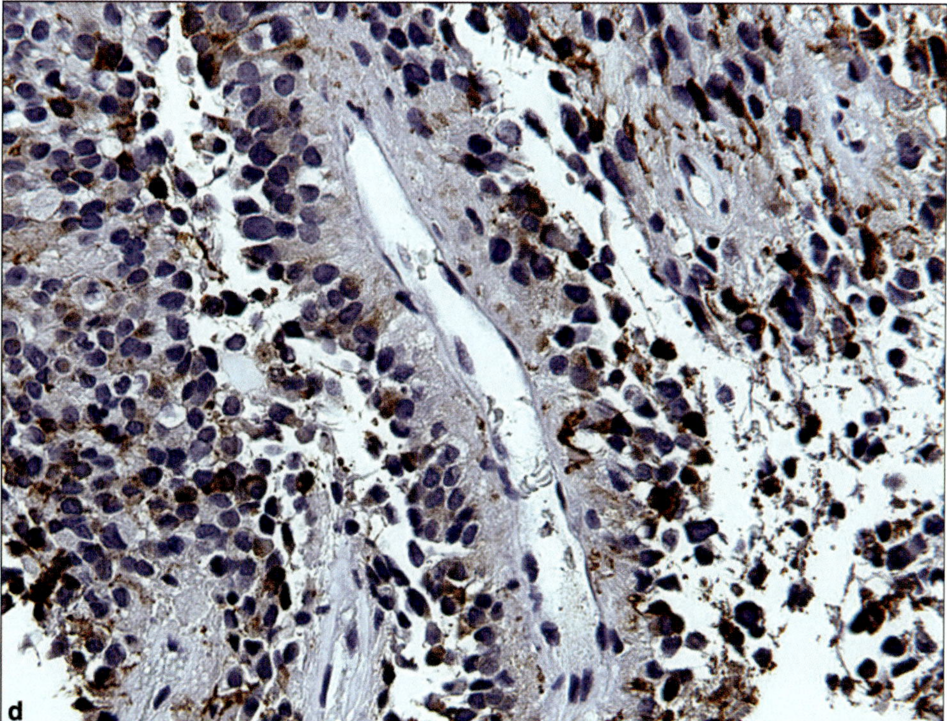

membrane antigen. Synaptophysin may be weakly immunopositive (Figure 3.54d). Proliferative activity, as determined by the MIB-1 labeling index and mitotic activity should be used in the attempt of assignment as either WHO Grade II or III although firm criteria do not exist.

WHO GRADE IV

Pineoblastoma

Clinical and Radiological Features

Unlike the previously described pineal parenchymal tumors, this tumor occurs mostly in the pediatric age group into early adulthood, although it may occur at any age. There is no sex predilection. Pineoblastomas may carry a genetic association when they occur as part of the either sporadic or familial trilateral retinoblastoma syndrome, defined as bilateral retinoblastoma with pineoblastoma (Amoaku et al., 1996; Bader et al., 1982; Tarkkanen et al., 1984).

The pace of symptom onset and interval to surgery may be considerably less than with pineocytomas, reflecting the malignant histology. The prognosis is poor especially when one considers the combination of an aggressive embryonal neoplasm with the notable difficulties encountered in the attempt at surgical resection. The pineoblastomas have a well-known propensity for remote CSF dissemination and even extracranial metastasis (Constantine et al., 2005; Herrick and Rubinstein, 1979; Schild et al., 1993). Neuroimaging indicates a large and relatively poorly demarcated solid mass with heterogeneous contrast enhancement.

Pathology

Histological evaluation will reveal a primitive embryonal neoplasm comparable to that in medulloblastoma or other similar primitive neuroectodermal tumors. They are densely cellular with increased nuclear–cytoplasmic ratios, markedly elevated mitotic activity, necrosis, with Homer Wright and Flexner–Wintersteiner (retinoblastic) rosettes (Figure 3.55). Rarely, a mixed

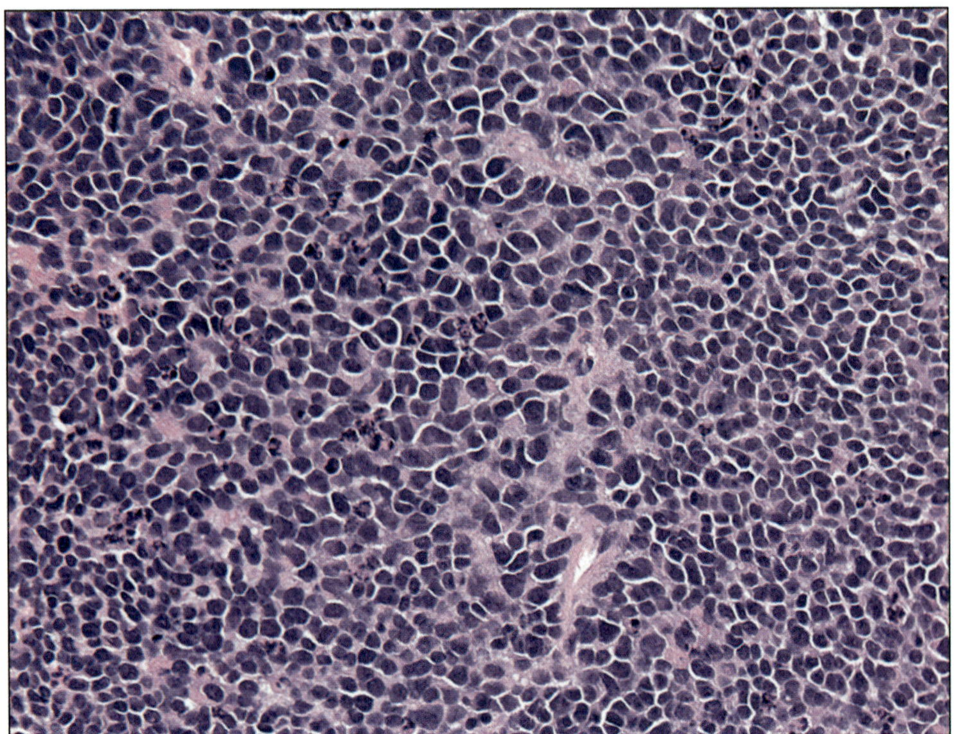

Figure 3.55. Characteristic features of a pineoblastoma, with crowded cells, Homer Wright rosettes, frequent mitoses and apoptotic cells.

pattern is present combining pineocytoma and pineoblastoma. Melanocytic, cartilaginous, and rhabdomyoblastic differentiation has been recorded, referred to as pineal anlage tumors (Berns and Pearl, 2006; Herrick and Rubinstein, 1979; Numoto, 1994).

Immunohistochemistry shows neuronal immunopositivity as the dominant diagnostic feature. GFAP immunostaining is generally noncontributory or signifying reactive astrocytosis.

REFERENCES

Amoaku WM, Willshaw HE, Parkes SE, Shah KJ, Mann JR. Trilateral retinoblastoma. A report of five patients. *Cancer* 1996; 78: 858–63.

Bader JL, Meadows AT, Zimmerman LE, Rorke LB, Voute PA, Champion LA, et al. Bilateral retinoblastoma with ectopic intracranial retinoblastoma: trilateral retinoblastoma. *Cancer Genet Cytogenet* 1982; 5: 203–13.

Berns S, Pearl G. Review of pineal anlage tumor with divergent histology. *Arch Pathol Lab Med* 2006; 130: 1233–5.

Chiechi MV, Smirniotopoulos JG, Mena H. Pineal parenchymal tumors: CT and MR features. *J Comput Assist Tomogr* 1995; 19: 509–17.

Constantine C, Miller DC, Gardner S, Balmaceda C, Finlay J. Osseous metastasis of pineoblastoma: a case report and review of the literature. *J Neurooncol* 2005; 74: 53–7.

Fevre-Montange M, Hasselblatt M, Figarella-Branger D, Chauveinc L, Champier J, Saint-Pierre G, et al. Prognosis and histopathologic features in papillary tumors of the pineal region: a retrospective multicenter study of 31 cases. *J Neuropathol Exp Neurol* 2006; 65: 1004–11.

Herrick MK, Rubinstein LJ. The cytological differentiating potential of pineal parenchymal neoplasms (true pinealomas). A clinicopathological study of 28 tumours. *Brain* 1979; 102: 289–320.

Jouvet A, Fauchon F, Liberski P, Saint-Pierre G, Didier-Bazes M, Heitzmann A, et al. Papillary tumor of the pineal region. *Am J Surg Pathol* 2003; 27: 505–12.

Jouvet A, Saint-Pierre G, Fauchon F, Privat K, Bouffet E, Ruchoux MM, et al. Pineal parenchymal tumors: a correlation of histological features with prognosis in 66 cases. *Brain Pathol* 2000; 10: 49–60.

Konovalov AN, Pitskhelauri DI. Principles of treatment of the pineal region tumors. *Surg Neurol* 2003; 59: 250–68.

Mena H, Rushing EJ, Ribas JL, Delahunt B, McCarthy WF. Tumors of pineal parenchymal cells: a correlation of histological features, including nucleolar organizer regions, with survival in 35 cases. *Hum Pathol* 1995; 26: 20–30.

Numoto RT. Pineal parenchymal tumors: cell differentiation and prognosis. *J Cancer Res Clin Oncol* 1994; 120: 683–90.

Parwani AV, Baisden BL, Erozan YS, Burger PC, Ali SZ. Pineal gland lesions: a cytopathologic study of 20 specimens. *Cancer* 2005; 105: 80–6.

Regis J, Bouillot P, Rouby-Volot F, Figarella-Branger D, Dufour H, Peragut JC. Pineal region tumors and the role of stereotactic biopsy: review of the mortality, morbidity, and diagnostic rates in 370 cases. *Neurosurgery* 1996; 39: 907–12; discussion 912–4.

Roncaroli F, Scheithauer BW. Papillary tumor of the pineal region and spindle cell oncocytoma of the pituitary: new tumor entities in the 2007 WHO Classification. *Brain Pathol* 2007; 17: 314–18.

Sasaki A, Horiguchi K, Nakazato Y. Pineal parenchymal tumor of intermediate differentiation with cytologic pleomorphism. *Neuropathology* 2006; 26: 212–17.

Schild SE, Scheithauer BW, Schomberg PJ, Hook CC, Kelly PJ, Frick L, et al. Pineal parenchymal tumors. Clinical, pathologic, and therapeutic aspects. *Cancer* 1993; 72: 870–80.

Tarkkanen A, Haltia M, Karjalainen K. Trilateral retinoblastoma. Pineoblastoma (ectopic intracranial retinoblastoma) associated with bilateral retinoblastoma. *Ophthalmic Paediatr Genet* 1984; 4: 1–6.

Embryonal Tumors

MEDULLOBLASTOMA

Clinical and Radiological Features

Medulloblastoma is the second most common brain tumor of childhood with astrocytomas as a whole being the most common (Surawicz et al., 1999). Approximately 400 new cases are reported in the United States each year with an annual incidence estimated to be 0.5 per 100,000 children less than 15 years of age and a peak age at presentation of 7 years. They are more common in males and Caucasians as compared with African Americans. Medulloblastoma may also occur in adulthood in which the vast majority occur between the ages of 21 and 40 years (Giordana et al., 1999).

The majority of childhood medulloblastomas arise in the cerebellar vermis and usually project into the fourth ventricle. Cerebellar hemispheric examples are more common in adulthood and are usually of the desmoplastic/nodular subtype.

The clinical presentation of medulloblastoma reflects the behavior of a malignant, invasive, and highly proliferative tumor, including truncal ataxia, obstructive hydrocephalus due to obliteration of the fourth ventricle, lethargy, headache, and morning nausea with vomiting.

Medulloblastomas appear as solid masses with variable but often intense contrast enhancement by CT and magnetic resonance imaging MRI scans (Figure 3.56). Cerebellar hemispheric examples may be misinterpreted as meningiomas or schwannomas. An important subtype of medulloblastoma is signified by a nodular pattern on MRI imaging, which is predictive of the subtype known as medulloblastoma with extensive nodularity (Giangaspero et al., 1999).

Grading Medulloblastomas

Chemotherapy and particularly radiation therapy have achieved great success in many cases of medulloblastoma, with survival rates as high 80% in specialized treatment centers (Packer et al., 1994). However, negative neurocognitive, endocrine, and other treatment effects as well as the risk of second malignancies are disturbingly common in long-term survivors. For these reasons, there has been heightened awareness of the importance of recognizing subtypes of medulloblastoma with differing prognoses, thus raising the possibility that some examples

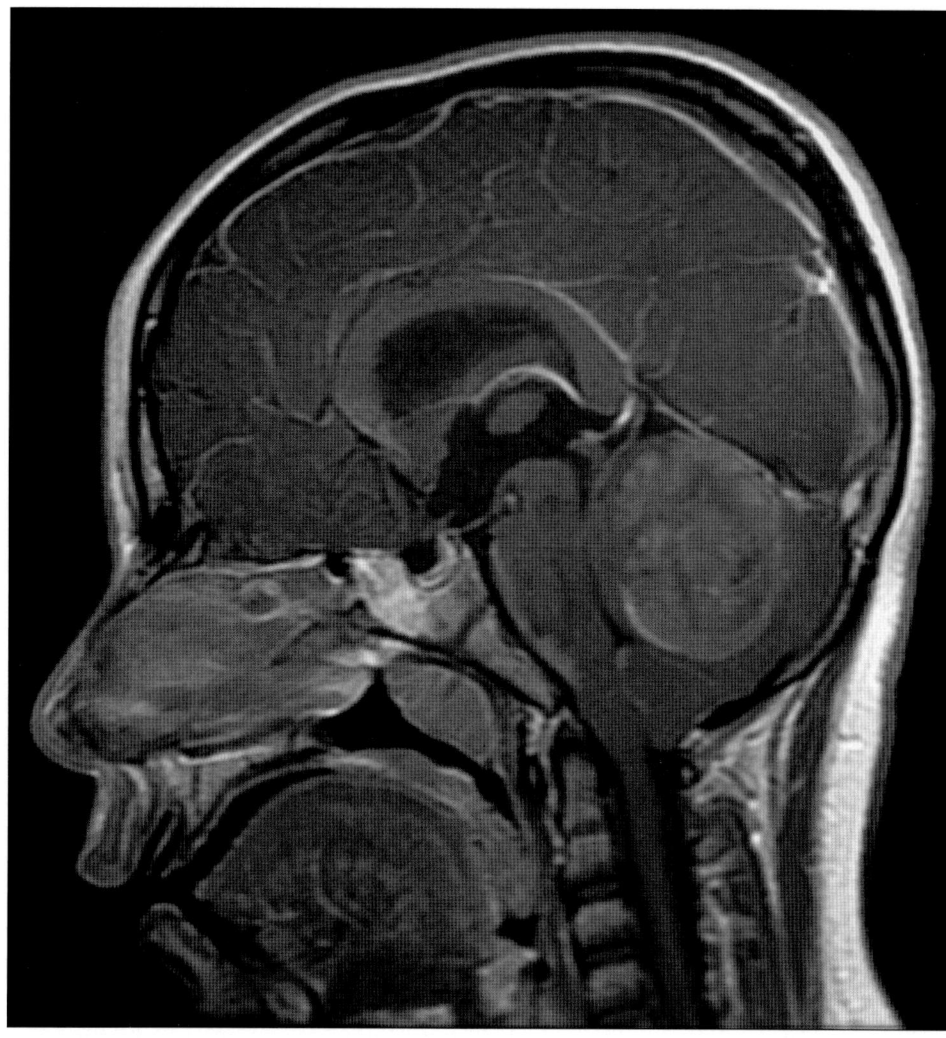

Figure 3.56. Medulloblastoma. A sagittal T1 contrast enhanced image shows an enhancing mass centered in the cerebellar vermis. The fourth ventricle is compressed. In young children, medulloblastomas tend to be centered in the midline near the roof of the fourth ventricle, whereas in older children and adults, medulloblastomas often arise from the cerebellar hemispheres. On CT images, greater than 90% of medulloblastomas have high attenuation, probably reflecting hypercellularity or a high nuclear-to-cytoplasmic ratio. Atypical teratoid rhabdoid tumors can have an identical appearance to medulloblastomas. Ependymomas can appear similar to medulloblastomas, but tend to be centered on the floor rather than the roof of the fourth ventricle.

could be successfully treated with less toxic therapy (Polkinghorn and Tarbell, 2007). Accordingly, classification methods have been proposed in the effort to both predict survival based on histological findings and assign less toxic therapy in cases with favorable histology (Eberhart et al., 2002).

Pathology

Grossly, medulloblastomas are fleshy or variegated tumors with focal hemorrhage. Cerebellar hemispheric examples may be more well circumscribed and firm.

The 2007 WHO classification of brain tumors lists the following types of medulloblastoma in addition to the classic form: desmoplastic/nodular; medulloblastoma with extensive nodularity; anaplastic; and large cell medulloblastoma.

Medulloblastomas of classic histology display the microscopic features of a primitive, largely undifferentiated neoplasm with densely packed cells containing nuclei which range from round to polygonal or molded forms and variable but generally scanty amounts of cytoplasm (Figure 3.57).

Figure 3.57. Classic medulloblastoma may contain an admixture of elements including pale islands (left) and denser areas with neuroblastic Homer Wright rosettes (arrow).

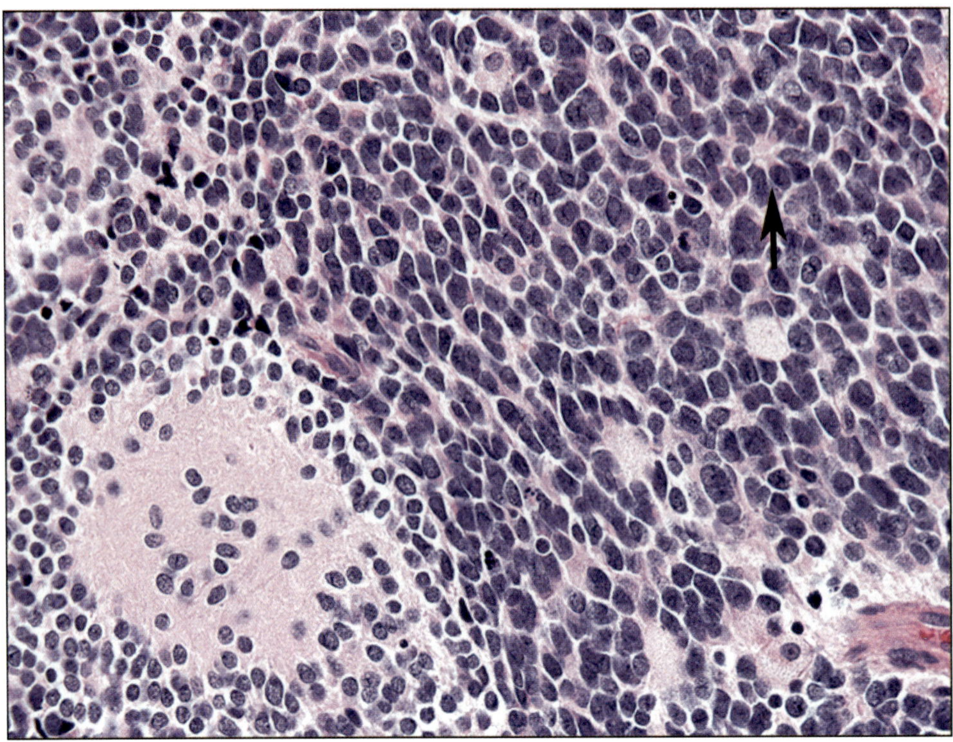

Neuroblastic Homer Wright rosettes are seen as evidence of neuronal differentiation but are present in less than 40% of cases. Adult medulloblastomas are believed to show less anaplasia as compared with pediatric examples (Rodriguez et al., 2007).

Medulloblastomas have undergone extensive characterization by markers for glial, neuronal, myogenic, and other forms a differentiation. The aforementioned neuronal immunophenotype in the pale islands of the desmoplastic/nodular medulloblastoma is important in confirming that variant; however, these immunohistochemical studies otherwise carry no prognostic importance.

Immunohistochemistry may confirm the existence of myogenic differentiation as rhabdomyoblasts or even strap cells (*medullomyoblastoma*) (Helton et al., 2004), identifiable by immunohistochemistry for desmin, myogenin, fast myosin, but not smooth muscle actin.

An analogous entity is the *melanocytic medulloblastoma* (Boesel et al., 1978; Dolman, 1988), recognizable as focal and otherwise undifferentiated pigmented cells, which may also show epithelial or tubular differentiation. Such areas are usually immunopositive for S-100 protein.

Desmoplastic/Nodular Medulloblastoma

This variant of medulloblastoma is characterized by pale islands forming reticulin-free nodules, which are surrounded by more densely packed and proliferative cells with hyperchromatic and moderately pleomorphic nuclei and the

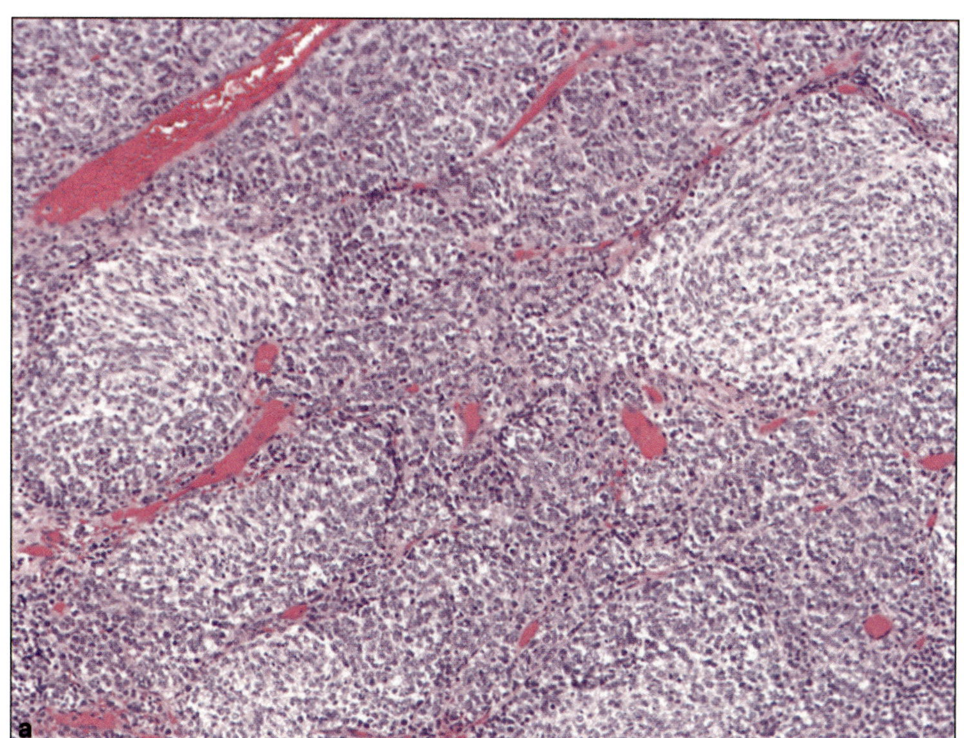

Figure 3.58. (a) Desmoplastic medulloblastoma shows numerous "pale island" consisting of relative separation of cells, (b) showing neuronal differentiation as compared with intervening regions of compact, poorly differentiated cells with increased proliferative index, and (c) reticulin deposition.

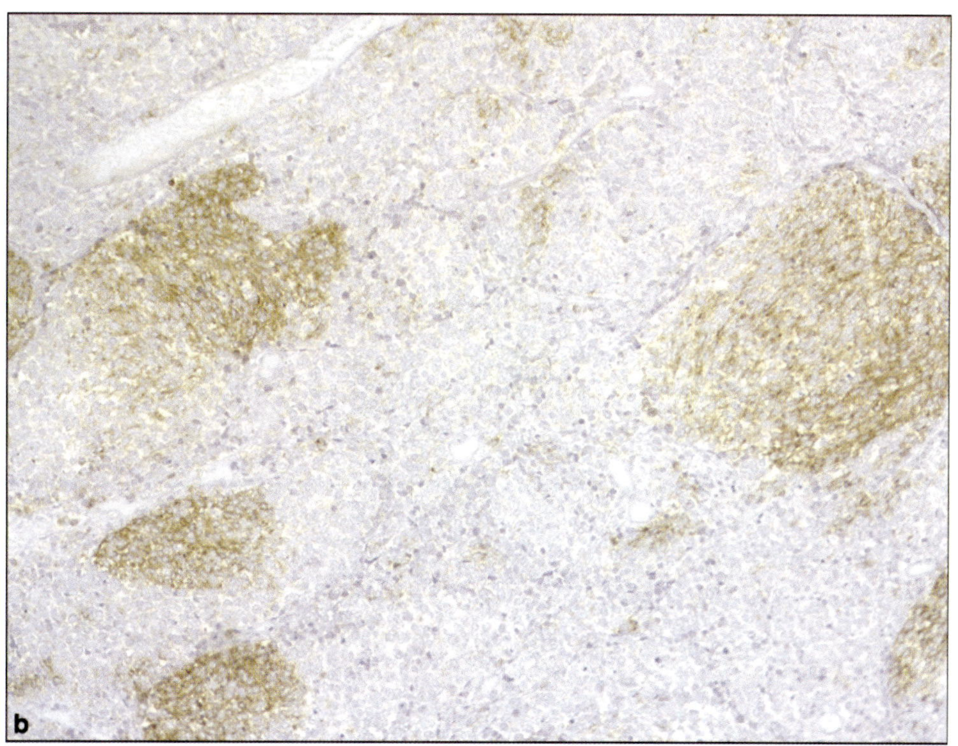

dense deposition of concentric and pericellular reticulin (Figure 3.58). The nodules lack significant mitotic or apoptotic activity and characteristically demonstrate reactivity for neuronal antigens such as synaptophysin and sometimes display recognizable cytological features of neuronal differentiation. The

Figure 3.58. *continued.*

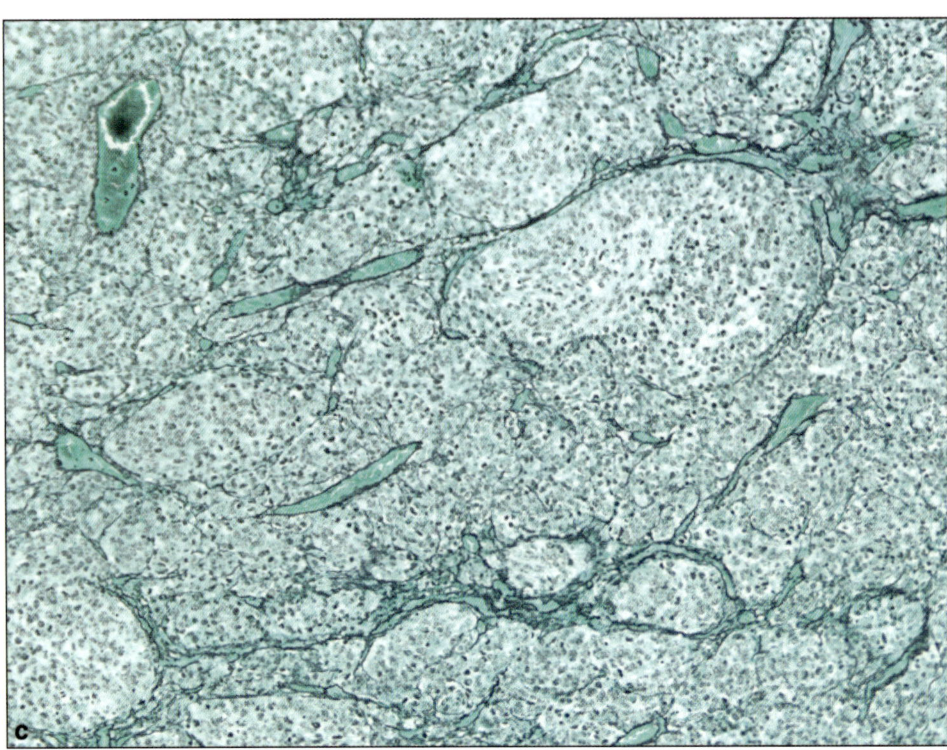

nodular appearance is the most central feature of the desmoplastic/nodular medulloblastoma, not the reticulin-rich zones.

Immunohistochemistry for the proliferative index will show a distinctive contrast between the perinodular dense areas with increased proliferation and the relatively nonproliferative pale islands of desmoplastic medulloblastomas.

Medulloblastoma with Extensive Nodularity

This variant typically occurs in infants and was previously termed "cerebellar neuroblastoma." It is characterized by unusually extensive nodule formation, usually recognizable by neuroimaging (Figure 3.59a,b). Microscopically, these nodular zones contains small neurocytic cells in a fibrillary background (Figure 3.59c) (Giangaspero et al., 1999). Such tumors may occasionally undergo even further differentiation to include ganglion cell formation.

Anaplastic Medulloblastoma

As described, medulloblastomas with marked nuclear pleomorphism and enlargement, nuclear moulding, and wrapping of one cell upon another represent anaplastic nuclear features in medulloblastomas (Figure 3.60). This variant also shows increased mitotic and apoptotic activity. Varying degrees of

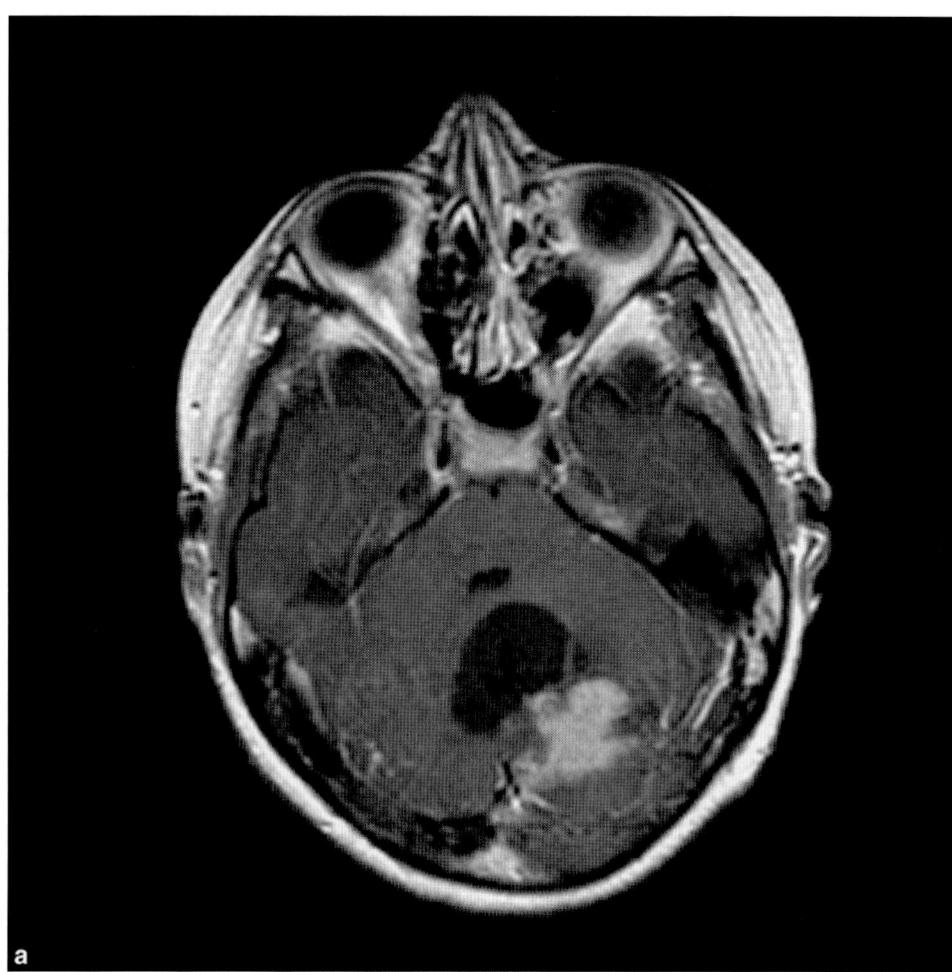

Figure 3.59. Medulloblastoma with extensive nodularity. MRI images showing mass in axial section with cystic component separate from the 4th ventricle (a) T1 with contrast enhancement and (b) T2. Images generously provided by Dr. Patrick Barnes, Department of Radiology, Lucile Packard Children's Hospital, Palo Alto, CA. (c) Microscopy shows streaming of "small" cells and scattered ganglionic differentiation in a neuropil-like background.

anaplasia may be present in the same specimen or worsen with recurrence. Anaplastic medulloblastomas require diffuse anaplasia to be present in all low-power microscopic fields. Vascular proliferation is not a pertinent finding in medulloblastoma and does not carry the same significance as in glial neoplasms.

Large Cell Medulloblastoma

This variant has a dismal prognosis in comparison with other variants of medulloblastoma due to a high incidence of subarachnoid spread, sometimes present at diagnosis (Figure 3.61). Approximately 2–4% of medulloblastomas will show a distinctive histologic pattern characterized by sheets of monomorphic cells with large round vesicular nuclei containing prominent nucleoli and a variable amount of faint or eosinophilic cytoplasm, more than is seen in frankly anaplastic cells in medulloblastoma (Figure 3.62). Coexistence of frank anaplasia and large cell morphology is common, to the extent that formal recognition of a combined form has been proposed. MYCC or MYCN amplification is associated with this subtype and accordingly with aggressive behavior and poor clinical outcome (Stearns et al., 2006).

Figure 3.59. *continued.*

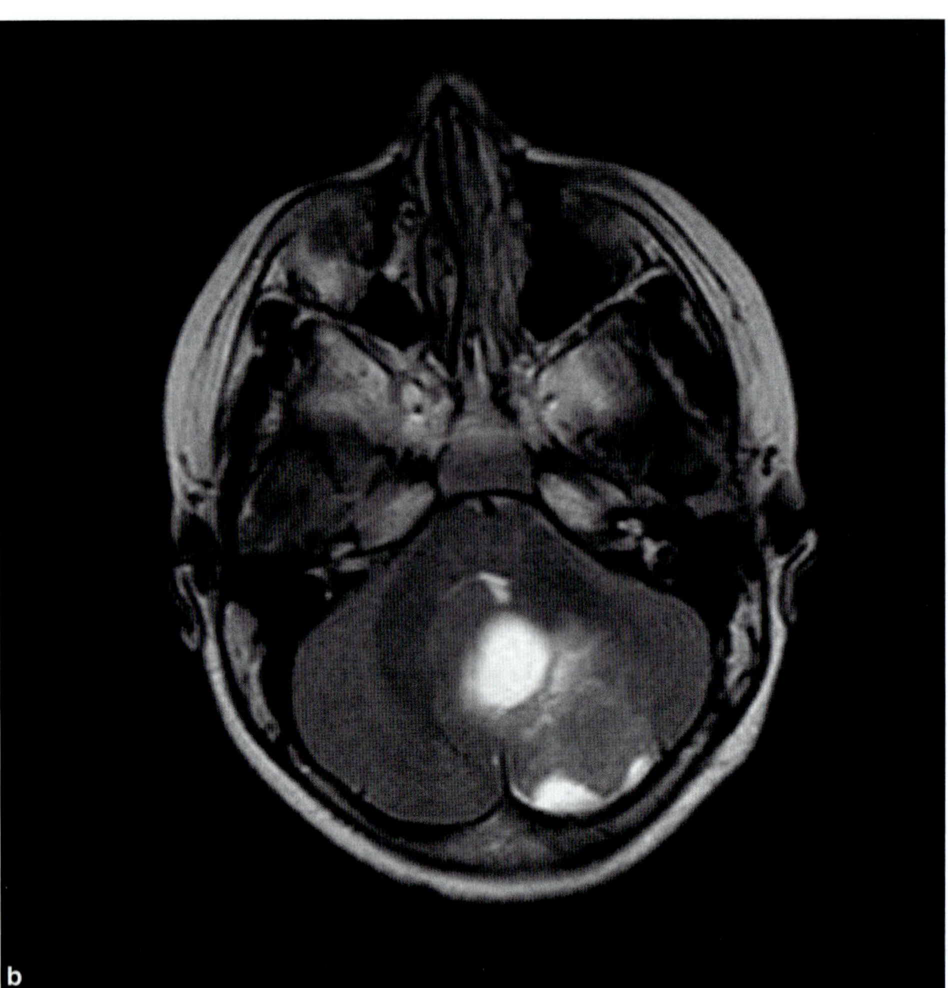

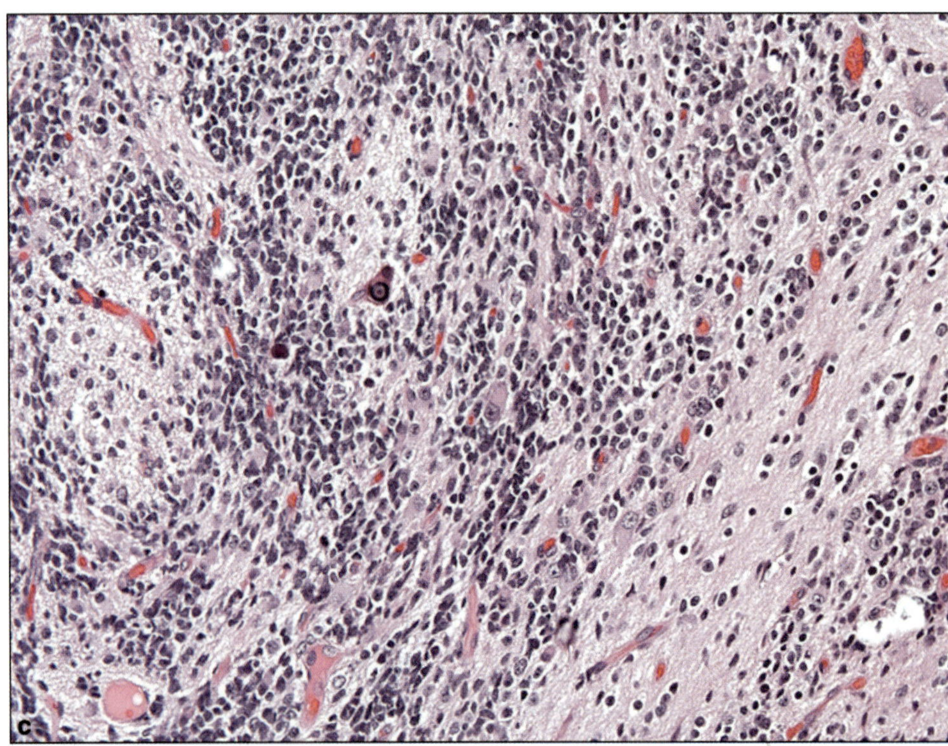

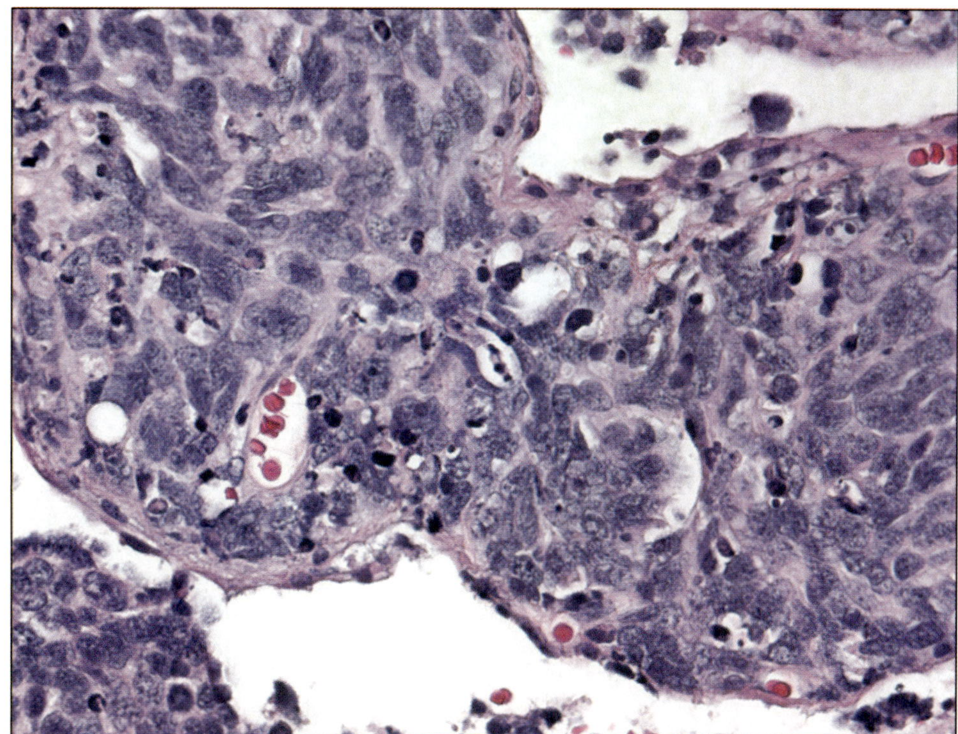

Figure 3.60. Anaplastic medulloblastoma. Severe anaplasia is defined as large cells, as large as three erythrocyte diameters, with diminutive cytoplasm, nuclear molding, nuclear wrapping, and conspicuous apoptotic and mitotic activity.

CNS PRIMITIVE NEUROECTODERMAL TUMOR

This group of tumors includes what was previously termed supratentorial primitive neuroectodermal tumor but now subsumes this entity, along with neuroblastoma and ganglioneuroblastoma, ependymoblastoma, and medulloepithelioma into this category. These are embryonal tumors with mostly undifferentiated cells analogous to medulloblastoma, with the potential of glial, neuronal, myogenic, or melanocytic differentiation. Tumors with only neuronal differentiation are called CNS neuroblastomas, and when ganglionic differentiation is present, CNS ganglioneuroblastomas (McLendon et al., 2007).

Clinical and Radiological Features

These tumors are predominantly found between early infancy and 20 years of age with a mean of 5.5 years. As in all other brain tumors and medulloblastomas, there is a male predominance. They occur most frequently within the hemispheres but may also be found in the spinal cord. Accordingly, they present with seizures or symptoms of rapidly increasing intracranial pressure or in the case of infants, an abnormal increase in head size (before closure of cranial sutures begins). Children less than 2 years of age at the time of diagnosis carry a poorer prognosis and the overall prognosis is worse than that of medulloblastoma.

Neuroimaging studies show features also analogous to those seen in medulloblastoma, namely inhomogeneous to homogeneous bright contrast

Figure 3.61. Radiographic image of large cell medulloblastoma at initial diagnosis, with extensive subarachnoid spread seen as contrast enhancement along surfaces of the cerebellum and brainstem.

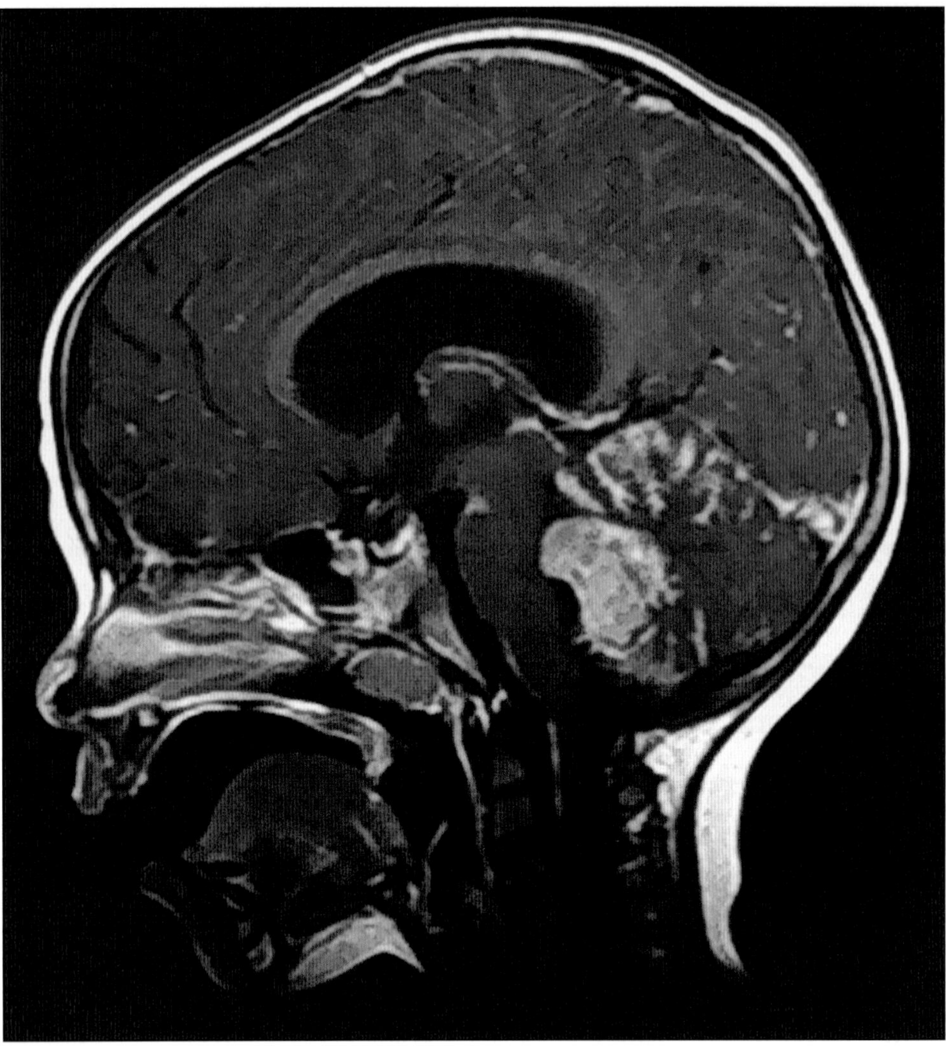

enhancement, sometimes cystic or showing evidence of necrosis. More than 50% show calcification.

Pathology

There is no uniform gross appearance to these tumor; however, necrosis or hemorrhage may frequently be grossly evident. They sometimes show relatively sharp demarcation between tumor and surrounding brain tissue.

Microscopically, these tumors are formed by primitive or poorly differentiated cells with increased nuclear cytoplasmic ratio and significant nuclear atypia (Figure 3.63). Neurocytic Homer Wright rosettes may be found. Sometimes a dense fibrillar background is noted containing cords or palisades of neurocytic cells.

A variety of neuronal, glial, and other epitopes of differentiation may be found in these tumors but they carry no particular diagnostic or prognostic significance. Similarly, the measurement of proliferative activity adds nothing to the diagnosis other than confirming the high proliferative percentage of cells in these tumors.

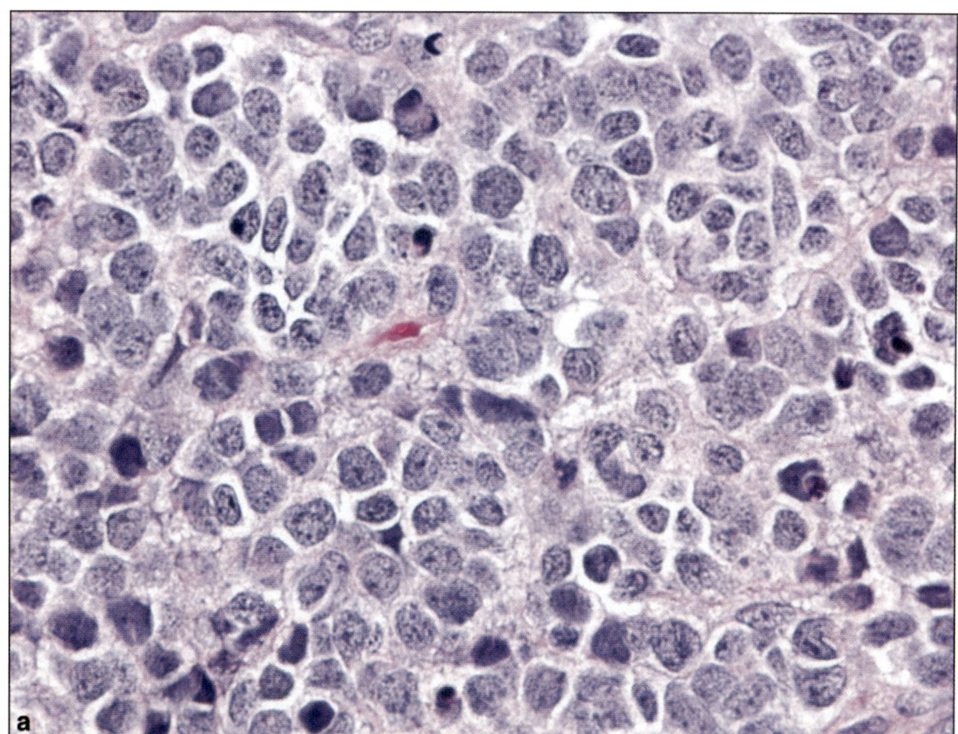

Figure 3.62. (a) Large cell medulloblastoma is a particular form of anaplasia in which cytoplasm is relatively abundant, and nuclei are round with prominent nucleoli. (b) FISH for Cmyc signified by the red signal, shows significant amplification.

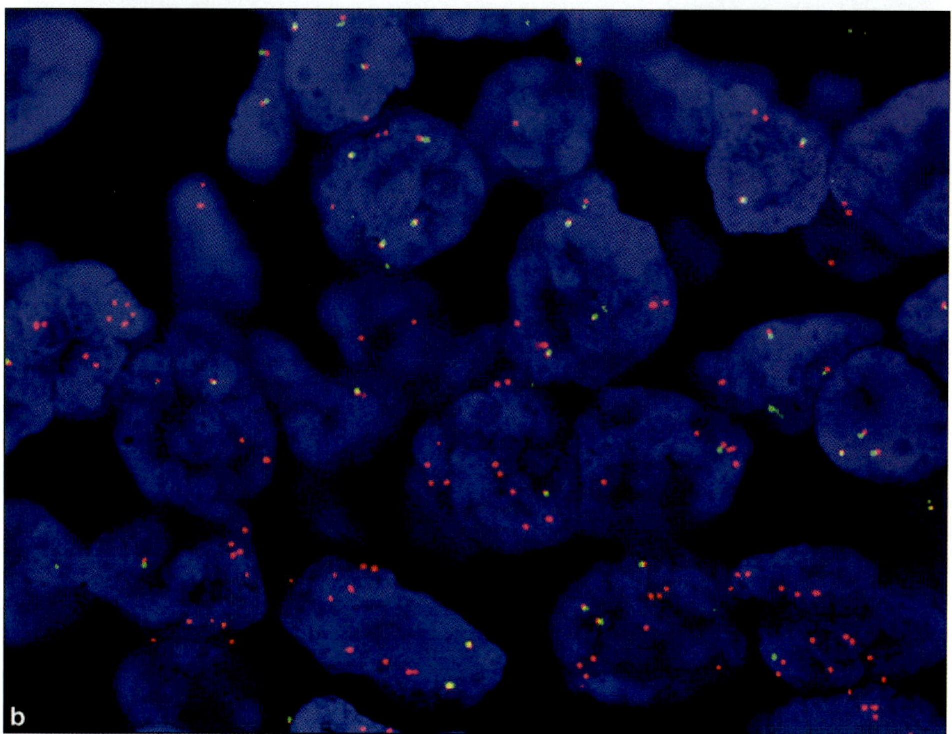

MEDULLOEPITHELIOMA

Clinical and Radiological Features

This extremely rare tumor constitutes the most primitive embryonal brain tumor yet recognized. They generally occur between 6 months and 5 years of age

Figure 3.63. CNS PNET.
(a) This MRI shows features
of a malignant neoplasm with
inhomogeneous increase in
T2 signal in a large
predominantly occipital lobe
mass.

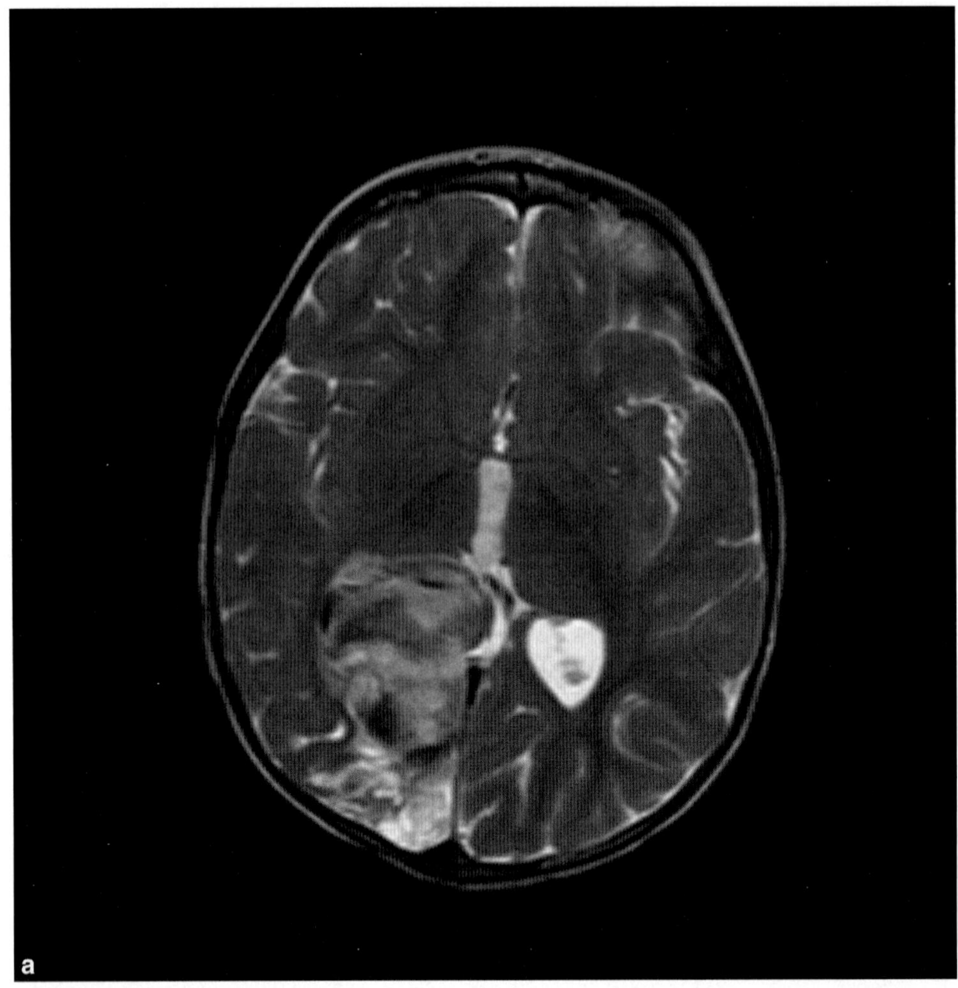

even with congenital occurrence, and mostly in the first 2 years of life (Molloy et al., 1996), They may arise in the supra- or infratentorial compartments but most commonly in a periventricular location. They may be very large at diagnosis and thus present with symptoms of severely increased intracranial pressure and ominously abnormal neurological findings. Neuroimaging characteristics are variable, usually with variable enhancement and iso- to hypodensity on CT or T1-weighted MR imaging.

Pathology

The histological appearance of medulloepithelioma bespeaks the primitive nature of this tumor since it recapitulates features of the embryonic neural tube (Figure 3.64). There is the diagnostically essential combination of the papillary, tubular, or trabecular arrangement of neuroepithelium, which is formed by pseudostratified cells. These take residence upon a prominent basement membrane, which stains positively with PAS or antibodies to collagen type IV.

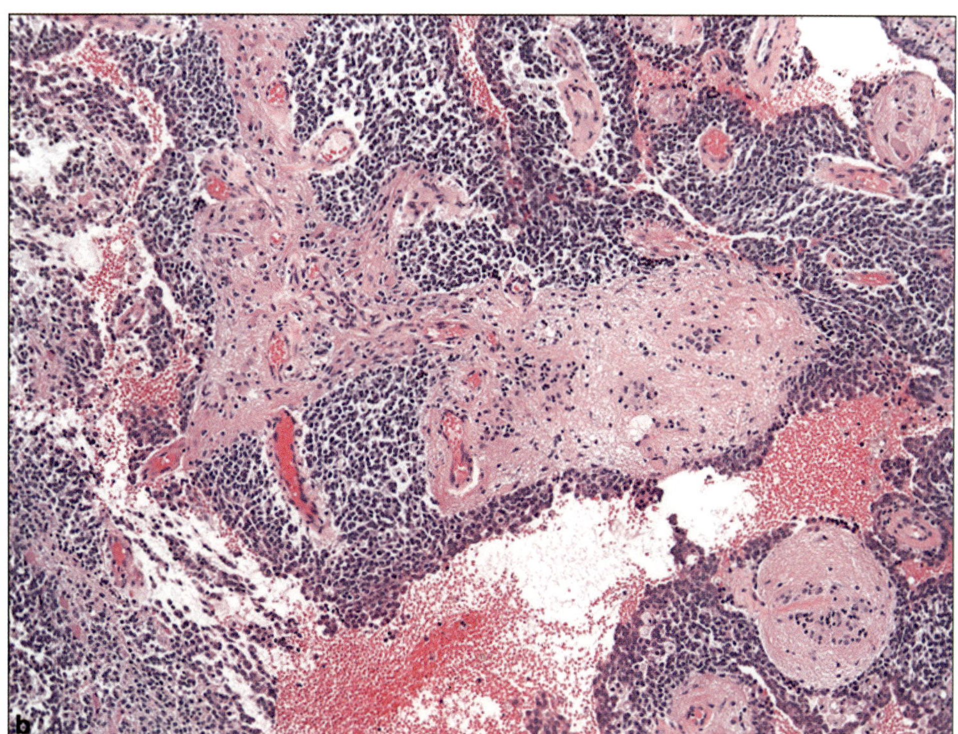

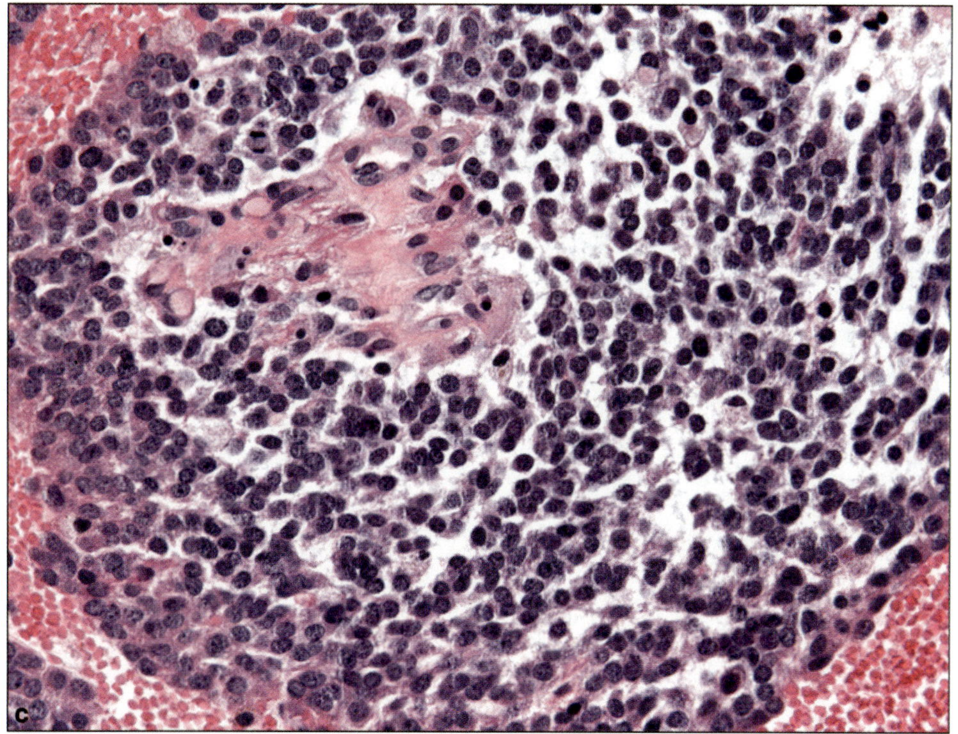

Figure 3.63. *continued* (b,c) Histological features are essentially indistinguishable from medulloblastoma or other CNS embryonal tumors. (d) Immunohistochemical analysis of CNS PNETs will typical disclose both (d) glial (GFAP) and (e) neuronal (synaptophysin) differentiation.

EPENDYMOBLASTOMA

Clinical and Radiological Features

This is a rare embryonal tumor of infants and young children that typically occur in supratentorial locations, sometimes in the periventricular

Figure 3.63. *continued.*

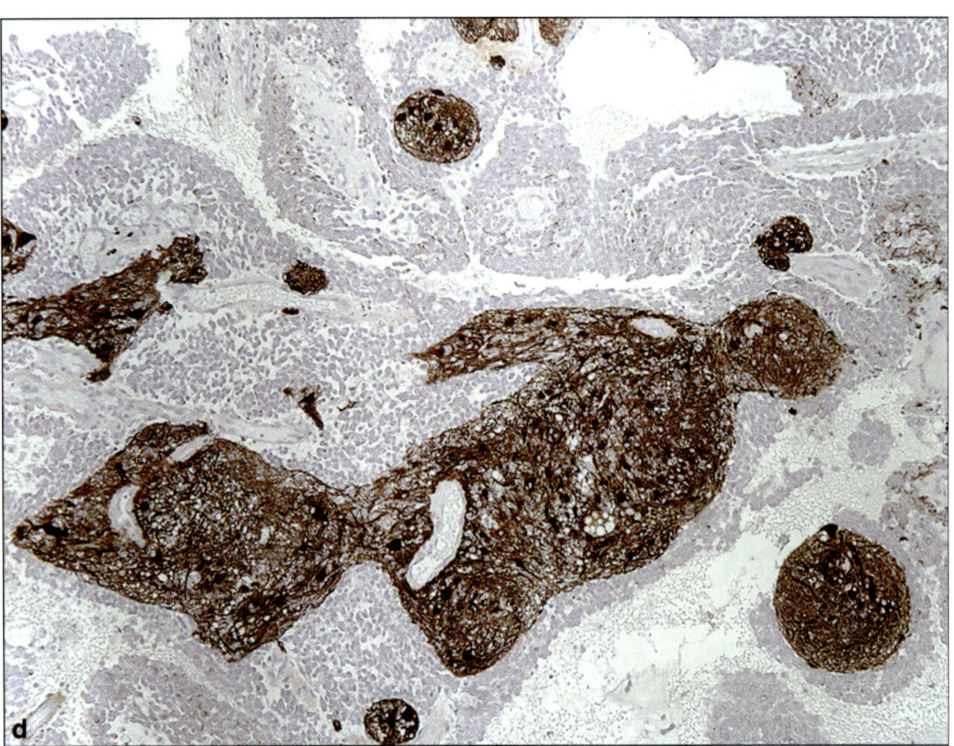

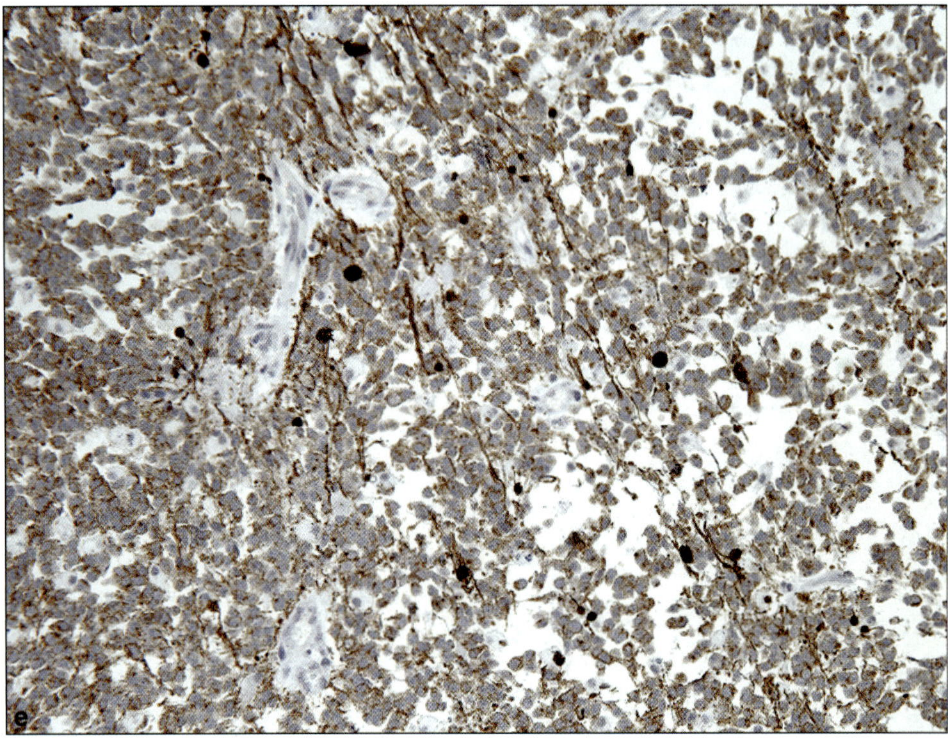

compartment (Liu et al., 1976; Mork and Rubinstein, 1985). Symptoms are referable to increased intracranial pressure and hydrocephalus. Radiological features are not separable from those of other supratentorial primitive neuro-ectodermal tumor (PNETs) (Dorsay et al., 1995).

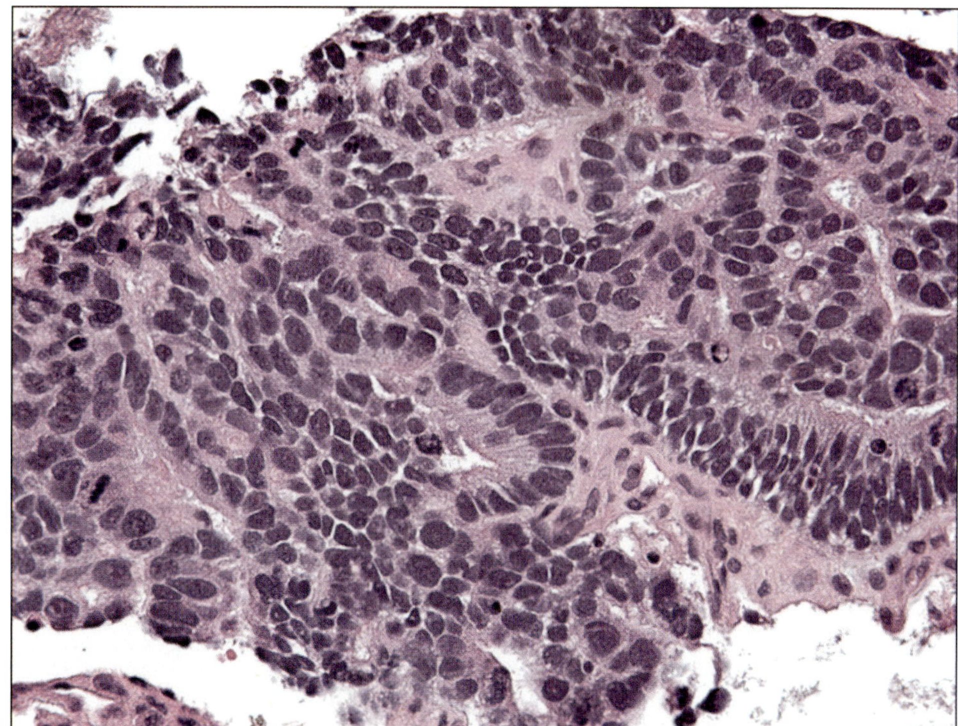

Figure 3.64. Medulloepithelioma. This is the most poorly differentiated of embryonal neoplasms of the CNS, resembling the neuroepithelium of the embryonic neural tube.

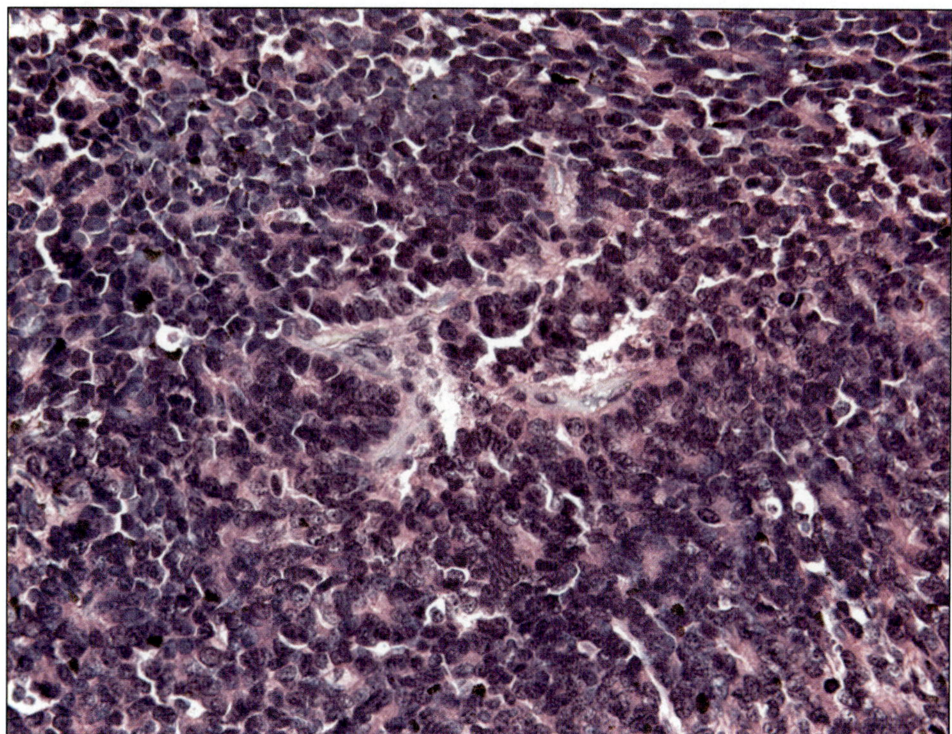

Figure 3.65. Ependymoblastoma, a primitive neoplasm with innumerable true ependymal rosettes and no perivascular pseudorosettes which are characteristic of ependymomas of all grades.

Pathology

The gross appearance of an ependymoblastoma is also that of an embryonal neoplasm, with a notable propensity for subarachnoid spread. The histological appearance is that of a mitotically active primitive neoplasm with numerous and multilayered ependymal rosettes (Figure 3.65). These are formed by tumor cells

Figure 3.66. AT/RT. This large hemispheric example shows extreme mass effect, inhomogeneous contrast enhancement with probable hemorrhage and necrosis. One-third may show CSF dissemination at diagnosis.

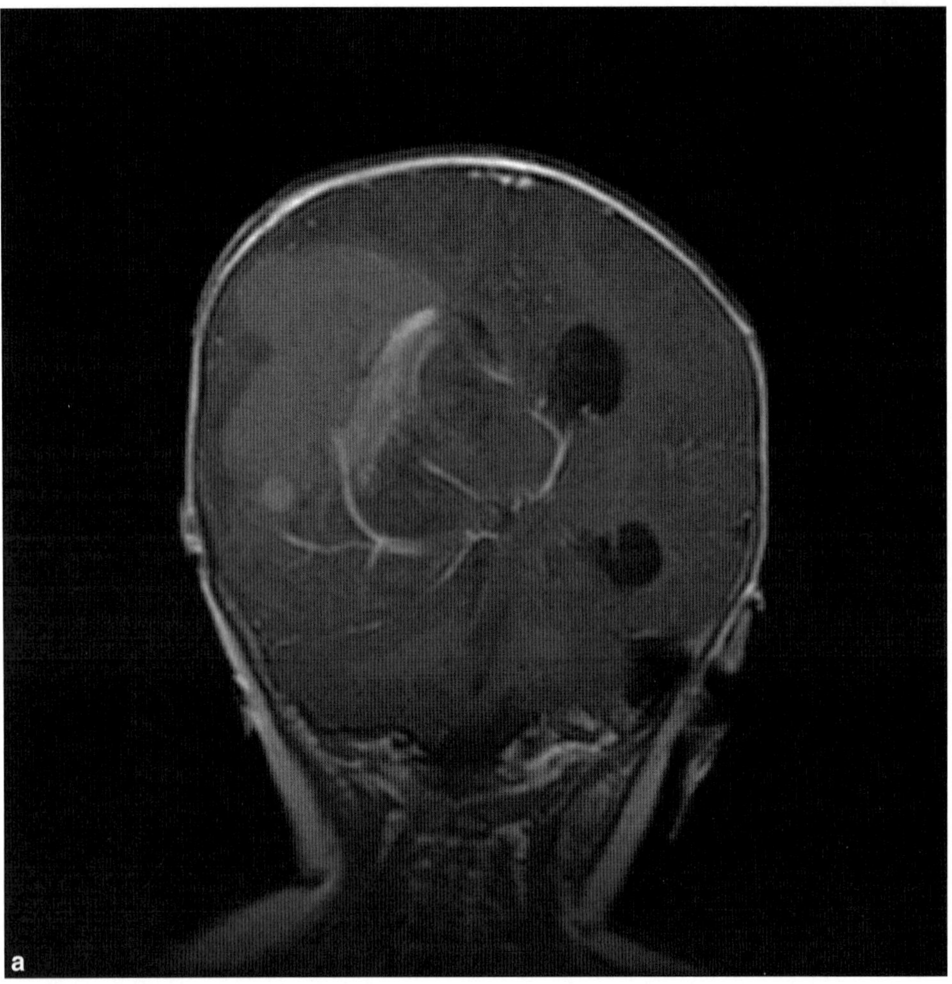

surrounding a small lumen with cilia or basal bodies at the apical surfaces of the cells and the nuclei in basal positions.

ATYPICAL TERATOID/RHABDOID TUMOR (AT/RT)

Clinical and Radiological Features

This is an aggressive and highly malignant neoplasm of young children occurring most often under the age of 3 years and rarely over the age of 6 years although examples of rare occurrence in adulthood, usually in the hemispheres, have been reported (Raisanen et al., 2005). Like most pediatric neoplasms, there is a male predominance. Occurrence before the age of 12 months should prompt consideration of the rhabdoid tumor predisposition syndrome due to the germline loss or inactivation of one allele of the *INI1* gene. This tumor carries a distinctly poor prognosis with a mean survival after surgery generally less than 1 year.

These tumors occur with somewhat greater frequency in the supratentorial compartment, in the hemispheres, or sometimes intraventricular in location. In the posterior fossa, they may appear to arise at the cerebellopontine angle or brainstem but because of their large size at diagnosis, they may seem to be

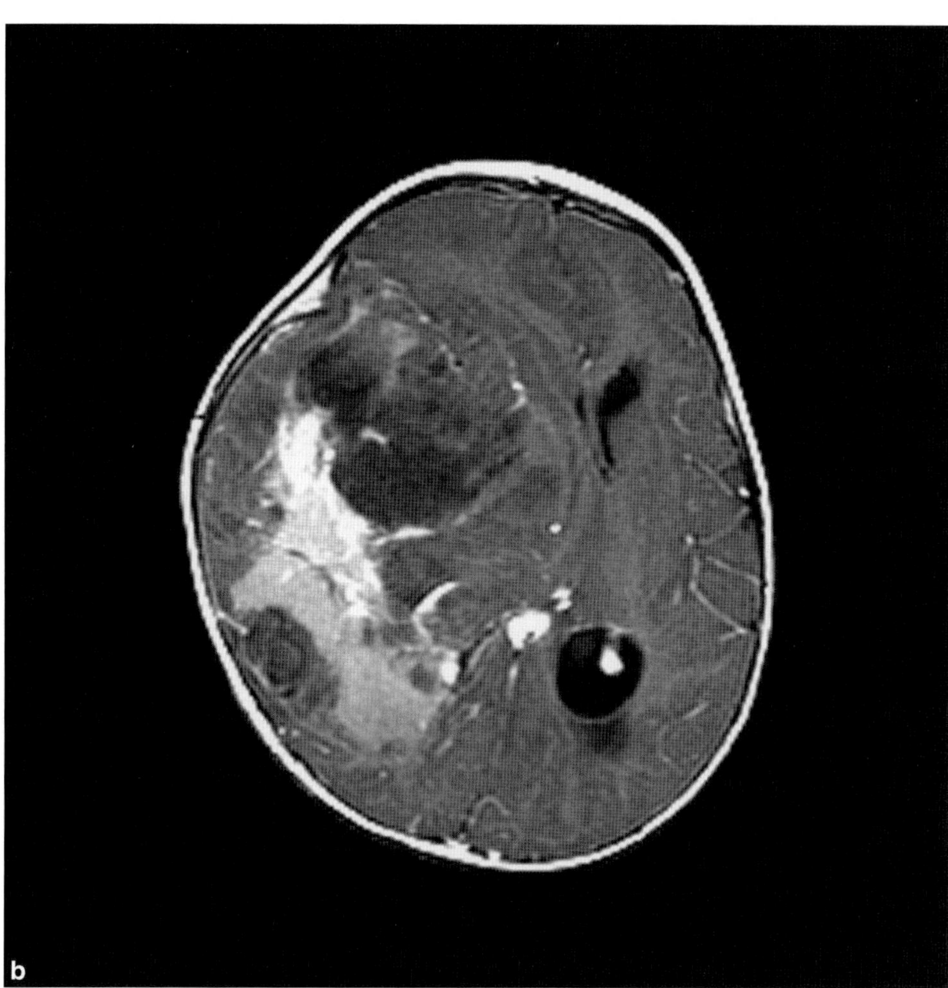

Figure 3.66. *continued.*

centered predominantly within a cerebellar hemisphere. The AT/RT has a well-known propensity for subarachnoid spread and this may be noted radiologically at diagnosis in at least 20% of cases (Hilden et al., 2004; Meyers et al., 2006). Primary paraspinal occurrence has also been noted.

Clinical signs and symptoms depend upon the age and location of the tumor but most commonly relate to the rapid increase in intracranial pressure or obstruction of CSF flow, producing lethargy, vomiting or failure to thrive. Headache and hemiplegia may be important signs in older children.

CT and MRI show features similar to other embryonal tumors, either of the posterior fossa or supratentorial compartment (Figure 3.66). They almost always show some degree of contrast enhancement.

Pathology

The gross appearance of an AT/RT bespeaks the highly malignant nature of the tumor whereby macroscopic foci of hemorrhage and necrosis may be noted. The AT/RT is dominated by variable features of a highly malignant embryonal neoplasm, with regions of necrosis and increased mitotic activity (Figure 3.67). Portions of the tumor may resemble "ordinary" medulloblastomas or CNS PNETs,

Figure 3.67. (a, b) Atypical teratoid rhabdoid tumor (AT/RT) shows a highly variable mixture of primitive neoplastic elements, many of which do not include any clue as to the focally rhabdoid nature of these tumors, (c) seen in the middle of this image, surrounded by poorly differentiated embryonal histology. (d) Higher power view of rhabdoid component.

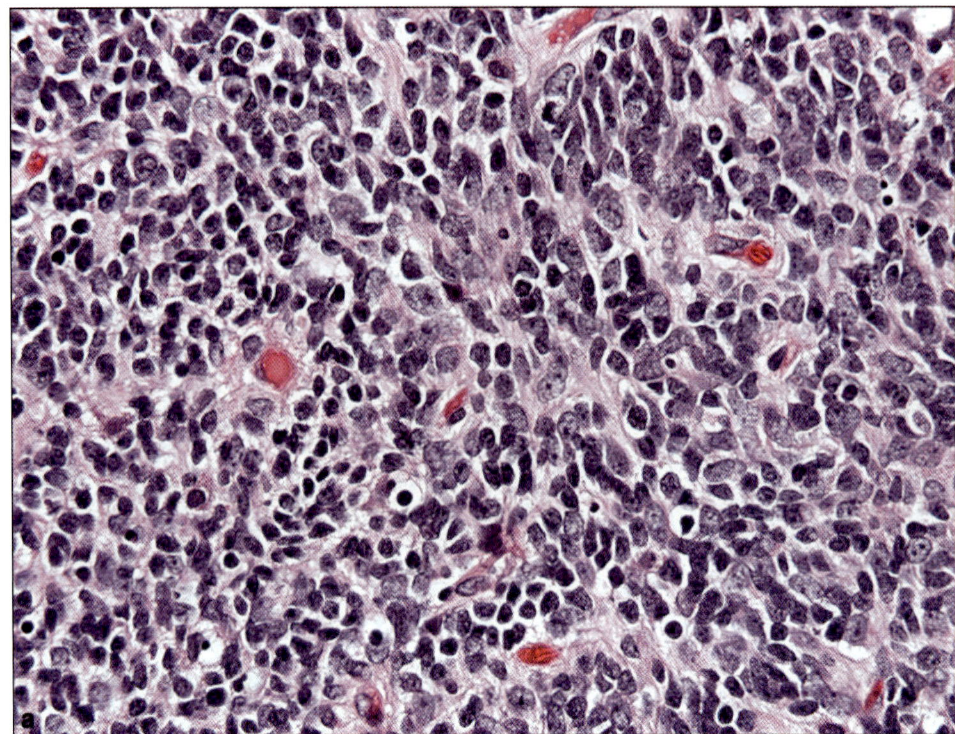

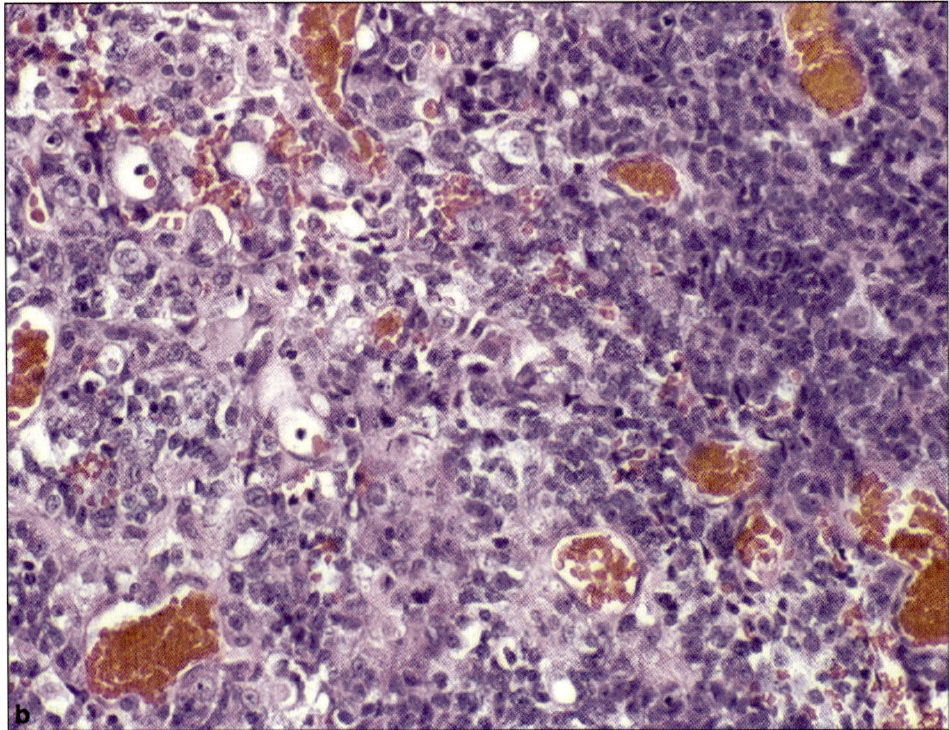

with sheets of crowded cells bearing markedly increased nuclear–cytoplasmic ratios and essentially no secondary differentiation. However, the definitional feature of this neoplasm is the presence of cells with rhabdoid features, consisting of an eosinophilic cytoplasmic body, sometimes seen to gently indent the nucleus. These and other cells in an AT/RT are enlarged, with spherical vesicular

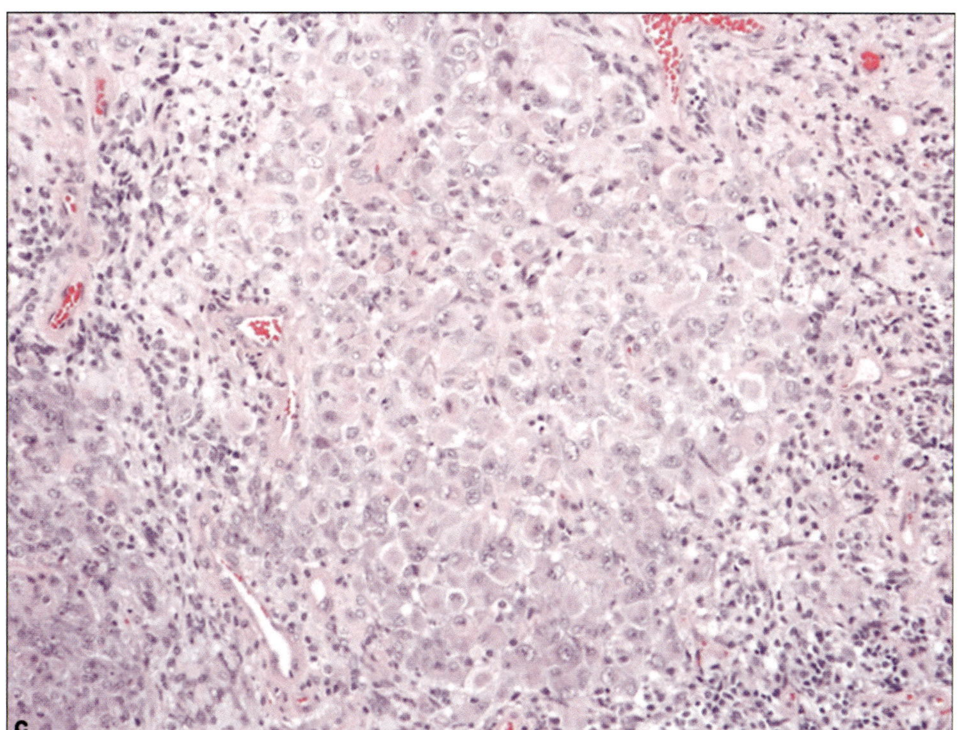

Figure 3.67. *continued.*

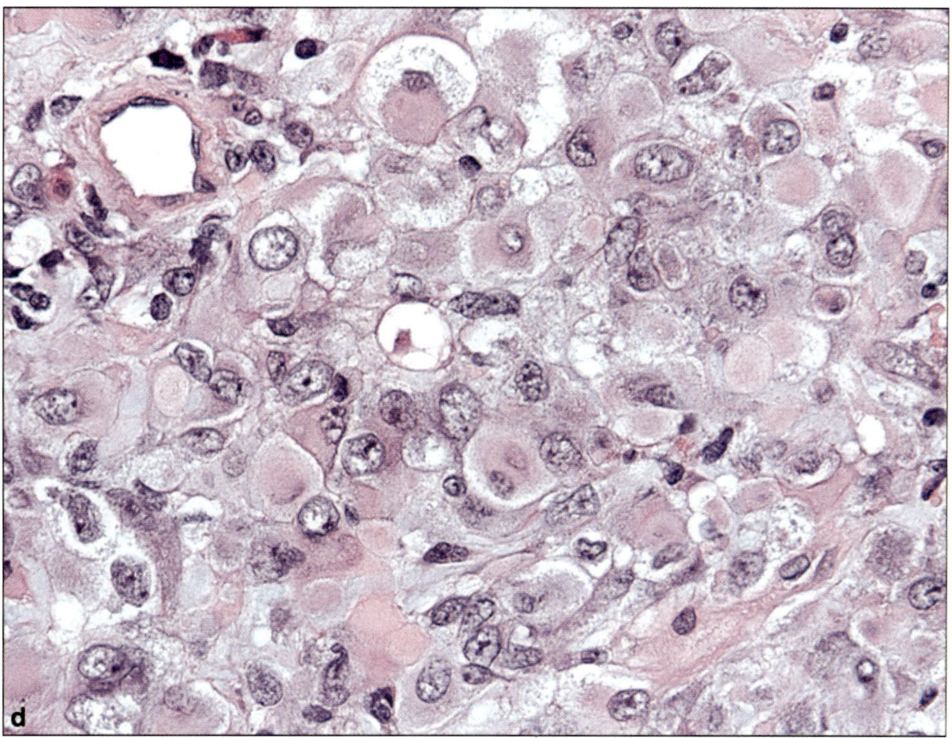

nuclei and prominent nucleoli and relatively abundant cytoplasm. Such rhabdoid inclusions may be highlighted by immunohistochemistry for vimentin. The ultrastructural appearance of these rhabdoid inclusions is quite distinctive, consisting of mass of whorled intermediate filaments (Bhattacharjee et al., 1997). The AT/RT may also show evidence of mesenchymal differentiation in

Figure 3.67. *continued*
(e) Immunohistochemistry
for GFAP shows both
immunopositive tumor cells
with clearly associated
atypical nuclei and reactive
astrocytes with inconspicuous
nuclei and slender processes,
a difficult distinction
in certain cases.
(f) Previously, extensive
immunophenotyping was
done to show
neuroectodermal, epithelial,
and mesenchymal elements of
an AT/RT, which has been
supplanted by
immunohistochemistry for
BAF47/SNF5 in which
negative staining in tumor
cells with positive
immunoreactivity for
endothelial cells serving as an
internal control, is diagnostic
of AT/RT.

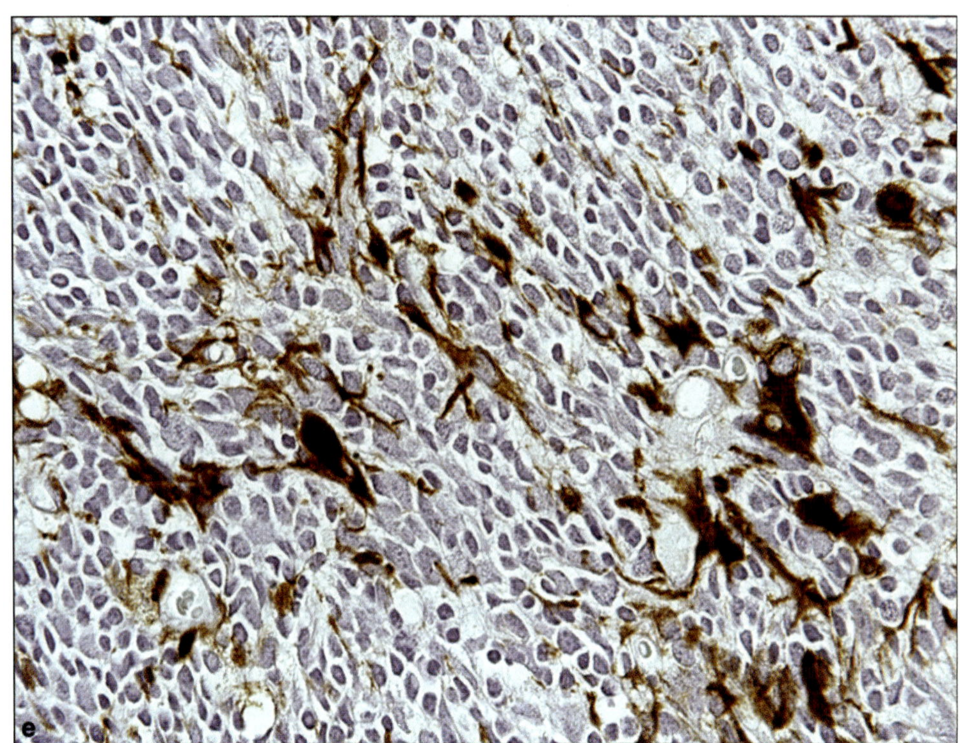

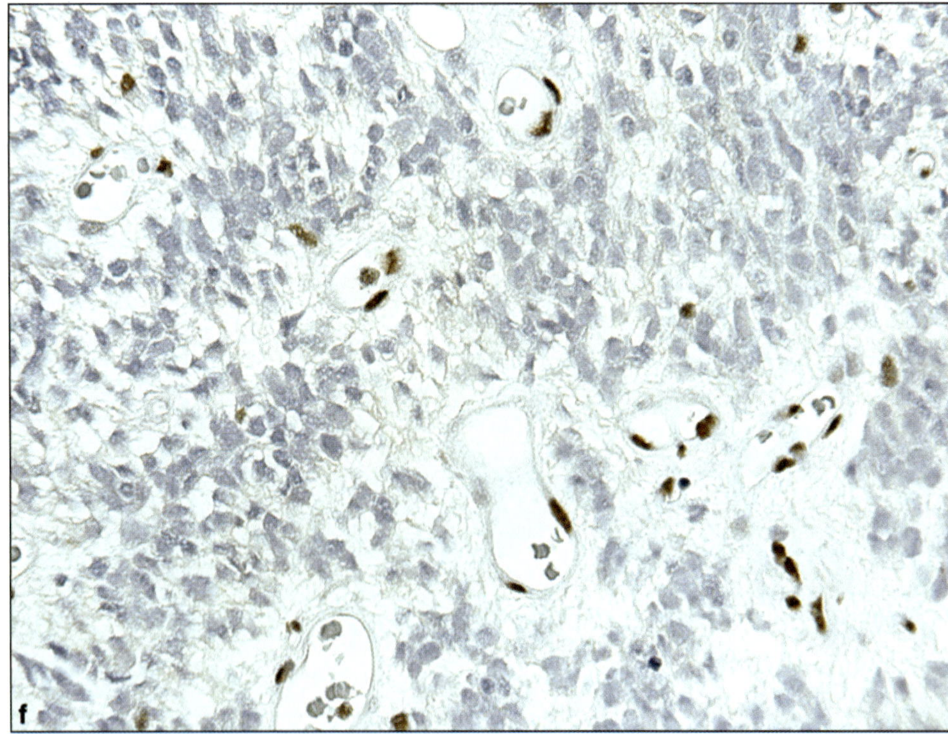

the form of spindle cells or a myxoid background, or less commonly epithelial differentiation, with papillary or glandular formation.

When the AT/RT was first described, a rather extensive battery of immunohistochemical stains was recommended in order to document combined

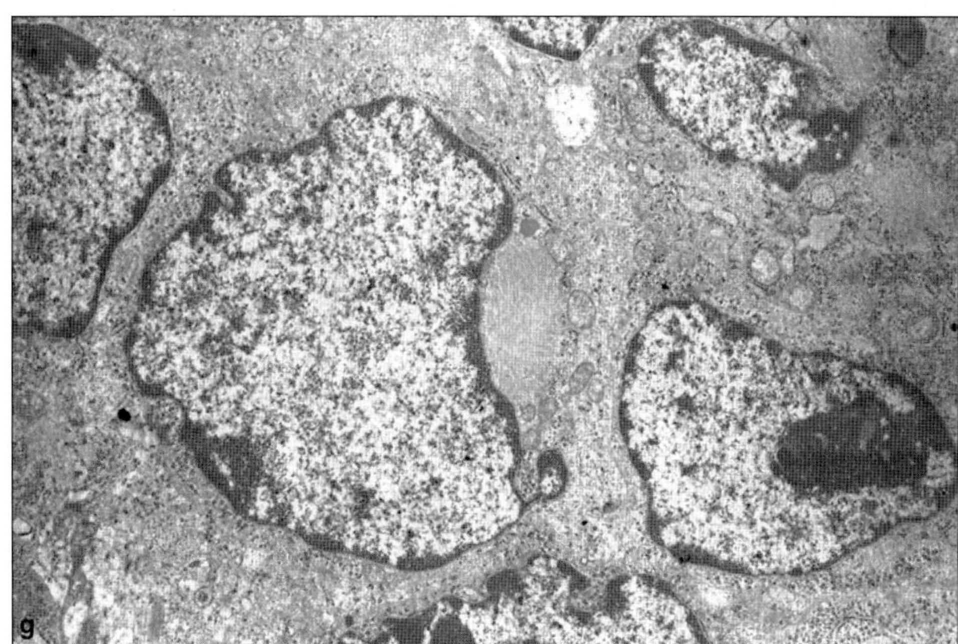

Figure 3.67. *continued*
(g) Electron microscopic appearance of cytoplasmic rhabdoid inclusions, an ovoid aggregate of filaments gently indenting the nucleus.

neuronal, glial, possible mesenchymal and epithelial differentiation, and by definition no reactivity for germ cell tumor elements (thus the term "teratoid") (Rorke et al., 1996). Such a diagnostic approach would typically involve antibodies to neurofilament, GFAP, smooth muscle actin, and EMA, and vimentin toward highlighting the rhabdoid inclusions. This approach has been superseded by the availability of an antibody to the INI1 protein whereby its immunohistochemical absence in a suspected AT/RT is diagnostic, along with characteristic immunopositivity for tumor blood vessels as an internal positive control. Current surgical neuropathology dictates that in order to avoid a serious pitfall in diagnosis, this antibody applied to embryonal tumors of diverse locations in young children because obvious rhabdoid elements may not be present.

REFERENCES

Bhattacharjee M, Hicks J, Langford L, Dauser R, Strother D, Chintagumpala M, et al. Central nervous system atypical teratoid/rhabdoid tumors of infancy and childhood. *Ultrastruct Pathol* 1997; 21: 369–78.

Boesel CP, Suhan JP, Sayers MP. Melanotic medulloblastoma. Report of a case with ultrastructural findings. *J Neuropathol Exp Neurol* 1978; 37: 531–43.

Dolman CL. Melanotic medulloblastoma. A case report with immunohistochemical and ultrastructural examination. *Acta Neuropathol* 1988; 76: 528–31.

Dorsay TA, Rovira MJ, Ho VB, Kelley J. Ependymoblastoma: MR presentation. A case report and review of the literature. *Pediatr Radiol* 1995; 25: 433–5.

Eberhart CG, Kepner JL, Goldthwaite PT, Kun LE, Duffner PK, Friedman HS, et al. Histopathologic grading of medulloblastomas: a Pediatric Oncology Group study. *Cancer* 2002; 94: 552–60.

Giangaspero F, Perilongo G, Fondelli MP, Brisigotti M, Carollo C, Burnelli R, et al. Medulloblastoma with extensive nodularity: a variant with favorable prognosis. *J Neurosurg* 1999; 91: 971–7.

Giordana MT, Schiffer P, Lanotte M, Girardi P, Chio A. Epidemiology of adult medulloblastoma. *Int J Cancer* 1999; 80: 689–92.

Helton KJ, Fouladi M, Boop FA, Perry A, Dalton J, Kun L, et al. Medullomyoblastoma: a radiographic and clinicopathologic analysis of six cases and review of the literature. *Cancer* 2004; 101: 1445–54.

Hilden JM, Meerbaum S, Burger P, Finlay J, Janss A, Scheithauer BW, et al. Central nervous system atypical teratoid/rhabdoid tumor: results of therapy in children enrolled in a registry. *J Clin Oncol* 2004; 22: 2877–84.

Liu HM, Boogs J, Kidd J. Ependymomas of childhood. I. Histological survey and clinicopathological correlation. *Childs Brain* 1976; 2: 92–110.

McLendon RE, Judkins AR, Eberhart CG, Fuller GN, Sarkar C, Ng HK. Central nervous system primitive neuroectodermal tumors. In: Louis DN, editor. *WHO Classification of Tumours of the Central Nervous System*. Lyon: International Agency for Research on Cancer, 2007.

Meyers SP, Khademian ZP, Biegel JA, Chuang SH, Korones DN, Zimmerman RA. Primary intracranial atypical teratoid/rhabdoid tumors of infancy and childhood: MRI features and patient outcomes. *AJNR Am J Neuroradiol* 2006; 27: 962–71.

Molloy PT, Yachnis AT, Rorke LB, Dattilo JJ, Needle MN, Millar WS, et al. Central nervous system medulloepithelioma: a series of eight cases including two arising in the pons. *J Neurosurg* 1996; 84: 430–6.

Mork SJ, Rubinstein LJ. Ependymoblastoma. A reappraisal of a rare embryonal tumor. *Cancer* 1985; 55: 1536–42.

Packer RJ, Sutton LN, Elterman R, Lange B, Goldwein J, Nicholson HS, et al. Outcome for children with medulloblastoma treated with radiation and cisplatin, CCNU, and vincristine chemotherapy. *J Neurosurg* 1994; 81: 690–8.

Polkinghorn WR, Tarbell NJ. Medulloblastoma: tumorigenesis, current clinical paradigm, and efforts to improve risk stratification. *Nat Clin Pract Oncol* 2007; 4: 295–304.

Raisanen J, Biegel JA, Hatanpaa KJ, Judkins A, White CL, Perry A. Chromosome 22q deletions in atypical teratoid/rhabdoid tumors in adults. *Brain Pathol* 2005; 15: 23–8.

Rodriguez FJ, Eberhart C, O'Neill BP, Slezak J, Burger PC, Goldthwaite P, et al. Histopathologic grading of adult medulloblastomas. *Cancer* 2007; 109: 2557–65.

Rorkej LB, Packer RJ, Biegel JA. Central nervous system atypical teratoid/rhabdoid tumors of infancy and childhood: definition of an entity. *J Neurosurg* 1996; 85: 56–65.

Stearns D, Chaudhry A, Abel TW, Burger PC, Dang CV, Eberhart CG. c-myc overexpression causes anaplasia in medulloblastoma. *Cancer Res* 2006; 66: 673–81.

Surawicz TS, McCarthy BJ, Kupelian V, Jukich PJ, Bruner JM, Davis FG. Descriptive epidemiology of primary brain and CNS tumors: results from the Central Brain Tumor Registry of the United States, 1990–1994. *Neuro Oncol* 1999; 1: 14–25.

TUMORS OF CRANIAL AND PARASPINAL NERVES

SCHWANNOMA

Clinical and Radiological Features

Schwannomas account for 8% of intracranial tumors, 85% of cerebellopontine angle masses, and almost one-third of spinal nerve root tumors (Urich and

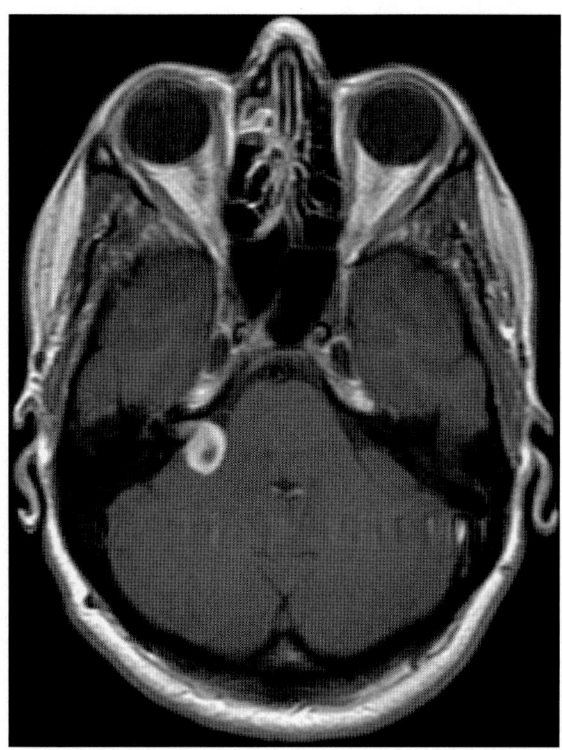

Figure 3.68. Vestibular schwannoma. An axial T1 MRI with contrast shows a right cerebellopontine angle mass. An intensely enhancing cerebellopontine angle mass, which extends into the internal auditory canal and does not display a dural tail is very characteristic of a nerve sheath tumor. The central area of poorer enhancement shown here is also common in the larger schwannomas. Rarely, an intracanalicular meningioma, lymphoma, or metastases could have a similar imaging appearance.

Tien, 1998) When symptoms occur, there are usually associated with corresponding cranial neuropathy or spinal radiculopathy, most likely sensory in nature. Approximately 90% are sporadic and solitary while 4% occur in patients with neurofibromatosis type 2 (NF2). A roughly equal percentage may be multiple but are unassociated with NF2 (Antinheimo et al., 2000). They occur most frequently in mid-adulthood with spinal examples more common in women. Intraparenchymal cerebral schwannomas are associated with a younger age and male predominance (Casadei et al., 1993). Schwannomas are assigned to WHO Grade I.

Most intracranial schwannomas arise in association with the eighth cranial nerve in the cerebellopontine angle. Bilateral examples are considered diagnostic of NF2. They are otherwise preferentially located in sensory rather than motor cranial nerves as well as in spinal sensory nerve roots. Intraparenchymal examples are presumed to be derived from unmyelinated Schwann cells, which invest the vasa nervorum that serve cerebral blood vessels.

Neuroimaging will reveal a well-circumscribed, sometimes cystic and heterogeneously contrast-enhancing mass (Figure 3.68). Vestibular schwannomas may be associated with enlargement of the internal auditory meatus and bone erosion.

Pathology

Schwannomas in all locations share a variety of histologic appearances, dominated by spindle cells forming two basic patterns: compact elongated cells with occasional nuclear palisading or Verocay bodies (Antoni A pattern) and a looser pattern with indistinct cell processes and delicate vacuolation (Antoni B

Figure 3.69. Schwannomas are usually recognizable by a variable admixture of microscopic appearances: (a) Dense Antoni A (left) and relatively hypocellular Antoni B (right) regions. Note the characteristic thick-walled vessels of a schwannoma. (b) Verocay bodies are closely aligned aggregates of parallel nuclei with adjacent anuclear areas.

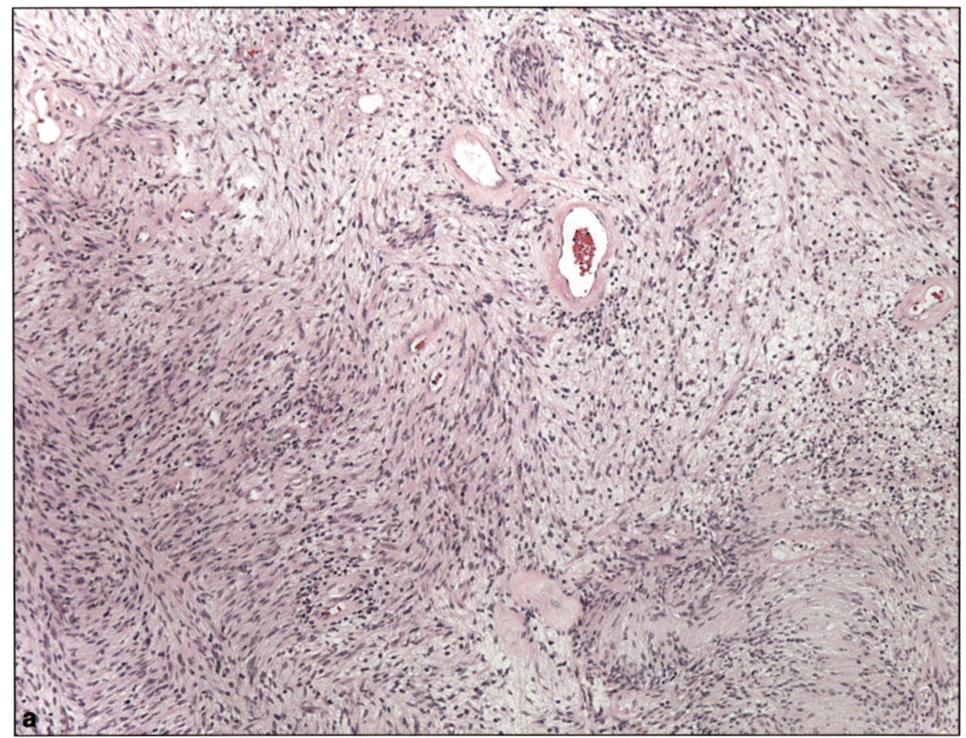

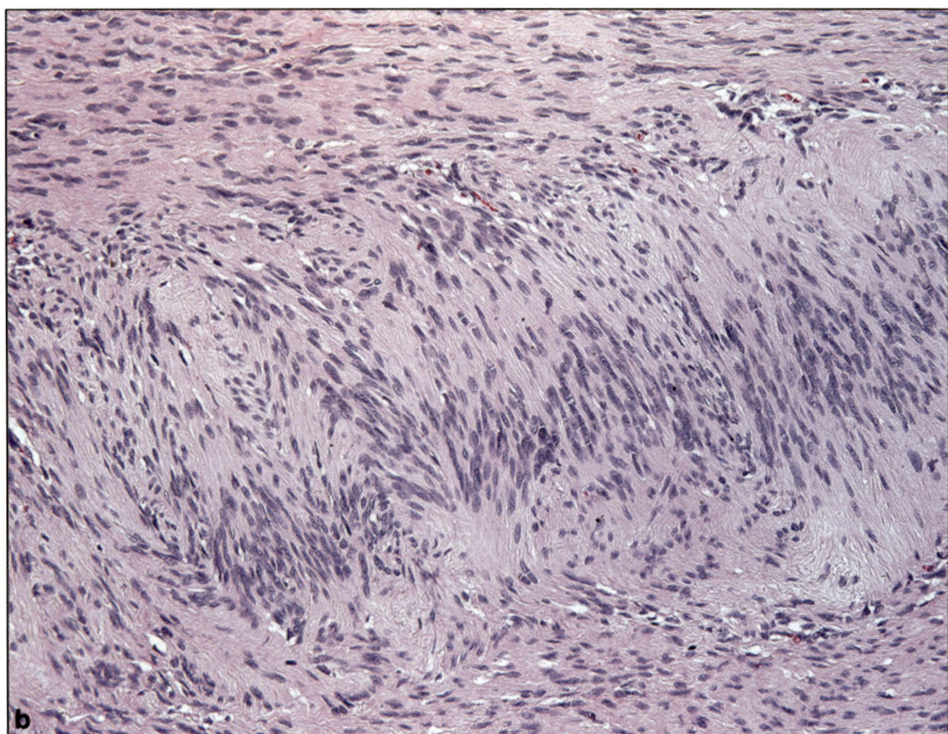

pattern) (Figure 3.69). The nuclei of neoplastic Schwann cells are gently undulating and may show nuclear vacuolation. The ends of the nuclei are classically described as tapered rather than blunt although a spectrum clearly exists in most tumors and as an isolated finding carries little discriminatory value. Significant

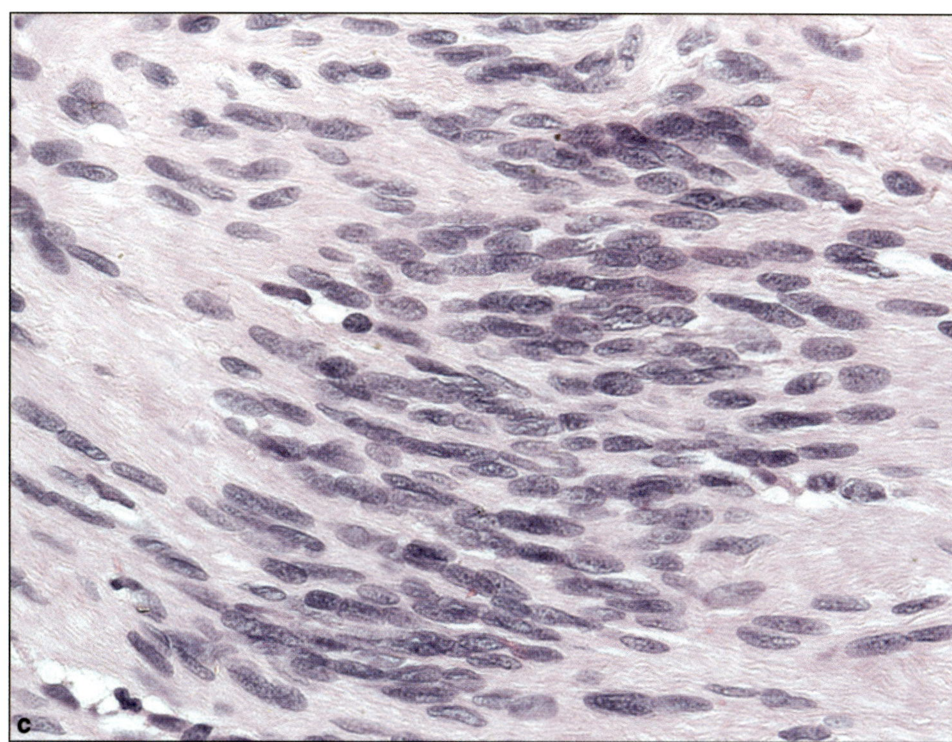

Figure 3.69. *continued* (c) Typical nuclei of a schwannoma display a slightly undulated contour with either tapered or rounded ends with a slightly vesicular change imparted by formalin fixation and paraffin embedding. (d) In some schwannoma resections involving peripheral nerve, the "parent" nerve may be seen compressed along the side of the mass (arrow).

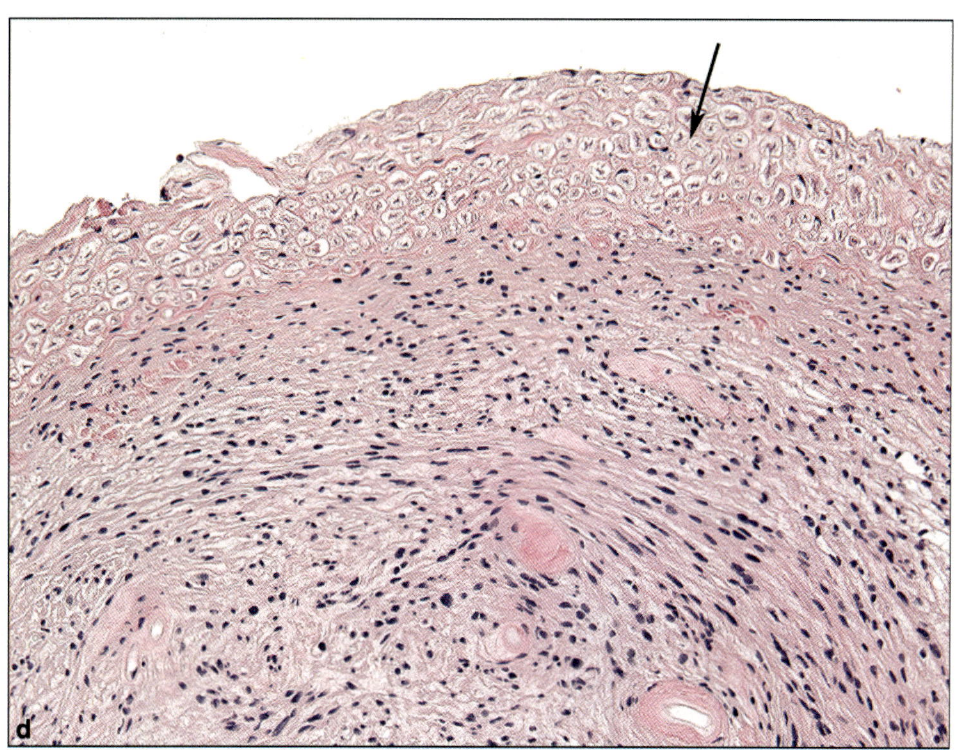

nuclear pleomorphism may occur including bizarre large nuclei representing the so-called ancient schwannoma, thus a feature of an indolent rather than aggressive tumor. Occasional mitotic figures may be seen.

A highly characteristic feature of schwannomas is thick-walled blood vessels, sometimes to the point of occlusion of the lumen through the extensive

Figure 3.69. *continued* (e) One of the most distinctive, if not specific, features of schwannomas is the thickened vascular walls with sometimes extreme hyaline sclerosis, seen here along with extensive myxoid degeneration. (f) Marked nuclear pleomorphism in an otherwise benign-appearing schwannoma signifies an indolent course, thus the term "ancient change."

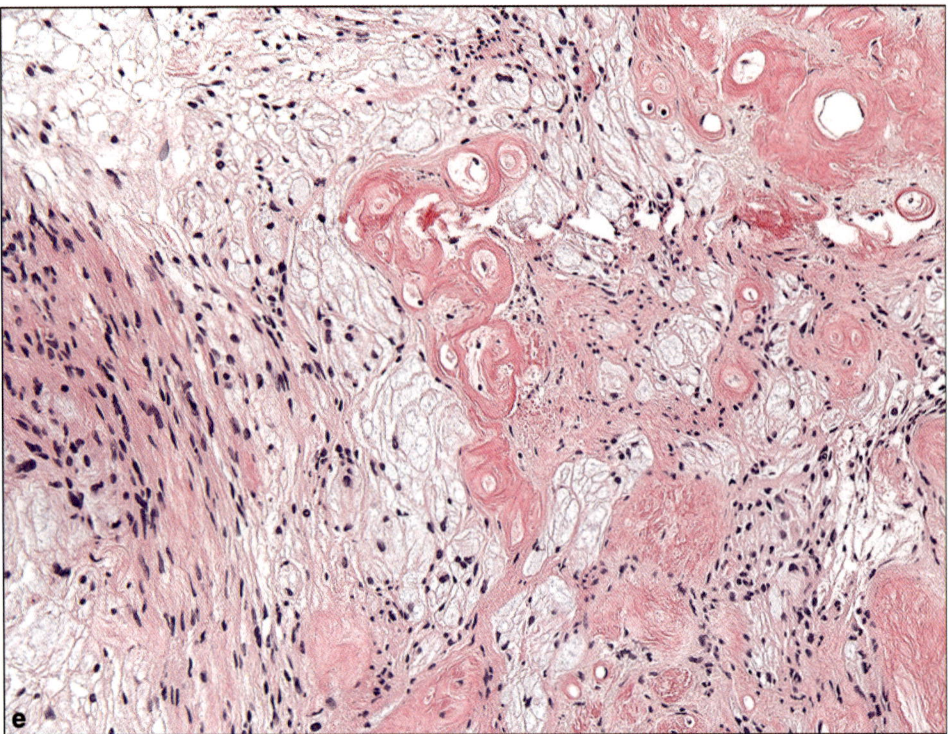

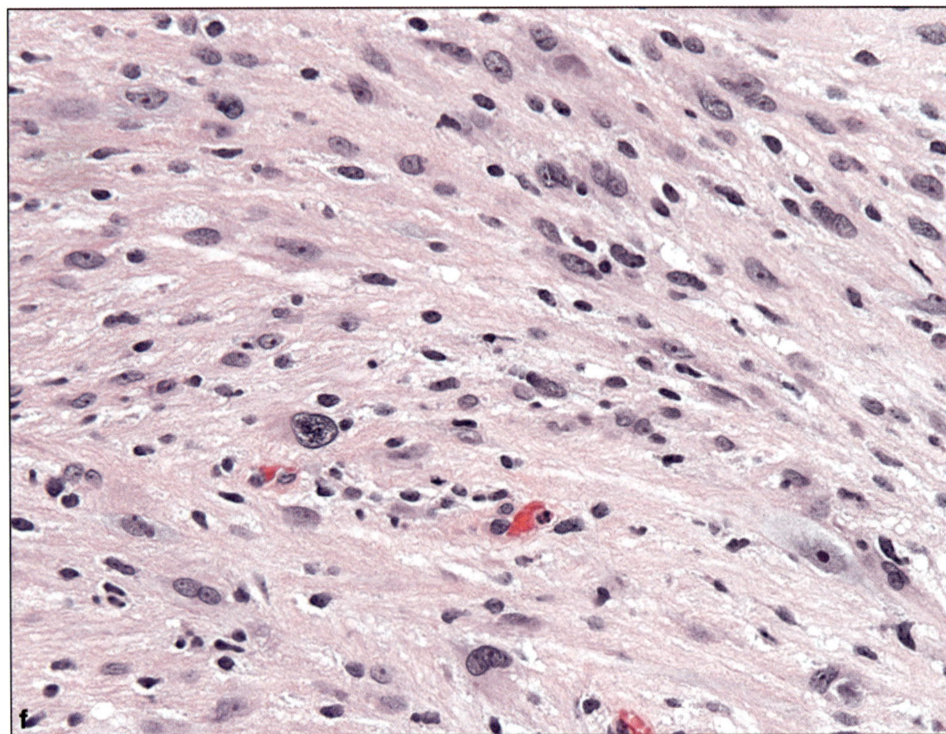

thickening and hyalinization. Verocay bodies are a highly useful but sometimes unapparent feature of schwannomas, particularly those of the eighth cranial nerve. In addition to immunohistochemistry, the reticulin stain will highlight pericellular reticulin deposition and correspondingly electron microscopy will reveal the lining of tumor cells by basal lamina.

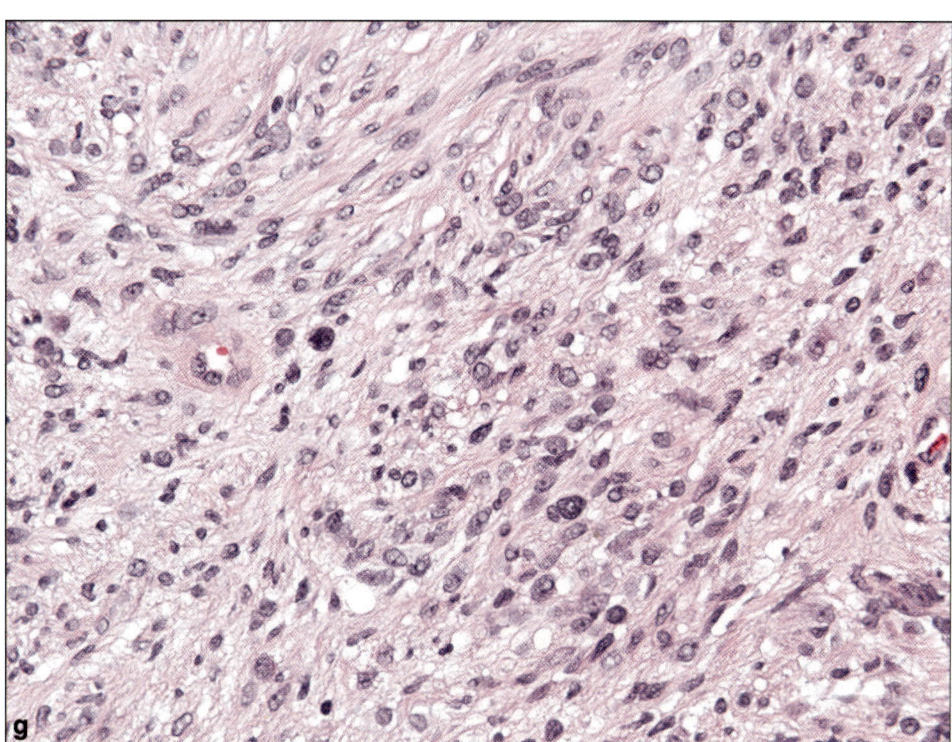

Figure 3.69. *continued*
(g) Some schwannomas show epithelioid features to the point of essentially lacking the appearance of a spindle cell tumor. (h) Unambiguous S-100 nuclear immunopositivity is a regular feature of all but the most poorly differentiated schwannoma.

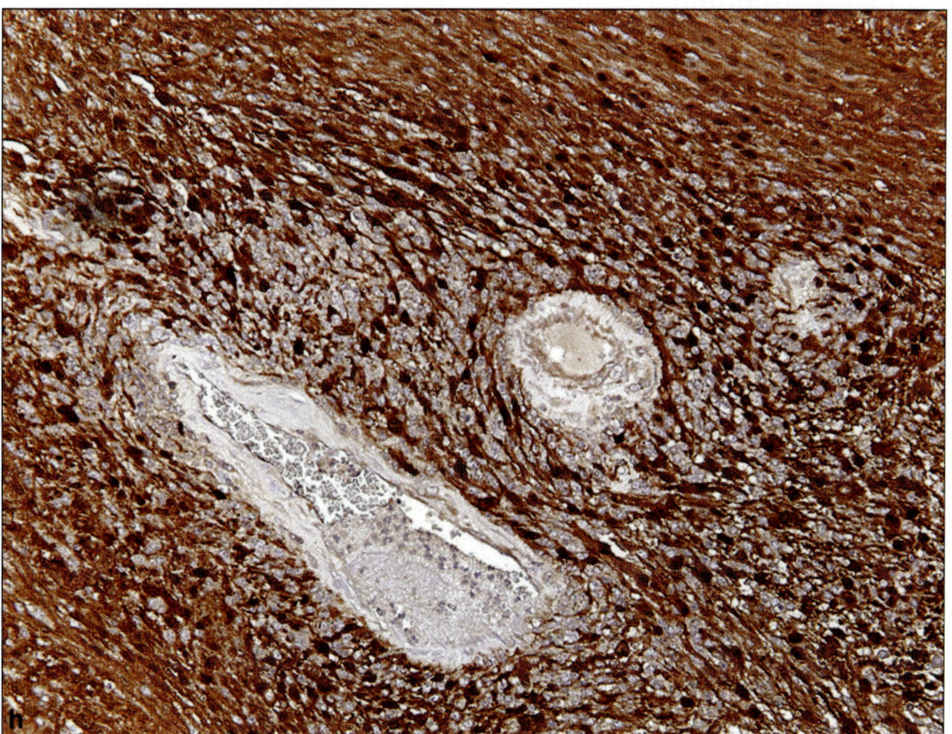

Schwannoma cells should be strongly and diffusely immunopositive for S-100 protein, may express Leu-7 and calretinin, and may focally express GFAP. Intra-lesional axons may be detected in small numbers by neurofilament immuno-histochemistry, particularly in NF2 or schwannomatosis-associated tumors (Wechsler et al., 2003).

Figure 3.70. Cellular schwannoma. Note the nuclear hyperchomasia and pleomorphism, and mitotic activity with a lack of well-formed Verocay bodies.

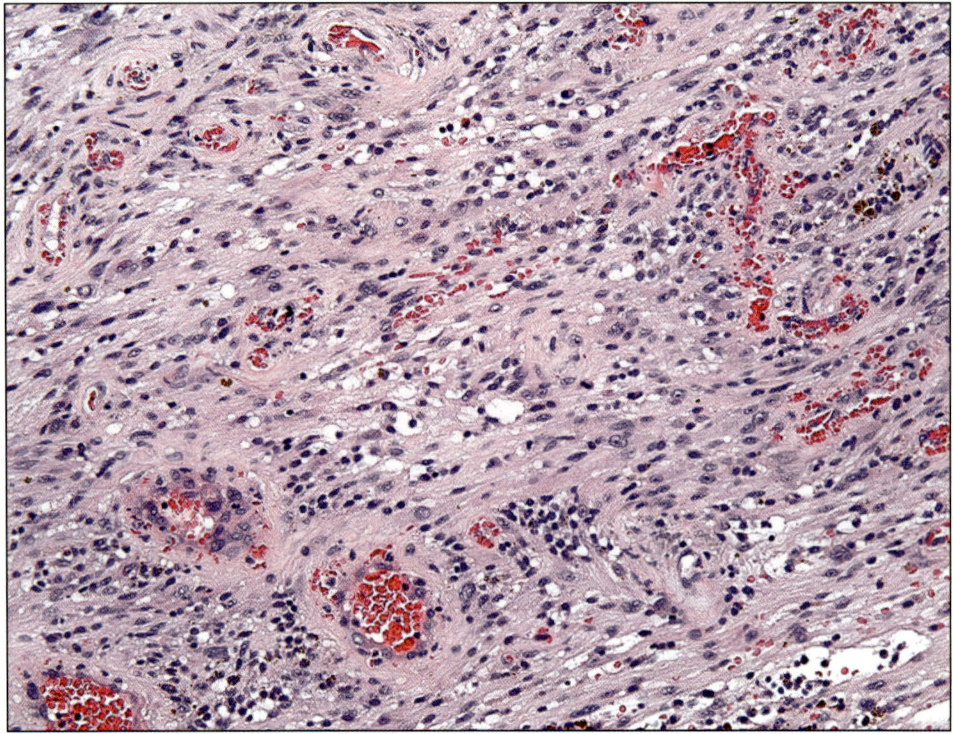

Cellular Schwannoma

The presence of predominantly Antoni A tissue and the nuclear zones of Verocay bodies yields a hypercellular appearance to this variant (Figure 3.70). They are more common in paravertebral locations in the pelvis, retroperitoneum, and mediastinum (Woodruff et al., 1981), although cranial nerves may be involved. Mitotic activity, although more common than in conventional schwannomas, is usually less than four per ten high-powered fields and should not be confused with the usually higher proliferative index seen in malignant peripheral nerve sheath tumors. Flow cytometry may show abnormalities in ploidy (Casadei et al., 1995). In spite of these abnormalities, cellular schwannomas should be considered more closely related to conventional schwannomas as no metastatic examples have been recorded and they almost never undergo malignant transformation.

Plexiform Schwannoma

These are most frequently encountered as a skin or subcutaneous tumor of an extremity, heads and neck, or trunk. They are not associated with NF1, have a low association with NF2, and have also been noted in non-NF2 patients with multiple schwannomas (schwannomatosis) (Iwashita and Enjoji, 1987). They are defined as schwannomas growing in a plexiform or multinodular manner, either with conventional or cellular histological features (Figure 3.71).

Melanotic Schwannoma

Schwannomas are rarely grossly pigmented and are composed of cells having the ultrastructure and immunophenotype of Schwann cells but containing

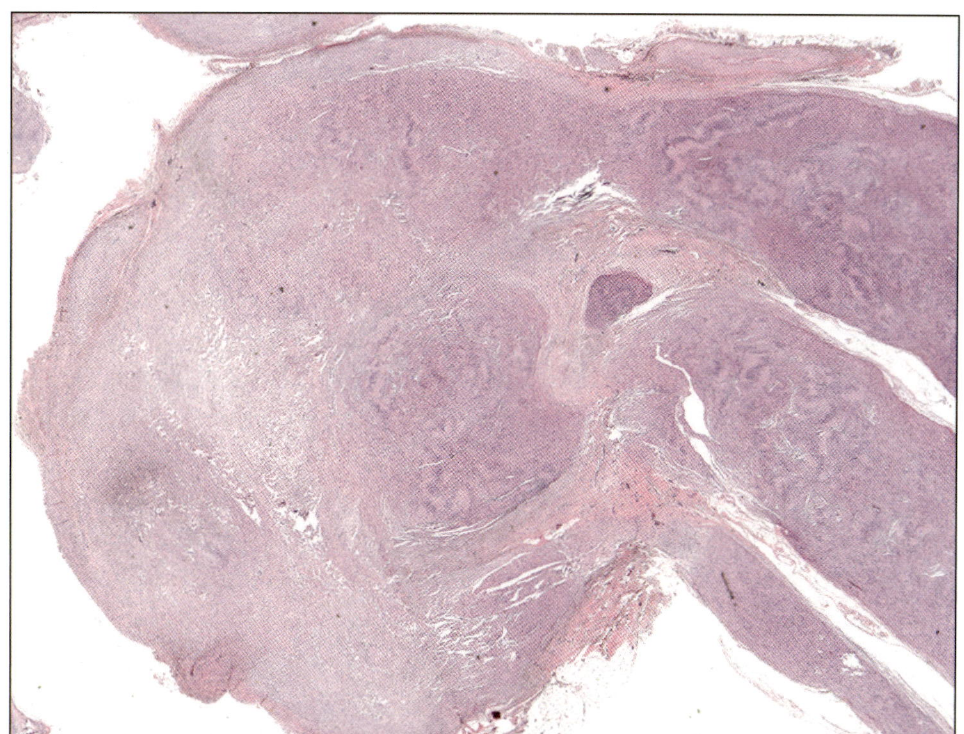

Figure 3.71. Plexiform is a term that may equally apply to wormlike masses comprising a schwannoma.

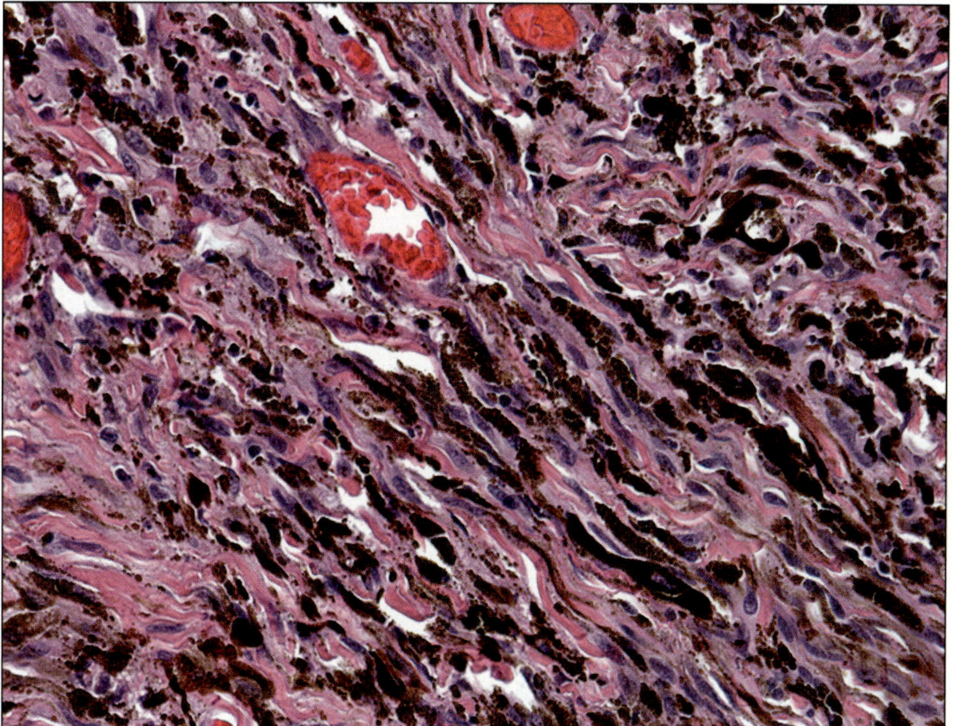

Figure 3.72. Melanotic schwannomas may be so densely pigmented as to obscure the nature of the underlying spindle cell proliferation.

melanosomes and showing immunoreactivity for melanoma markers (Figure 3.72). They may show conspicuous psammomatous calcification. In 50% of such examples, the patients have the Carney complex, an autosomal dominant disorder characterized by lentiginous facial pigmentation, cardiac myxoma, and endocrine abnormalities. Cytological atypia of may be seen, including hyperchromasia and macronucleoli. Bleaching of the tissue section prior to immunohistochemistry may be required in order to plainly reveal the immunophenotype.

NEUROFIBROMA

Clinical Features

Neurofibromas are composed of a mixture of three cell types, including Schwann cells, perineurial like cells, and fibroblasts. They may be multiple and present as a plexiform subtype in association with NF1; however, neurofibromas occur most commonly as sporadic solitary nodules. Neurofibromas correspond to WHO Grade I.

Neurofibromas occur most commonly as a painless subcutaneous nodule or circumscribed mass involving a peripheral nerve. They are seen as neurosurgical specimens when involving spinal roots but are essentially unknown in cranial nerves. Multiple or plexiform variants are characteristic of NF1 for which the presence of two or more of the following signs establishes the diagnosis:

1. Six or more café au lait macules (1.5 cm or larger in postpubertal individuals, 0.5 cm or larger in prepubertal individuals).
2. Two or more neurofibromas of any type or one or more plexiform neurofibromas.
3. Freckling of arm pits or groin.
4. Pilocytic astrocytoma of optic pathway.
5. Two or more Lisch nodules (iris hamartomas).
6. Dysplasia/absence of the sphenoid bone or dysplasia/thinning of long bone cortex.
7. First-degree relative with NF1.

Pathology

Grossly, *cutaneous neurofibromas* are nodular or polypoid relatively well-circumscribed masses involving skin and subcutaneous tissue. *Peripheral nerve neurofibromas* are well-circumscribed fusiform masses. *Plexiform neurofibromas* are traditionally determined by gross diagnosis, appearing as a multinodular mass composed of a tangle of wormlike cords.

Neurofibromas exhibit a wide range of microscopic appearances; however, they tend to include areas composed of well-spaced spindle cells with ovoid or elongated nuclei and poorly defined cytoplasm (Figure 3.73). There may be a variable matrix of collagen, sometimes showing a fragmented appearance reminiscent of "shredded carrots" (Figure 3.72). Mast cells are a regular feature. There may also be scattered lymphocytic infiltrates. Some examples contain discrete parallel arrays of spindle cells reminiscent of pressure receptors, referred to as pseudo-Meissnerian corpuscles. Others may show conspicuous and multiple aggregates of spindle cells showing Schwannian

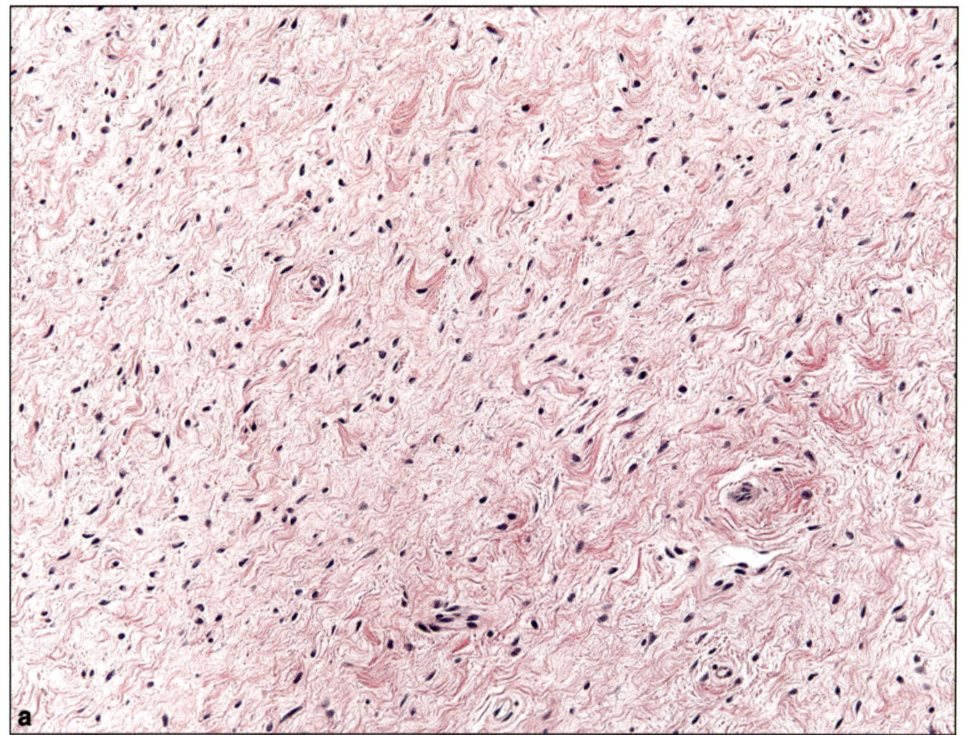

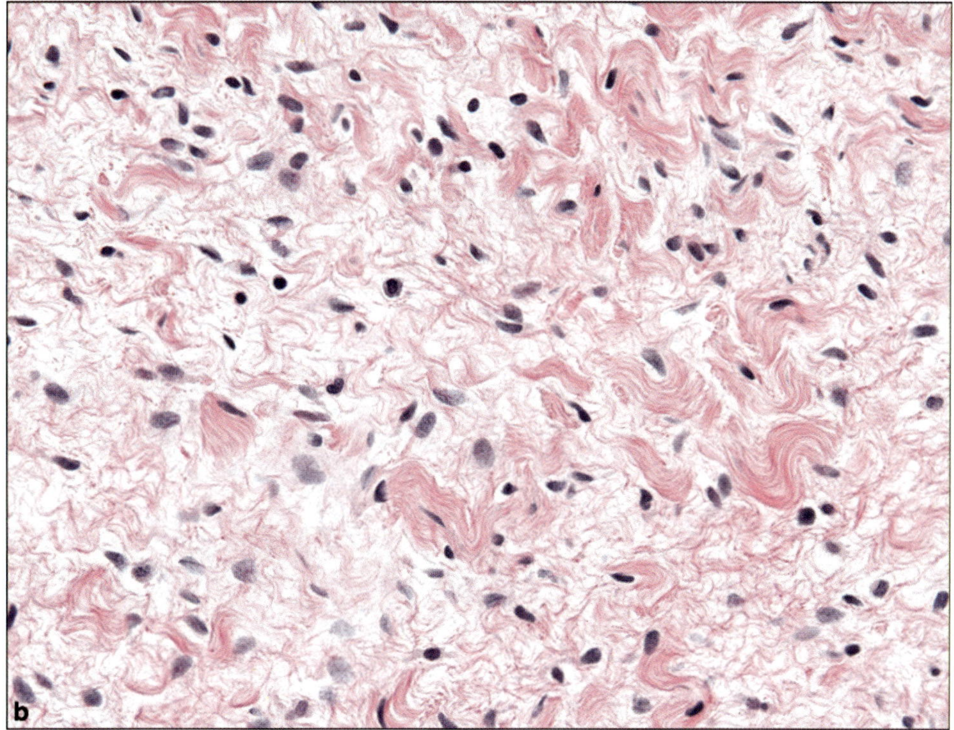

Figure 3.73. Neurofibromas show a very wide range of microscopic appearances because of their heterogeneous cellular composition with variable amounts of myxoid stroma or fibrous component, including (a, b) interspersed small strands of fibrous tissue resembling "shredded carrots," and (c) pseudo-Meissnerian corpuscles recapitulating the appearance of pressure receptors. Note the propensity to invade adipose tissue. (d) Neurofibroma with schwannoma-like nodules represents significant focal proliferation of Schwann cell elements, and provides an instructive contrast between the characteristic immunopositivity of Schwann cell nuclei for (e) S-100 and

differentiation, thus allowing the diagnosis of *neurofibroma with schwannoma-like nodules*. Neurofibromas may contain numerous atypical nuclei, termed *atypical neurofibroma*, or increased cellularity (*cellular neurofibroma*) although without significant increase in mitotic activity. Neither of these subtypes has been shown to carry a worse prognosis.

Figure 3.73. *continued.*

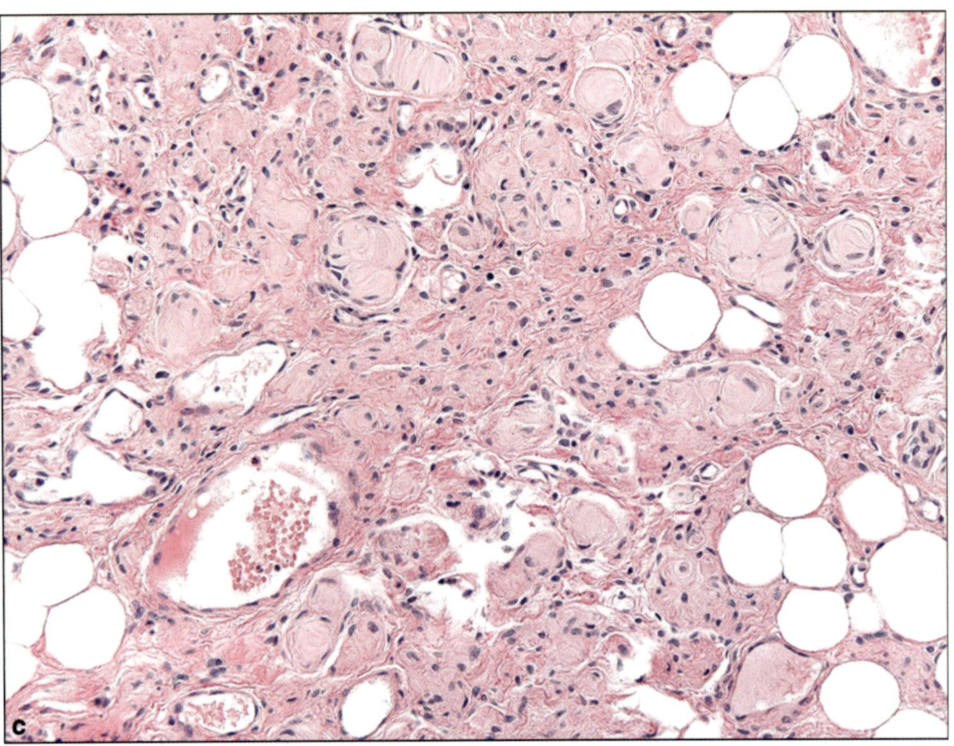

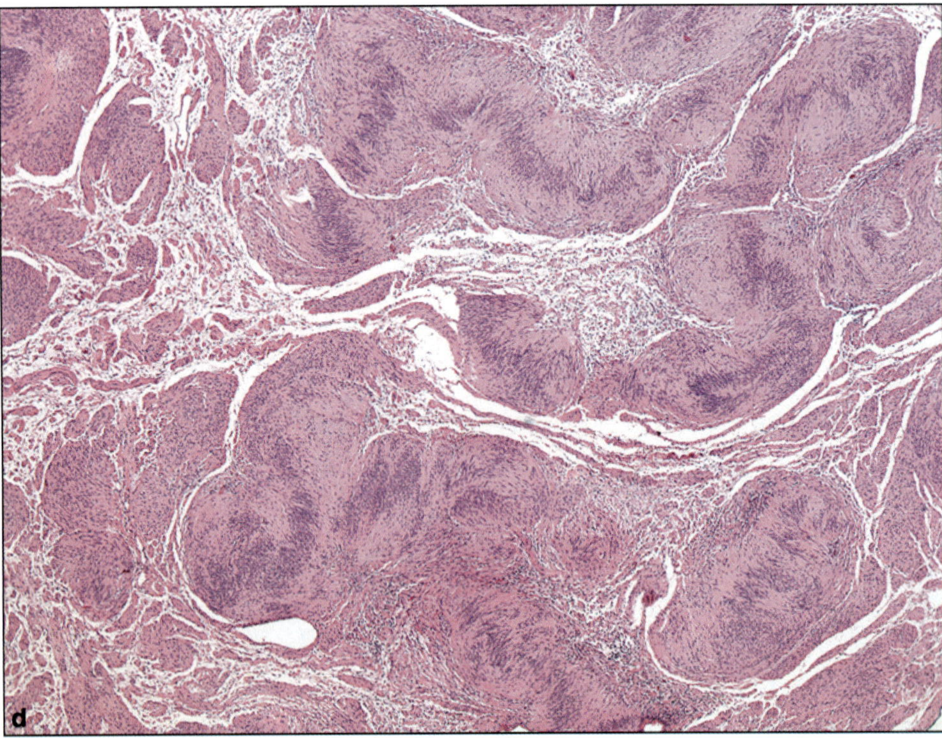

Immunohistochemistry may reveal that only a subset of cells is S-100 protein positive. CD34 may also be detected. The notion that the presence of neurofilament-positive fibers within a neurofibroma may help to distinguish them from schwannomas has been challenged, whereby these may be found in both examples (Nascimento and Fletcher, 2007).

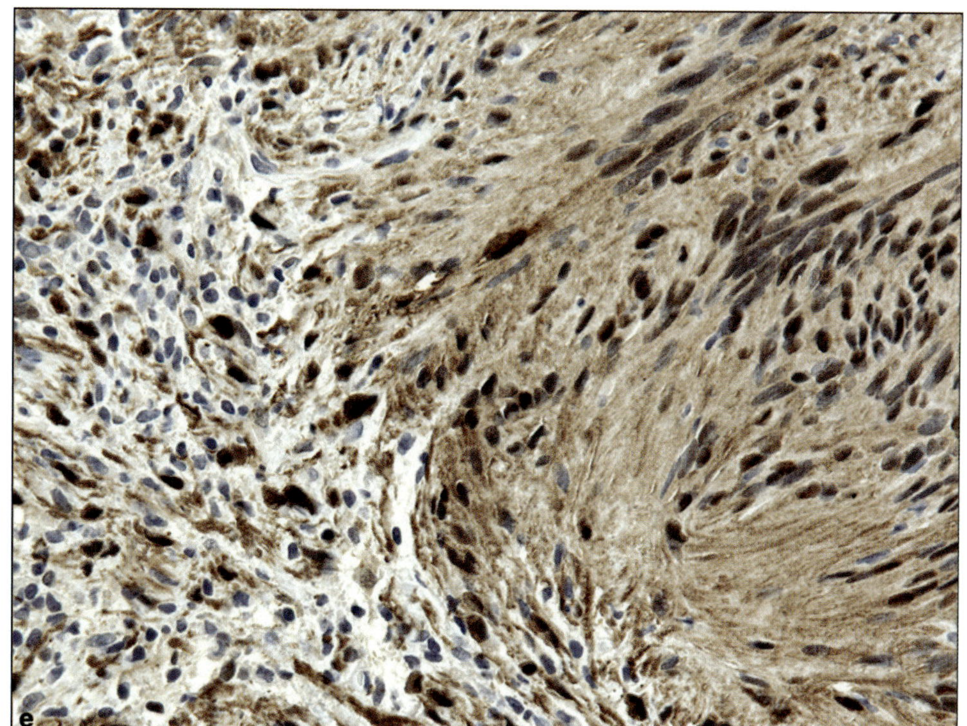

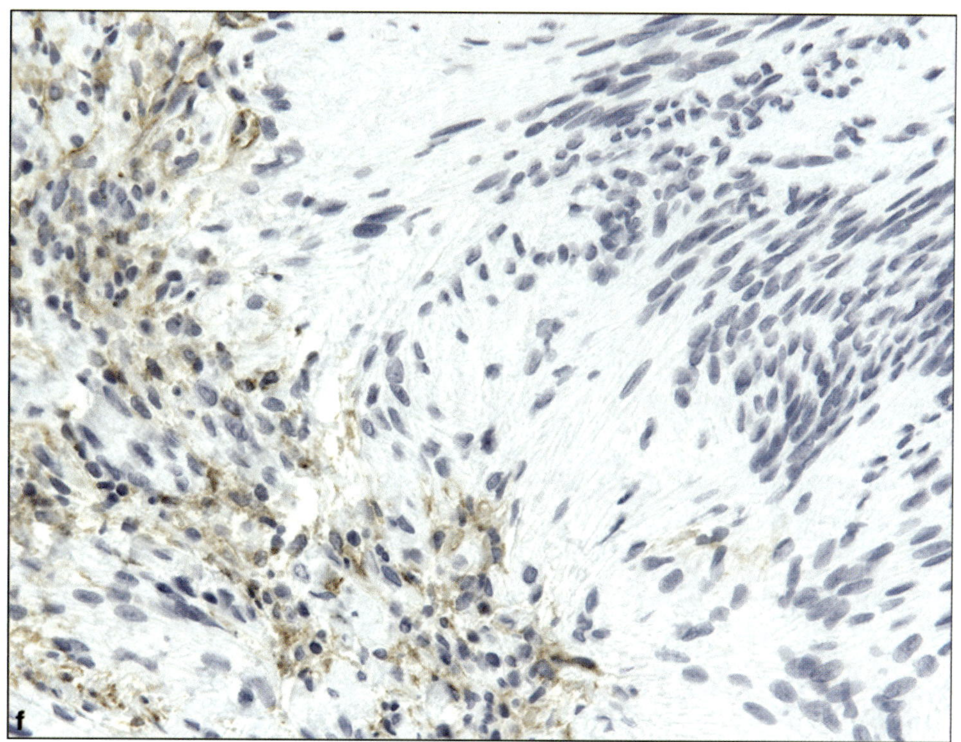

Figure 3.73. *continued* (f) CD34 positivity for neurofibroma stromal elements.

Plexiform Neurofibroma

Clinical Features

This is an uncommon but highly characteristic type of neurofibroma that preferentially involves large nerves. It occurs exclusively in NF1, although there is some debate over this point since rare examples of been reported in patients lacking other manifestations of NF1(McCarron and Goldblum, 1998). Plexiform neurofibromas have a propensity for malignant transformation, estimated to be approximately 10% over a lifetime. They may develop during the first 1 or 2 years of life as a single subcutaneous swelling with ill-defined margins. Later in life, they may cause a severe disfigurement, sometimes being even life-threatening when occurring in the head or neck region.

Pathology

These tangled, wormlike masses tend to reflect the degree of complexity in parent nerves such that highly branched nerves exemplified by paraspinal plexuses or number of fascicles in large caliber nerves like the sciatic results in the greatest degree of complexity. The mucin-rich stroma creates a glistening or translucent quality to the cut surface. The microscopic appearance of plexiform neurofibromas does not differ significantly from ordinary neurofibromas although the low-power examination will often highlight the curled and intersecting tumorous nerve bundles.

PERINEURIOMA

Clinical Features

There are two types of perineurioma: *intraneural* and *soft tissue*. Both types are associated with monosomy of chromosome 22. *Intraneural perineuriomas* were previously considered a form of hypertrophic neuropathy but are now recognized is an unusual cause of peripheral nerve sheath enlargement. Intraneural perineuriomas present in adolescents or early adulthood and cause progressive muscle weakness with variable muscle atrophy. Peripheral nerves and the extremities are more frequently involved although cranial nerve lesions have been rarely reported.

Soft tissue perineuriomas are not associated with nerves and are also quite rare. They occur predominately in the adult females with local mass effect within deep soft tissues. The general prognosis is favorable for perineuriomas, although rare instances of malignant transformation have been reported (Fukunaga, 2001; Hirose et al., 1998; Karaki et al., 1999). *Malignant perineuriomas* arising in the soft tissue are usually not associated with a peripheral nerve.

Pathology

Intraneural perineuriomas cause a segmental enlargement of the affected nerves by a tubular or fusiform mass resulting in significant enlargement.

Microscopically, they are formed by neoplastic perineurial cells proliferating throughout the nerve, forming concentric layers or whorls the around nerve fibers known as pseudo-onion bulbs, and forming vague fascicles (Figure 3.74).

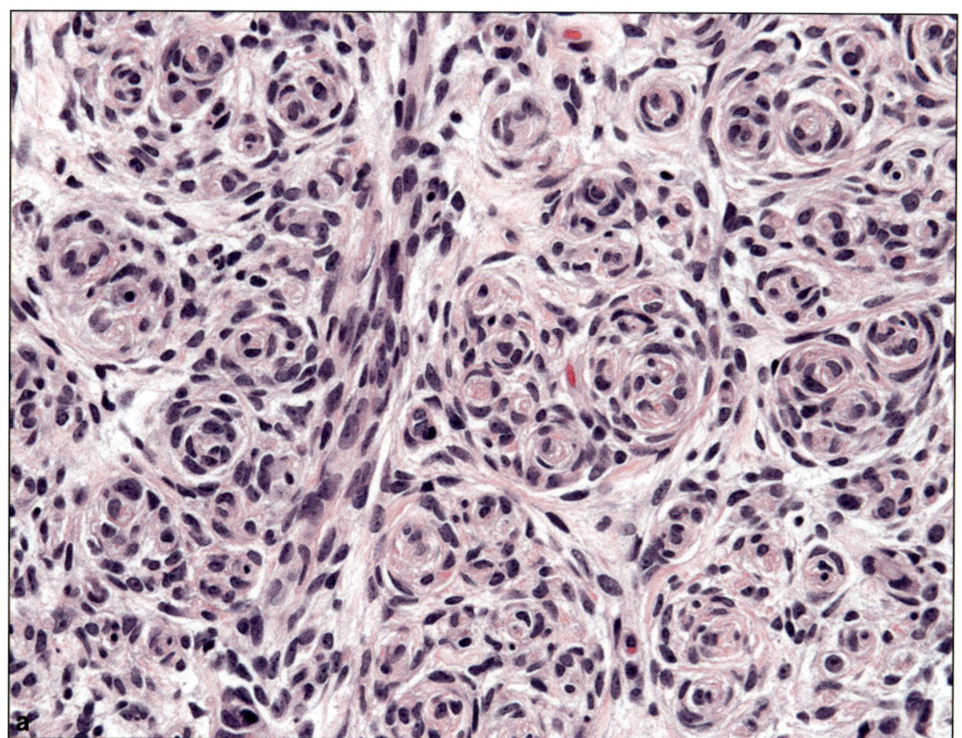

Figure 3.74. (a) Intraneural perineuriomas show numerous onion bulblike structures, with (b) immunopositivity for EMA in the dominant cellular component and (c) S-100 positivity within the centers.

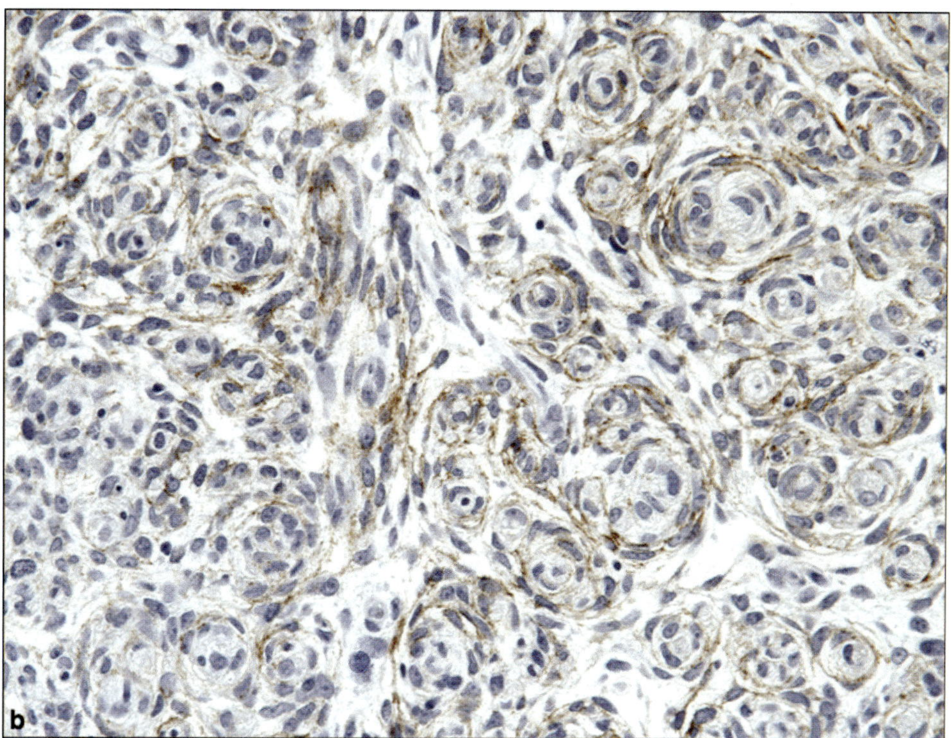

The proliferative process may extend into the perineurium. Axonal stains may show one or more axons at the center of the pseudo-onion bulb. Extensive hyalinization may also occur.

Soft tissue perineuriomas are composed of wavy spindle cells with thin cytoplasmic processes in layers and embedded in whorls of collagen fibers

Figure 3.74. *continued.*

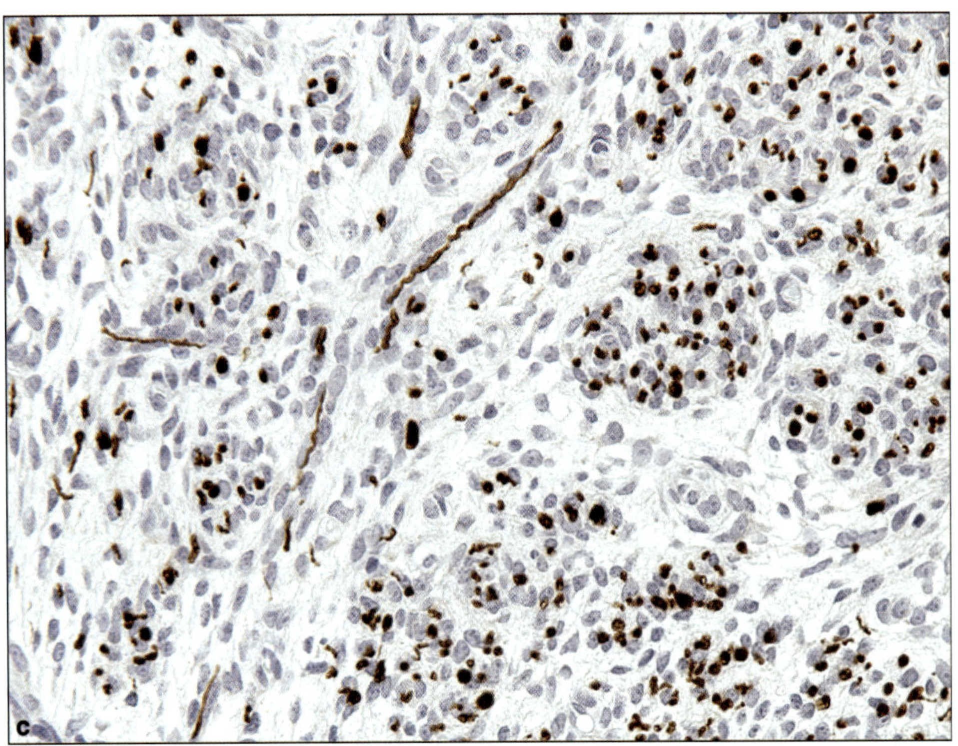

Figure 3.75. Soft tissue perineuriomas are spindle-cell tumors, sometimes with a vague storiform pattern.

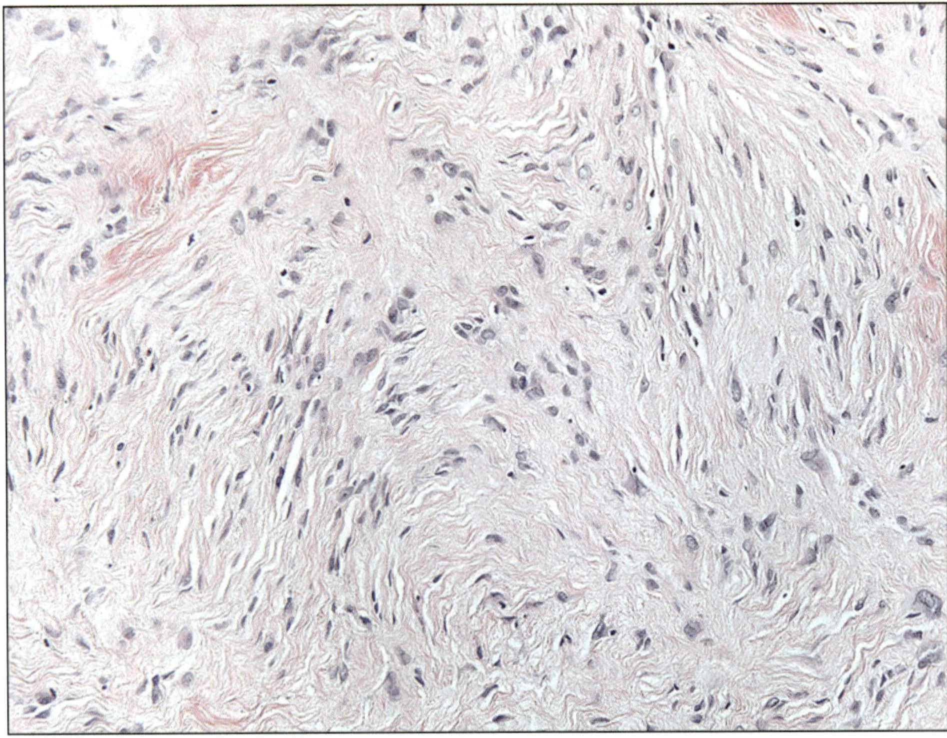

(Figure 3.75). A storiform pattern may be recognized. Mitotic figures are usually scant. "Degenerative atypia" represented by pleomorphic or hyperchromatic nuclei and nuclear cytoplasmic inclusions may be seen in tumors of long duration (Hornick and Fletcher, 2005). There may be extensive collagenous change, noted in examples occurring in the fingers of young males (Fetsch and

Miettinen, 1997). Malignant soft tissue perineuriomas show invasive growth characterized by hypercellularity, hyperchromasia, and sometimes brisk mitotic activity, resulting in WHO grade II and if variable necrosis is noted, warrants a WHO grade of III.

The hallmark of perineuriomas is the characteristic immunoreactivity for EMA in both normal and neoplastic perineurial cells. Other components of the lesion may be delineated such as Schwann cells by S-100 immunostaining and axons by neurofilament or silver impregnation techniques. EMA reactivity is usually preserved to some extent in malignant examples.

MALIGNANT PERIPHERAL NERVE SHEATH TUMOR

Clinical and Radiological Features

Malignant peripheral nerve sheath tumors (MPNSTs) affect young and middle-aged adults with a slight female predominance. Pediatric examples account for 13% of cases in one series (Ducatman et al., 1984). NF1 is associated with between 50% and 60% of MPNSTs. Ionizing radiation, either therapeutic or through occupational exposure, may contribute to the development of a MPNST, with a latency following irradiation averaging between 15 and 18 years with a range of 4–41 years.

MPNSTs are usually found in large- and medium-sized nervous of the buttock with the sciatic nerve being the most frequently affected, and in addition the thigh, brachial plexus, upper arm, and paraspinal nerves (Figure 3.76).

Wide resection is the treatment of choice with postoperative radiation therapy. Recurrence depends upon the extent of surgical resection. In the lower extremity and buttock, 40% may recur whereas over two-thirds recur in paraspinal locations. There is an overall metastatic rate of approximately 30–40% but is high as 65%, particularly in lesions arising in the lower extremity or buttock (Hruban et al., 1990). Mortality from tumor is

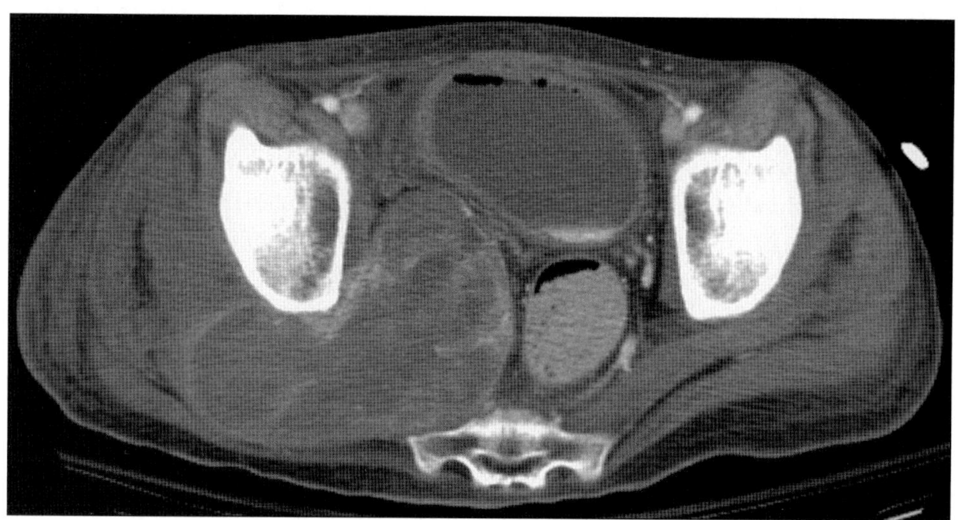

Figure 3.76. Malignant peripheral nerve sheath tumor. A contrast-enhanced axial CT shows a heterogeneously enhancing 12 cm mass in the greater sciatic notch, which is intimately associated with the sciatic nerve.

found in approximately two-thirds of patients and the presence of tumor at the resection margin figure greatly in predicting local recurrence and thus survival.

Pathology

The gross appearance of an MPNST may suggest that it has arisen in a large nerve in either a solitary or plexiform neurofibroma. They are globoid or fusiform and surrounded by a fibrous pseudocapsule of varying thickness. They display a firm opaque consistency on cut section with areas of necrosis grossly recognizable in the majority of cases. Pathologic sampling under ideal circumstances should allow for revealing the associated nerve or neurofibroma and the specimen should be treated with the goal of identifying resection margins.

MPNSTs show a wide diversity of histologic appearances as well as features that allow for grading. Generally speaking, they show features of a malignant spindle cell tumor composed of tightly packed cells with variable amounts of eosinophilic cytoplasm. Nuclei are elongated but in contrast to "benign" nerve sheath tumors, the nuclei are enlarged, hyperchromatic, and crowded. These findings may be especially useful in distinguishing a *low grade MPNST* from a cellular neurofibroma (Figure 3.77). It should be noted that finding of some mitotic activity may not be a reliable observation in distinguishing MPNST from lower grade tumors although the majority of MPNSTs exhibit a high mitotic index (Figure 3.78). In certain instances, it is possible to recognize a malignant transition from prior surgical resections or in the primary lesion of a transformation from a benign nerve sheath tumor such as neurofibroma, schwannoma, or ganglioneuroma/ganglioneuroblastoma to MPNST.

MPNSTs show histologic patterns reminiscent of fibrosarcoma or even a malignant fibrous histiocytoma. Pathologic patterns include storiform, loose whorls, nuclear palisading, perivascular crowding of tumor cells, and myxoid or edematous backgrounds in some cases. Some lesions may be highly vascular. And others may show heterologous mesenchymal elements including rhabdomyoblasts, benign or malignant cartilage and bone, melanotic, carcinomatous, or neuroendocrine elements. Areas of geographic necrosis are usually present and mitotic figures are typically abundant. Direct soft tissue and intraneural extension is common. Grading criteria are as follows: WHO Grade II MPNSTs (low-grade MPNST) are distinguished from cellular neurofibromas by increased cellularity, nuclear size greater than three times that of neurofibroma cells, and hyperchromasia. WHO Grade III examples show a higher degree of mitotic activity and atypical features, and WHO Grade IV lesions are those containing necrosis. Approximately 5% of MPNSTs are the epithelioid variant, which shows no association with NF1 and can arise in benign schwannomas.

MPNST with mesenchymal differentiation include the so-called *malignant Triton tumor*, defined as MPNST with rhabdomyosarcomatous differentiation. It is estimated that 60% of patients with malignant Triton tumor have NF1. *MPNST with*

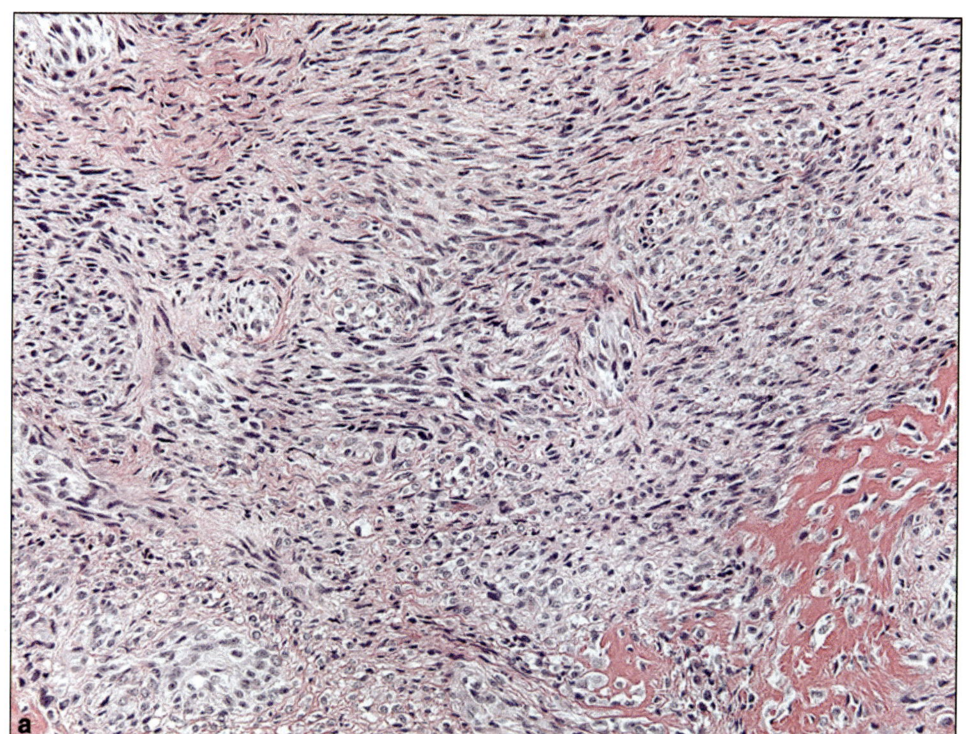

Figure 3.77. Low-grade MPNSTs are characterized by distinctly increased cellularity, nuclear size (>3 of neurofibroma nuclei), hyperchromasia, and occasional mitotic activity.

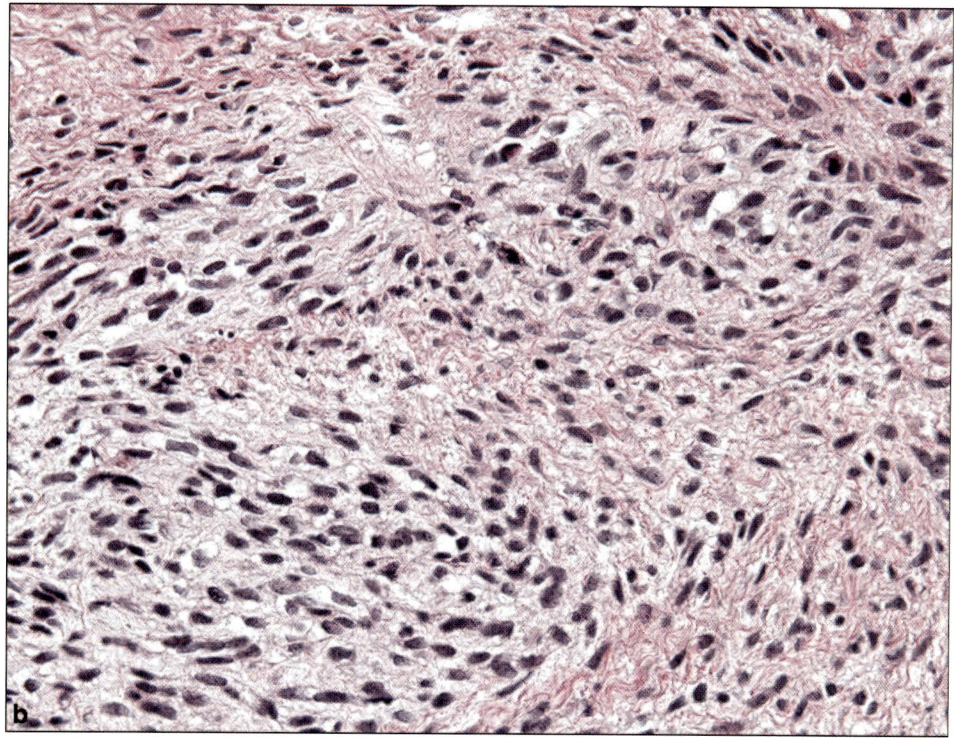

glandular differentiation by definition includes benign glandular epithelium resembling that of the intestine, frequently accompanied by endocrine differentiation.

Judging from the great heterogeneity histologic differentiation and degrees of malignancy, immunohistochemistry can be of use in excluding entities commonly placed on the differential diagnosis of MPNST. Cytokeratin may be seen

Figure 3.78. (a) High-grade MPNSTs are cellular malignancies with brisk mitotic activity, with a plethora of histological variations and forms of differentiation including a herringbone pattern of growth. (b) The presence of necrosis, present in the left portion of this photomicrograph, allows for a distinction between WHO Grads III and IV MPNST.

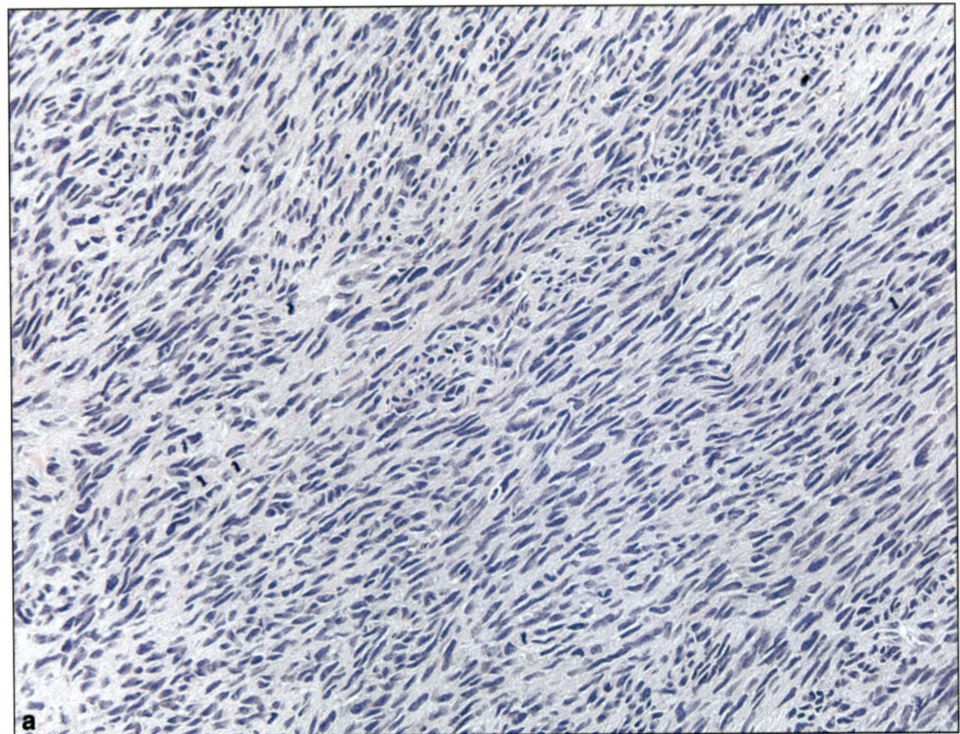

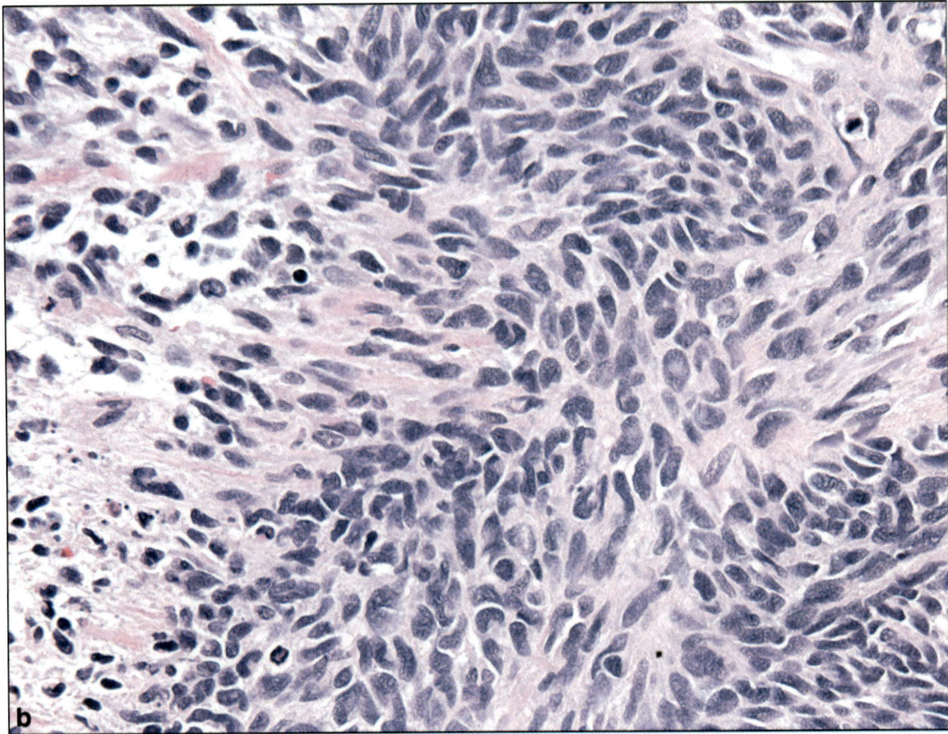

in epithelioid or synovial sarcoma and only focally in the glandular variant of MPNST, along with carcinoembryonic antigen (CEA). Twenty percent of schwannomas may show GFAP immunopositivity but this is rarely present in an MPNST although it is negative in other sarcomas. Similarly, S-100 protein is present in almost all "benign" nerve sheath tumors and present in approximately 50–70% of MPNSTs depending on the degree of dedifferentiation.

Aside from the grading of MPNSTs, histologic subtypes may have a bearing upon prognosis, with the perineurial MPNST being less aggressive and MPNST with mesenchymal or glandular differentiation showing distinctly poor prognoses.

TRAUMATIC NEUROMA

Clinical Features

Common clinical circumstances producing traumatic neuromas include brachial plexus avulsion injury from shoulder dystocia occurring in some vaginal deliveries, and other forms of either complete transection or crush injury of nerves, sometimes postsurgically or after seemingly insignificant trauma.

Pathology

These appear grossly as the firm nodular masses with an associated nerve. Histologic preparations will often reveal a transition from a relatively intact nerve to the neuromatous component, which is composed of small nodules of proliferating Schwann cells in a collagenous matrix (Figure 3.79). Close inspection will reveal bundles of regenerating axons within the Schwannian nodules. The stroma may be mucinous. The scarring reaction may include regional adipose or skeletal muscle tissue.

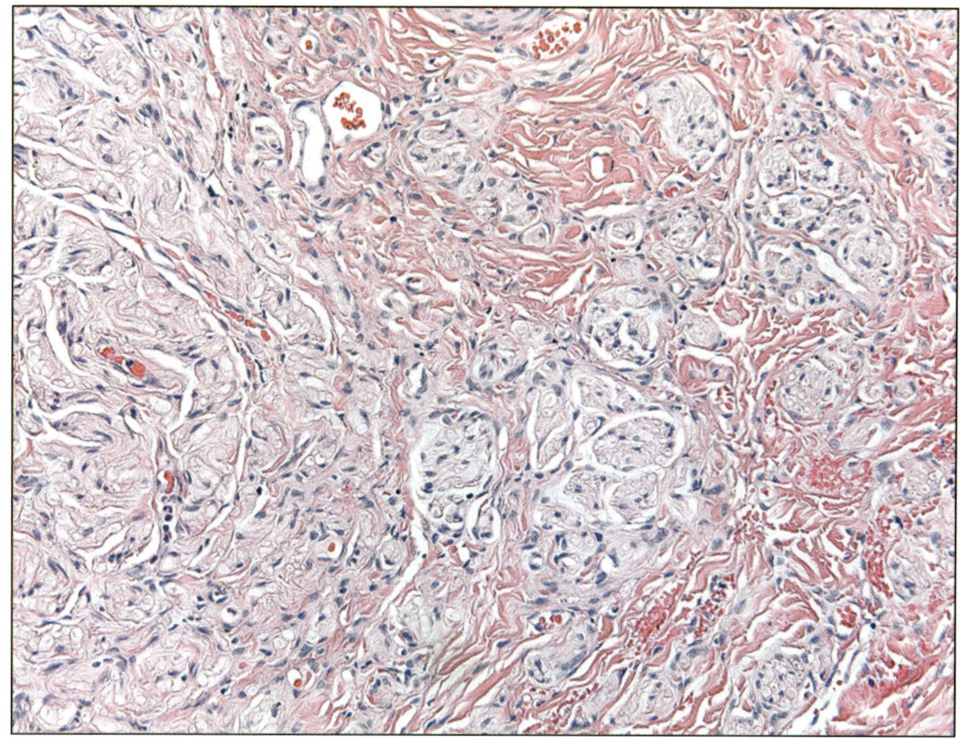

Figure 3.79. Traumatic neuromas contain distinctive loose aggregates of proliferating Schwann cells intimately associated with axonal sprouting, in a variably dense fibrotic background.

REFERENCES

Antinheimo J, Sankila R, Carpen O, Pukkala E, Sainio M, Jaaskelainen J. Population-based analysis of sporadic and type 2 neurofibromatosis-associated meningiomas and schwannomas. *Neurology* 2000; 54: 71–6.

Casadei GP, Komori T, Scheithauer BW, Miller GM, Parisi JE, Kelly PJ. Intracranial parenchymal schwannoma. A clinicopathological and neuroimaging study of nine cases. *J Neurosurg* 1993; 79: 217–22.

Casadei GP, Scheithauer BW, Hirose T, Manfrini M, Van Houton C, Wood MB. Cellular schwannoma. A clinicopathologic, DNA flow cytometric, and proliferation marker study of 70 patients. *Cancer* 1995; 75: 1109–19.

Ducatman BS, Scheithauer BW, Piepgras DG, Reiman HM. Malignant peripheral nerve sheath tumors in childhood. *J Neurooncol* 1984; 2: 241–8.

Fetsch JF, Miettinen M. Sclerosing perineurioma: a clinicopathologic study of 19 cases of a distinctive soft tissue lesion with a predilection for the fingers and palms of young adults. *Am J Surg Pathol* 1997; 21: 1433–42.

Fukunaga M. Unusual malignant perineurioma of soft tissue. *Virchows Arch* 2001; 439: 212–14.

Hirose T, Scheithauer BW, Sano T. Perineurial malignant peripheral nerve sheath tumor (MPNST): a clinicopathologic, immunohistochemical, and ultrastructural study of seven cases. *Am J Surg Pathol* 1998; 22: 1368–78.

Hornick JL, Fletcher CD. Soft tissue perineurioma: clinicopathologic analysis of 81 cases including those with atypical histologic features. *Am J Surg Pathol* 2005; 29: 845–58.

Hruban RH, Shiu MH, Senie RT, Woodruff JM. Malignant peripheral nerve sheath tumors of the buttock and lower extremity. A study of 43 cases. *Cancer* 1990; 66: 1253–65.

Iwashita T, Enjoji M. Plexiform neurilemmoma: a clinicopathological and immuno-histochemical analysis of 23 tumours from 20 patients. *Virchows Arch A Pathol Anat Histopathol* 1987; 411: 305–9.

Karaki S, Mochida J, Lee YH, Nishimura K, Tsutsumi Y. Low-grade malignant perineurioma of the paravertebral column, transforming into a high-grade malignancy. *Pathol Int* 1999; 49: 820–5.

McCarron KF, Goldblum JR. Plexiform neurofibroma with and without associated malignant peripheral nerve sheath tumor: a clinicopathologic and immunohistochemical analysis of 54 cases. *Mod Pathol* 1998; 11: 612–17.

Nascimento AF, Fletcher CD. The controversial nosology of benign nerve sheath tumors: neurofilament protein staining demonstrates intratumoral axons in many sporadic schwannomas. *Am J Surg Pathol* 2007; 31: 1363–70.

Urich H, Tien RD. Tumors of the cranial, spinal and peripheral nerve sheaths. In: Bigner DD, McLendon RE, Bruner JM, Russell DS, editors. *Russell and Rubinstein's Pathology of Tumors of the Nervous System*. London, New York: Arnold, Oxford University Press, 1998.

Wechsler J, Lantieri L, Zeller J, Voisin MC, Martin-Garcia N, Wolkenstein P. Aberrant axon neurofilaments in schwannomas associated with phacomatoses. *Virchows Arch* 2003; 443: 768–73.

Woodruff JM, Godwin TA, Erlandson RA, Susin M, Martini N. Cellular schwannoma: a variety of schwannoma sometimes mistaken for a malignant tumor. *Am J Surg Pathol* 1981; 5: 733–44.

TUMORS OF THE MENINGES

Meningiomas

Clinical and Radiological Features

Meningiomas are defined as meningeal tumors arising from meningothelial arachnoid cells, typically arising at the inner surface of the dura mater. They show a staggering diversity of locations, growth patterns, and histologic variations such that in both the neuroanatomical and histological senses they are the great mimicker of many other pathological entities.

Meningiomas account for approximately 30% of all primary brain tumors and are thus the single most common "brain" tumor, excluding glioblastoma as the most common glioma, in persons over the age of 35 years (Claus et al., 2005). In middle-aged adults, meningiomas are distinctly more common in females (Longstreth et al., 1993). Spinal meningiomas are also more common in women (Cohen-Gadol et al., 2003), accounting for almost 90% in some series among the older patients (Gezen et al., 2000).

Meningiomas are also recognized in childhood and represent the most common dural or leptomeningeal based neoplasm in this age group. Pediatric meningiomas may be characterized by large size at diagnosis, cyst formation, intraparenchymal location and high-grade histology, aggressive behavior, particularly in the clear cell and papillary variants (Perry and Dehner, 2003; Rushing et al., 2005). Unlike in adults, there is a male predilection in pediatric meningiomas. Pediatric meningiomas are also within the spectrum of postirradiation tumors.

Multiple meningiomas are a cardinal feature of NF2 and occur in half of NF2 patients (Louis et al., 1995). Forty percent of pediatric patients with meningioma have NF2 (Perry and Dehner, 2003).

The vast majority of meningiomas arise in obvious association with the dura in intracranial, intraspinal, or orbital locations. Intraventricular meningiomas may occur, arising in the tela choroidea at the base of the choroid plexus. Most spinal meningiomas are in the thoracic region. Meningiomas have also been reported in nonneural tissue such as the lung (Maiorana et al., 1996; Picquet et al., 2005; van der Meij et al., 2005) and temporal bone (Kuzeyli et al., 1996; Marcelissen et al, 2008; O'Reilly et al., 1998).

Radiographically, meningiomas typically are well-circumscribed dural-based masses with homogeneous contrast enhancement (Figure 3.80). A small tapering portion at the edge is often referred to as the "dural tail." A cystic component is not uncommon.

Pathology

The gross pathology of meningiomas reflects their usually discrete globular appearance in association with dura. An *en plaque* variant, usually found over the sphenoid wing, is a flattened mass without formation of the usual globular mass. The external surface of most meningiomas is cobblestoned or bosselated

Figure 3.80. (a) An axial T1 contrast-enhanced MRI study shows a homogeneously enhancing extracerebral mass compressing the frontal lobe. The mass displays dural tails, which are suggestive, but not diagnostic of meningioma. Conversely, they are not often seen in pediatric meningiomas. A dural blood vessel is seen supplying the core of the meningioma; pial vessels typically supply the surface of meningiomas. Visualization of cortical vessels interposed between meningioma and brain parenchyma can help localize meningiomas to the extraaxial space. (b) A coronal T1 contrast-enhanced MRI in a different patient shows similar homogeneous enhancement in a mass centered within the middle cranial fossa, extending into the cavernous sinus and encircling the carotid artery. Meningiomas tend to cause narrowing of the cavernous carotid artery whereas pituitary adenomas do not. Meningiomas can be difficult to distinguish by neuroimaging from metastases, from pituitary adenomas in the sellar region, and from schwannomas in the cerebellopontine angle or spinal roots.

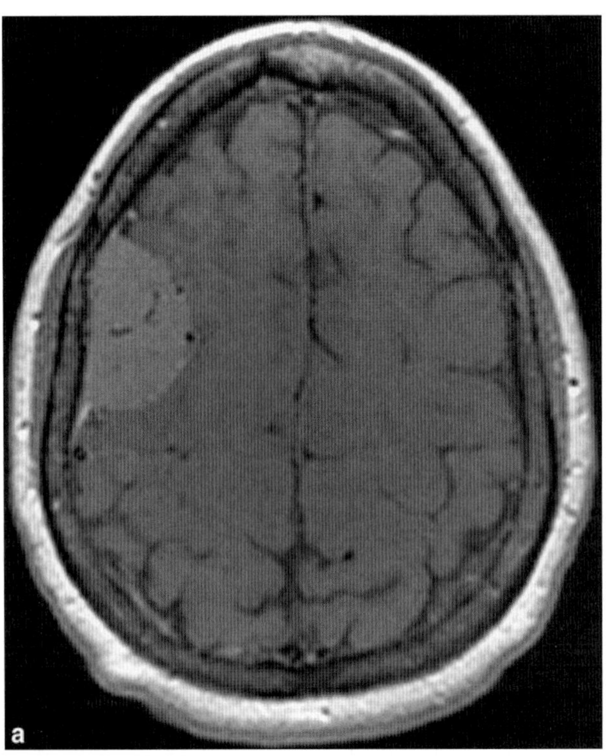

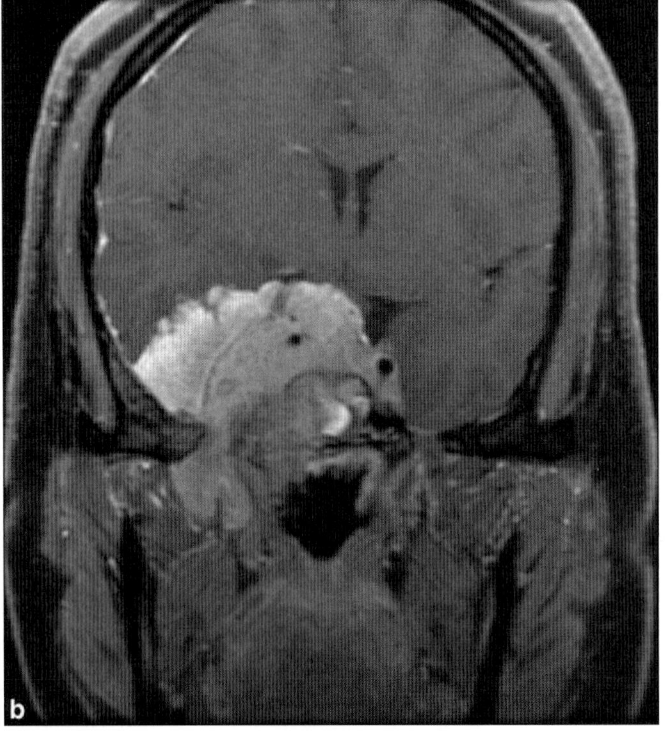

and may be appreciated in cut section as well. Fibrous meningiomas are known to be exceptionally smooth and well demarcated. Lipidic or xanthomatous change may be signified by a yellow–orange color. Secretory meningiomas may have a glistening mucoid cut surface. An unusual form of meningothelial

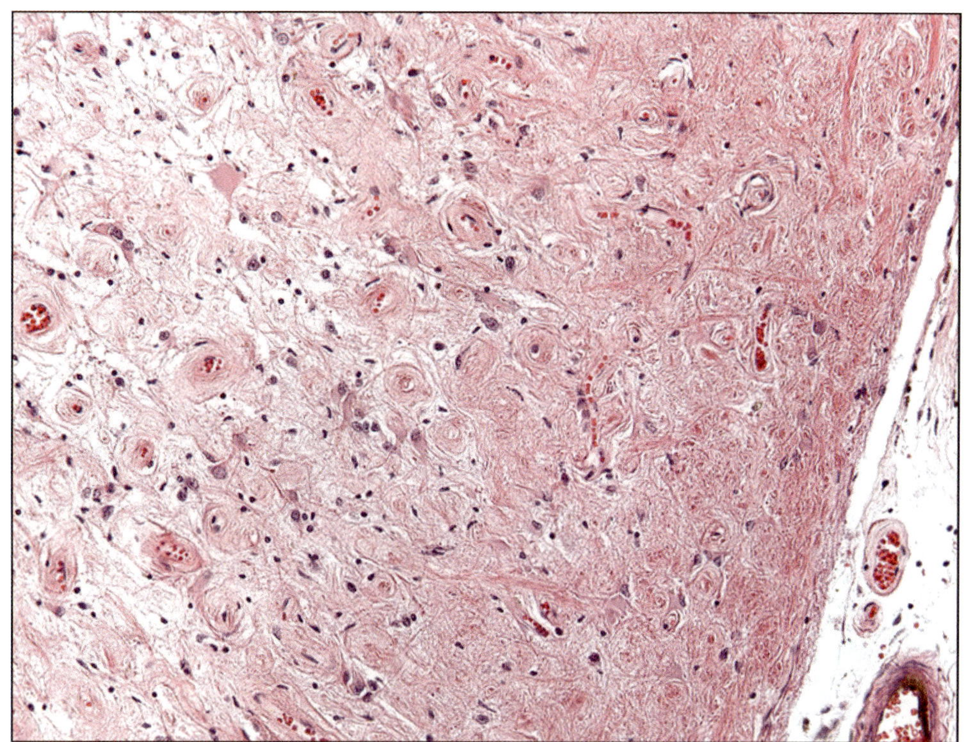

Figure 3.81. Meningioangiomatosis. Cortical blood vessels are surrounded by spindle cells with associated gliosis, and atypical neuronal changes in some examples.

cell proliferation is represented by meningioangiomatosis, a lesion of presumed hamartomatous origin that is commonly associated with seizures, with a male predominance. It occasionally occurs combined with meningioma. It is recognized as a plaquelike firm cerebral mass, most often involving the temporal and frontal lobes. The microscopic pathology includes a wide spectrum of changes, but the essential features are intracortical and leptomeningeal collections of small blood vessels with perivascular spindle cells (Figure 3.81), and varying degrees of gliosis, hyalinization, and calcification. Entrapped neurons may show unusual changes, including granulovacuolar degeneration and neurofibrillary tangles (Perry et al., 2005).

Immunohistochemistry

The standard immunohistochemical marker in meningioma is EMA, present in the vast majority of meningiomas (Schnitt and Vogel, 1986). However, EMA immunoreactivity is less consistent in atypical and malignant forms. The characteristic intermediate filament of meningiomas is vimentin, which is a reliable if not entirely discriminatory marker in all meningiomas. S-100 protein may be present focally and in a cytoplasmic staining pattern without classic nuclear positivity in approximately 40% of meningiomas. As noted below, CEA shows the cytoplasmic inclusions in secretory meningiomas.

One study indicates that p63 may be used to distinguish characteristically immunonegative WHO Grade I meningiomas from often p63-positive WHO Grades II and III meningiomas (Rushing et al., 2008).

Proliferative Indices in Meningiomas

Just as gliomas show a progression in grade closely linked to their proliferative indices, the mitotic index in meningiomas is related to the risk of recurrence and invasion or even metastatic spread. Mitotic figures are rare, meaning far less than one per ten high-powered fields in WHO Grade I examples, average approximately five per ten high-powered fields in atypical meningiomas and approximately nineteen per ten high-powered fields in malignant meningiomas (Hsu et al., 1994). The MIB-1 proliferative index is also useful with average percentages of 3.8%, 7.2%, and 14.7% in benign, atypical, and anaplastic meningiomas, respectively (Maier et al., 1997).

The challenge for the diagnostic pathologist is in identifying examples of "benign" meningiomas with an increased propensity for recurrence, since as a group there is a recurrence rate of 7–25%. A meningioma without diagnostic features of atypicality (WHO Grade II) but with a proliferative index of greater than 4% may be designated as a *meningioma with increased proliferative potential* and thus signifying a need for close clinical follow-up. The absence of progesterone receptors has also been linked with poor outcome along with a high mitotic index and malignant grade (Perry et al., 1999).

Some studies suggest that meningiomas associated with NF2 have a higher mitotic index and more aggressive behavior than sporadic meningiomas (Antinheimo et al., 1997; Perry et al., 2001).

WHO GRADE I

Meningothelial

This is the most common and classic variant of meningioma. Cells form lobules or swirling fascicles of cells in a syncytial background, in which cell borders cannot be discerned, but rather the background exists as a delicate interwoven web of cellular processes (Figure 3.82). Whorls of varying size are usually identifiable. These specimens show the classic nuclear features of meningiomas, which may be seen in other types as well, namely ovoid nuclei with optically empty nuclear pseudoinclusions. Multinucleation or nuclear "degenerative" atypia may be seen in WHO Grade I meningiomas (Figure 3.83).

Some meningiomas may lack conspicuous whorls, and when collagen bands and "staghorn" vessels are noted may raise suspicion for solitary fibrous tumor/hemangiopericytoma (Figure 3.84) (page 206). Immunohistochemical demonstration of EMA in the former and CD34 in the latter should clarify the distinction. Most meningiomas represent the opportunity to use cytological preparations for intraoperative consultation, either as a squash preparation or particularly the touch preparation in displaying meningothelial whorls (Figure 3.85).

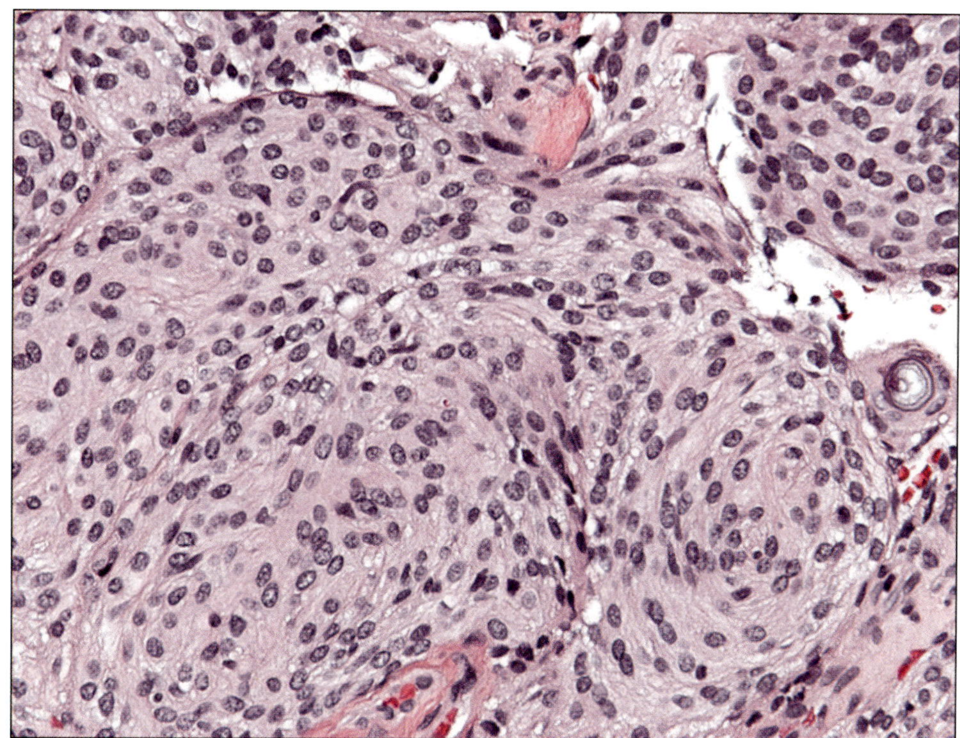

Figure 3.82. Meningothelial meningioma, representing the most classic appearance of meningiomas, with whorls, intranuclear inclusions, and a syncytial background.

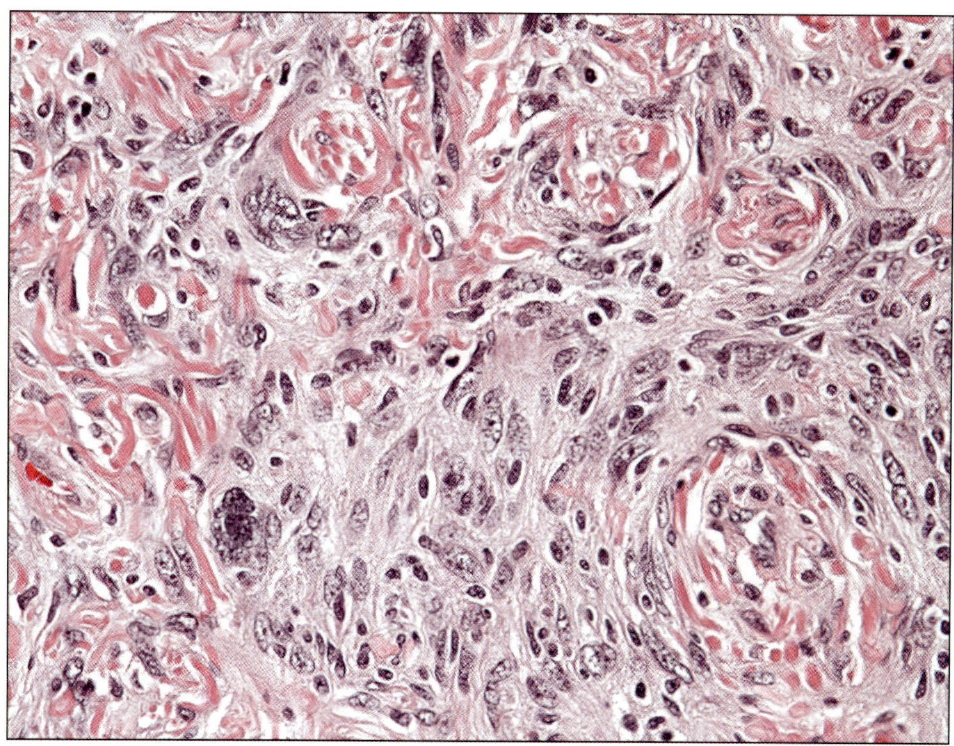

Figure 3.83. Some otherwise completely benign meningiomas may show nuclear pleomorphism or multinucleate cells, which should not be misinterpreted as signifying potentially aggressive behavior.

Fibrous (Fibroblastic)

The fibrous meningioma shows broad fascicles of elongated spindle cells with variable amounts of intercellular collagen deposition (Figure 3.86). Classical whorls may be inconspicuous. Mineralization of the collagen

Figure 3.84.
Hemangiopericytoma-like
meningioma.

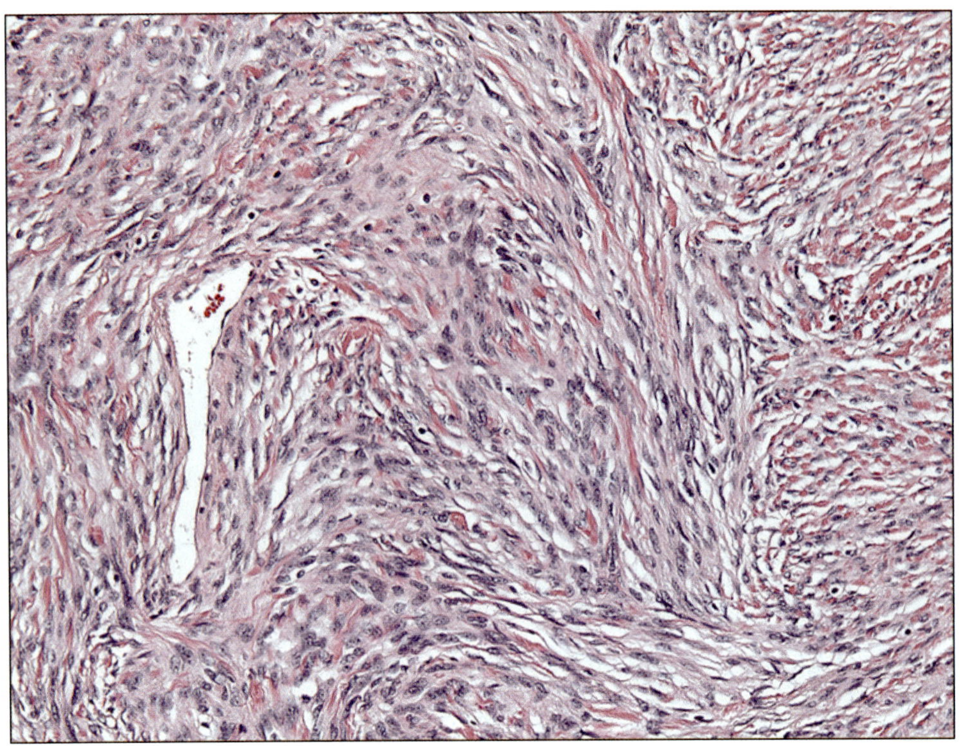

Figure 3.85. Squash
preparations are often clearly
diagnostic of meningiomas
because of the presence of
cellular whorls that readily
exfoliate.

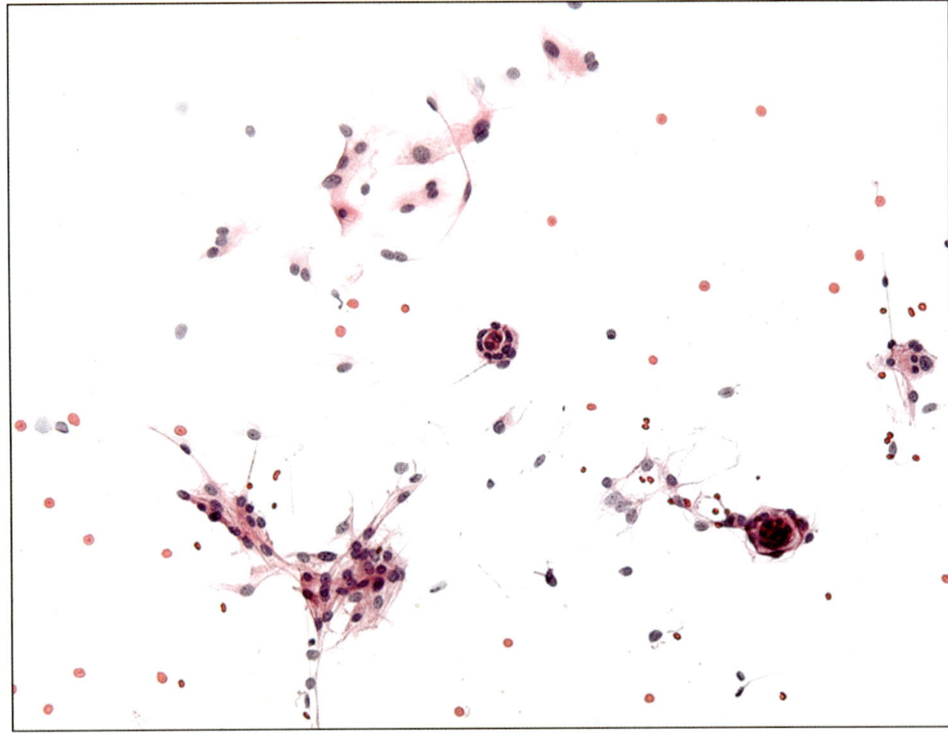

bands may be present. Psammoma bodies are rare. Immunohistochemical staining for epithelial membrane (EMA) may be weak. These
tumors may be difficult to distinguish from schwannoma or solitary fibrous
tumor.

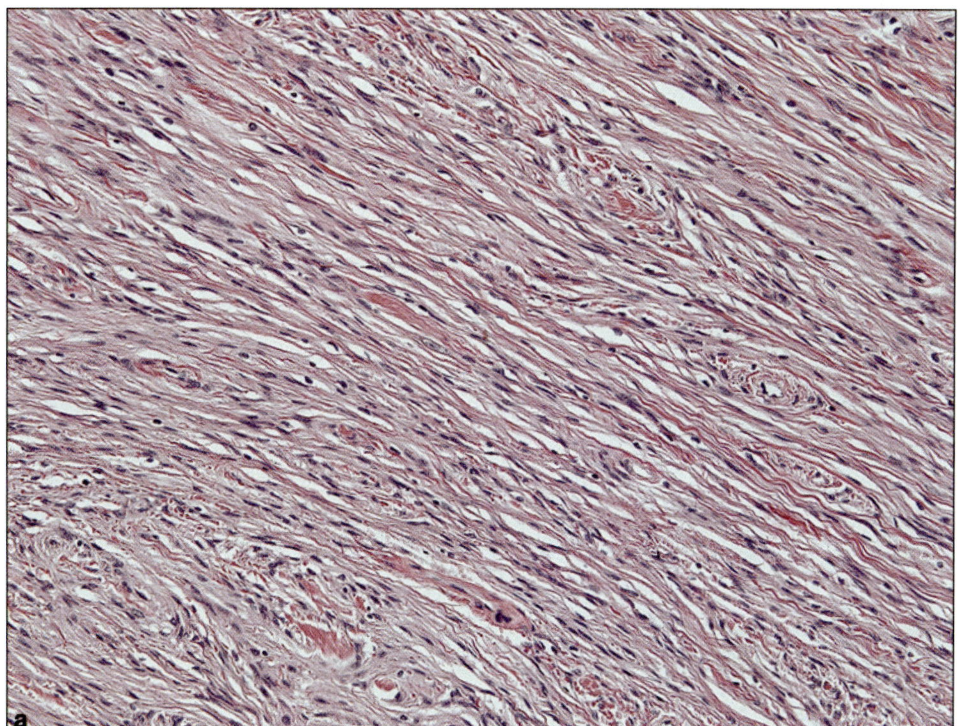

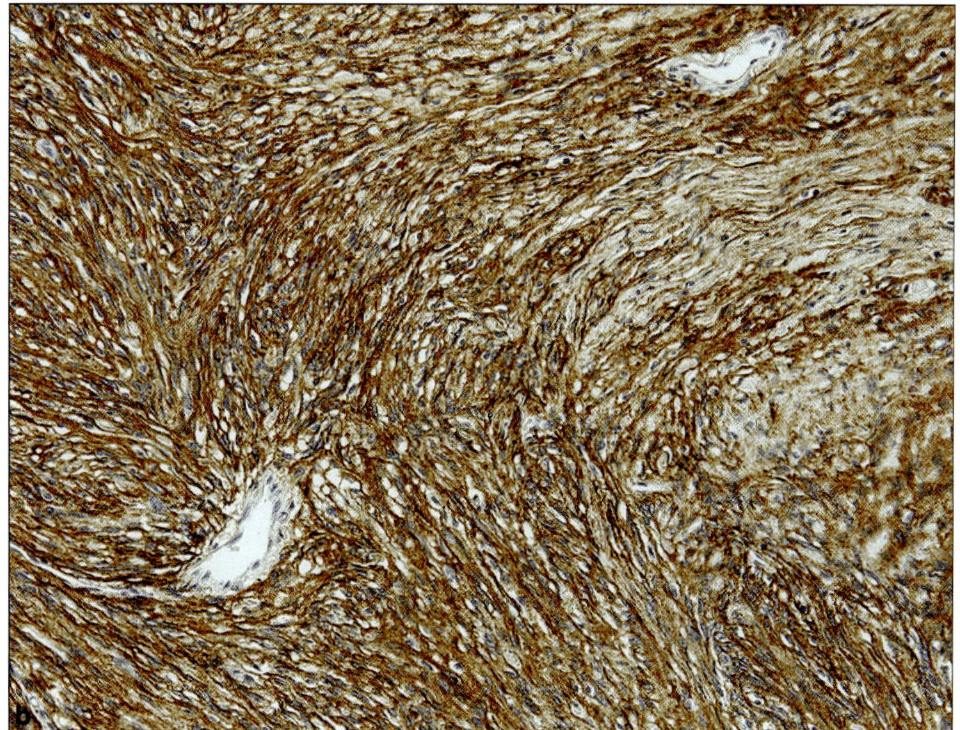

Figure 3.86. (a) Fibrous (fibroblastic) meningiomas may closely mimic other spindle cell tumors, (b) but EMA immunopositivity provides diagnostic support.

Transitional (Mixed)

The transitional meningioma combines mixed elements of different subtypes, most commonly the meningothelial and fibrous types (Figure 3.87). Whorls and psammoma bodies may be readily found.

Figure 3.87. Transitional (mixed) meningiomas contain elements of both meningothelial and fibrous meningioma.

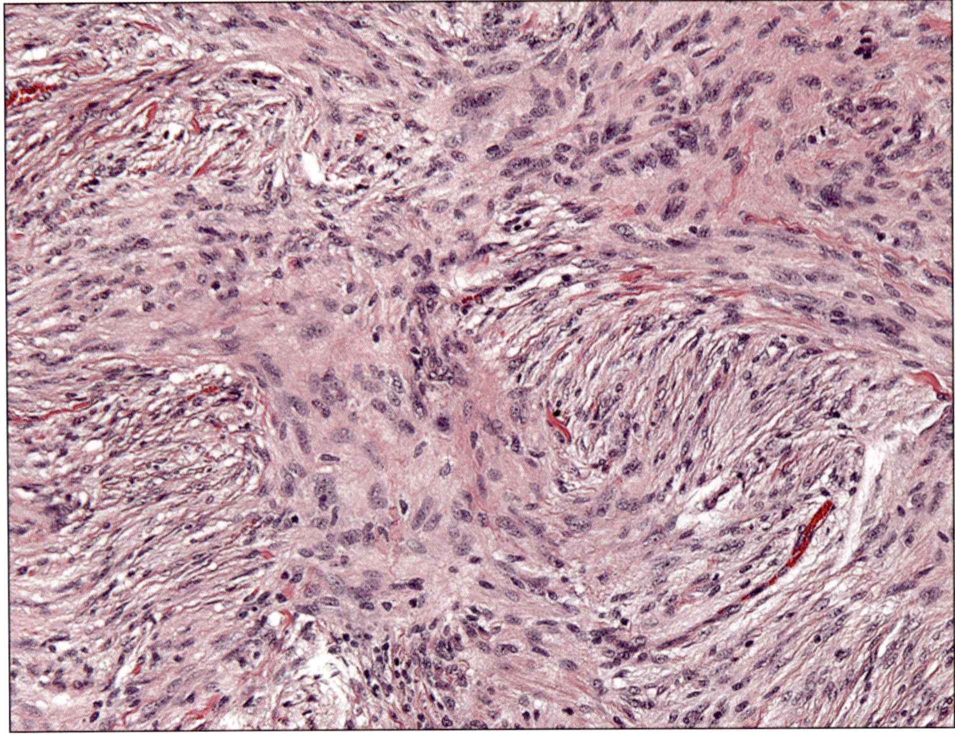

Figure 3.88. Psammomatous meningioma.

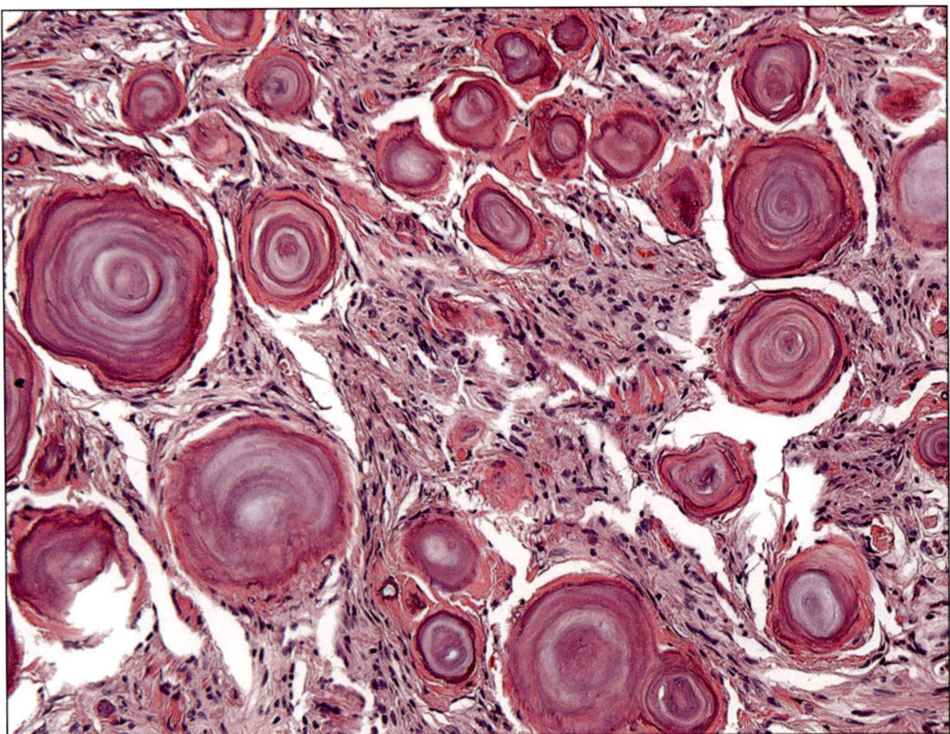

Psammomatous

The psammomatous meningioma shows innumerable and often back-to-back psammoma bodies, defined as concentric laminated calcified structures (Figure 3.88). The density of psammomatous meningiomas for these structures

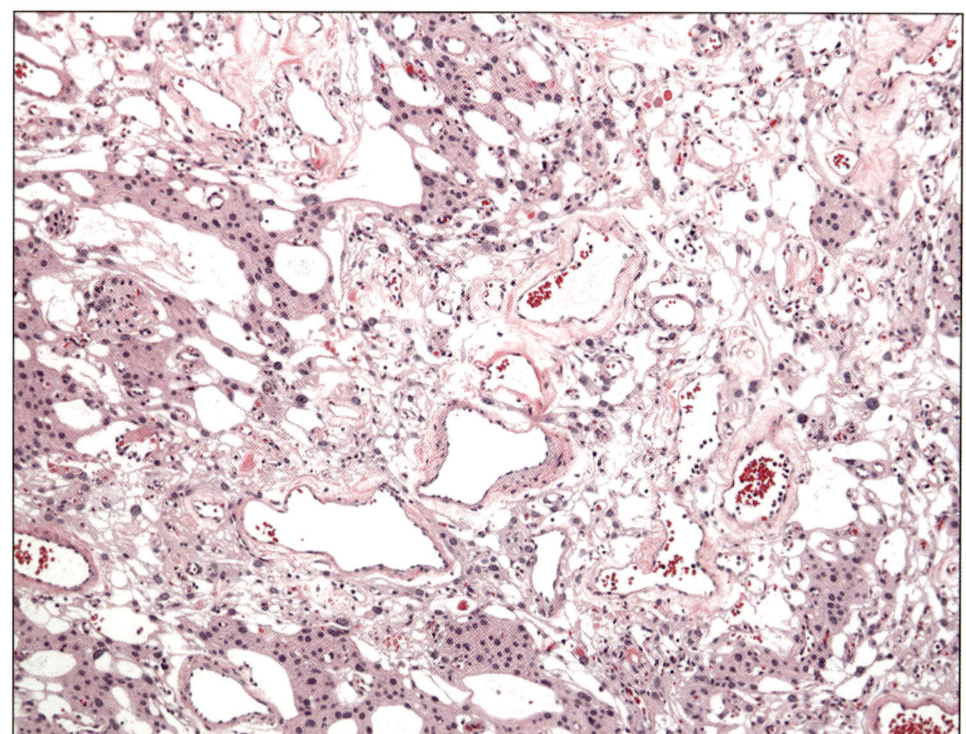

Figure 3.89. Microcystic meningiomas often contain prominent vasculature as seen in angiomatous meningiomas.

may even obscure recognition of the meningothelial cells. These may be more common among intraspinal meningiomas and in the olfactory grooves.

Angiomatous

These meningiomas contain conspicuous vascular elements, often dominated by ectatic vessels and with frequent hyaline change. Features of microcystic meningioma are frequently coexistent in these tumors.

Microcystic

The microcystic meningioma displays mucin-containing microcysts of varying sizes along with vacuolated cells and sometimes xanthomatous cells with scattered pleomorphic nuclei and hyalinized blood vessels (Figure 3.89). This type of meningioma may lack classic meningothelial features although careful microscopic scrutiny of the entire specimen will often reveal small foci of ordinary meningothelial meningioma.

Secretory

The secretory meningioma more closely resembles the meningothelial or transitional types but contains the distinctive feature of discrete eosinophilic and strongly PAS-positive cytoplasmic inclusions (Figure 3.90).

Figure 3.90. (a) The secretory meningioma contains vacuoles of varying sizes with eosinophilic material that is both CEA and (b) EMA immunopositive.

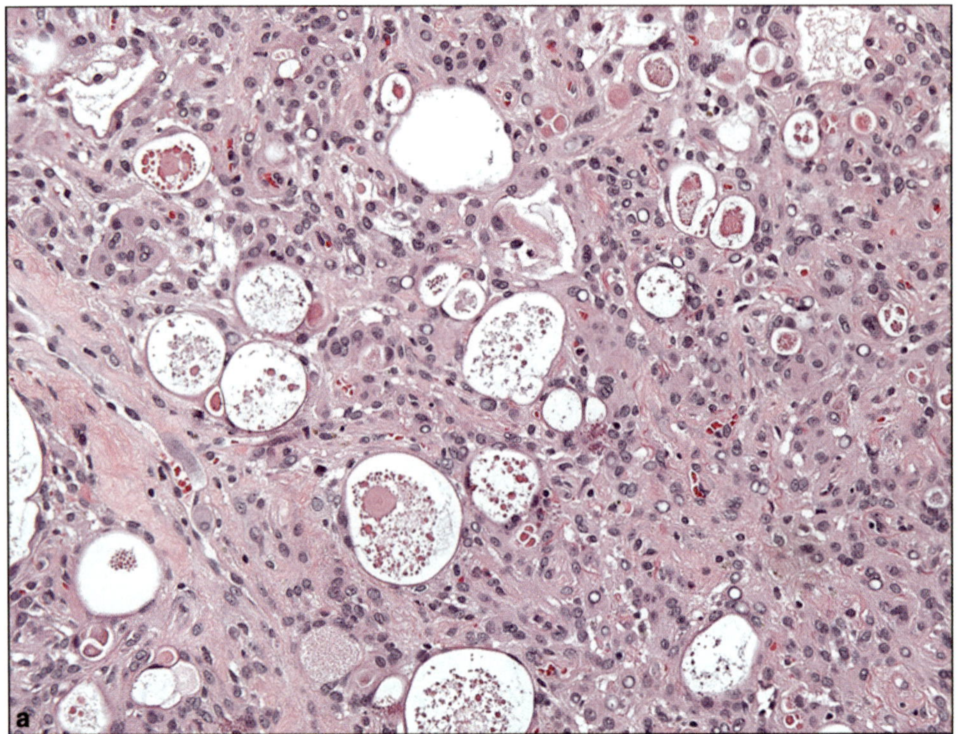

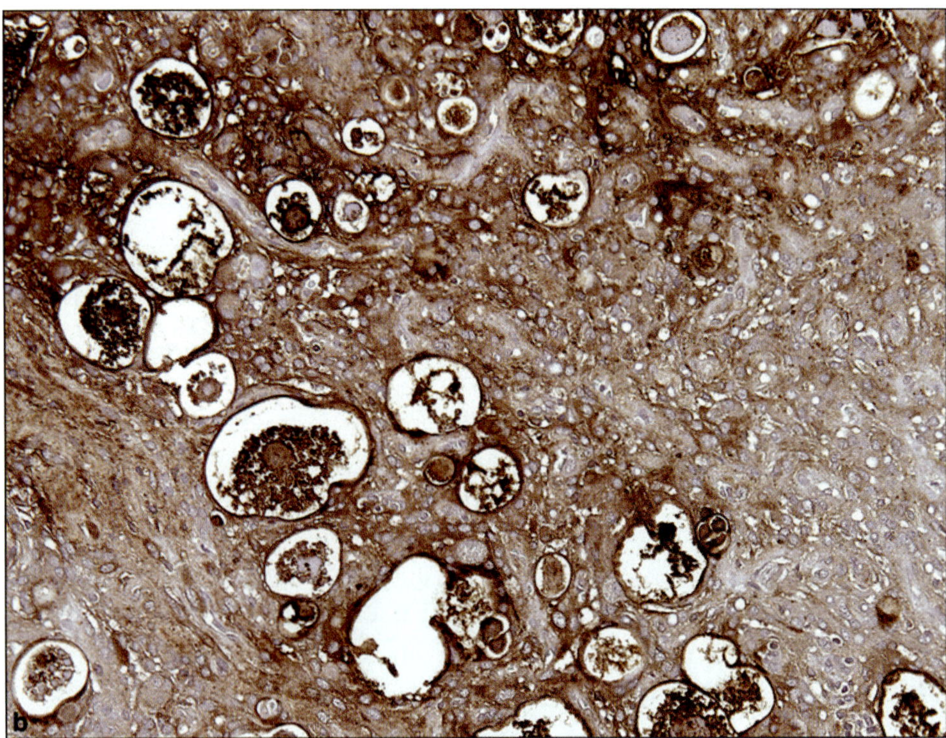

These are typically strongly immunopositive for EMA and CEA. At the ultra-structural level these intracytoplasmic inclusions are seen to be microvilli-lined spaces with proteinaceous contents. The secretory meningioma is a subtype that is recognized as more frequently infiltrated by mast cells (Tirakotai et al., 2006).

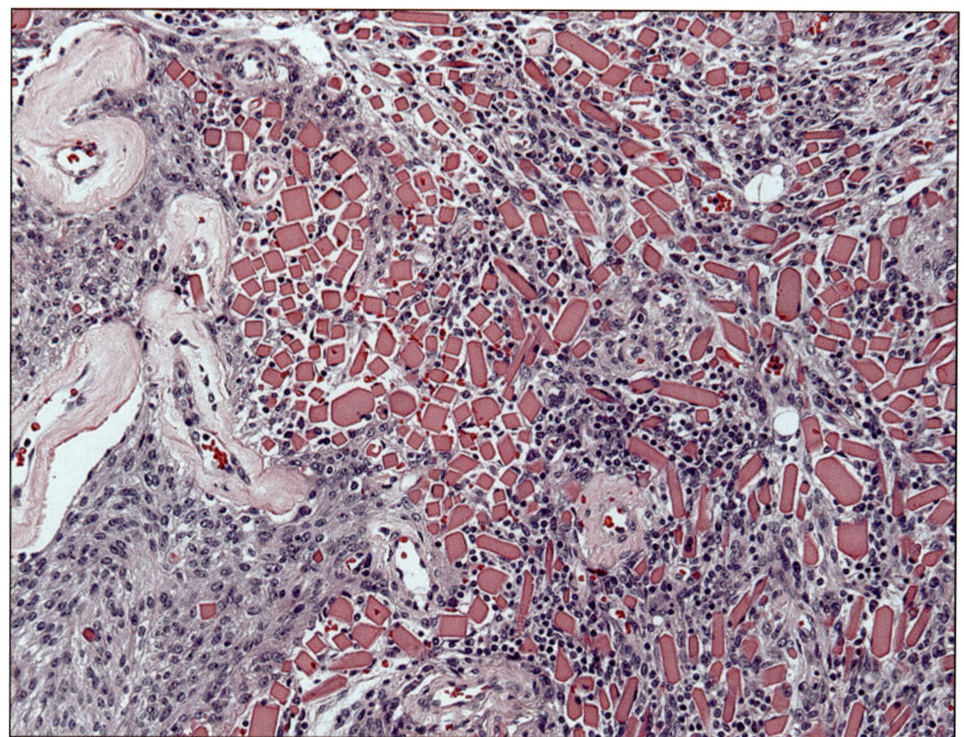

Figure 3.91. This unusual example of a meningioma contains a prominent plasma cell infiltrate in which many of the cells show a crystalline aggregation of intracytoplasmic immunoglobulin analogous to that of Mott cells seen in other lesions with plasma cells.

Lymphoplasmacyte-Rich

These extremely rare tumors may show massive infiltration by lymphocytes and plasma cells, often with Russell bodies (Figure 3.91). Some putative examples may in fact represent primary inflammatory lesions, including plasma cell granuloma or Rosai–Dorfman disease. The lymphocytic infiltrate may be so extensive as to obscure the underlying meningothelial proliferation. Immuno-histochemistry for EMA may be of limited usefulness since plasma cells are also EMA-immunopositive.

Metaplastic

Metaplastic meningiomas are recognized by the WHO as those with widespread mesenchymal components, which may include bony, cartilaginous, lipomatous, myxoid, sclerosing (Figure 3.92), or xanthomatous changes, individually or in combination.

WHO GRADE II

Chordoid

These are typically large, supratentorial tumors with an increased rate of recurrence, thus the WHO Grade II assignment. An infrequent association with Castleman's disease has been cited (Kepes et al., 1988). Chordoid meningiomas show ribbons or trabeculae of cells, often vacuolated, in an abundant mucoid matrix background (Figure 3.93). Careful inspection of these lesions may show

Figure 3.92. Examples of metaplastic meningiomas include (a) myxoid and (b) sclerosing meningioma.

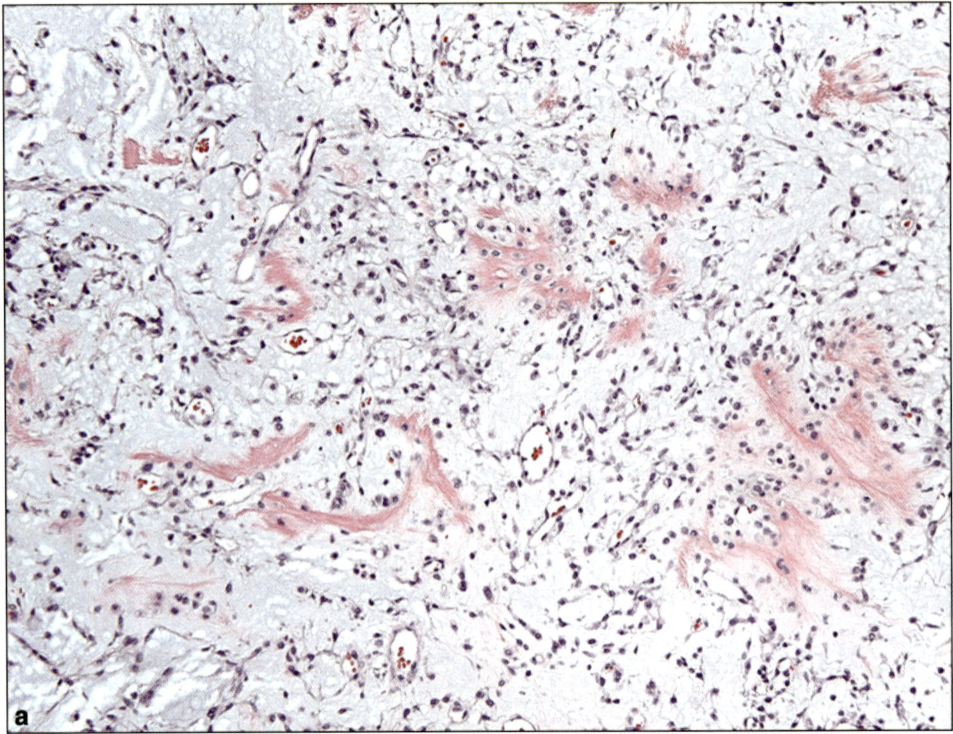

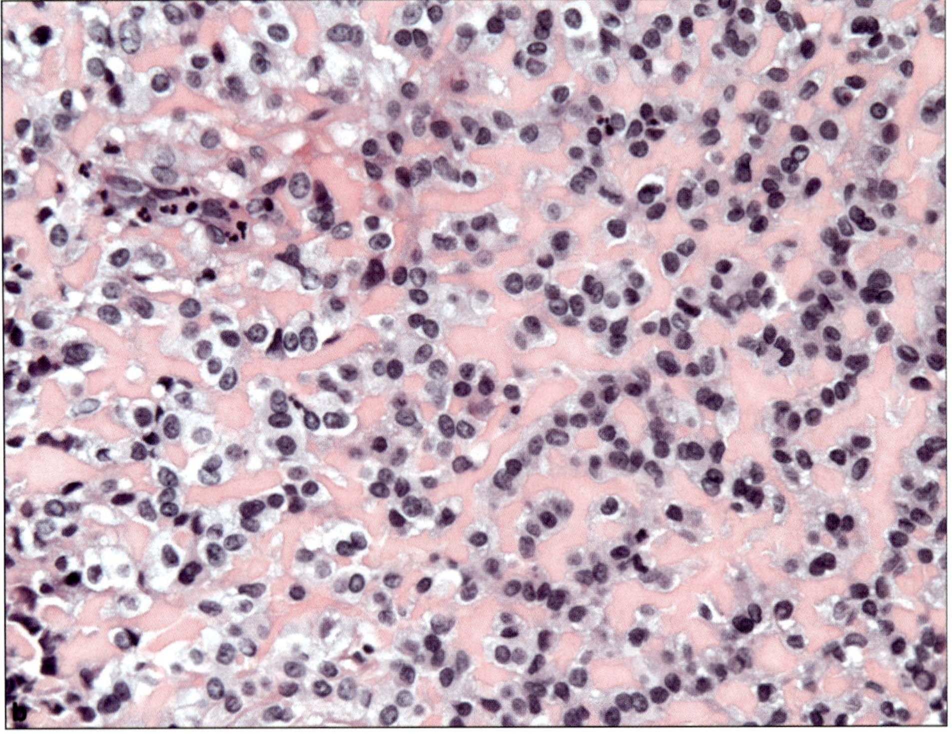

more typical meningothelial elements. Mononuclear inflammatory cell infiltrates may be focally prominent. Immunohistochemistry for EMA may be used to distinguish these from actual chordomas, which are typically EMA -negative and diffusely S-100-immunopositive.

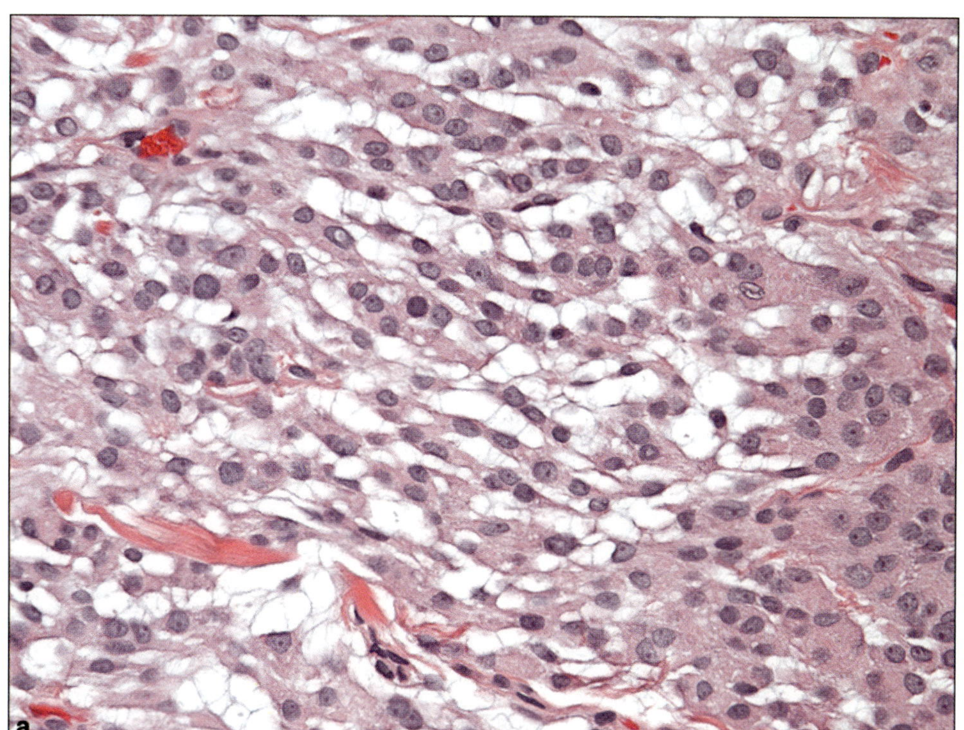

Figure 3.93. Chordoid meningiomas have been described in two forms, including (a) the usual appearance of ribbons of cells closely resembling the pattern of chordomas and (b) a form with prominent spindle-cell formation.

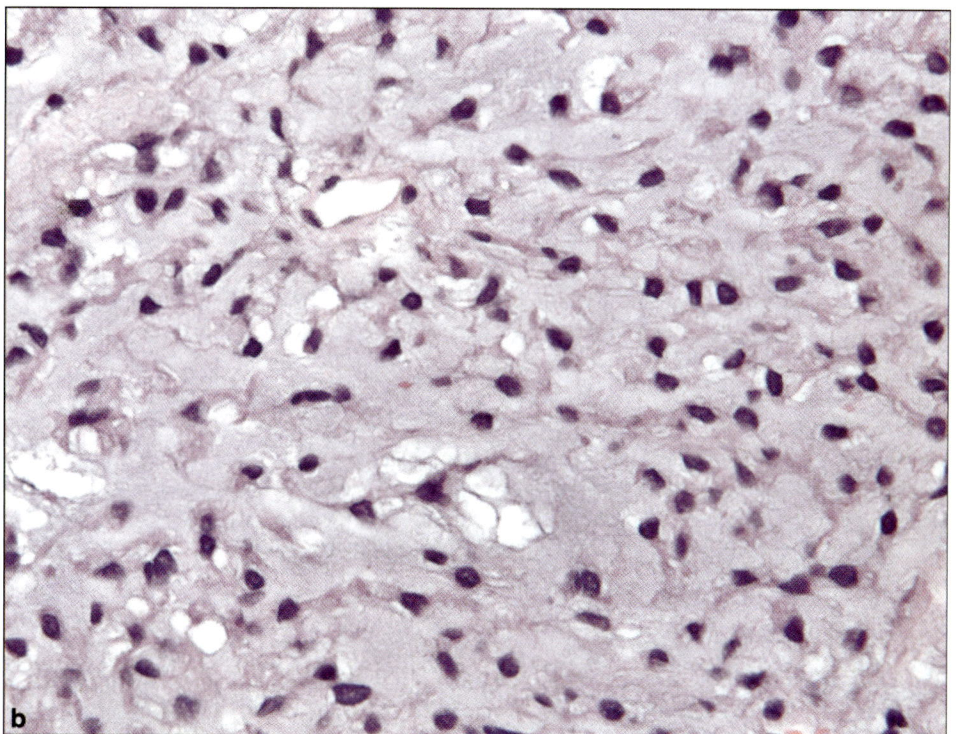

Clear Cell

The clear cell meningioma is more common at the cerebellopontine angle and cauda equina. It has been reported more frequently in pediatric and young adult patients. Because of a tendency for aggressive behavior and occasional CSF dissemination, this tumor is assigned to WHO Grade II.

Figure 3.94. (a) Clear cell meningiomas often lack any hint of obvious meningothelial differentiation, with clear cells often distributed between strands of collagen. (b) EMA immunopositivity can be a valuable observation in excluding other clear cell tumors of the CNS.

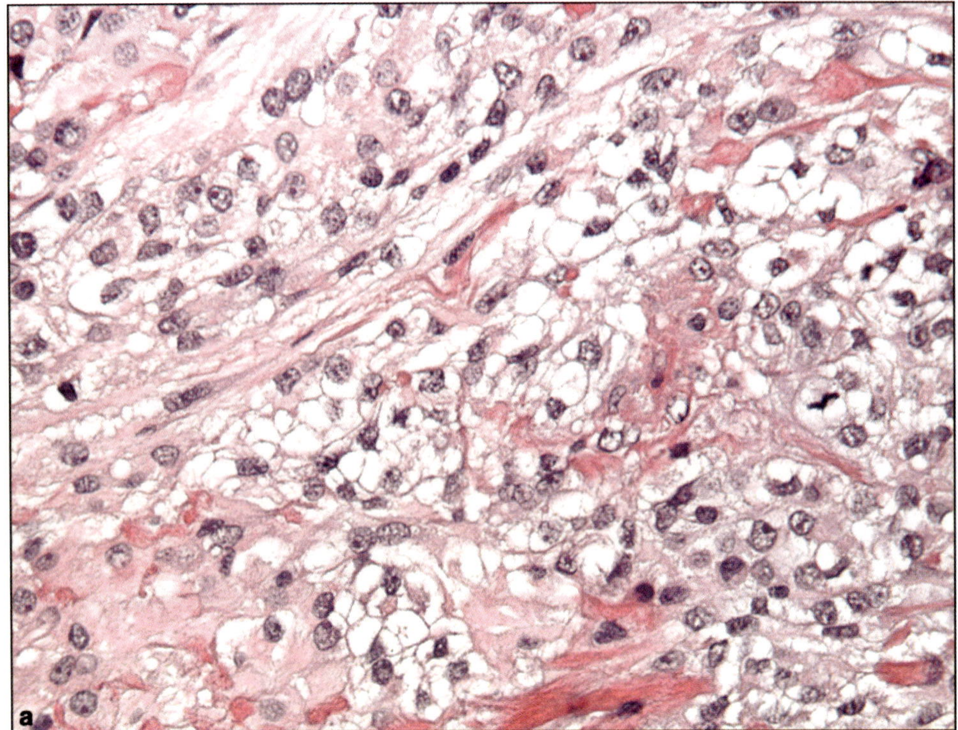

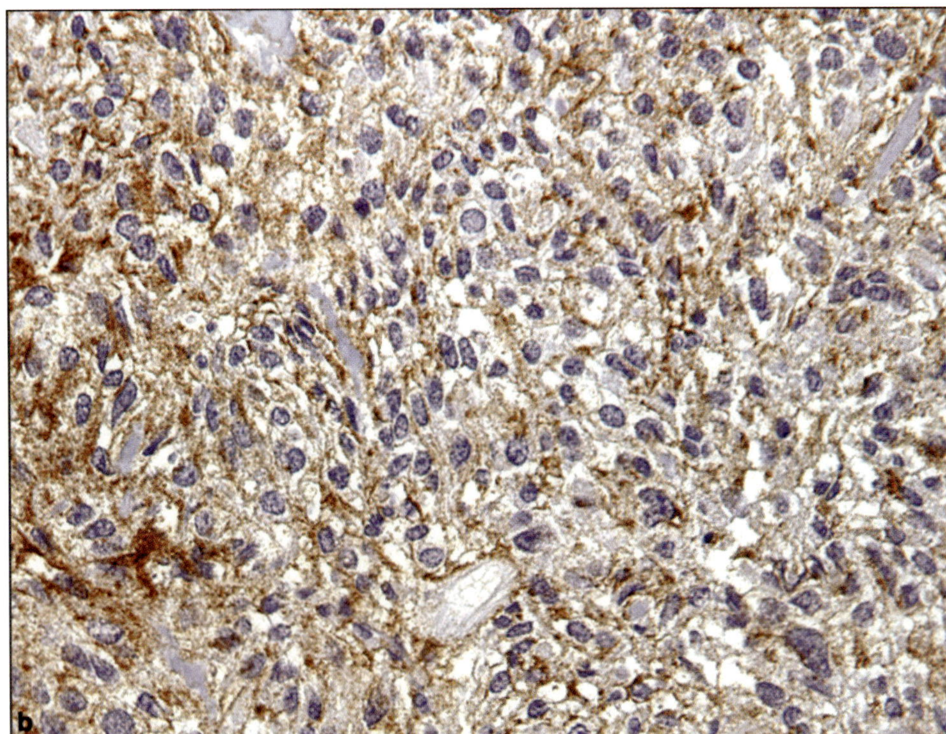

Histologically, this type of meningioma may be especially difficult to recognize as a meningothelial tumor because of the patternless array of clear cells in a collagenous background (Figure 3.94). Cells are typically glycogen-rich and thus PAS-positive. Whorl formation and psammoma bodies are essentially nonexistent.

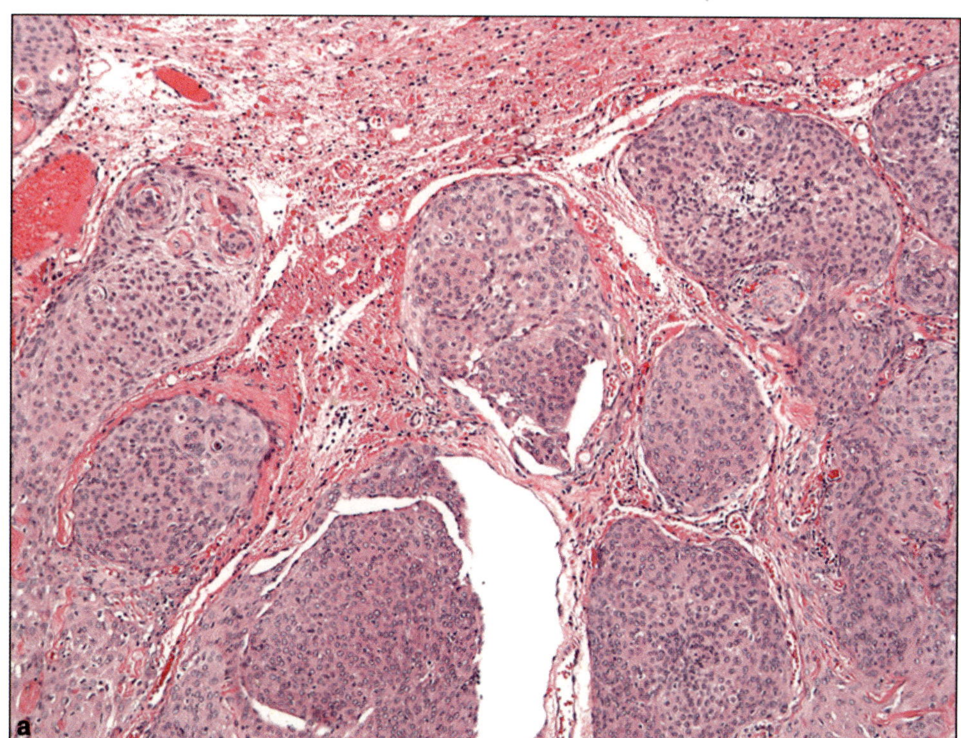

Figure 3.95. The determination of true brain invasion is important toward diagnosing WHO Grade II meningioma, and can be aided by immunostaining of brain tissue in the section for GFAP. (a) Some WHO Grade I meningiomas show pushing pattern upon adjacent brain by nodules of tumor. (b) highlighted by GFAP immunostaining.

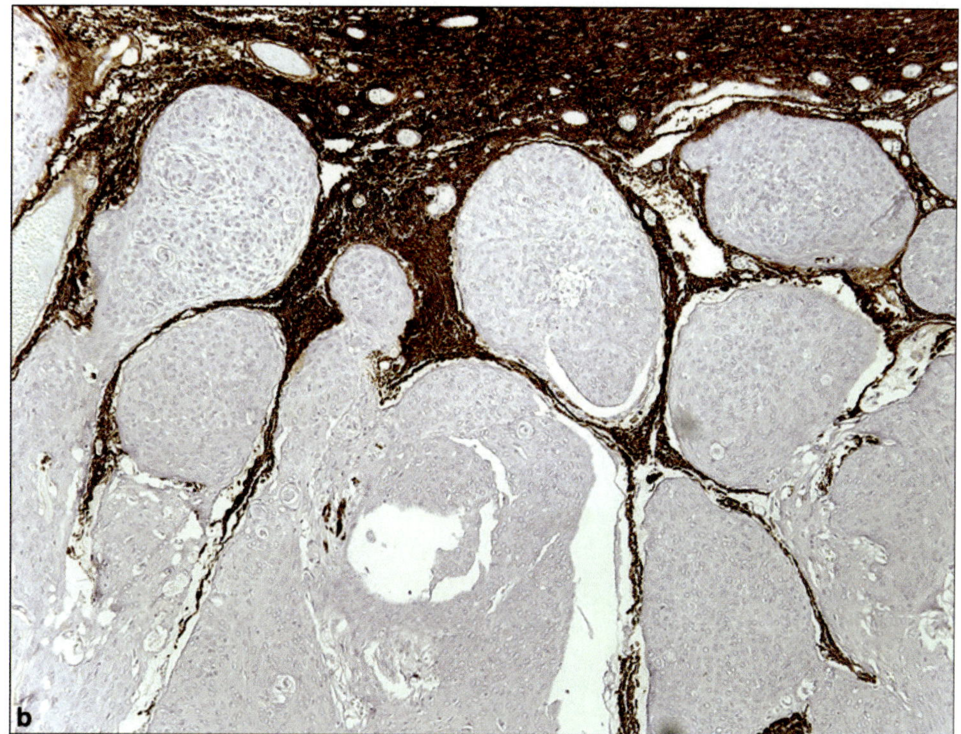

Atypical

Meningiomas, which otherwise lack clear cell or chordoid designations, may be assigned a WHO grade of II if certain histologic features are noted either singly or in combination. A mitotic count of four to twenty mitotic figures

Figure 3.95. *continued*
(c) True brain invasion is seen as individual meningioma cell invasion into brain parenchyme, (d) also demonstrated by GFAP immunohistochemistry.

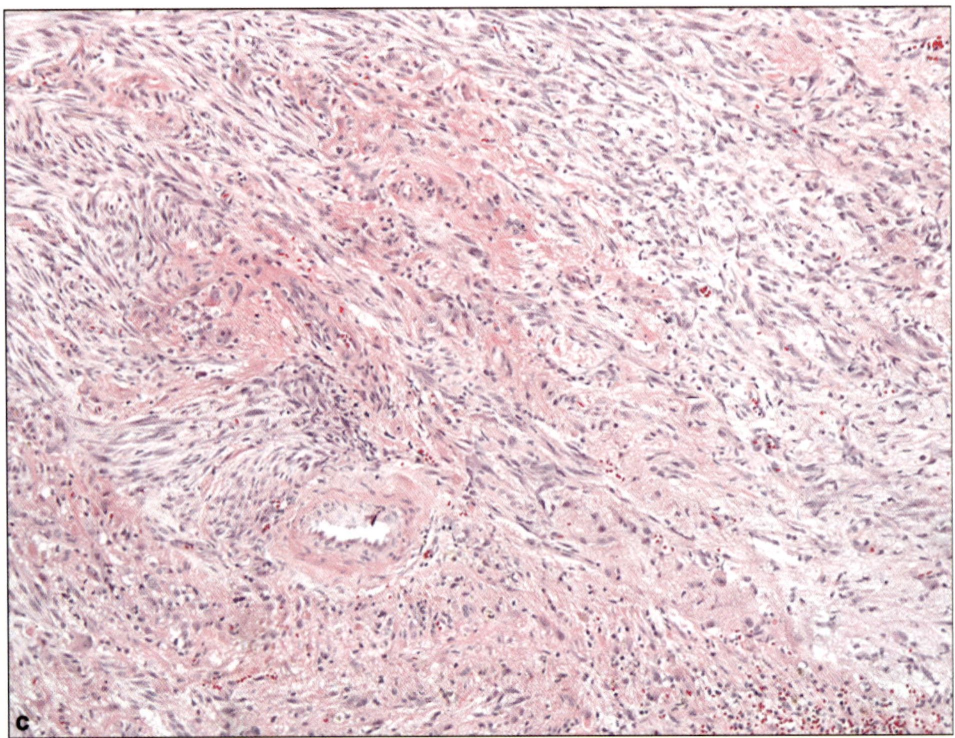

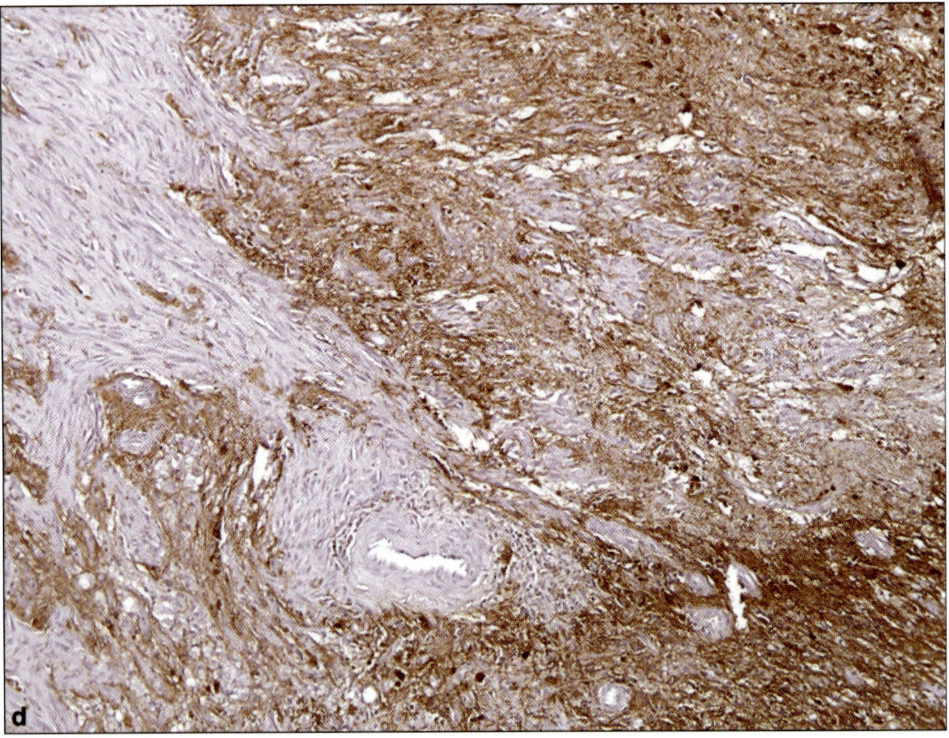

per ten high-powered fields is diagnostic of atypical WHO Grade II meningioma. The method in counting the mitotic figures should involve finding the ten consecutive high-powered fields with the highest number of mitotic figures.

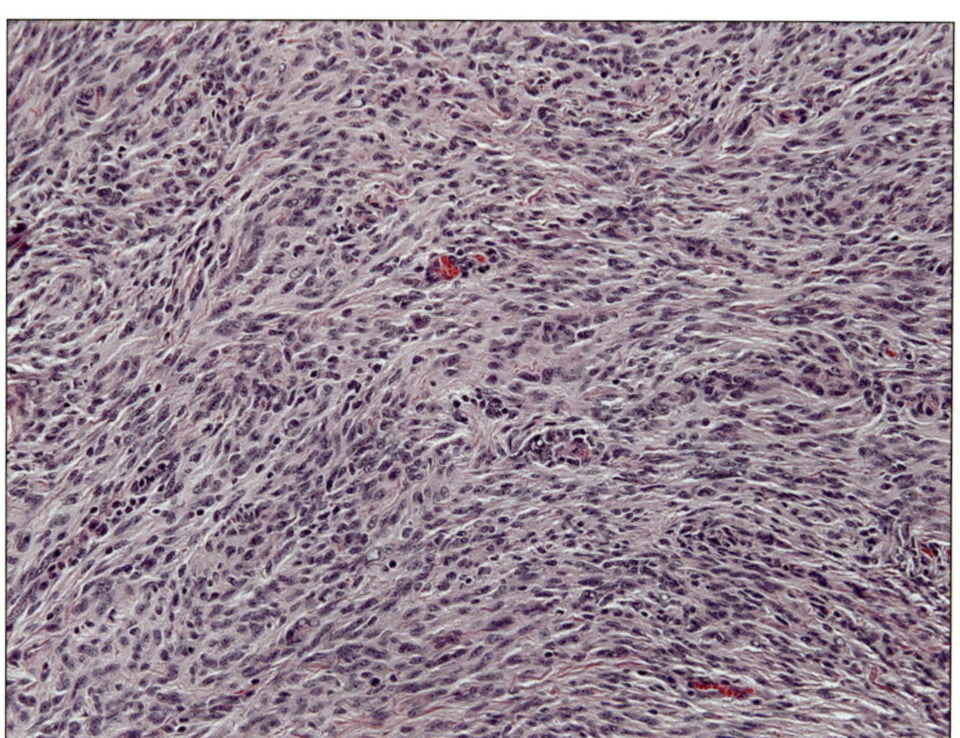

Figure 3.96. Patternless pattern in atypical meningioma.

Brain invasion is also diagnostic of WHO Grade II meningioma. Rarely, meningioma infiltrates brain as small aggregates or single cells. This diagnosis may be aided by the use of GFAP immunohistochemistry, which highlights brain tissue, occasionally entrapped between the fingers or lobules of infiltrating meningioma (Figure 3.95). The presence of at least three of the following histological features will also suffice to diagnose atypical WHO Grade II meningioma: sheeting architecture or patternless pattern (Figure 3.96), hypercellularity, macronucleoli, and small cell formation, and spontaneous or "geographic" necrosis, unlike that seen as a consequence of tumor embolization (Figure 3.97).

WHO GRADE III

Papillary

This rare type of meningioma tends to occur in the pediatric age group and has a marked tendency for recurrence. Local brain invasion, remote metastases to the lung, and death due to disease are unusually prominent features of this type of meningioma. For these reasons, they are designated as WHO Grade III. The histological pattern consists of a perivascular pseudo-papillary arrangement of cells, which may not be clearly recognizable as meningothelial in origin (Figure 3.98). Immunohistochemical detection of EMA or electron microscopy may be helpful in confirming the diagnosis (Al-Sarraj et al., 2001) by demonstrating the characteristic ultrastructural markers of meningioma: interdigitating cell processes, desmosomes, and intermediate filaments.

Figure 3.97. Embolization of meningiomas results in clearly recognizable intravascular foreign material. Resulting necrosis should not be considered spontaneous as this is one feature of some atypical meningiomas.

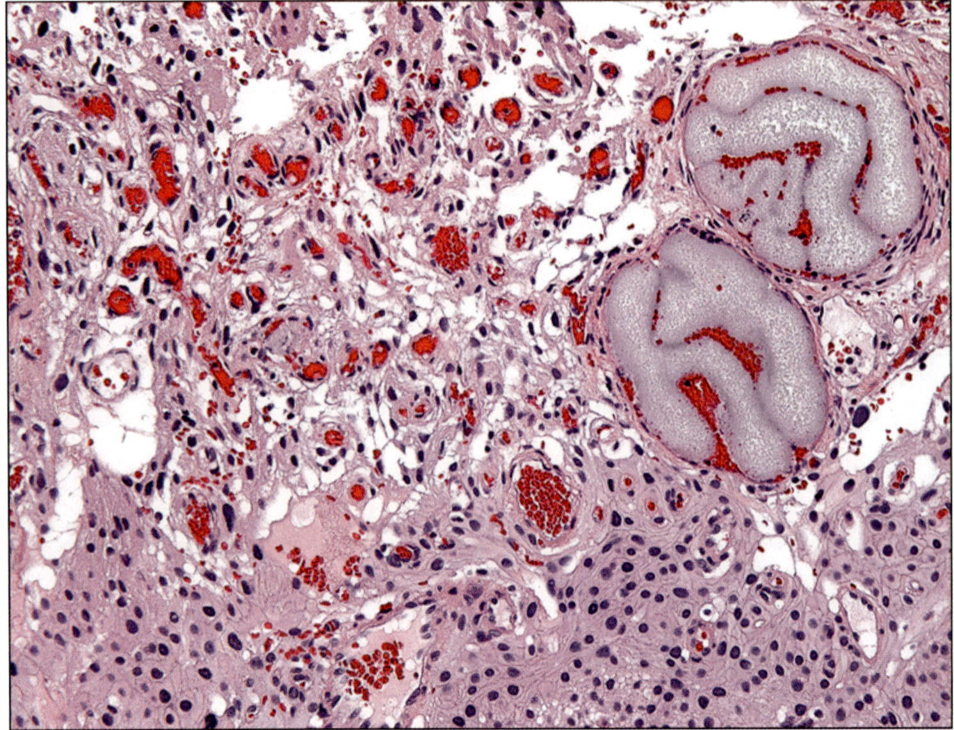

Figure 3.98. Papillary meningioma, WHO Grade III.

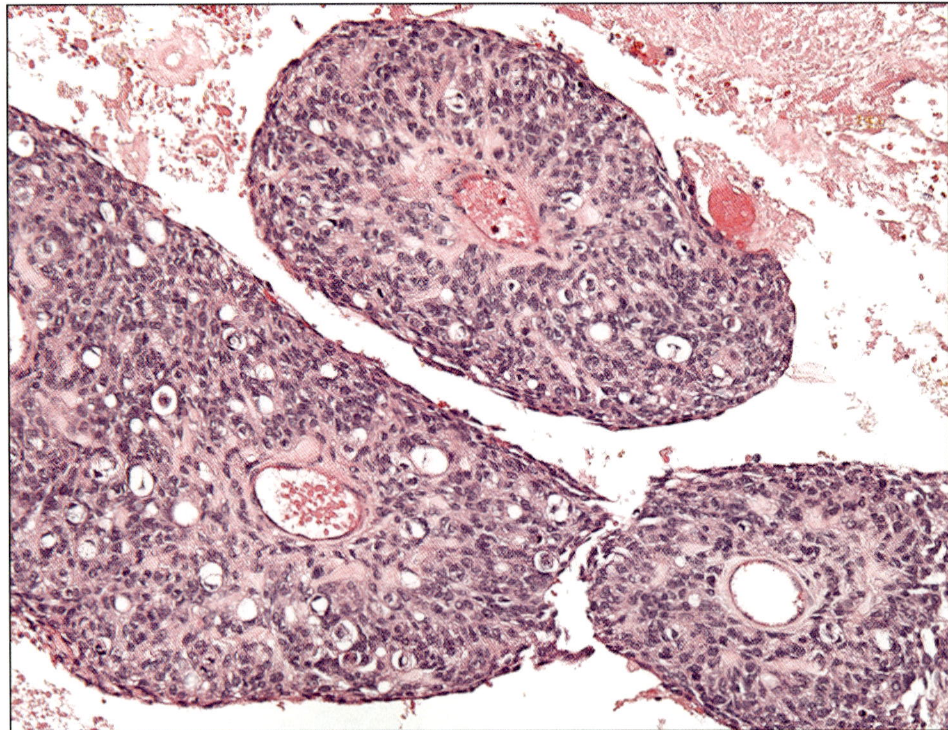

Rhabdoid

Rhabdoid meningiomas are also uncommon and are known for frequent recurrence and an aggressive clinical course, prompting the WHO grade of III (Perry et al., 1998). Rhabdoid cells are present, defined as plump cells with eccentric displacement of the nuclei by eosinophilic cytoplasmic masses (Figure 3.99).

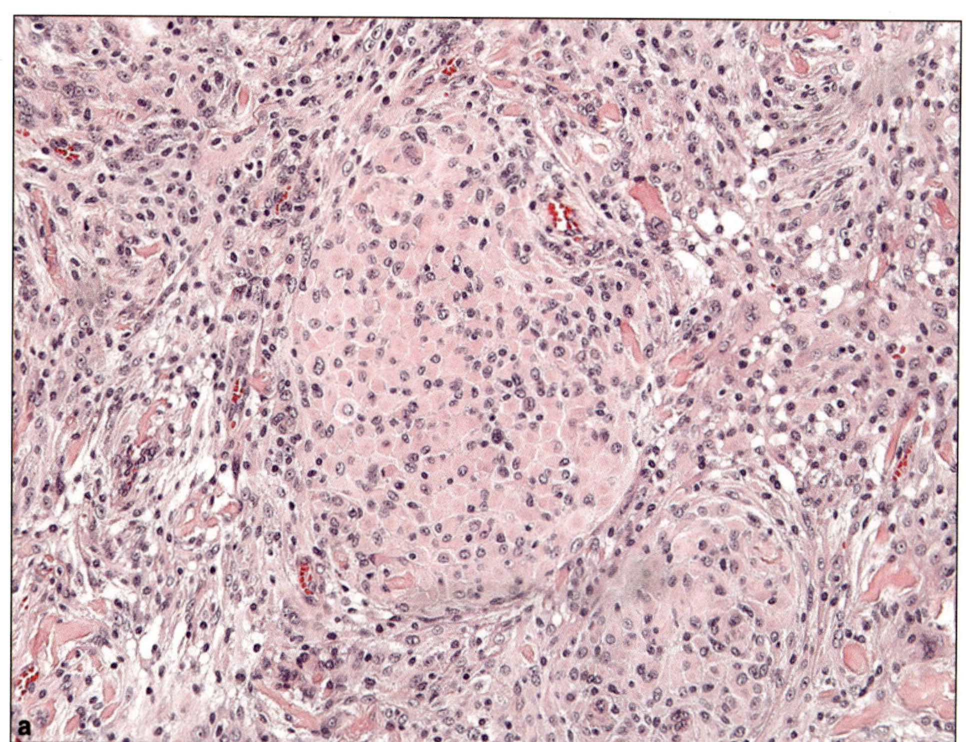

Figure 3.99. (a) Rhabdoid meningioma, in which rhabdoid features may be focal, but are usually accompanied by other atypical features. (b) Immunohistochemistry for vimentin, the characteristic intermediate filament of meningiomas, may highlight rhabdoid cells.

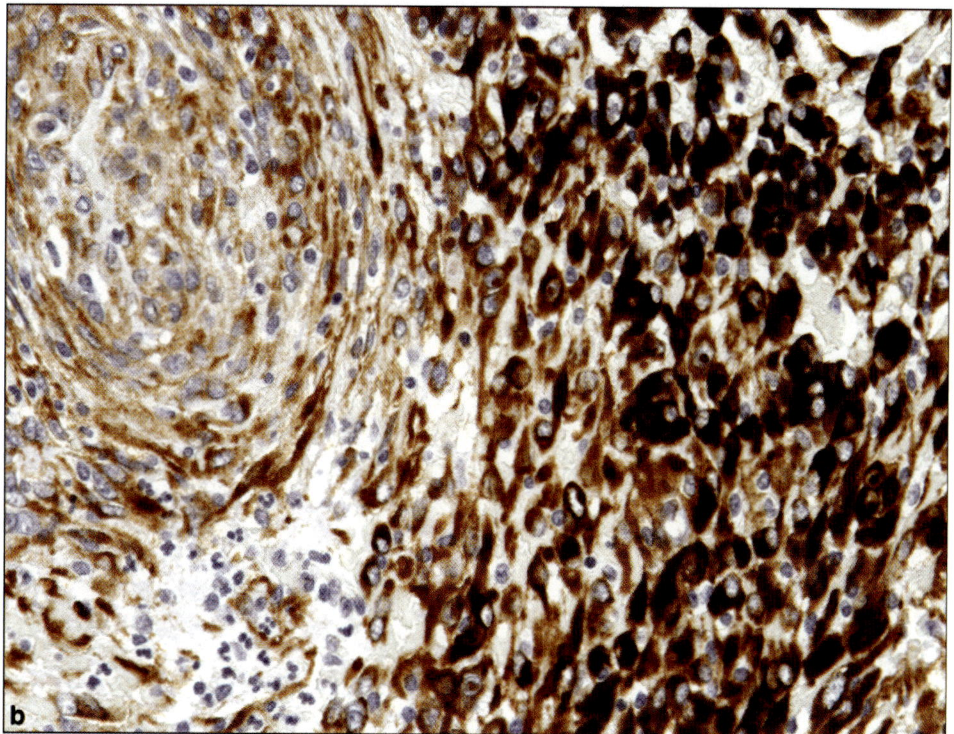

Careful scrutiny of some meningiomas may show small foci of rhabdoid cells. In the context of an otherwise WHO Grade I meningioma, the significance of this differentiation is unknown although retrospective analysis of recurrent rhabdoid meningiomas showed minor or unapparent rhabdoid elements in the primary specimens.

Figure 3.100. (a) Anaplastic (malignant) meningiomas are sometimes not easily recognizable as meningiomas because of carcinomatous or sarcomatous differentiation, (b) with a significant number of mitotic figures.

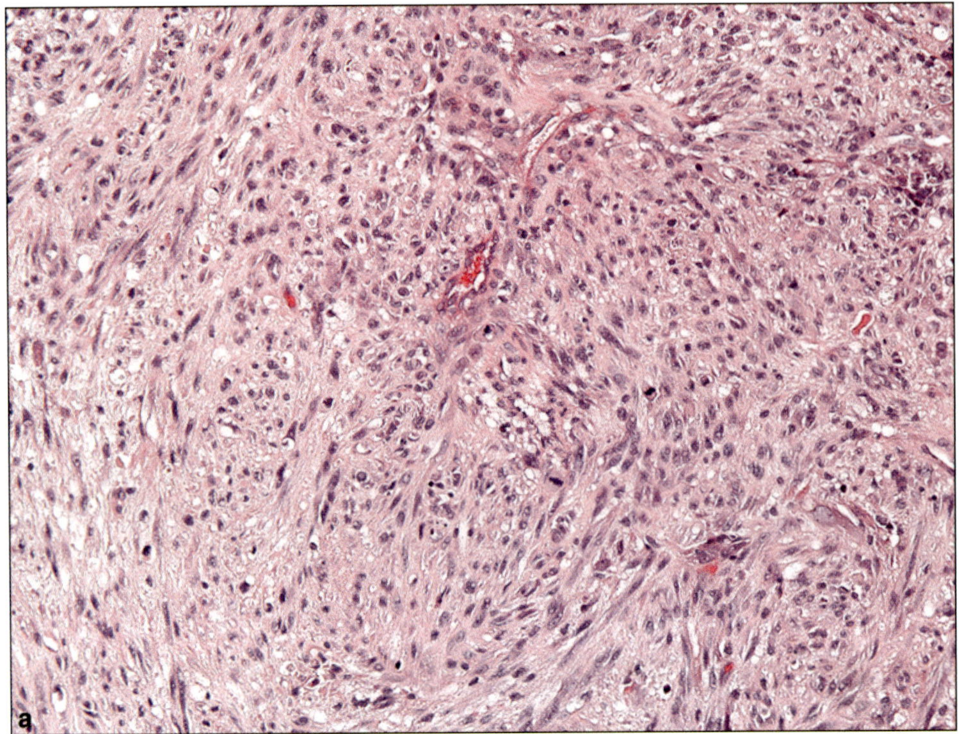

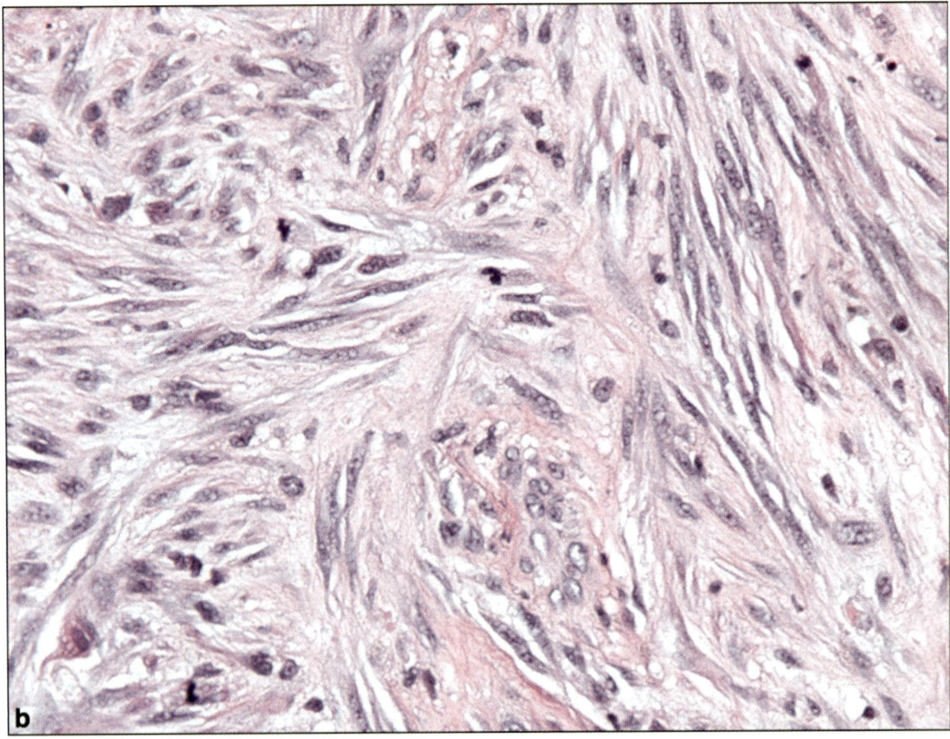

Anaplastic Meningioma

In addition to the papillary and rhabdoid types of WHO Grade III meningiomas, those with greater than twenty mitotic figures per ten high-powered fields or significant loss of meningothelial differentiation accompanied by frank evidence of carcinomatous, sarcomatous, or malignant melanocytic differentiation are malignant, WHO grade III lesions (Figure 3.100) (Perry et al., 1999).

REFERENCES

Al-Sarraj S, King A, Martin AJ, Jarosz J, Lantos PL. Ultrastructural examination is essential for diagnosis of papillary meningioma. *Histopathology* 2001; 38: 318–24.

Antinheimo J, Haapasalo H, Haltia M, Tatagiba M, Thomas S, Brandis A, et al. Proliferation potential and histological features in neurofibromatosis 2-associated and sporadic meningiomas. *J Neurosurg* 1997; 87: 610–14.

Claus EB, Bondy ML, Schildkraut JM, Wiemels JL, Wrensch M, Black PM. Epidemiology of intracranial meningioma. *Neurosurgery* 2005; 57: 1088–95; discussion 1088–95.

Cohen-Gadol AA, Zikel OM, Koch CA, Scheithauer BW, Krauss WE. Spinal meningiomas in patients younger than 50 years of age: a 21-year experience. *J Neurosurg* 2003; 98: 258–63.

Gezen F, Kahraman S, Canakci Z, Beduk A. Review of 36 cases of spinal cord meningioma. *Spine* 2000; 25: 727–31.

Hsu DW, Pardo FS, Efird JT, Linggood RM, Hedley-Whyte ET. Prognostic significance of proliferative indices in meningiomas. *J Neuropathol Exp Neurol* 1994; 53: 247–55.

Kepes JJ, Chen WY, Connors MH, Vogel FS. "Chordoid" meningeal tumors in young individuals with peritumoral lymphoplasmacellular infiltrates causing systemic manifestations of the Castleman syndrome. A report of seven cases. *Cancer* 1988; 62: 391–406.

Kuzeyli K, Duru S, Baykal S, Usul H, Ceylan S, Akturk F. Primary intraosseous meningioma of the temporal bone in an infant. A case report. *Neurosurg Rev* 1996; 19: 197–9.

Longstreth WT, Jr., Dennis LK, McGuire VM, Drangsholt MT, Koepsell TD. Epidemiology of intracranial meningioma. *Cancer* 1993; 72: 639–48.

Louis DN, Ramesh V, Gusella JF. Neuropathology and molecular genetics of neurofibromatosis 2 and related tumors. *Brain Pathol* 1995; 5: 163–72.

Maier H, Wanschitz J, Sedivy R, Rossler K, Ofner D, Budka H. Proliferation and DNA fragmentation in meningioma subtypes. *Neuropathol Appl Neurobiol* 1997; 23: 496–506.

Maiorana A, Ficarra G, Fano RA, Spagna G. Primary solitary meningioma of the lung. *Pathologica* 1996; 88: 457–62.

Marcelissen TA, de Bondt RB, Lammens M, Manni JJ. Primary temporal bone secretory meningioma presenting as chronic otitis media. *Eur Arch Otorhinolaryngol* 2008; 265: 843–6.

O'Reilly RC, Kapadia SB, Kamerer DB. Primary extracranial meningioma of the temporal bone. *Otolaryngol Head Neck Surg* 1998; 118: 690–4.

Perry A, Cai DX, Scheithauer BW, Swanson PE, Lohse CM, Newsham IF, et al. Merlin, DAL-1, and progesterone receptor expression in clinicopathologic subsets of meningioma: a correlative immunohistochemical study of 175 cases. *J Neuropathol Exp Neurol* 2000; 59: 872–9.

Perry A, Dehner LP. Meningeal tumors of childhood and infancy. An update and literature review. *Brain Pathol* 2003; 13: 386–408.

Perry A, Giannini C, Raghavan R, Scheithauer BW, Banerjee R, Margraf L, et al. Aggressive phenotypic and genotypic features in pediatric and NF2-associated meningiomas: a clinicopathologic study of 53 cases. *J Neuropathol Exp Neurol* 2001; 60: 994–1003.

Perry A, Kurtkaya-Yapicier O, Scheithauer BW, Robinson S, Prayson RA, Kleinsch-midt-DeMasters BK, et al. Insights into meningioangiomatosis with and without meningioma: a clinicopathologic and genetic series of 24 cases with review of the literature. *Brain Pathol* 2005; 15: 55–65.

Perry A, Scheithauer BW, Stafford SL, Abell-Aleff PC, Meyer FB. "Rhabdoid" menin-gioma: an aggressive variant. *Am J Surg Pathol* 1998; 22: 1482–90.

Perry A, Scheithauer BW, Stafford SL, Lohse CM, Wollan PC. "Malignancy" in men-ingiomas: a clinicopathologic study of 116 patients, with grading implications. *Cancer* 1999; 85: 2046–56.

Picquet J, Valo I, Jousset Y, Enon B. Primary pulmonary meningioma first suspected of being a lung metastasis. *Ann Thorac Surg* 2005; 79: 1407–9.

Rushing EJ, Olsen C, Man YG. Correlation of p63 immunoreactivity with tumor grade in meningiomas. *Int J Surg Pathol* 2008; 16: 38–42.

Rushing EJ, Olsen C, Mena H, Rueda ME, Lee YS, Keating RF, et al. Central nervous system meningiomas in the first two decades of life: a clinicopathological analysis of 87 patients. *J Neurosurg* 2005; 103: 489–95.

Schnitt SJ, Vogel H. Meningiomas. Diagnostic value of immunoperoxidase staining for epithelial membrane antigen. *Am J Surg Pathol* 1986; 10: 640–9.

Tirakotai W, Mennel HD, Celik I, Hellwig D, Bertalanffy H, Riegel T. Secretory men-ingioma: immunohistochemical findings and evaluation of mast cell infiltration. *Neurosurg Rev* 2006; 29: 41–8.

van der Meij JJ, Boomars KA, van den Bosch JM, van Boven WJ, de Bruin PC, Seldenrijk CA. Primary pulmonary malignant meningioma. *Ann Thorac Surg* 2005; 80: 1523–5.

LYMPHOMAS AND HEMATOPOIETIC NEOPLASMS

MALIGNANT LYMPHOMAS

Clinical and Radiological Features

Malignant lymphomas may occur in the brain either as primary CNS lym-phoma (PCNSL) or in the setting of systemic lymphoma. The incidence of PCNSL has risen dramatically in recent decades, mostly in males and at least in part attributable to the spread of acquired immunodeficiency syndrome (AIDS) (Cote et al., 1996) as well as immunocompromise due to organ transplantation but also as a more common diagnosis in the older population. In the context of immunodeficiency, Epstein–Barr virus (EBV) is associated with essentially all PCNSLs.

T-cell lymphomas are reportedly more common in some Asian countries, with the proportion of T-cell lymphomas of the CNS (T-CNSL) over 16% in Korea (Choi et al., 2003) and above 8% in Japan (Bataille et al., 2000). The reasons for these discrepancies remain unknown. The majority of T-CNSL arise in immunocompe-tent individuals (Louis and International Agency for Research on Cancer, 2007).

A variety of symptoms are associated with PCNSL, usually beginning with focal neurologic deficits or signs of increased intracranial pressure. The duration of symptoms vary widely but averages a few months prior to diagnosis.

Transplant associated PCNSL occurs with an interval averaging between 2 and 3 years after transplantation (Penn and Porat, 1995). Ocular uveal examples may precede the later development of PCNSL (Akpek et al., 1999).

PCNSL occurs more commonly in the supratentorial compartment and has a distinct propensity for periventricular growth. Multiple lymphomas occur in 25–50% of the cases, which is particularly common in patients with AIDS. Bilateral and symmetric spread is typical. Meningeal spread or involvement of the venous sinuses of the dura may also be seen, and examples of primary leptomeningeal lymphoma are also noted (Shenkier, 2005); however these locations may indicate intracranial involvement of systemic lymphoma, particularly when no parenchymal lesions are noted.

An important form of CNS lymphoma is in the form of intravascular dissemination, or intravascular lymphomatosis, with little to no parenchymal spread but consequences attributable to microvascular occlusion.

PCNSLs appear as isodense to hyperintense lesions in T2-weighted MRI studies and are strongly enhancing with contrast media (Figure 3.101). PCNSL may also present as a ring-enhancing lesion, resembling high-grade glial neoplasms or in the context of AIDS, a toxoplasmosis abscess, sometimes even as a coexistent process (Stenzel et al., 2004). As discussed below, treatment with steroids may induce rapid lysis and radiographic disappearance of the tumor.

Pathology

B-Cell Lymphomas The vast majority of CNS lymphomas are classified as diffuse large B-cell lymphomas. Only approximately 2–3% of CNS lymphomas are thought to be T-cell derived although this may reflect their under-recognition (Dulai et al., 2008). The most common pattern is the angiocentric proliferation of neoplastic lymphocytes although single-cell infiltration may also be seen (Figure 3.102). The blastic cells are typically characterized by large nuclei with distinct nucleoli. It may be confusing at the cytological level when a mixed population of lymphocytes is present, occasionally including a large component of reactive CD4- or CD8-positive T lymphocytes. The perivascular arrangement of cells results in the deposition of concentric bands of reticulin, which is highlighted with the corresponding stain. When necrosis is present, there is usually perivascular preservation of intact lymphoma cells. Reactive astrocytes and microglial activation may be common.

The neoplastic B-lymphocytes usually express pan-B–cell markers such as CD 20, CD19, and CD 79a. Immunohistochemistry also carries the advantage of highlighting the enlarged atypical B cells in a background of sometimes more numerous benign T cells, and the same phenomenon may be demonstrated with Ki-67 immunolabeling.

The effect of prior corticosteroid therapy may be dramatic both in radiologically evident shrinkage to virtual disappearance of the tumor or tumors, but

Figure 3.101. Primary CNS lymphoma. (a) An axial T1 contrast-enhanced MR image shows intense homogeneous enhancement of masses adjacent to the left frontal horn and right atria. (b) An axial T2 MR image shows that the masses have relatively low signal compared to the cortex and extensive surrounding vasogenic edema. The relatively low signal on T2-weighted MR images is likely related to the high nuclear to cytoplasmic ratio of lymphoma. As illustrated by this case, primary CNS lymphoma often involves the basal ganglia and periventricular white matter. In immunocompetent patients, lymphoma typically displays intense homogeneous enhancement (a), whereas in immunocompromised patients, there is often ring enhancement. The areas of poor central enhancement in immunocompromised patients correspond to areas of necrosis.

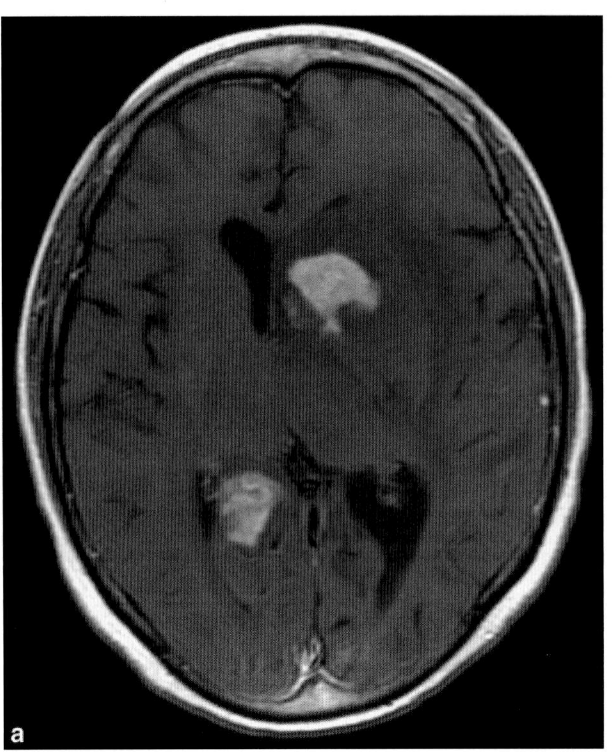

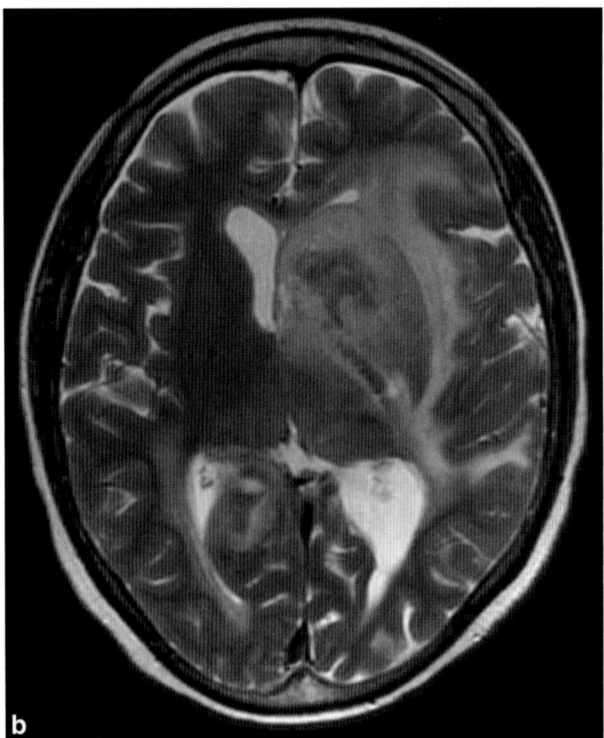

also in the histologic appearance of the biopsy sample. All that may remain are large numbers of macrophages, reactive astrocytes, reactive nonneoplastic lymphocytes, and if residual neoplastic B cells exist in the specimen, they may be detected by anti-B–cell markers (Figure 3.103). Cellular lysis and necrosis of

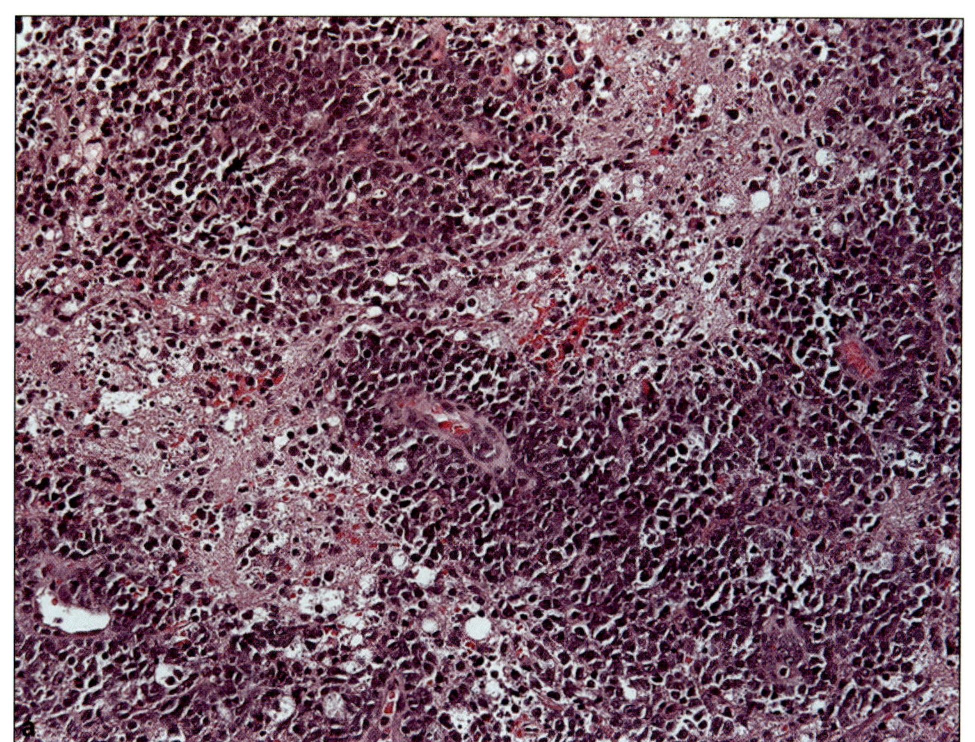

Figure 3.102. Primary CNS B-cell lymphoma, demonstrating (a) a malignant neoplasm with the tendency for necrosis that spares perivascular infiltrates. (b) Lymphomas may also mimic infiltrating gliomas.

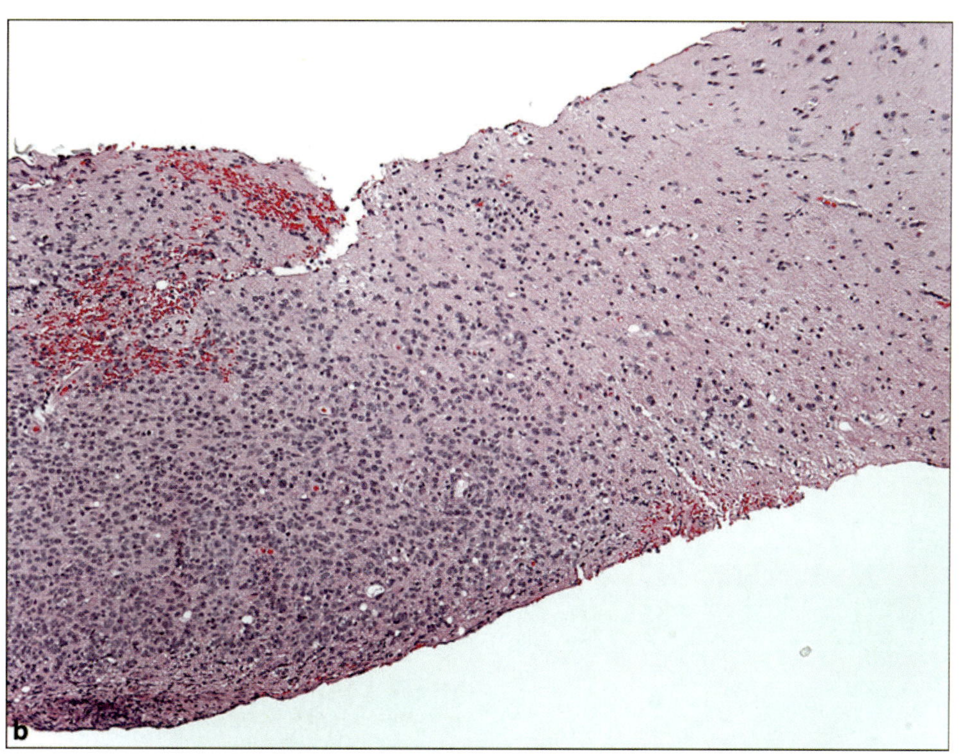

neoplastic B cells may lead to a residuum of CD20 positivity as strong but circumstantial evidence of the recent presence of viable tumor cells in a manner analogous to that which has been described in nodal lymphoma (Figure 3.104).

Figure 3.102. *continued*
(c) A squash preparation will reveal monotonous and dyscohesive neoplastic lymphocytes. Note the presence of scattered macrophages, which may be seen in lymphomas partially treated with corticosteroids. (d) Immunohistochemistry for CD20 will highlight the neoplastic B cells, and (e) a photomicrograph of the same field stained with anti-CD3 will show a sometimes prominent reactive T-cell infiltrate.

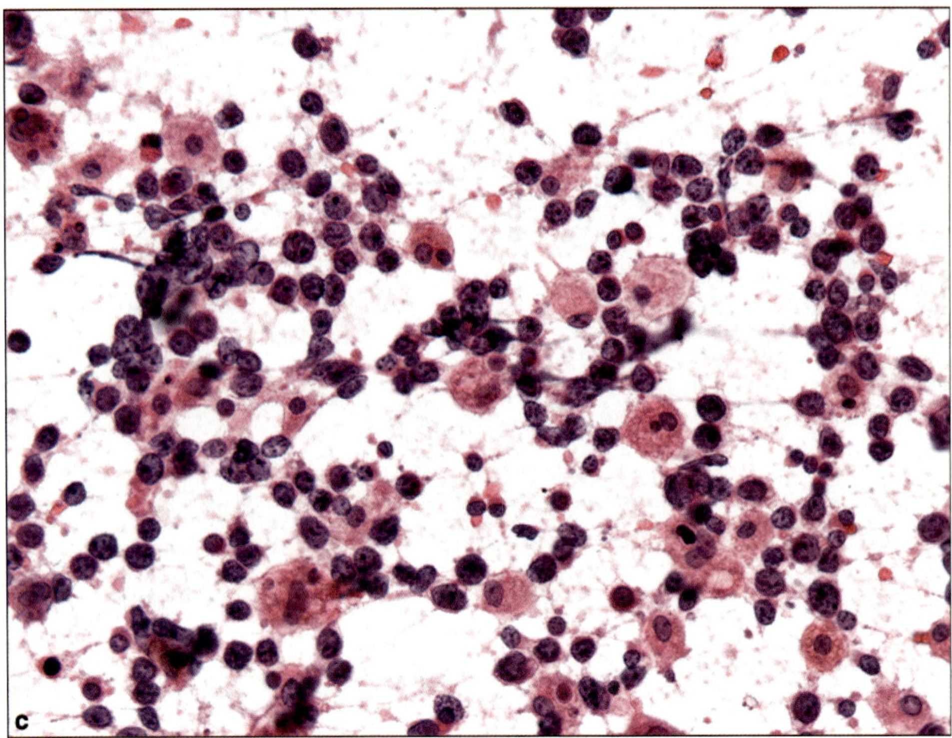

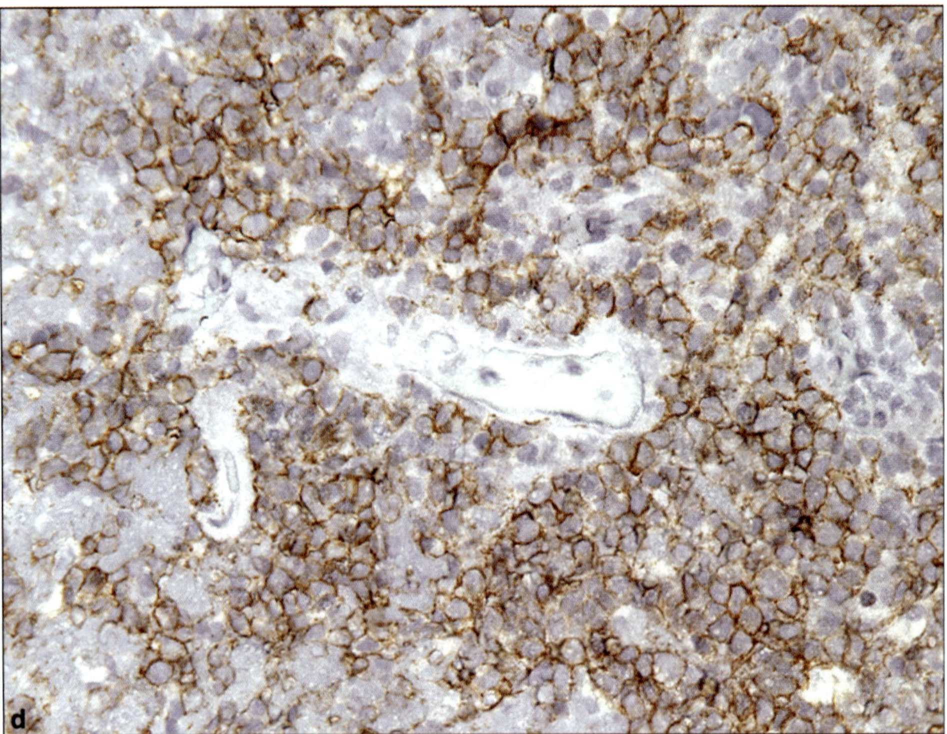

Much less frequently, low-grade histology may be present including that of *lymphoplasmacytic lymphoma*. Another distinctive manifestation of B-cell lymphoma is as a *marginal zone B-cell lymphoma* analogous to the lymphomas of the mucosa-associated lymphoid tissue (MALT) type. These typically present as

Figure 3.102. *continued.*

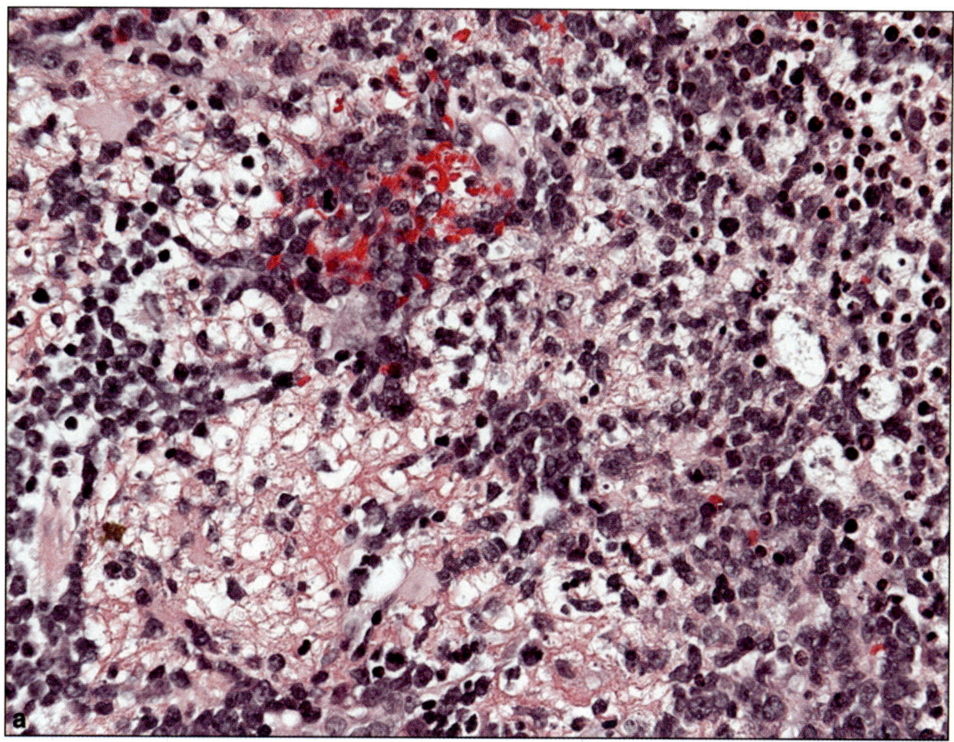

Figure 3.103. (a) Lymphomas undergoing recent exposure to corticosteroid therapy will reflect ongoing lysis of neoplastic B cells, leaving macrophages, activated microglia and astrocytes, and reactive T cells.

a dural-based mass mimicking meningioma (Tu et al., 2005). The cytological features are those of a low-grade lymphoma with small lymphocytes, some bearing irregular nuclei and variable plasmacytic differentiation. These tumors may contain foci of follicular differentiation as well as large deposits of amyloid.

Figure 3.103. *continued*
(b) Some areas with extensive necrosis will nevertheless show (c) preservation of concentric perivascular bands of reticulin, which is characteristic of CNS lymphomas.

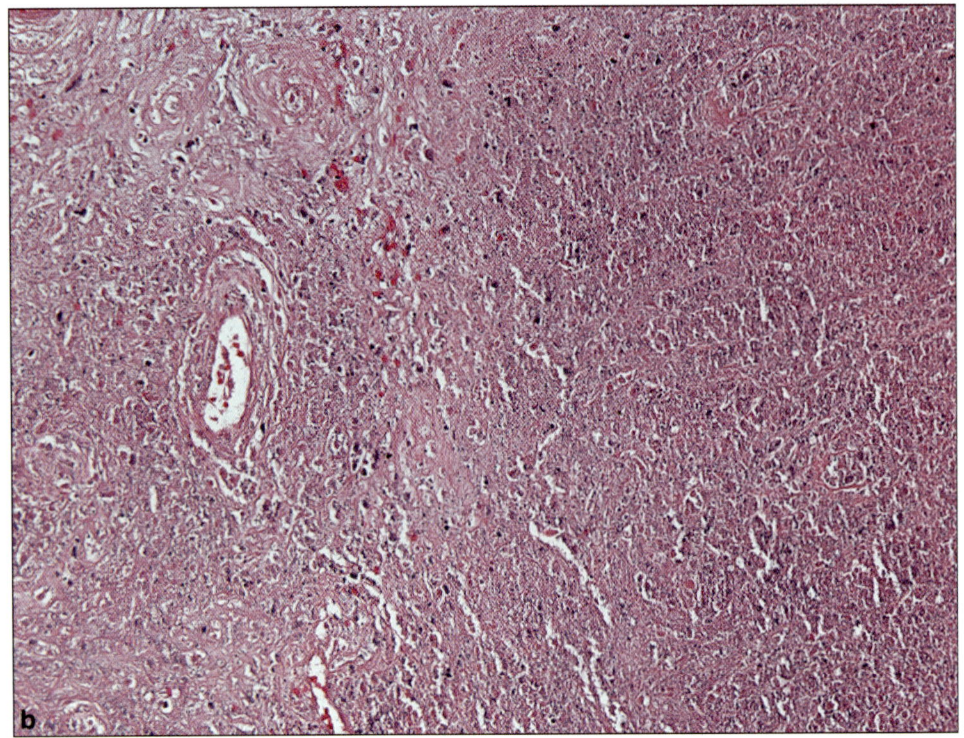

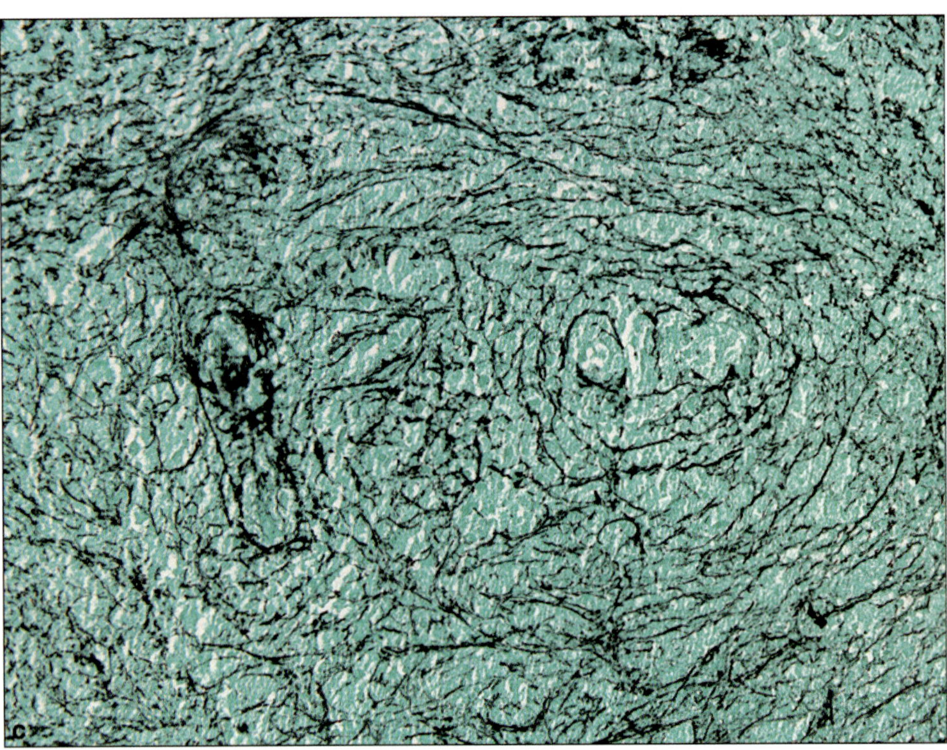

Plasmacytomas may involve cranial bone or meninges as an unusual manifestation of multiple myeloma but the extraosseous form typically manifests as nodular or plaquelike dural mass, capable of regional brain invasion (Figure 3.105) (Patriarca et al., 2001; Schluterman et al., 2004).

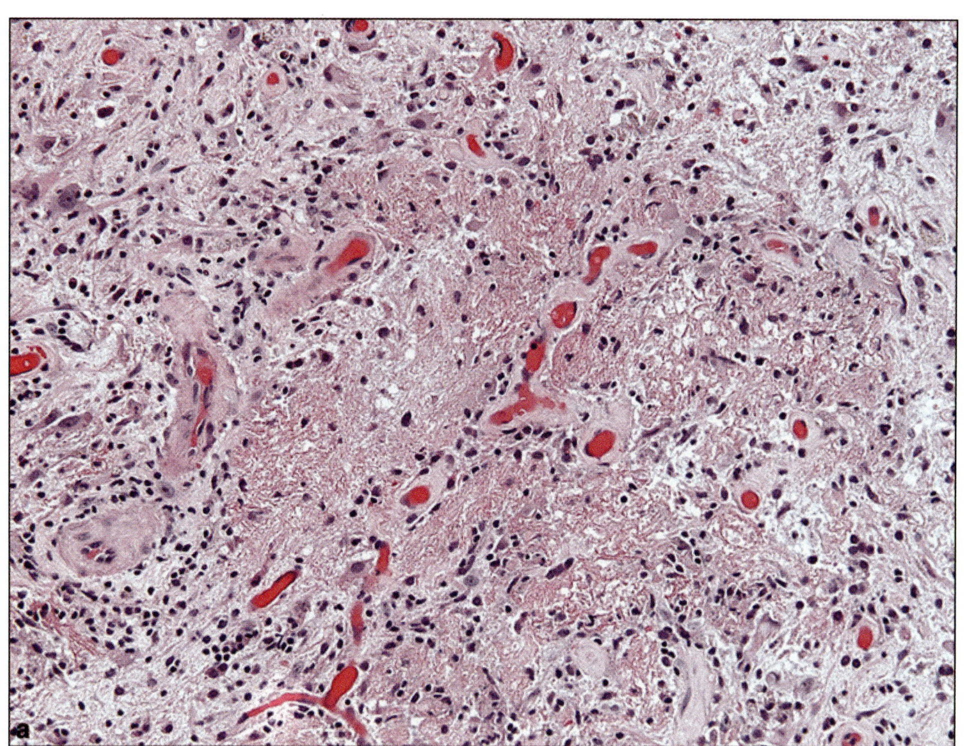

Figure 3.104. (a) An example of steroid-treated primary CNS B-cell lymphoma, with (b) preservation of specific B-cell CD20 immunoreactivity, (c) confirmed by a lack of staining for the necrotic B-cells and identification of remaining reactive T-cells with anti-CD3.

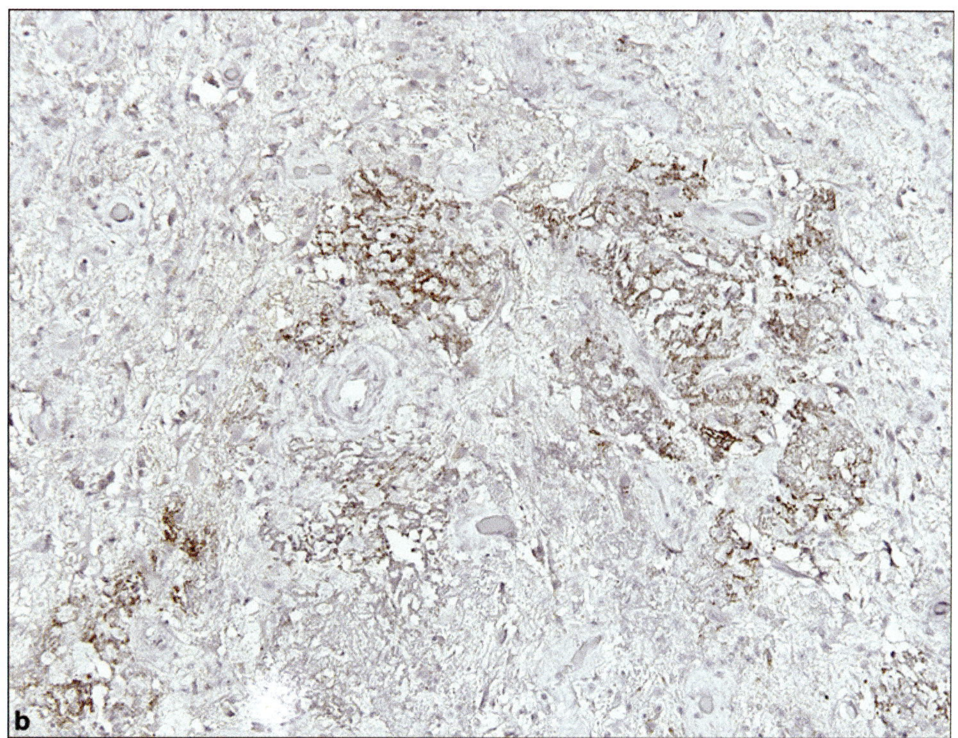

Intravascular (angiotropic) B-cell lymphoma often manifests as a rapidly progressive change in mental status with dementia and multifocal neurological deficits (Chapin et al., 1995; Liszka et al., 1994). The presence of single or small clusters of intravascular, neoplastic lymphocytes, typically in small- and medium-sized vessels, may be very subtle but highlighted with antibodies to B cell markers (Figure 3.106) (Ponzoni and Ferreri, 2006).

Figure 3.104. *continued.*

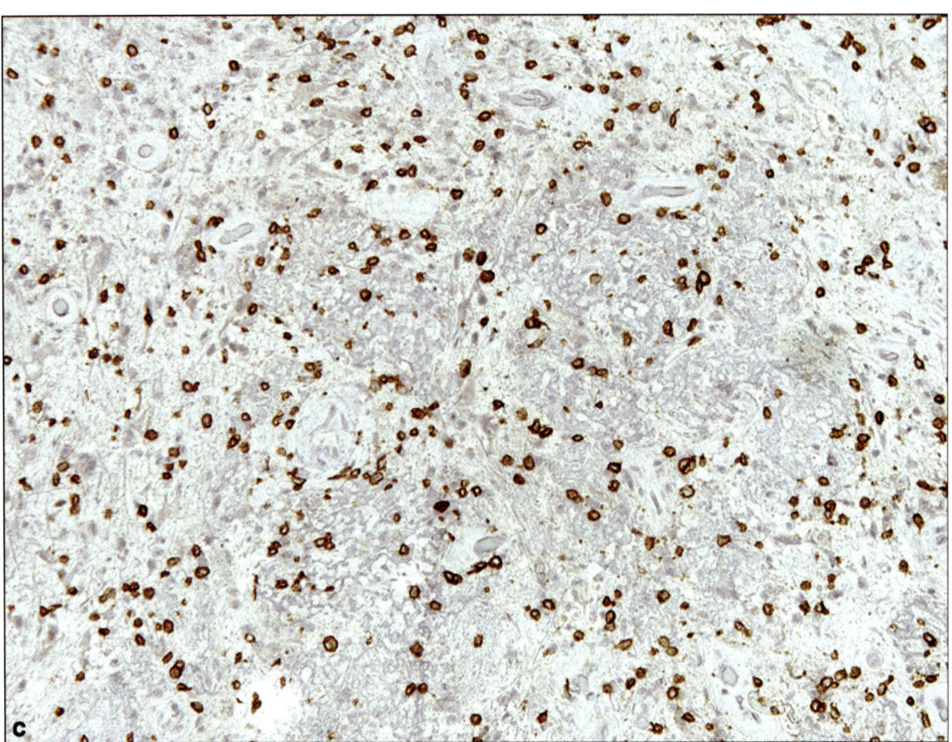

A number of other B-cell lymphomas or preneoplastic lymphoproliferative lesions have been described in the brain. Lymphomas include *follicular lymphoma* (Beriwal et al., 2003), *Burkitt's lymphoma* (Monabati et al., 2002), and *precursor B-cell lymphoblastic lymphoma* (Abla et al., 2004).

Lymphomatoid granulomatosis is almost always seen with concurrent pulmonary involvement, and presents with multifocal punctate or linear lesions (Figure 3.107a) (Patsalides et al., 2005; Tateishi et al., 2001). The condition is often seen in the context of immunodeficiency and is strongly associated with EBV infection (Mizuno et al., 2003). The histologic features consist of a mixed inflammatory infiltrate with atypical B cells (Figure 3.107b), which are positive for EBV, preferably demonstrated by in situ hybridization, or by immunohistochemistry.

A separate EBV–driven process is *posttransplant lymphoproliferative disease (PTLD)* in which lesions represent a spectrum ranging from polyclonal lymphoid populations to malignant lymphoma. These are categorized into early forms and as reactive plasmacytic hyperplasia, then to polymorphic PTLD, monomorphic PTLD of both B-cell and T-cell origins and Hodgkin lymphoma or a Hodgkin lymphoma–like PTLD (Harris et al., 2001). The onset of symptoms may be as early as 3 months after transplant to several years with a mean of 31 months (Castellano-Sanchez et al., 2004).

T-Cell Lymphoma T-cell lymphomas may occur as solitary or multiple brain masses and are apparently more common in males although large series do not exist because of the apparent rarity of the disorder. In most respects, they share

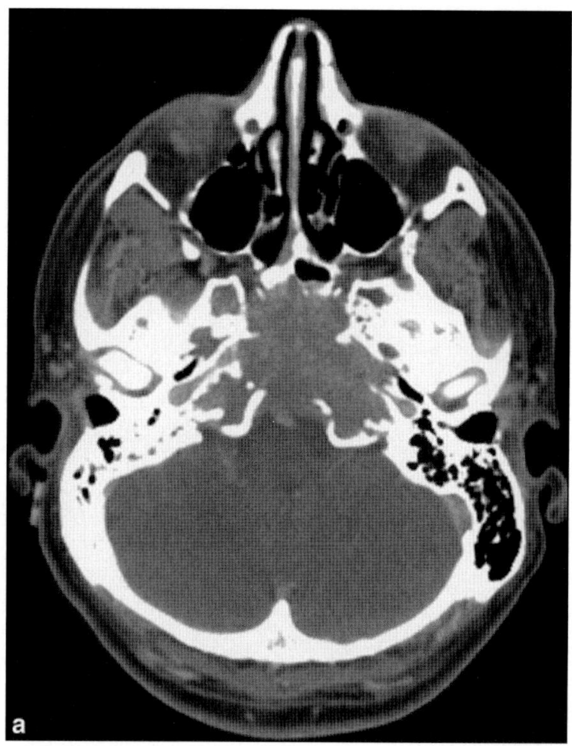

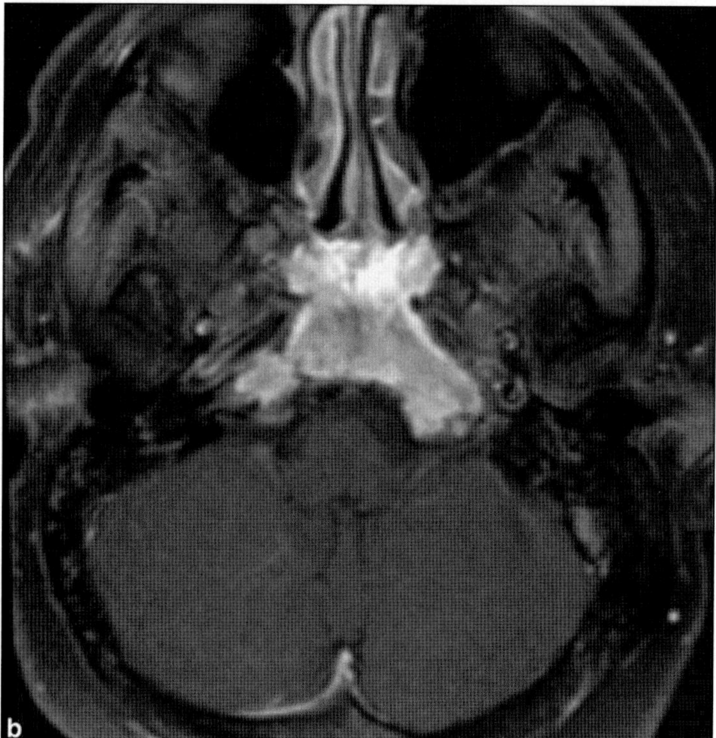

Figure 3.105. Plasmacytoma. (a) An axial CT-contrast-enhanced image shows a purely lytic central skull base mass with non-sclerotic margins. (b) On T1 contrast-enhanced MR, the mass displays homogenous enhancement. Plasmacytomas are generally purely lytic on CT images and have relatively low signal on T2 MR. The purely lytic nature of plasmacytomas is thought to be because they secrete osteoclast stimulating factor. Skull base metastasis, nasopharyngeal carcinoma, and intraosseous meningiomas are masses that could have a similar appearance on imaging. Chordomas and chondrosarcomas occur in this location, but can usually be distinguished from plasmacytomas based on their lower attenuation on CT images and higher attenuation on T2 MR images. The relatively high attenuation on CT and low signal on T2 MR of plasmacytomas is thought to reflect their high cellularity. Imaging is important in making the clinically important distinction between a single plasma cell-containing mass (plasmacytoma) and multiple lesions, which if present, would constitute multiple myeloma.

Figure 3.105. *continued* (c) Typical microscopic appearance of plasmacytoma, with sheets of monotonous or mildly pleomorphic cells with plasmacytoid features.

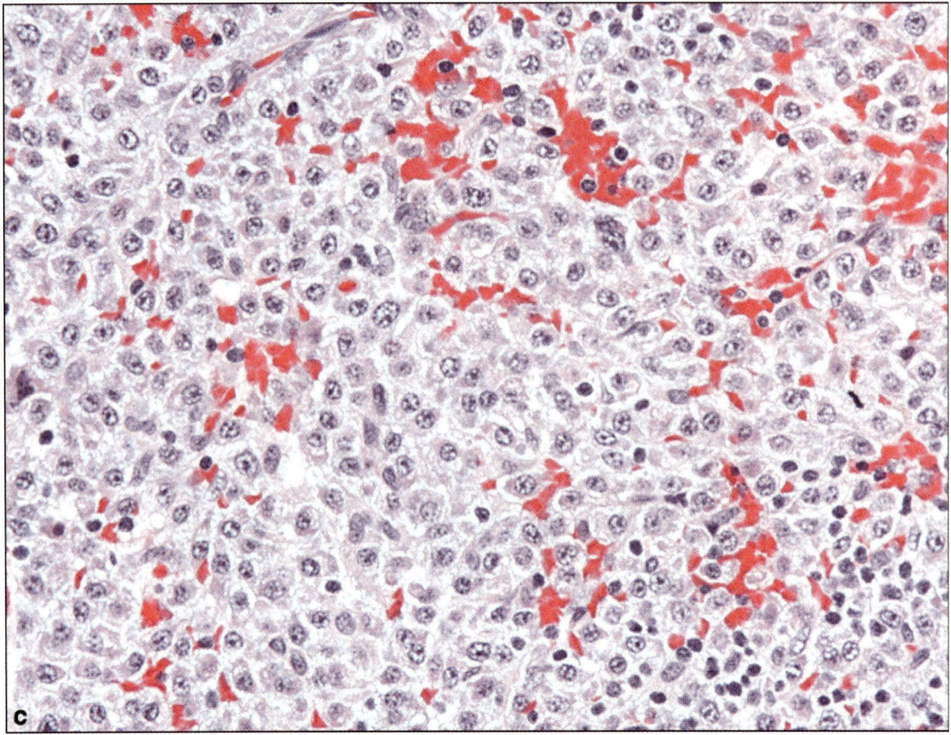

Figure 3.106. (a) MRI showing multifocal contrast-enhancing lesions signifying intravascular B-cell lymphoma.

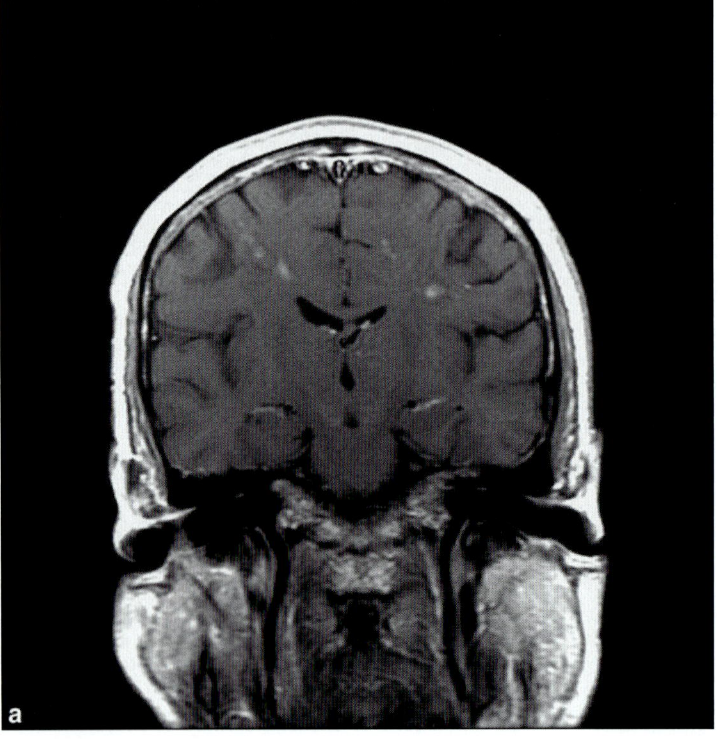

features with primary CNS B-cell lymphomas (Shenkier et al., 2005). Some cases may exhibit histologic features either suggestive of a reactive T-cell infiltrate or possibly a T-cell–rich B-cell lymphoma (Dulai et al., 2008). Molecular studies indicating clonal populations may be of particular importance in distinguishing these entities (Liu et al., 2003).

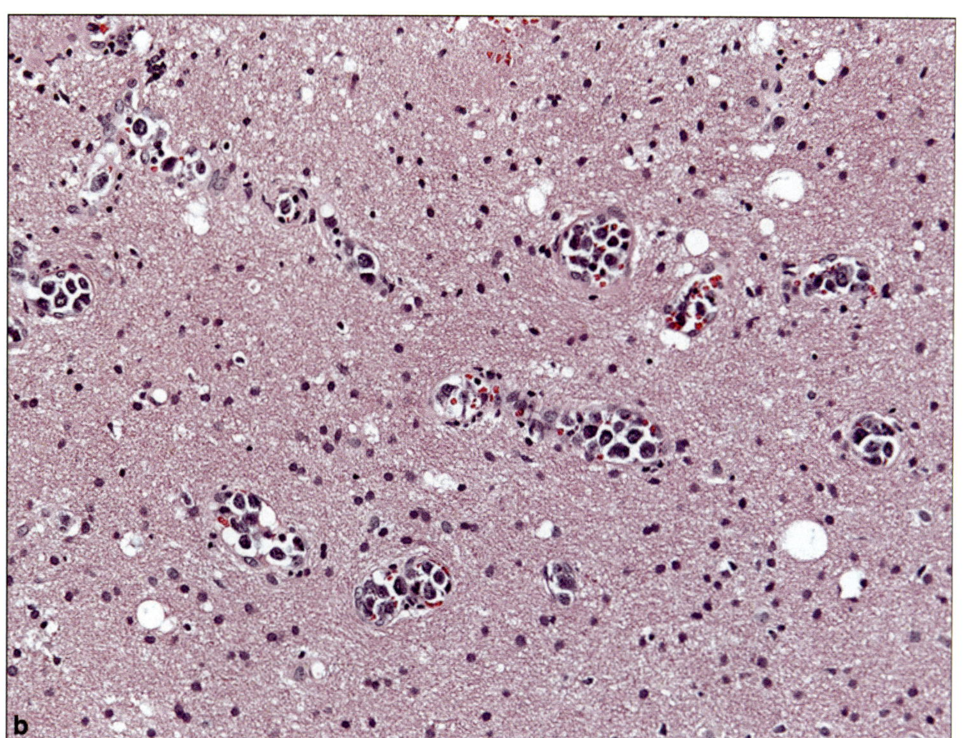

Figure 3.106. *continued*
(b) H&E and
(c) CD20-stained
intravascular B-cell
lymphoma.

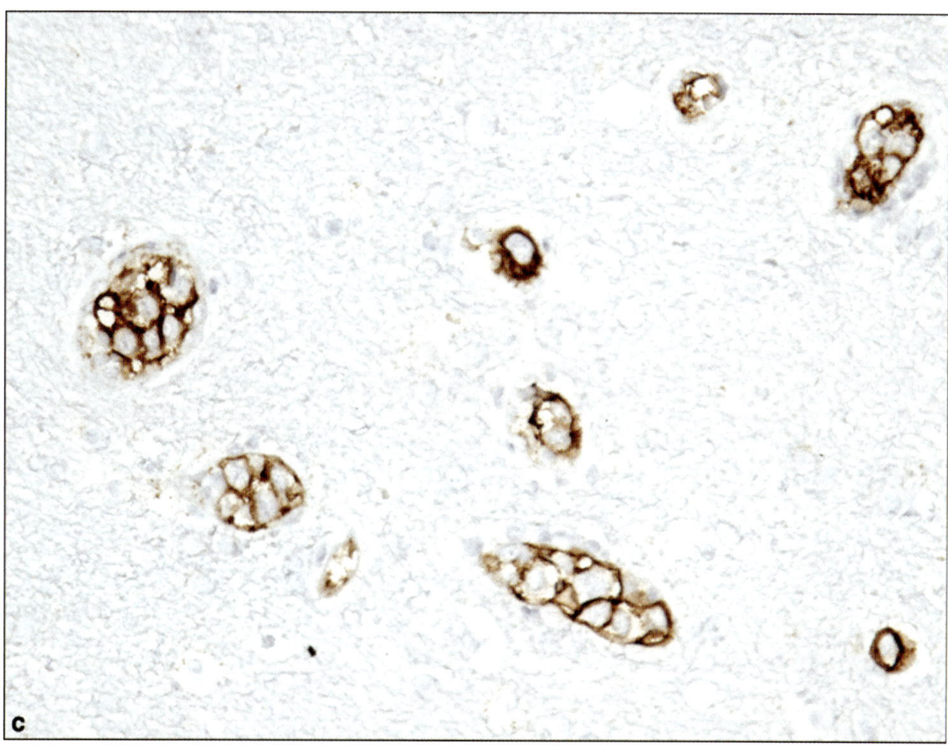

Anaplastic Large Cell Lymphoma This neoplasm is characterized by large atypical CD30-positive cells mostly of T-cell origin (Figure 3.108). Some tumors may be anaplastic lymphoma kinase (ALK 1) positive (George et al., 2003).

Figure 3.107.
(a) Lymphomatoid granulomatosis. A sagittal T1-weighted MR image shows numerous enhancing cerebral nodules with surrounding edema. The majority of nodules are within the gray matter or at the gray–white matter junction. Some of the nodules may be associated with hemorrhage or mineralization. The enhancement pattern reported with lymphomatoid granulomatosis is quite variable and includes leptomeningeal, perivascular, cranial nerve, gray matter and white matter.
(b) Lymphomatoid granulomatosis, with a mixed perivascular and parenchymal inflammatory infiltrate, characteristically immuno-hybridization or in situ hybridization positive for EBV, with a vague perivascular granulomatous morphology.

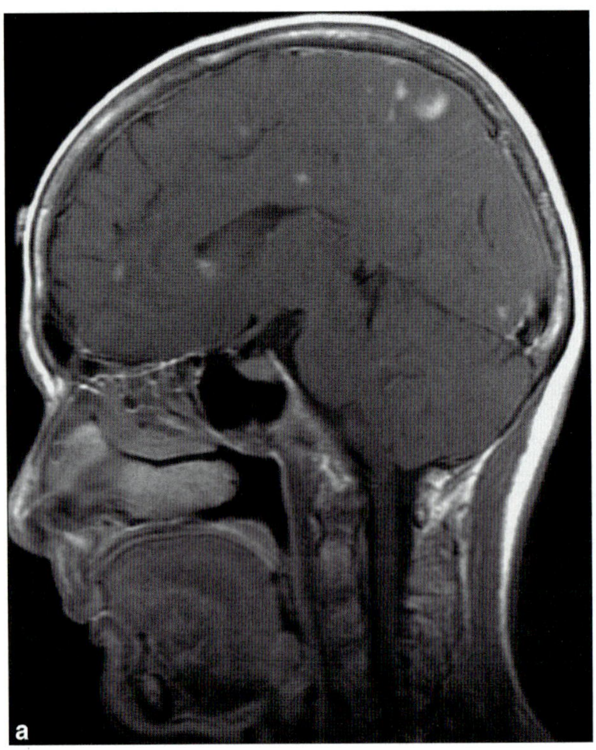

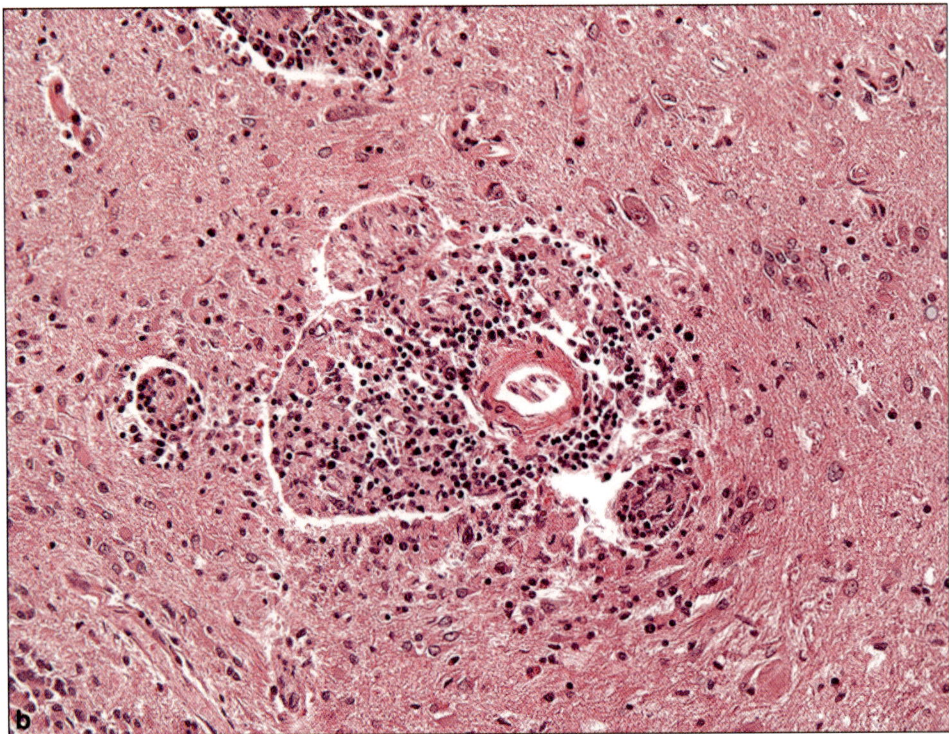

Hodgkin Disease CNS involvement, often dural or leptomeningeal-based (Deckert-Schluter et al., 1998), typically occurs late in the course of the disease. There are exceptional examples of primary intraparenchymal CNS Hodgkin disease (Herrlinger et al., 2000) Diagnosis requires the identification of Reed–Sternberg cells.

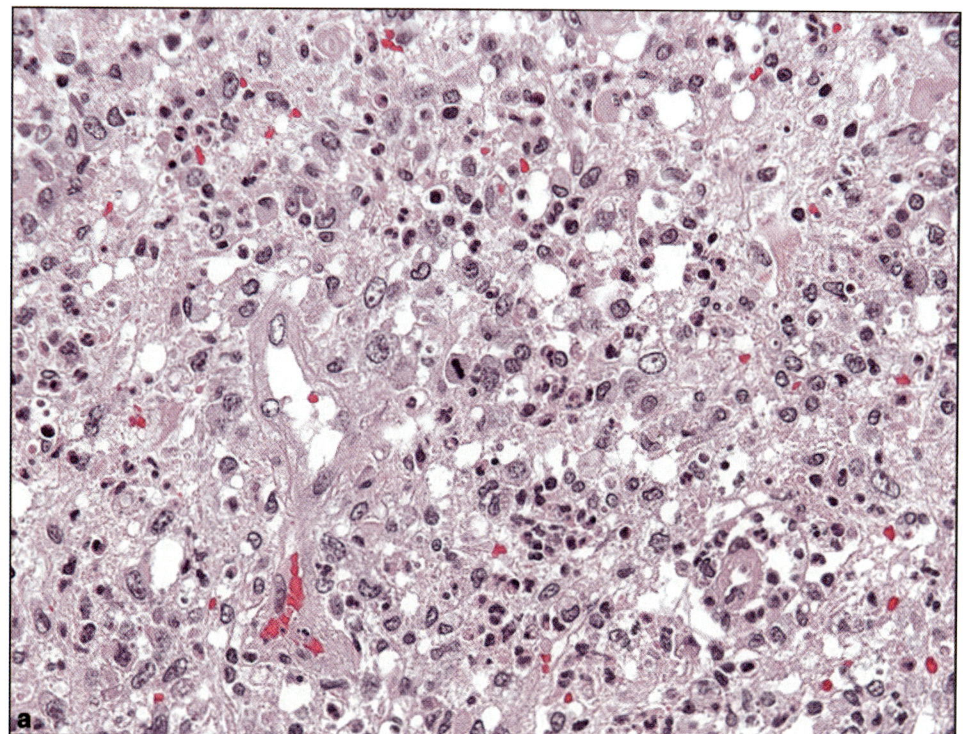

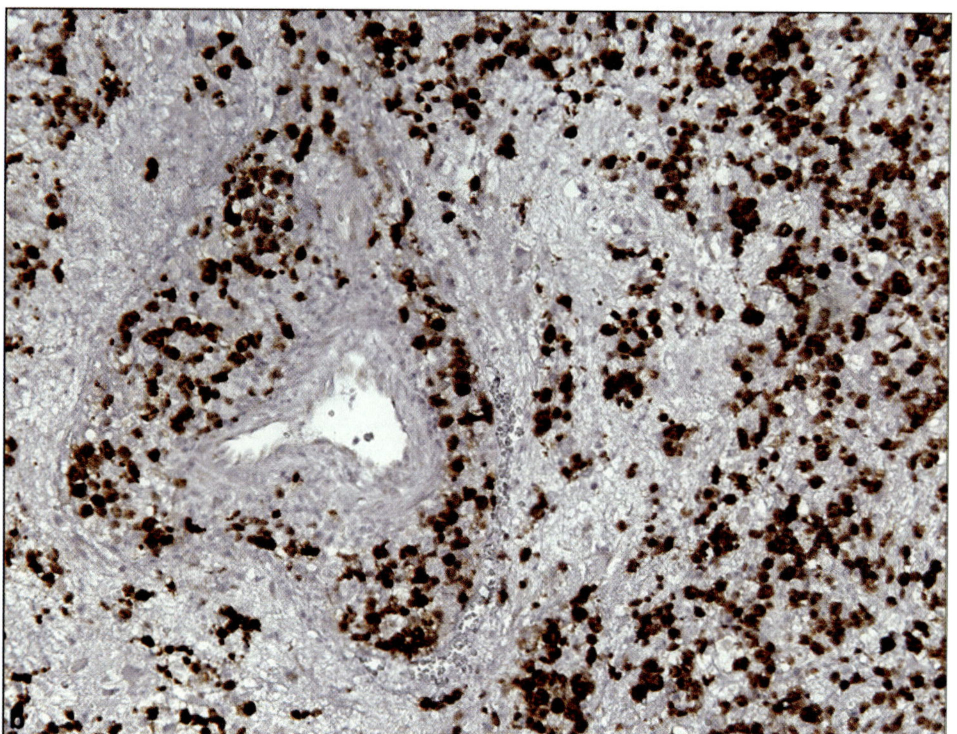

Figure 3.108. (a) Anaplastic large cell lymphoma is a poorly differentiated neoplasm of heterogeneous elements, with immunophenotyping showing (b) CD30 positivity and (c) numerous atypical T-cells with anti-CD3.

ROSAI–DORFMAN DISEASE

This lesion most commonly affects young adults, but all ages may be affected. Extranodal CNS involvement may be seen with or without concomitant lymph node involvement in the meninges as a mass lesion mimicking meningioma, or

Figure 3.108. *continued.*

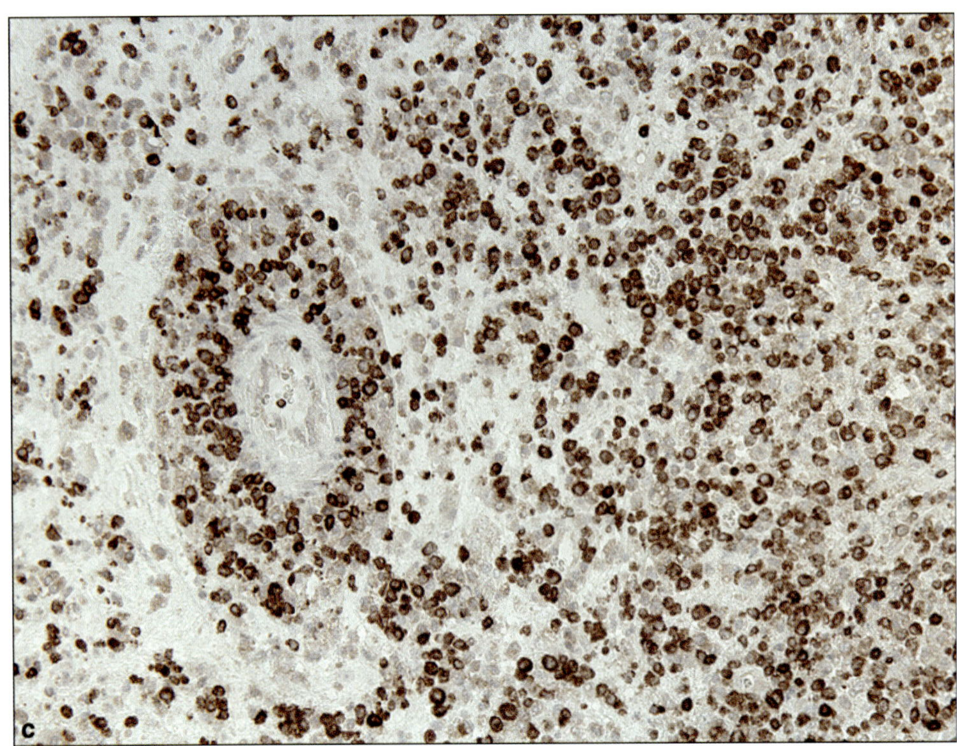

Figure 3.109.
Rosai–Dorfman disease,
composed of a
lymphoplasmacytic
proliferation with prominent
aggregates of histiocytes,
often multinucleated and
showing emperipolesis:
intracytoplasmic lymphocytes
in histiocyte,

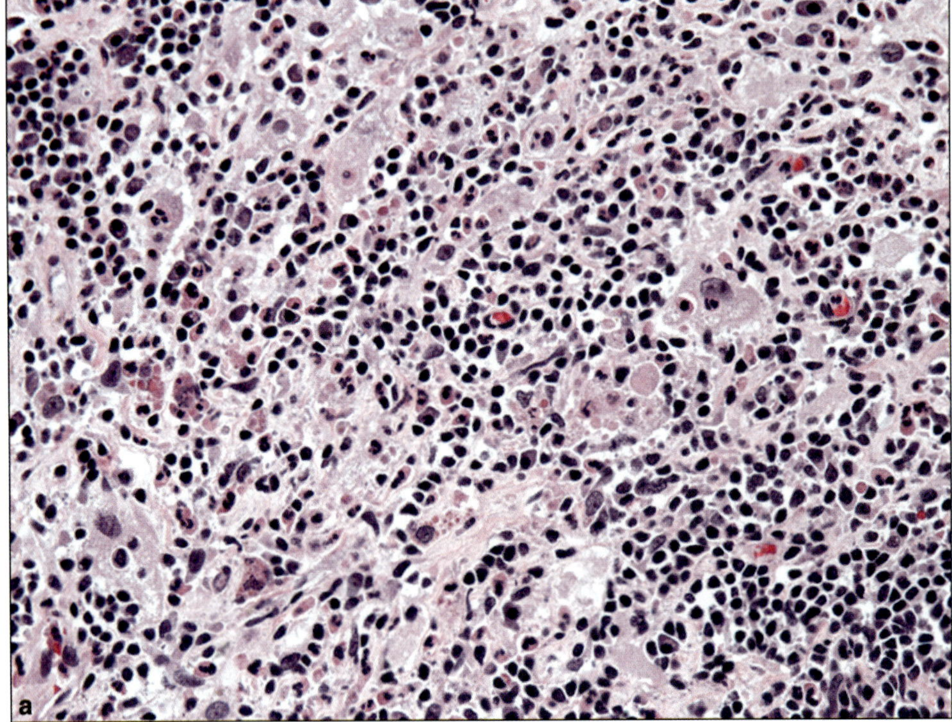

rarely in the sellar region or the brain parenchyma (Andriko et al., 2001; Juric et al., 2003). Excision is usually curative.

The histopathology of Rosai–Dorfman disease is that of a lympho-plasmacytic proliferation with prominent aggregates of histiocytes, often multi-nucleated (Figure 3.109). The phenomenon of emperipolesis may be seen

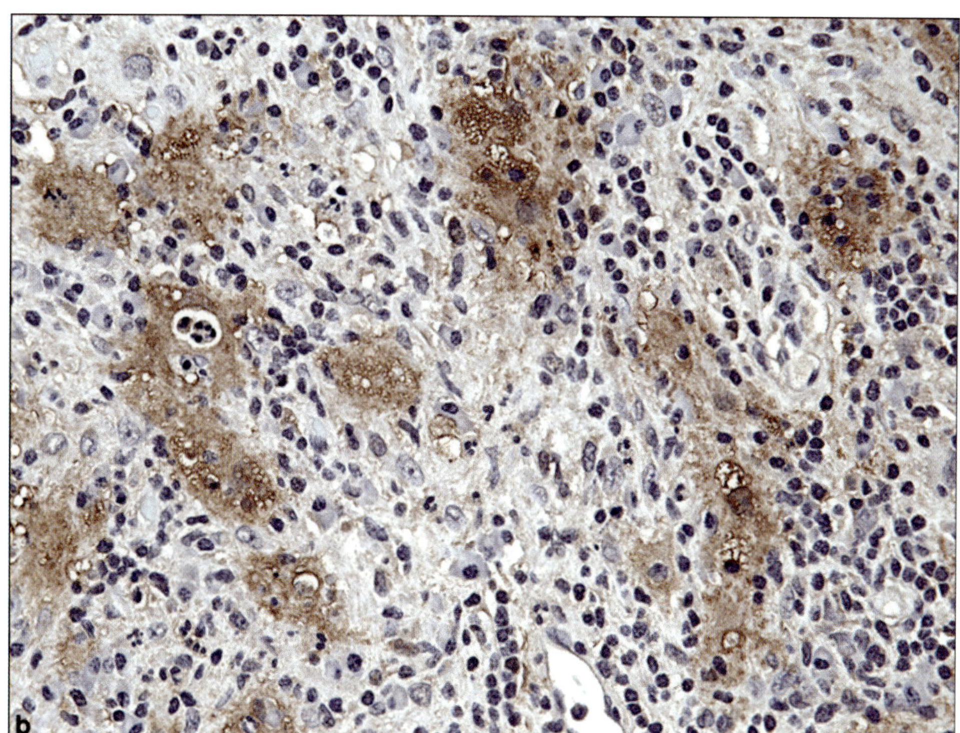

Figure 3.109. *continued* (b) highlighted by S-100 immunohistochemistry.

consisting of intracytoplasmic lymphocytes in histiocytes. The histiocytes are S-100 protein immunopositive, which aids in distinguishing this from other lymphohistiocytic lesions.

CNS INVOLVEMENT BY LEUKEMIA

Before the advent of now well-established protocols for chemotherapy in leukemia, involvement of the CNS was common in approximately 70% of patients with acute lymphocytic leukemia and approximately 50% of patients with acute myelogenous leukemia. Intracranial leukemia exists as a diffuse meningeal infiltrate or as a mass lesion. They are usually hyperdense by neuroimaging. One distinctive entity is *granulocytic sarcoma*, also known as extramedullary myeloid tumor or chloroma because of the green color historically associated with the gross specimen. These most often involves the dura with the capability of brain invasion (Barnett and Zussman, 1986).

Histologically, they are composed of myeloblasts and neutrophils and neutrophil precursors. In imprints, the myeloblasts and neutrophils are positive for myeloperoxidase (Harris, 2001).

REFERENCES

Abla O, Naqvi A, Ye C, Bhattacharjee R, Shago M, Abdelhaleem M, et al. Leptomeningeal precursor B-cell lymphoblastic lymphoma in a child with minimal bone marrow involvement. *J Pediatr Hematol Oncol* 2004; 26: 469–72.

Akpek EK, Ahmed I, Hochberg FH, Soheilian M, Dryja TP, Jakobiec FA, et al. Intra-ocular-central nervous system lymphoma: clinical features, diagnosis, and outcomes. *Ophthalmology* 1999; 106: 1805–10.

Andriko JA, Morrison A, Colegial CH, Davis BJ, Jones RV. Rosai-Dorfman disease isolated to the central nervous system: a report of 11 cases. *Mod Pathol* 2001; 14: 172–8.

Barnett MJ, Zussman WV. Granulocytic sarcoma of the brain: a case report and review of the literature. *Radiology* 1986; 160: 223–5.

Bataille B, Delwail V, Menet E, Vandermarcq P, Ingrand P, Wager M, et al. Primary intracerebral malignant lymphoma: report of 248 cases. *J Neurosurg* 2000; 92: 261–6.

Beriwal S, Hou JS, Miyamoto C, Garcia-Young JA. Primary dural low grade BCL-2 negative follicular lymphoma: a case report. *J Neurooncol* 2003; 61: 23–5.

Castellano-Sanchez AA, Li S, Qian J, Lagoo A, Weir E, Brat DJ. Primary central nervous system posttransplant lymphoproliferative disorders. *Am J Clin Pathol* 2004; 121: 246–53.

Chapin JE, Davis LE, Kornfeld M, Mandler RN. Neurologic manifestations of intravascular lymphomatosis. *Acta Neurol Scand* 1995; 91: 494–9.

Choi JS, Nam DH, Ko YH, Seo JW, Choi YL, Suh YL, et al. Primary central nervous system lymphoma in Korea: comparison of B- and T-cell lymphomas. *Am J Surg Pathol* 2003; 27: 919–28.

Cote TR, Manns A, Hardy CR, Yellin FJ, Hartge P. Epidemiology of brain lymphoma among people with or without acquired immunodeficiency syndrome. AIDS/Cancer Study Group. *J Natl Cancer Inst* 1996; 88: 675–9.

Deckert-Schluter M, Marek J, Setlik M, Markova J, Pakos E, Fischer R, et al. Primary manifestation of Hodgkin's disease in the central nervous system. *Virchows Arch* 1998; 432: 477–81.

Dulai MS, Park CY, Howell WD, Smyth LT, Desai M, Carter DM, et al. CNS T-cell lymphoma: an under-recognized entity? *Acta Neuropathol* 2008; 115: 345–56.

George DH, Scheithauer BW, Aker FV, Kurtin PJ, Burger PC, Cameselle-Teijeiro J, et al. Primary anaplastic large cell lymphoma of the central nervous system: prognostic effect of ALK-1 expression. *Am J Surg Pathol* 2003; 27: 487–93.

Harris N, Swerdlow SH, Frizzera G, Knowles DM. Post-transplant lymphoproliferative disorder. In: *Tumours of Haematopoietic and Lymphoid Tissues*. Lyon: IARC Press, 2001.

Herrlinger U, Klingel K, Meyermann R, Kandolf R, Kaiserling E, Kortmann RD, et al. Central nervous system Hodgkin's lymphoma without systemic manifestation: case report and review of the literature. *Acta Neuropathol (Berl)* 2000; 99: 709–14.

Juric G, Jakic-Razumovic J, Rotim K, Zarkovic K. Extranodal sinus histiocytosis (Rosai-Dorfman disease) of the brain parenchyma. *Acta Neurochir (Wien)* 2003; 145: 145–9; discussion 149.

Liszka U, Drlicek M, Hitzenberger P, Machacek E, Mayer H, Stockhammer G, et al. Intravascular lymphomatosis: a clinicopathological study of three cases. *J Cancer Res Clin Oncol* 1994; 120: 164–8.

Liu D, Schelper RL, Carter DA, Poiesz BJ, Shrimpton AE, Frankel BM, et al. Primary central nervous system cytotoxic/suppressor T-cell lymphoma: report of a unique case and review of the literature. *Am J Surg Pathol* 2003; 27: 682–8.

Louis DN, International Agency for Research on Cancer. *WHO Classification of Tumours of the Central Nervous System*. Lyon: International Agency for Research on Cancer, 2007.

Mizuno T, Takanashi Y, Onodera H, Shigeta M, Tanaka N, Yuya H, et al. A case of lymphomatoid granulomatosis/angiocentric immunoproliferative lesion with long clinical course and diffuse brain involvement. *J Neurol Sci* 2003; 213: 67–76.

Monabati A, Rakei SM, Kumar P, Taghipoor M, Rahimi A. Primary burkitt lymphoma of the brain in an immunocompetent patient. Case report. *J Neurosurg* 2002; 96: 1127–9.

Patriarca F, Zaja F, Silvestri F, Sperotto A, Scalise A, Gigli G, et al. Meningeal and cerebral involvement in multiple myeloma patients. *Ann Hematol* 2001; 80: 758–62.

Patsalides AD, Atac G, Hedge U, Janik J, Grant N, Jaffe ES, et al. Lymphomatoid granulomatosis: abnormalities of the brain at MR imaging. *Radiology* 2005; 237: 265–73.

Penn I, Porat G. Central nervous system lymphomas in organ allograft recipients. *Transplantation* 1995; 59: 240–4.

Ponzoni M, Ferreri AJ. Intravascular lymphoma: a neoplasm of 'homeless' lymphocytes? *Hematol Oncol* 2006; 24: 105–12.

Schluterman KO, Fassas AB, Van Hemert RL, Harik SI. Multiple myeloma invasion of the central nervous system. *Arch Neurol* 2004; 61: 1423–9.

Shenkier TN. Unusual variants of primary central nervous system lymphoma. *Hematol Oncol Clin North Am* 2005; 19: 651–64, vi.

Shenkier TN, Blay JY, O'Neill BP, Poortmans P, Thiel E, Jahnke K, et al. Primary CNS lymphoma of T-cell origin: a descriptive analysis from the international primary CNS lymphoma collaborative group. *J Clin Oncol* 2005; 23: 2233–9.

Stenzel W, Pels H, Staib P, Impekoven P, Bektas N, Deckert M. Concomitant manifestation of primary CNS lymphoma and Toxoplasma encephalitis in a patient with AIDS. *J Neurol* 2004; 251: 764–6.

Tateishi U, Terae S, Ogata A, Sawamura Y, Suzuki Y, Abe S, et al. MR imaging of the brain in lymphomatoid granulomatosis. *AJNR Am J Neuroradiol* 2001; 22: 1283–90.

Tu PH, Giannini C, Judkins AR, Schwalb JM, Burack R, O'Neill BP, et al. Clinicopathologic and genetic profile of intracranial marginal zone lymphoma: a primary low-grade CNS lymphoma that mimics meningioma. *J Clin Oncol* 2005; 23: 5718–27.

GERM CELL TUMORS

Clinical and Radiological Features

The vast majority of CNS germ cell tumors occur below the age of 25 years with a peak incidence that coincides with puberty and are more common in males. Pineal region germ cell tumors are more frequently found in boys with the opposite tendency in suprasellar examples. Pineal and suprasellar germ cell tumors may occur simultaneously or sequentially. CNS germ cell tumors epitomize the variable incidence of certain neoplasms according to geographic location. They are far more prevalent in Pacific Asia, particularly Japan, but this trend is also evidenced by series from Taiwan and Korea (Nomura, 2001).

Like other extragonadal germ cell tumors, CNS forms tend to occur in the midline. Most occur in the vicinity of the third ventricle, most commonly in the pineal gland followed by the suprasellar region. CNS germ cell tumors may also occur in an intraventricular, diffuse periventricular, or deep cortical gray matter location. Extremely large congenital teratomas may occur, either occupying much of the intracranial space or in the form of sacrococcygeal teratomas. CNS germ cell tumors do not carry WHO grade designations.

A wide variety of clinical manifestations may be seen with CNS germ cell tumors depending on their location and rate of growth. Examples arising in the pineal gland cause obstructive hydrocephalus at the level of the aqueduct of Sylvius, with paralysis of upward gaze and convergence occurring due to compression of the superior colliculi of the midbrain tegmentum, known as Parinaud syndrome. Suprasellar mass lesions may produce visual defects or endocrine manifestations of a disrupted hypothalamic–pituitary axis. Endocrine abnormalities such as precocious puberty have been associated with pineal germ cell tumors (Matsutani et al., 1997).

Neuroimaging will usually raise suspicion of a germ cell tumor in the appropriate clinical setting with any mass of the pineal or suprasellar region in a child (Figure 3.110a). There is an interesting tendency for some CNS germ cell tumors in Asians to form away from the midline (Figure 3.110b) (Masuzawa et al., 1986; Okamoto et al., 2002; Rushing et al., 2006; Sato et al., 2003). They usually show prominent contrast enhancement. As with other teratomas, a marked cystic component with calcification and fat may be seen. Choriocarcinoma is well known for their hemorrhagic tendency. It is important to realize that some CNS germ cell tumors may show a predominant pattern of infiltration rather than mass effect, particularly into subcortical gray matter.

Gross Pathology

Germinomas are usually soft friable tumors and hemorrhage should suggest the additional presence of choriocarcinoma or more malignant elements. A myxoid element may suggest yolk sac tumor. Benign teratomas are marked by the same bizarre admixture of gross elements such as fat, cartilage, bone, and or even teeth and hair as are seen in gonadal teratomas.

GERMINOMA

Pathology

This is the most common CNS germ cell tumor in a pure form (Bjornsson et al., 1985). The microscopic appearance is indistinguishable from ordinary seminomas or dysgerminomas of the testis or ovary, respectively (Figure 3.110c–e). The tumor is composed of primitive large cells in sheets and lobules separated by fibrovascular trabeculae. The tumor cells contain large spherical nuclei and prominent and characteristically angular nucleoli. The cytoplasm is faint, vacuolated, and lacy. The fibrovascular septae often contain variable

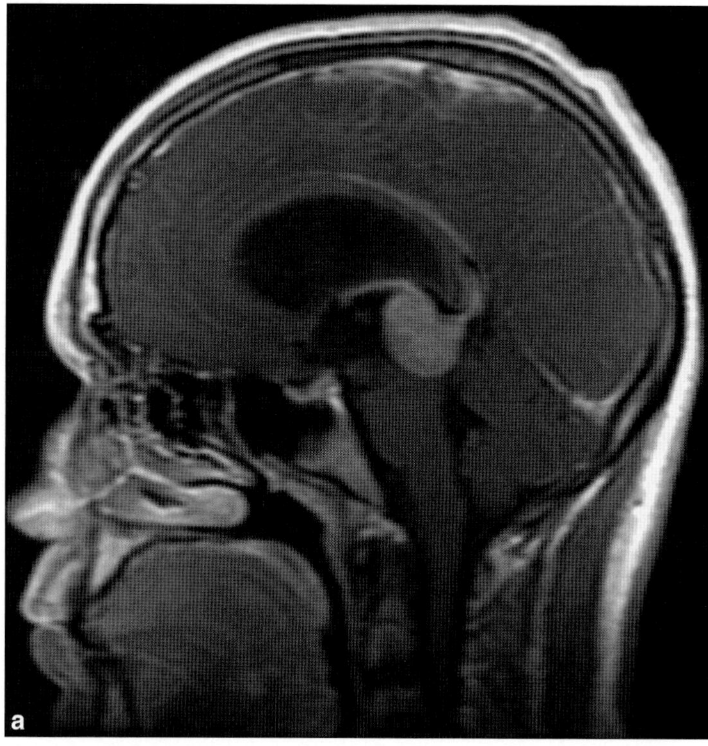

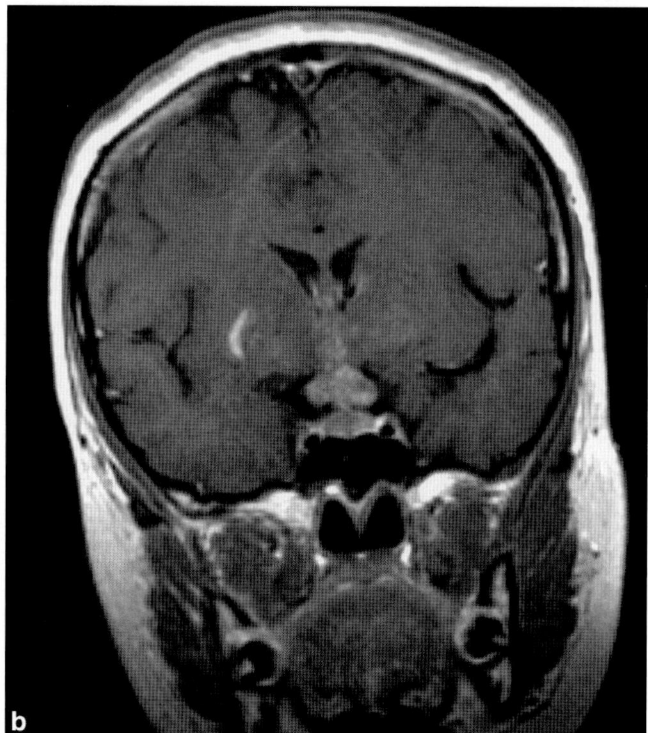

Figure 3.110. Germinoma. (a) A sagittal T1 MR with contrast enhancement shows a homogeneously enhancing pineal region mass that is compressing the tectum. There is hydrocephalous, presumably because of compression of the sylvian aqueduct. (b) A coronal T1 MR image with contrast enhancement shows a suprasellar germinoma. A cora T1 mi image with contra enhancem shows suprasella germinon There is an interesting tendency for some germinomas to occur outside the midline in Asian patients. Pineal region germinomas are much more common in males, whereas suprasellar germinomas or more common in females. Germinomas tend to demonstrate more uniform enhancement than other germ cell tumors. Germ cell tumors tend to engulf the pineal gland as opposed to pineoblastomas and pineocytomas, which tend to centrifugally disperse the gland. If a germinoma is suspected, the entire neuraxis should be imaged because of the high frequency of CSF tumor seeding.

numbers of benign small lymphocytes, usually a mixed T-cell population. Their presence is so variable that they may not be present in small biopsies or they may predominate to the point of obscuring the germ cell tumor population, thus posing a potential diagnostic pitfall (Mueller et al., 2007). Other examples

Figure 3.110. *continued* (c) Germinomas are histologically identical to seminomas or dysgerminomas, composed of large cells with vacuolated or lacy cytoplasm, and round nuclei with prominent and angular nucleoli. (d) Germinomas are regularly accompanied by varying degrees of lymphocytic inflammation, mostly as bands dividing large nest of germinoma cells, but in some instance may obscure the underlying presence of these cells.

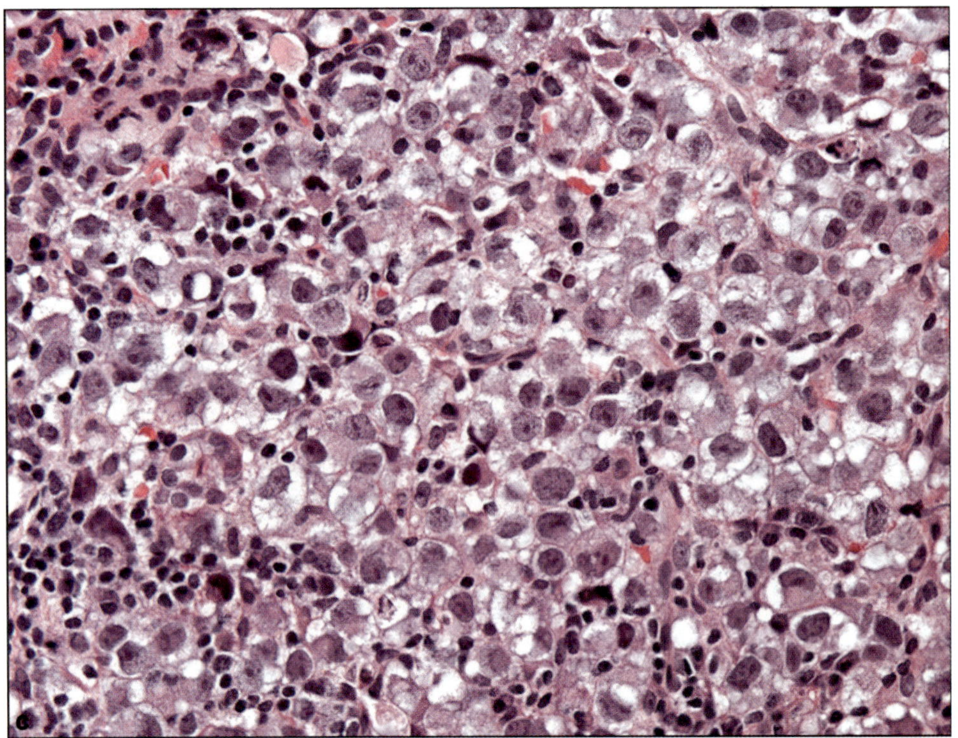

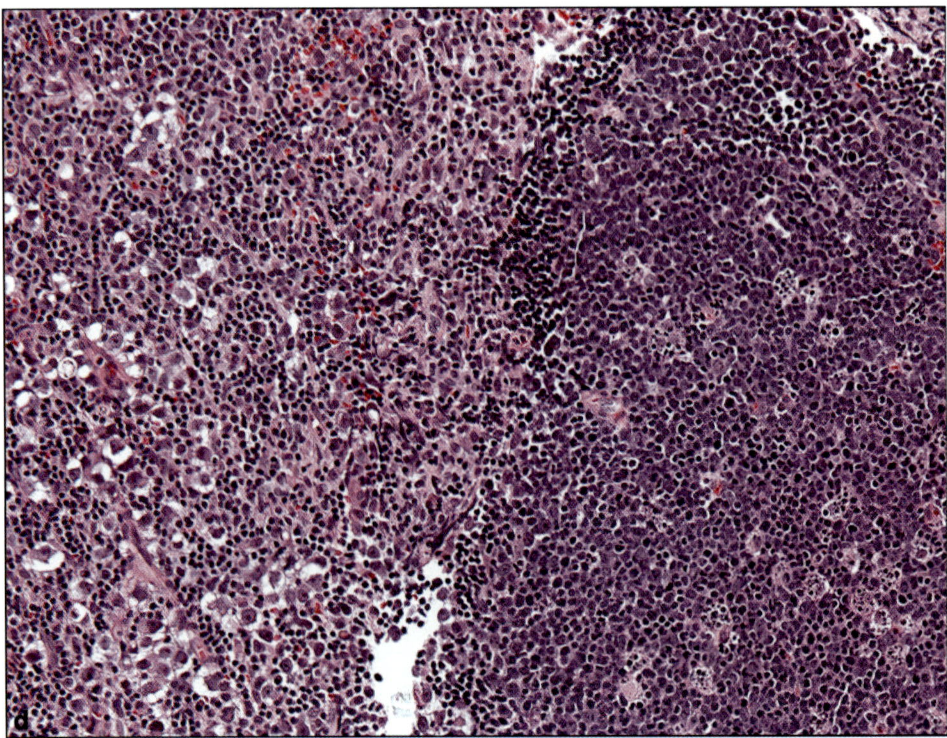

of lymphocytic proliferation include lymphoplasmacytic or germinal center differentiation.

Immunohistochemically, germinomas show strong cell membrane staining for c-kit (Nakamura et al., 2005) and slightly less commonly, placental alkaline phosphatase (PLAP) (Bjornsson et al., 1985; Felix and Becker, 1990).

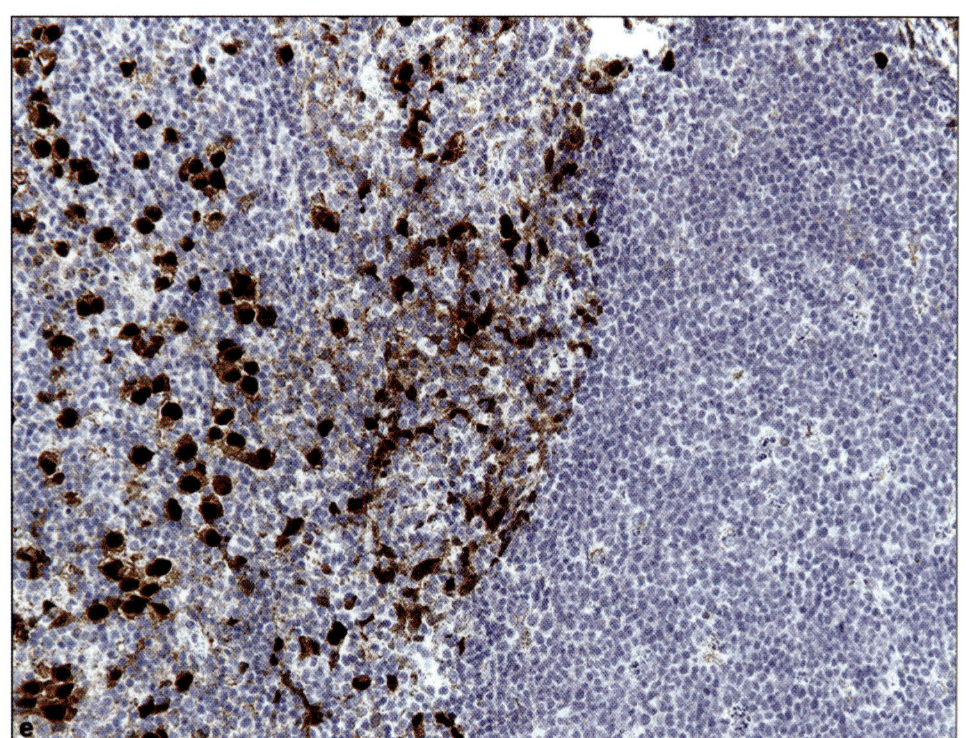

Figure 3.110. *continued* (e) OCT4 immunohistochemistry is the superior method of identifying germinoma cells.

A preferable immunostain for germinoma is OCT4, which shows nuclear reactivity (Hattab et al., 2005). Germinomas might also show focal immuno-positivity for cytokeratins (Felix and Becker, 1990; Ho and Liu, 1992). They may also show syncytiotrophoblastic differentiation with β–human chorionic gonadotropin (HCG) immunopositivity. These examples are currently believed to behave similar to pure germinomas and should not prompt variation in diagnosis.

EMBRYONAL CARCINOMA

Pathology

CNS embryonal carcinoma is exceedingly rare. They are composed of sheets or cords of primitive cells (Figure 3.111), forming abortive papillary and glandular structures with large nuclei and prominent nucleoli. The cells sometimes form "embryoid" bodies composed of disks of cells with cystic cavities resembling early embryos. They may be immunopositive for cytokeratin, CD30, as well as PLAP and OCT 4.

YOLK SAC TUMOR (ENDODERMAL SINUS TUMOR)

Pathology

This primitive neoplasm features differentiation resembling yolk sac endoderm. The cells show a sinusoidal growth pattern of variable cellularity

Figure 3.111. (a) Embryonal carcinoma, with (b) CD30 immunopositivity.

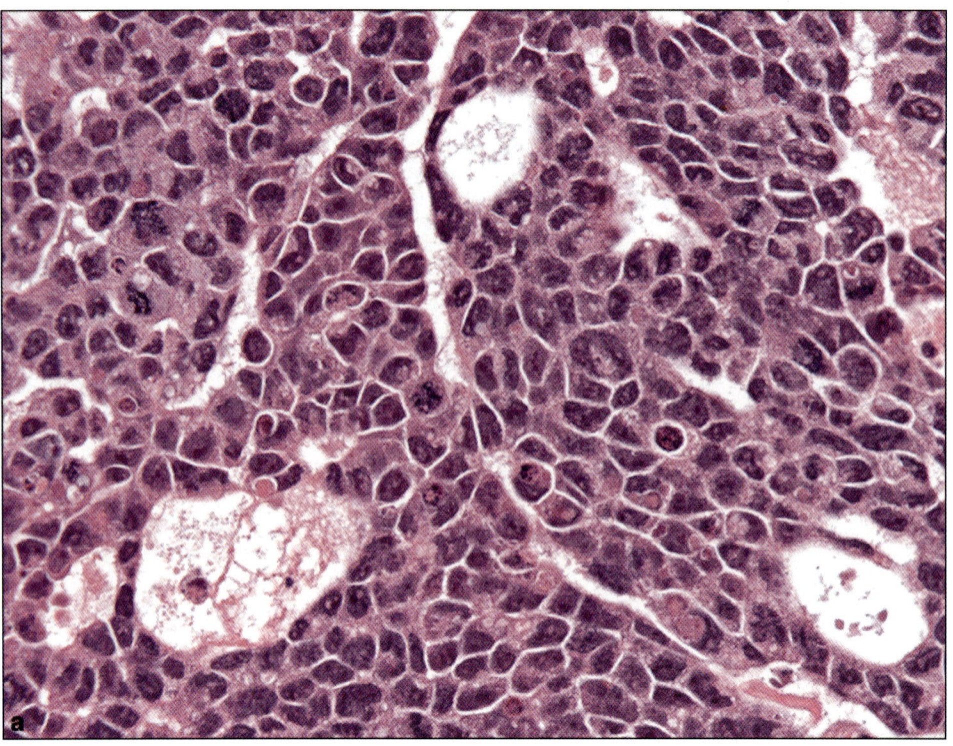

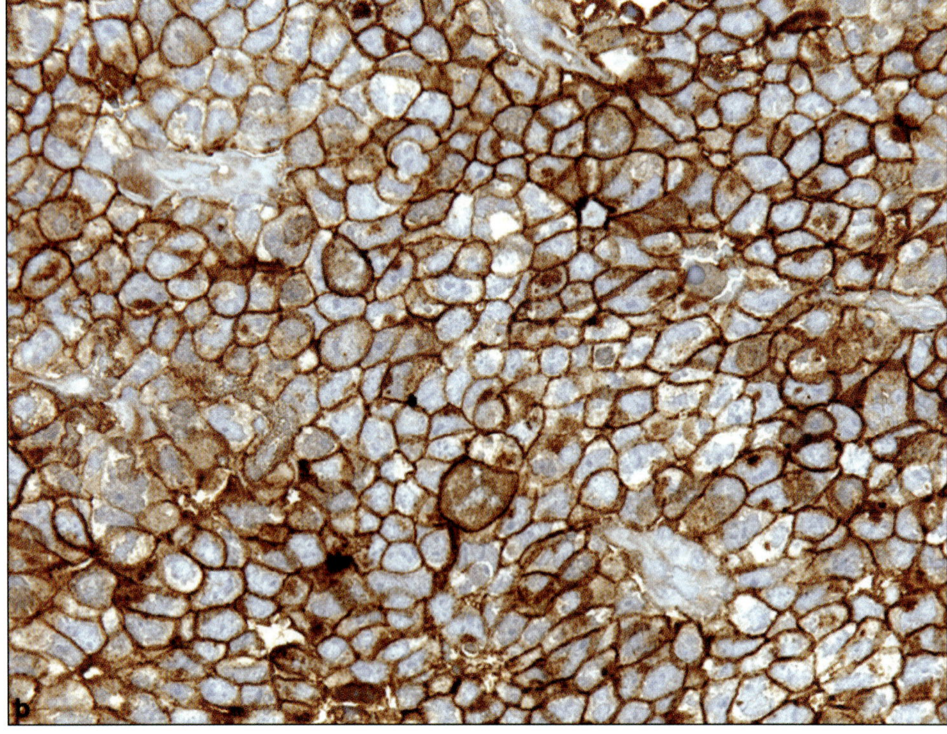

in a myxoid matrix. Epithelioid elements may produce sheets of cells but more commonly produce a reticular pattern composed of sinusoidal channels lined by epithelium (Figure 3.112). When these form a fibrovascular projection into such a space, they represent a Schiller–Duval body. Other

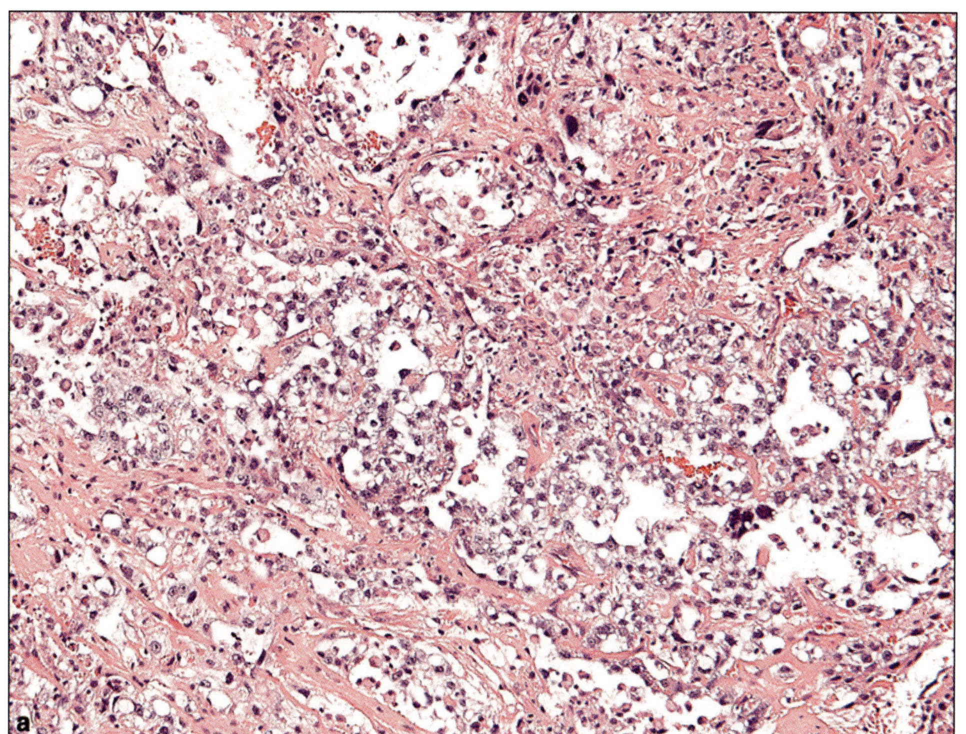

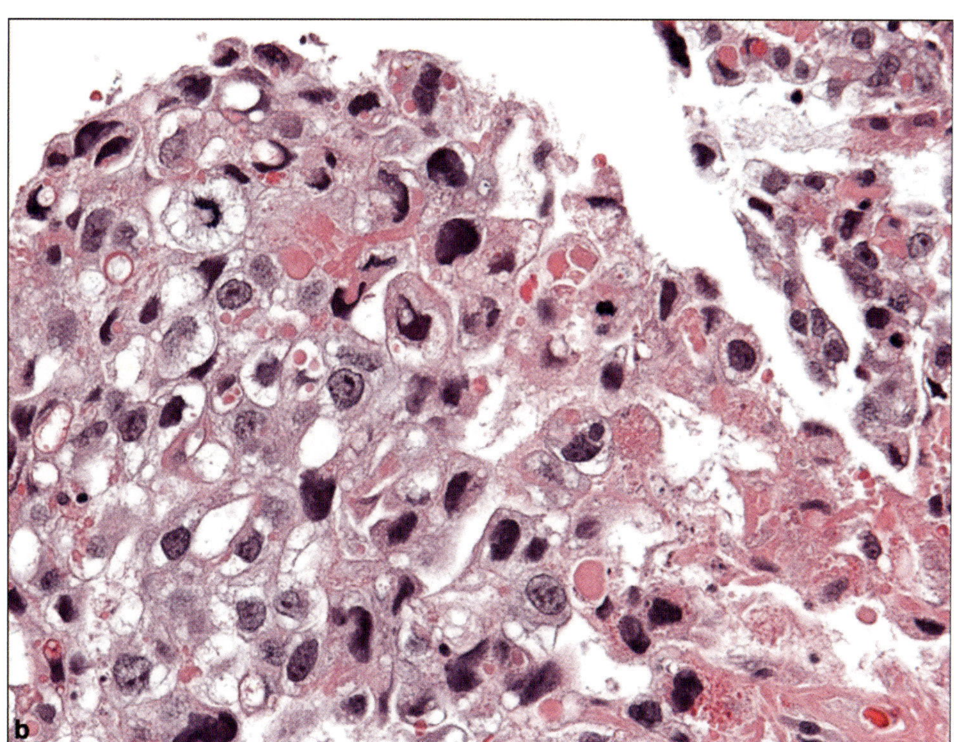

Figure 3.112. Yolk sac tumor (endodermal sinus tumor). (a) The most common pattern includes cystic spaces with a sinusoidal growth pattern. (b) Solid growth patterns may also be observed,

forms of differentiation include enteric-type glands with goblet cells or hepatocellular differentiation. Brightly eosinophilic, diastase-resistant PAS, and alpha-fetoprotein (AFP)-positive hyaline globules either in cytoplasm or the stroma is considered diagnostic of yolk sac tumor. AFP is considered the

Figure 3.112. *continued*
(c) in which eosinophilic cytoplasmic globules are PAS positive.
(d) Alpha fetoprotein is the diagnostic immunostain.

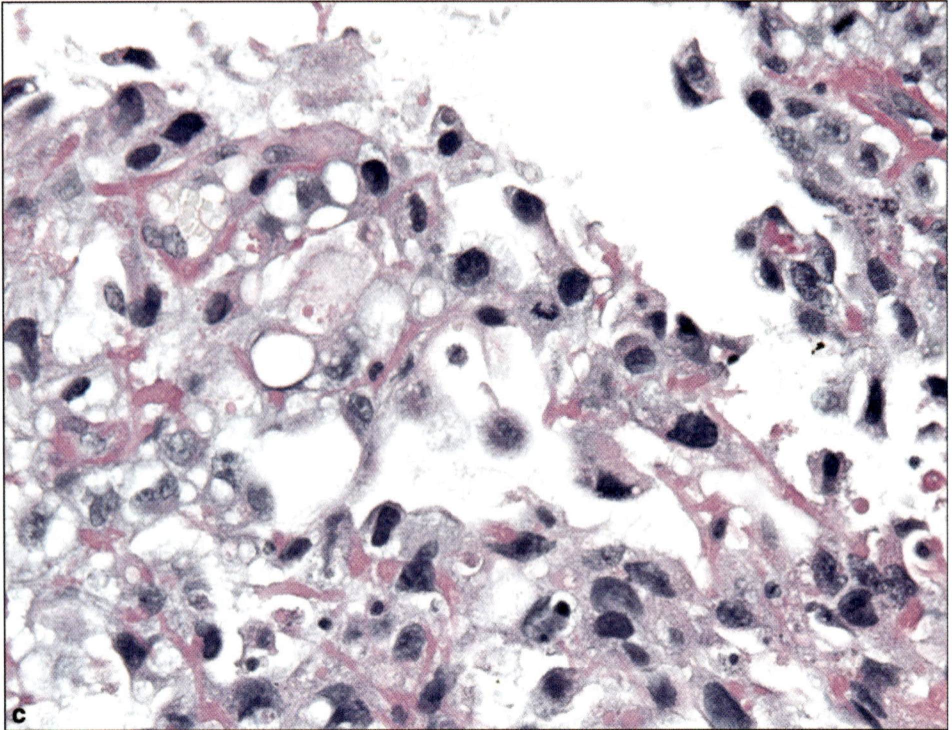

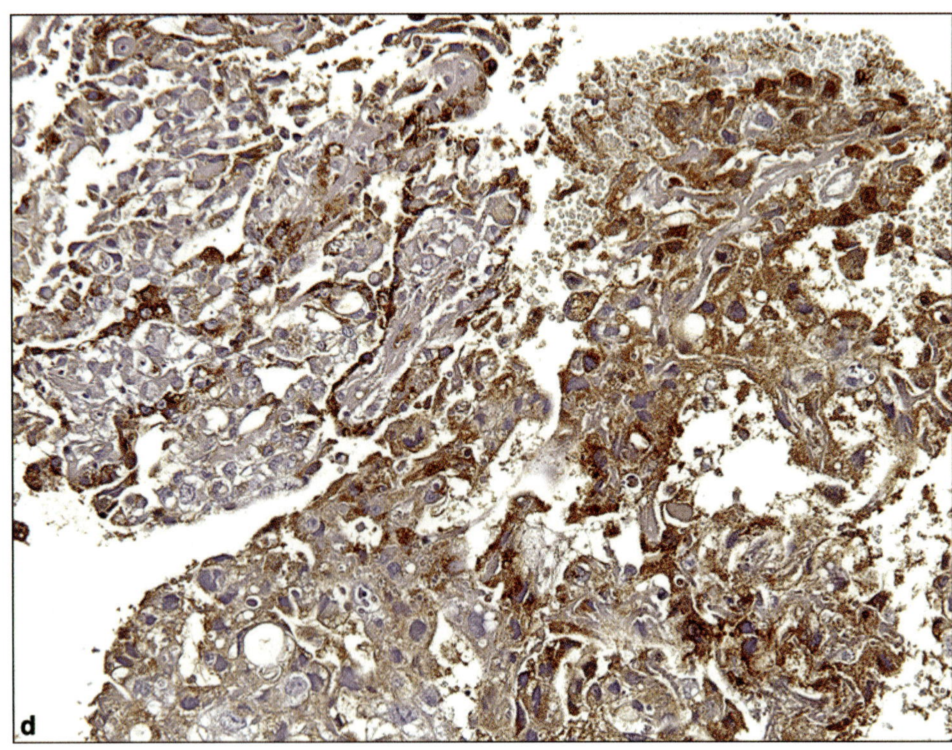

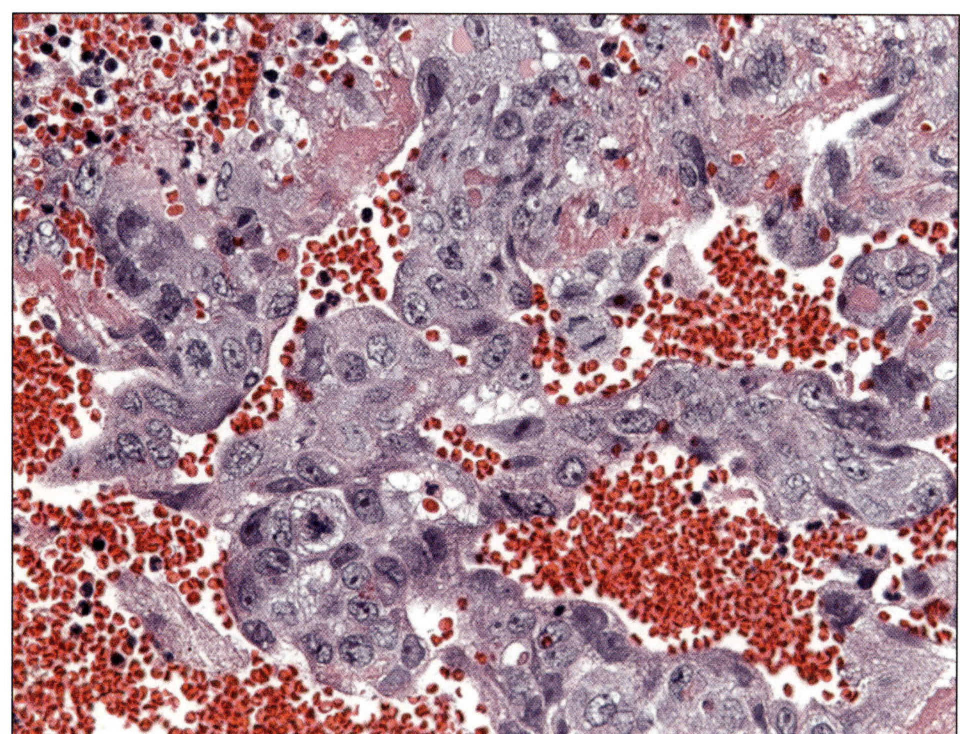

Figure 3.113. The cyto- and syncytiotrophoblastic giant cell elements of choriocarcinoma, with prominent vasculature.

diagnostic immunostains, which allows distinction from other primitive CNS germ cell tumors.

CHORIOCARCINOMA

Pathology

This tumor displays the combined elements of cytotrophoblastic as well as syncytiotrophoblastic giant cell elements (Figure 3.113). Such giant cells may show wildly pleomorphic and giant cell forms of differentiation. These tumors are also characterized by ectatic blood vessels and a marked propensity for hemorrhage. Syncytiotrophoblastic giant cells are β-HCG-immunopositive.

TERATOMA

Teratomas must include elements derived from ectodermal, endodermal, and mesodermal lines of differentiation.

Mature

Mature teratomas have fully differentiated elements without unusual proliferative activity. Frequent elements include brain, choroid plexus, and benign epithelial structures, representing ectodermal derivatives. Mesodermal components may include cartilage, bone, fat, and skeletal and smooth muscle. Endodermal derivatives may be the most difficult to identify, represented by epithelial lined tissues sometimes including rare goblet cells, highlighted by a mucin stain.

Figure 3.114. Immature teratomas are often diagnosed by the presence of poorly differentiated neuroepithelial (upper right) and mesenchymal elements.

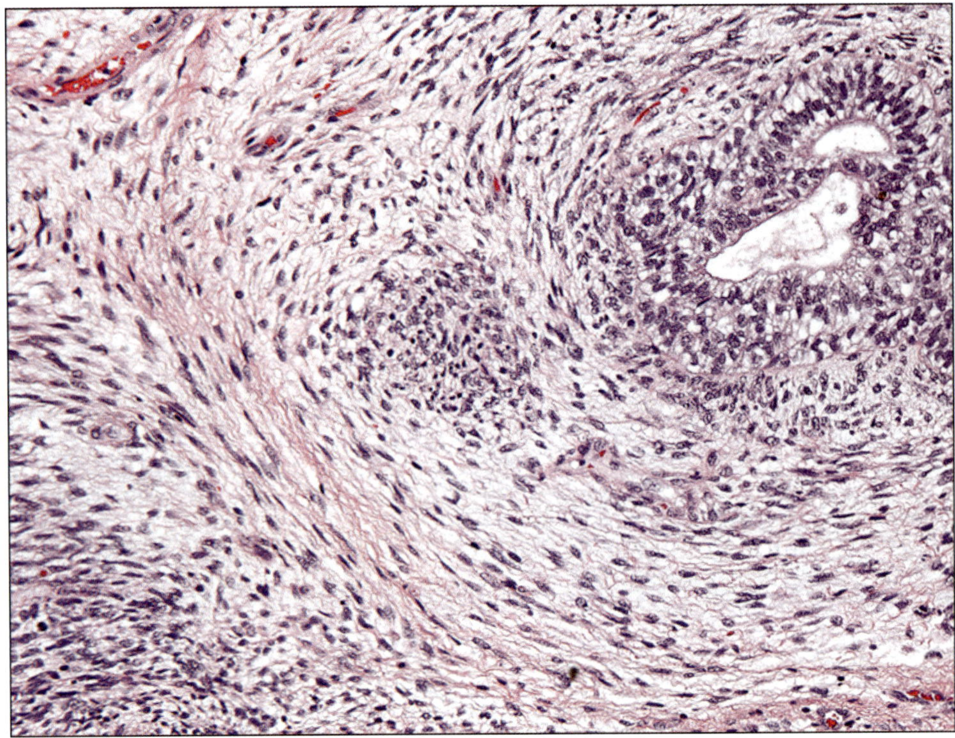

Immature

The immature teratoma is comparable to the mature form except for relatively undifferentiated and proliferative elements, commonly manifested as primitive mesenchyme or structures resembling the embryonic neuroepithelial canal or neural tube (Figure 3.114). Varying degrees of differentiation may be noted amongst primitive elements. The designation immature teratoma must be made even if the immature elements represent a small minority of the tumor.

TERATOMA WITH MALIGNANT TRANSFORMATION

Malignant teratomas contain frankly carcinomatous, either as squamous or adenocarcinoma, or sarcomatous differentiation, commonly seen as rhabdomyosarcoma or as otherwise undifferentiated sarcoma (Bjornsson et al., 1985; Rueda-Pedraza et al., 1987).

MIXED GERM CELL TUMOR

Pathology

This entity is second only to germinomas in incidence among CNS germ cell tumors. The most common combination of elements is pure germinoma with immature teratoma or other germ cell tumor elements. The identification of the most primitive element is important in assigning a prognosis.

REFERENCES

Bjornsson J, Scheithauer BW, Okazaki H, Leech RW. Intracranial germ cell tumors: pathobiological and immunohistochemical aspects of 70 cases. *J Neuropathol Exp Neurol* 1985; 44: 32–46.

Felix I, Becker LE. Intracranial germ cell tumors in children: an immunohistochemical and electron microscopic study. *Pediatr Neurosurg* 1990; 16: 156–62.

Hattab EM, Tu PH, Wilson JD, Cheng L. OCT4 immunohistochemistry is superior to placental alkaline phosphatase (PLAP) in the diagnosis of central nervous system germinoma. *Am J Surg Pathol* 2005; 29: 368–71.

Ho DM, Liu HC. Primary intracranial germ cell tumor. Pathologic study of 51 patients. *Cancer* 1992; 70: 1577–84.

Masuzawa T, Shimabukuro H, Nakahara N, Iwasa H, Sato F. Germ cell tumors (germinoma and yolk sac tumor) in unusual sites in the brain. *Clin Neuropathol* 1986; 5: 190–202.

Matsutani M, Sano K, Takakura K, Fujimaki T, Nakamura O, Funata N, et al. Primary intracranial germ cell tumors: a clinical analysis of 153 histologically verified cases. *J Neurosurg* 1997; 86: 446–55.

Mueller W, Schneider GH, Hoffmann KT, Zschenderlein R, von Deimling A. Granulomatous tissue response in germinoma, a diagnostic pitfall in endoscopic biopsy. *Neuropathology* 2007; 27: 127–32.

Nakamura H, Takeshima H, Makino K, Kuratsu J. C-kit expression in germinoma: an immunohistochemistry-based study. *J Neurooncol* 2005; 75: 163–7.

Nomura K. Epidemiology of germ cell tumors in Asia of pineal region tumor. *J Neurooncol* 2001; 54: 211–17.

Okamoto K, Ito J, Ishikawa K, Morii K, Yamada M, Takahashi N, et al. Atrophy of the basal ganglia as the initial diagnostic sign of germinoma in the basal ganglia. *Neuroradiology* 2002; 44: 389–94.

Rueda-Pedraza ME, Heifetz SA, Sesterhenn IA, Clark GB. Primary intracranial germ cell tumors in the first two decades of life. A clinical, light-microscopic, and immunohistochemical analysis of 54 cases. *Perspect Pediatr Pathol* 1987; 10: 160–207.

Rushing EJ, Sandberg GD, Judkins AR, Vezina G, Kadom N, Myseros JS, et al. Germinoma: unusual imaging and pathological characteristics. Report of two cases. *J Neurosurg* 2006; 104: 143–8.

Sato K, Nagayama T, Fujimura M, Okamoto K, Kamiya M, Nakazato Y. A case of germinoma in the septum pellucidum manifesting as amnesia and hemiparesis. *Acta Neurochir (Wien)* 2003; 145: 923–5; discussion 926.

NONNEOPLASTIC MASSES AND CYSTS

AMYLOIDOMA (PRIMARY SOLITARY AMYLOIDOSIS)

Clinical and Radiological Features

Amyloidomas occur more frequently in men between the fifth and seventh decades of life. They are rare mass lesions that occur in many diverse sites including the brain, base of skull, cranial nerves, or spinal epidural space, causing back pain and possibly a compressive myelopathy or radiculopathy.

Elsewhere in the brain, they present as single or multiple mass lesions with little or no mass effect on surrounding structures.

There is typically no association with a plasma cell dyscrasia or malignancy since they may possibly originate in the microglial processing of plasma proteins (Cohen et al., 1992); however, because of the occasional involvement of the spinal column by multiple myeloma, diagnostic measures should be taken to exclude systemic or plasma cell dyscrasia. MRI indicates a hypointense lesion on T1- and T2-weighted imaging with contrast enhancement (Figure 3.115a) (Gandhi et al., 2003).

Pathology

Amyloidomas have been described with varying amounts of chronic inflammation as well as in circumstances in which virtually no inflammation is noted. Microscopy typically reveals amorphous or globular acellular masses, birefringent with polarized light (Figure 3.115b). The presence of otherwise typical plasma cells within a mixed chronic inflammatory infiltrate should not be considered suspicious for a plasma cell malignancy. However, if this consideration persists, immunostaining and in situ hybridization may be used to reveal the presence of clonality in the plasma cell infiltrate.

NASAL GLIAL HETEROTOPIA (NASAL "GLIOMA")

Clinical and Radiological Features

The term nasal "glioma" is misleading since these are heterotopic and not neoplastic. Nasal glial heterotopia refers to heterotopic neural tissue, usually in the region of the nasal bridge or root or within the nasopharynx. This lesion usually manifests as a polypoid mass in the perinatal period but may also be diagnosed in adulthood (Penner and Thompson, 2003). Unlike a nasal encephalocele, nasal gliomas are usually firm and noncompressible. They are more common in males. Surgical excision is curative.

Radiographic analysis is important because a connection with the central nervous system may be demonstrated in a small minority. They may be distinguished from encephaloceles by generally intact underlying bone in the absence of herniated brain contents (Figure 3.116a) (Younus and Coode, 1986). However, this finding should prompt consideration of a nasal encephalocele, thus requiring a different surgical approach.

Pathology

The gross specimen may range from a few millimeters to several centimeters in diameter. Microscopic analysis shows a benign admixture of glial cells of different morphologies including gemistocytic and fibrous types, gangliocytic cells of varying morphology, and ependymal cells in a neuropil or fibrillar background

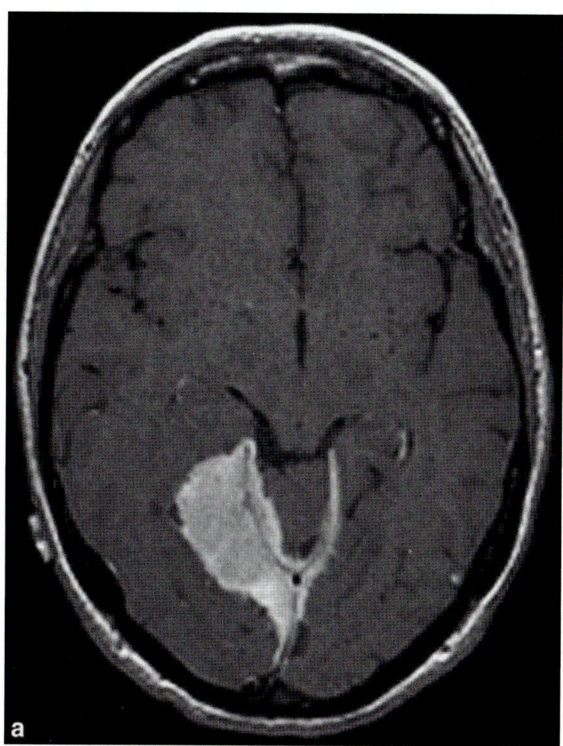

Figure 3.115. Amyloidoma. (a) Axial T1-weighted contrast-enhanced MR image shows an intensely enhancing extracerebral mass extending along the tentorium cerebelli and falx cerebri. The imaging appearance of this amyloidoma overlaps with that of a meningioma. (b) Mass of acellular congophilic globular material typical of an amyloidoma, with adjacent plasma cell proliferation of the dura. The patient had no other evidence of a plasma cell dyscrasia, and, plasma cells are sometimes not present in amyloidomas.

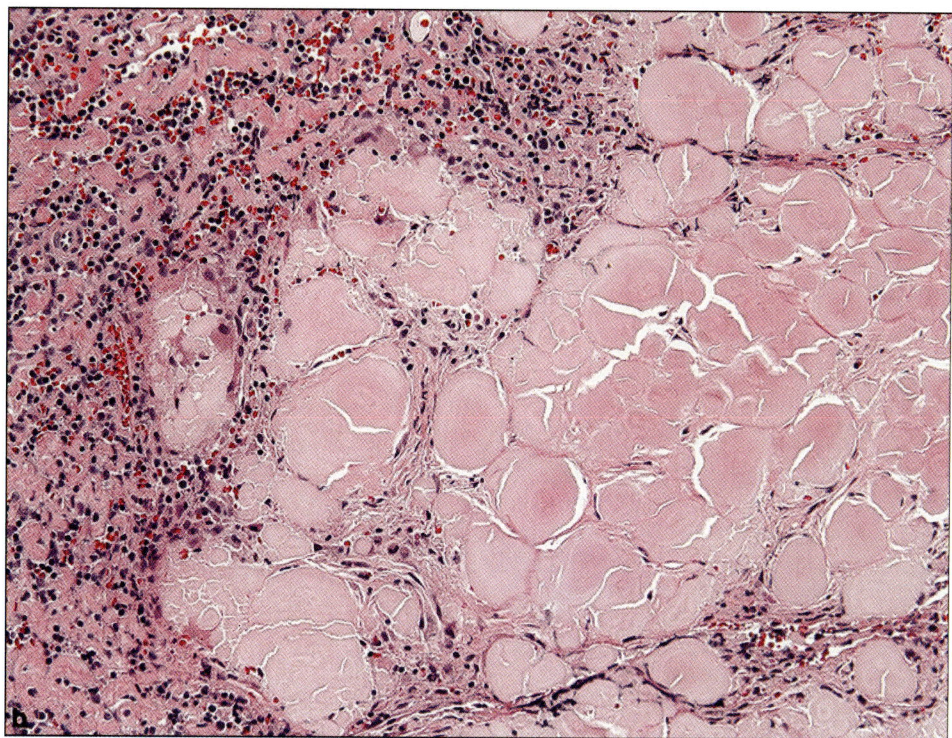

(Figure 3.116b). Microcalcifications and a variable chronic inflammatory infiltrate may also be present. They contain no immature or undifferentiated elements as would be seen in olfactory neuroblastoma and lack diverse elements seen in teratomas.

Figure 3.116. (a) Nasal cerebral heterotopia (nasal "glioma"). A sagittal T2 MR-image shows a heterogeneous mass within the nasal cavity. The mass appears sequestered and isolated from the subarachnoid space. By imaging, encephaloceles, dermoid cysts, and nasal polyps could appear similar to nasal cerebral heterotopia. (b) Nasal gliomas consist of benign neural elements, seen subjacent to respiratory epithelium in this resection.

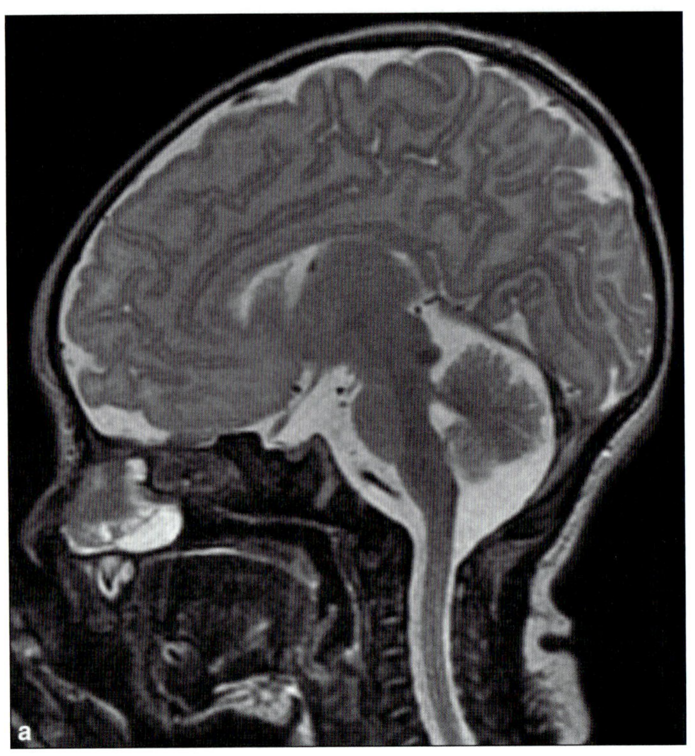

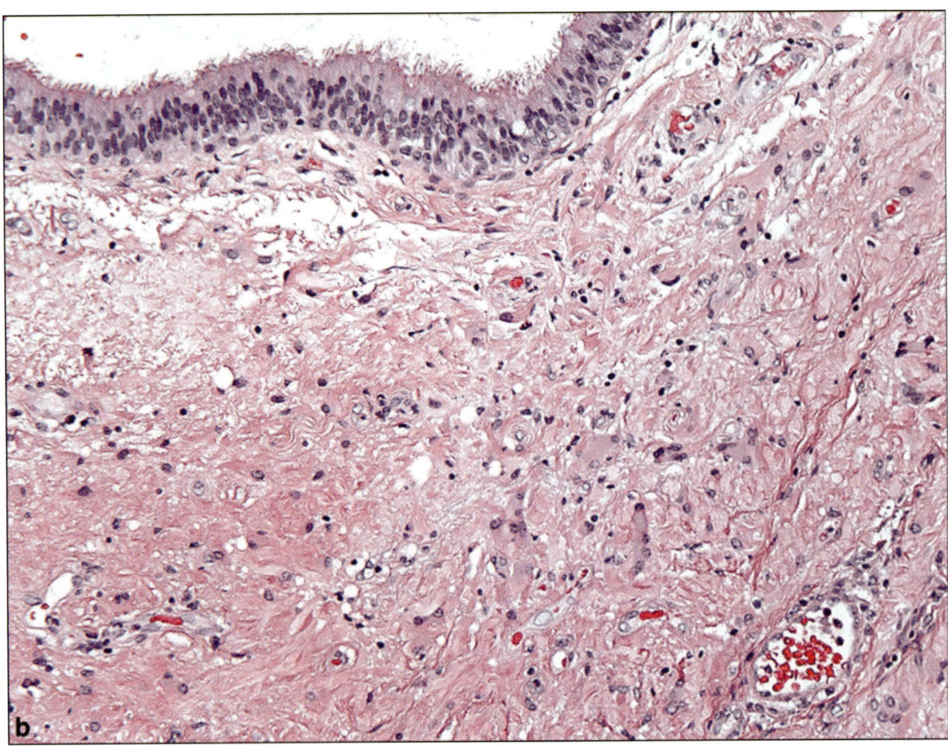

HYPOTHALAMIC HAMARTOMA

Clinical and Radiological Features

These are rare developmental tumors originating in the tuber cinereum and are associated with seizures or pituitary dysfunction because of their

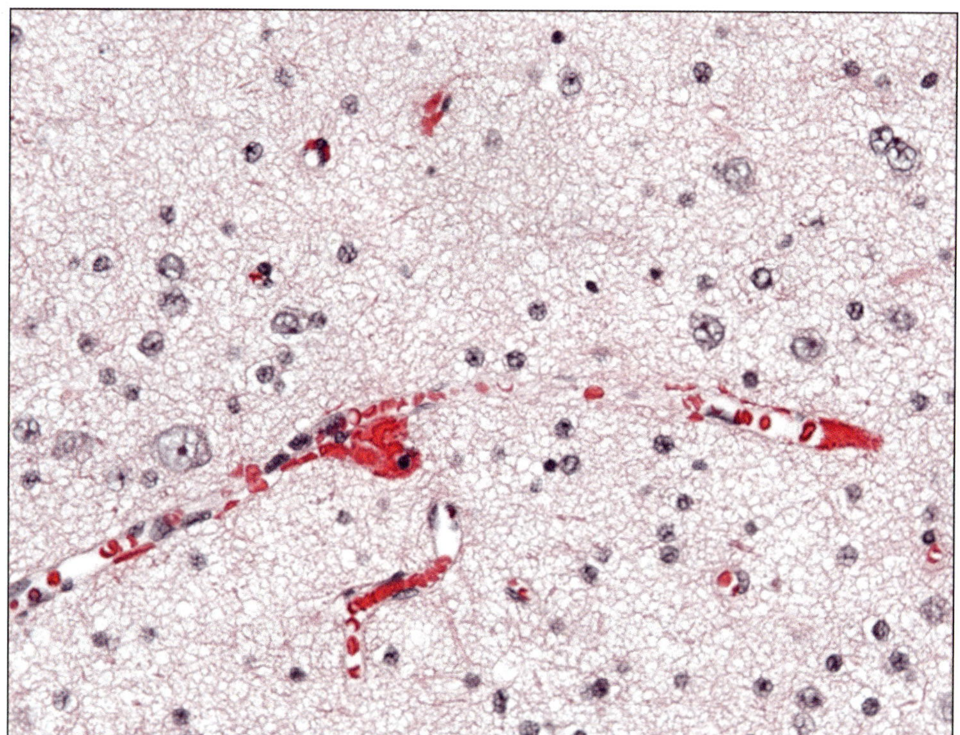

Figure 3.117. Hypothalamic hamartomas, a hypocellular lesion with disorganized arrangement of otherwise normal appearing neurons and glial cells.

hypothalamic location. They are classically associated with gelastic seizures, resulting in involuntary laughter, central precocious puberty, and developmental delay (Maixner, 2006). They typically appear as noncontrast-enhancing masses with the density of gray matter (Valdueza et al., 1994).

Pathology

The microscopic features of these tumors include nodular foci of normal-appearing neurons, which form the predominant cellular elements, with astrocytes and oligodendroglial elements (Figure 3.117). There is an increase in the astrocytic component with age. Overtly dysplastic ganglion cells are not typically seen (Coons et al., 2007).

CYSTS

A wide variety of benign cysts may be seen in all regions of the nervous system, including cranial or spinal nerves. However, it is important to recall that certain neoplasms may frequently show cystic change, particularly *pilocytic astrocytomas, gangliogliomas, hemangioblastomas, pleomorphic xanthoastrocytomas, craniopharyngiomas,* and occasionally *meningiomas* or large *schwannomas.*

Arachnoid and Meningeal Cysts

Clinical and Radiological Features

These lesions are seen in both children and adults, are more frequent in males, and result in a focal collection of cerebrospinal fluid. They may occur

Figure 3.118. Arachnoid cyst.
(a) Example in the pineal region. A sagittal T2 MR image shows a cystic mass centered in the quadrigeminal cistern. There is displacement of the cerebellar vermis inferiorly and displacement of the pineal gland anteriorly. The corpus callosum is thinned, and the lateral ventricles enlarged, presumably by obstruction at the Sylvian aqueduct. This arachnoid cyst, confirmed by pathology, is isointense to CSF on all sequences. The quadrigeminal cistern is an uncommon, but well-recognized, location for arachnoid cysts.
(b) Microscopy of the collapsed arachnoid cyst demonstrating the arachnoid cell lining, with clearly recognizable features such as nuclear inclusions and psammoma body formation.

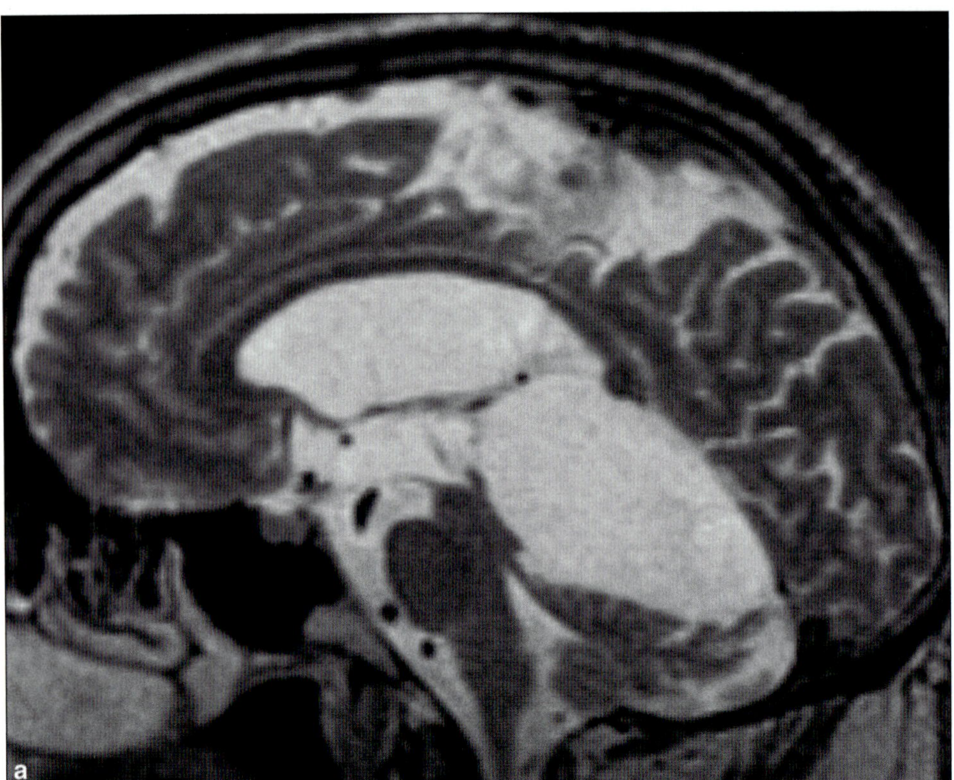

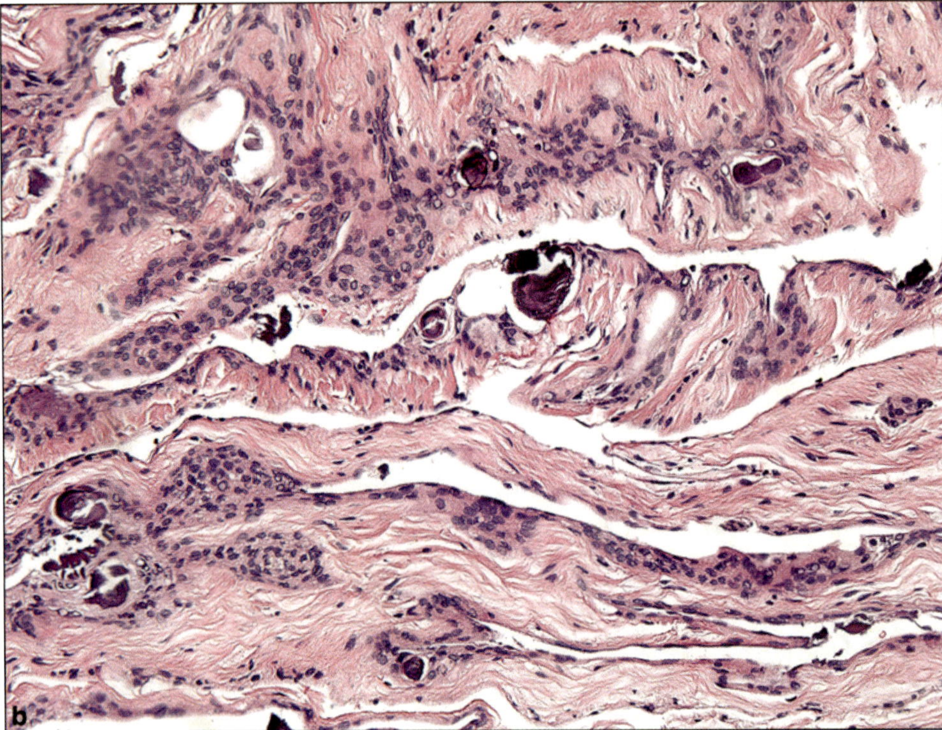

throughout the neuroaxis but favored locations include the Sylvian fissure, the left middle fossa, rarely in the sellar region, the cerebellopontine angle in the posterior fossa, or in association with the thoracic spine (Passero et al., 1990; Wester, 1999). The distinctive radiographic finding in these lesions is cystic contents showing the signal characteristics of cerebrospinal fluid with displacement of the adjacent brain and remodeling of the adjacent skull (Figure 3.118a).

Meningeal cysts are most commonly encountered as a diverticulum of spinal meninges and thus usually retain a connection with the subarachnoid space through a slender pedicle from the dura. They are typically situated in the posterior midline of the spine.

Pathology

Arachnoid cells may be seen lining a cyst wall of varying thickness depending on the degree of associated collagen formation (Figure 3.118b).

Colloid Cyst of the Third Ventricle

Clinical and Radiological Features

This unusual lesion occurs as a unilocular cyst in the anterior third ventricle near the foramen of Munro. Patients may present with the consequences of obstruction of cerebrospinal fluid flow, or chronic headaches, and under the unusual circumstance of a ball valve effect, abrupt loss of consciousness, coma, or even death may occur. By imaging, colloid cysts appear as well circumscribed nonenhancing cysts of the anterior third ventricle (Figure 3.119a).

Surgical excision is curative, and endoscopic drainage is also an option. Some lesions may even be followed radiographically when discovered incidentally and are asymptomatic.

Pathology

The intact specimen will appear as a tense cyst with translucent wall and mucoid contents although the usual appearance of the surgical specimen is that of a collapsed thin-walled cyst. Microscopy shows a distinctive epithelial lining composed of mucin-producing or ciliated epithelial cells that may be pseudostratified (Figure 3.119b). Proteinaceous contents may form filamentous aggregates. Although superfluous to the diagnosis in most cases, immunohistochemistry will reveal the presence of EMA and cytokeratin in the lining cells.

Dermoid and Epidermoid Cysts

Clinical and Radiological Features

These cysts derive from displaced embryonic ectoderm or through the iatrogenic introduction of dermal epithelium in percutaneous procedures including lumbar puncture. According to their embryonic origin, they are most commonly found in the meninges or ventricles and are particularly common to the cerebellopontine angle or in the region of the pituitary gland. The locations of dermoid cysts are considered more restricted and are more typically in the midline. These

Figure 3.119. Classic colloid cyst. (a) A coronal T1 MR image shows a subcentimeter high-intensity colloid cyst in the roof of the third ventricle between the columns of the fornix and near the foramen of Monro. There is mild ventriculomegaly. Approximately two-thirds of colloid cysts will have high signal on T1 MR images, which is likely related to cholesterol content. Because colloid cysts typically occur next the foramen of Monro, they have a propensity to cause hydrocephalus. (b) The colloid cyst wall is composed of ciliated epithelial cells ranging from pseudostratified to simpler arrangements.

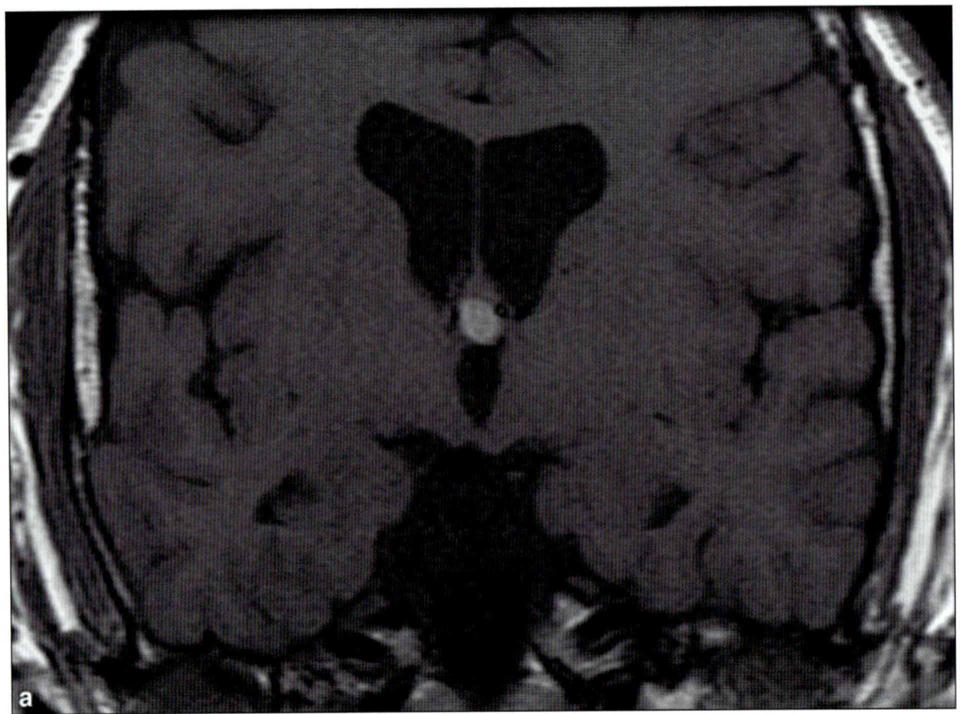

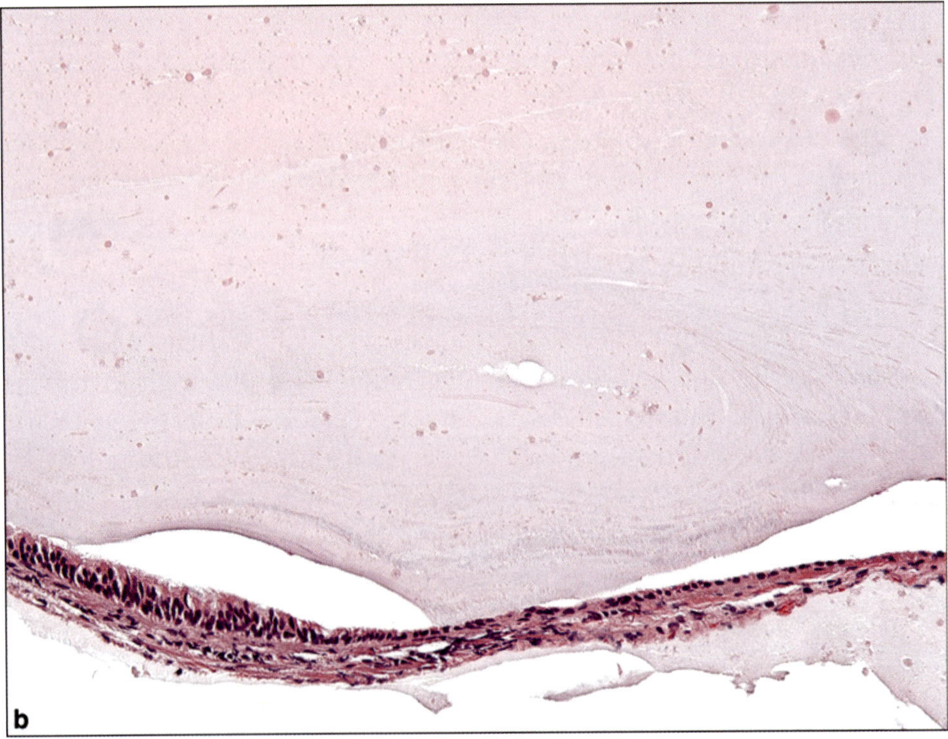

lesions become clinically apparent through mass effect or by leakage of their contents into cerebrospinal fluid, resulting in a sterile chemical meningitis.

With radiographic imaging, epidermoid cysts are isointense with CSF in T1-weighted MR images (Figure 3.120a–c) whereas dermoid cyst contents tend to be either hypo- or hyperintense.

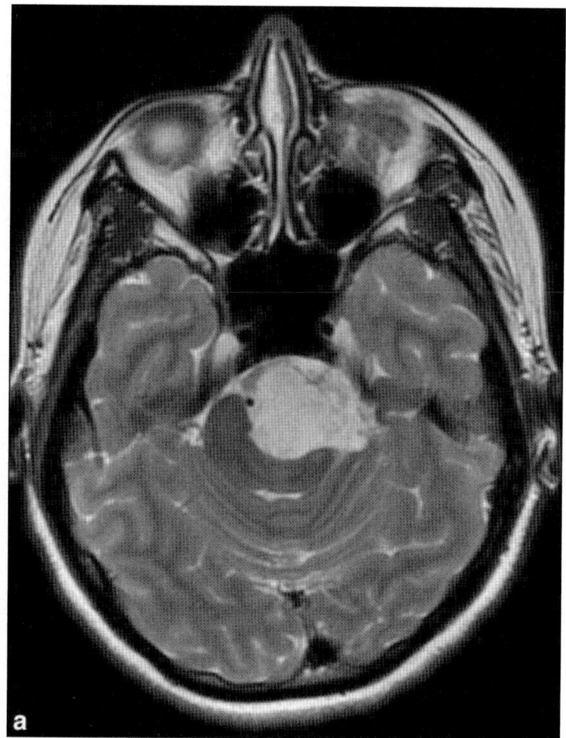

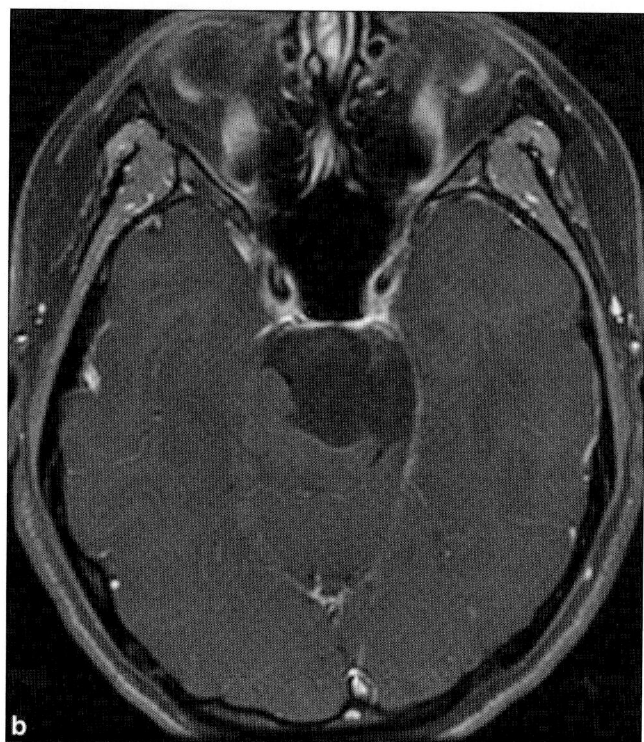

Figure 3.120. Epidermoid cyst. (a) An axial T2 MR image shows a very high signal in a left cerebellopontine angle mass, which is compressing the pons. (b) The axial T1 MR image shows no enhancement.

Total removal of these lesions results in a favorable outlook, however, even the smallest residual amount may be all that is necessary for regrowth. Malignant transformation has been documented for both epidermoid and dermoid cysts (Cannon et al., 1998; Gluszcz, 1962; Goldman and Gandy, 1987).

Figure 3.120. *continued*
(c) A diffusion-weighted MR image shows extensive diffusion restriction within the mass. Prior to the advent of diffusion-weighted imaging, it could be difficult to distinguish epidermoid from arachnoid or neuroenteric cysts. However, with diffusion-weighted images, epidermoid cysts have high signal (restrict diffusion), whereas arachnoid cysts have very low signal (do not restrict diffusion).
(d) Stratified keratinizing squamous epithelial wall of an epidermoid cyst. A dermoid cyst would show an identical lining with the addition of adnexal appendages.

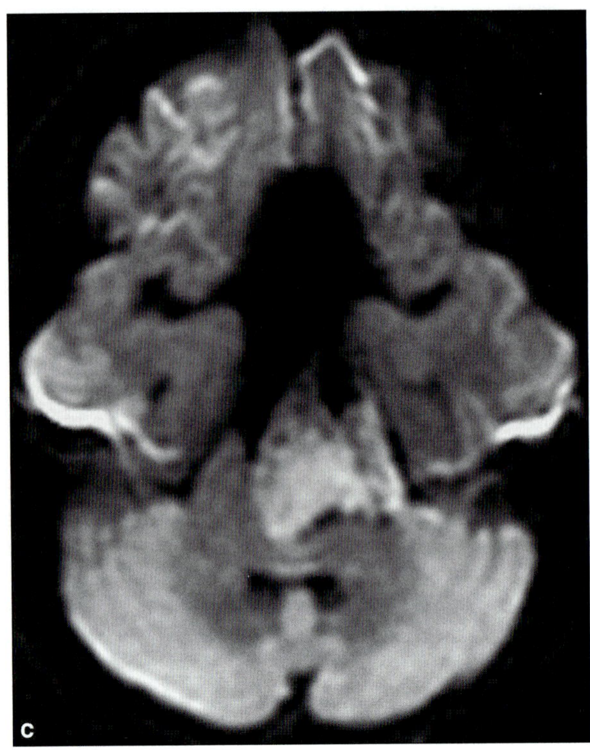

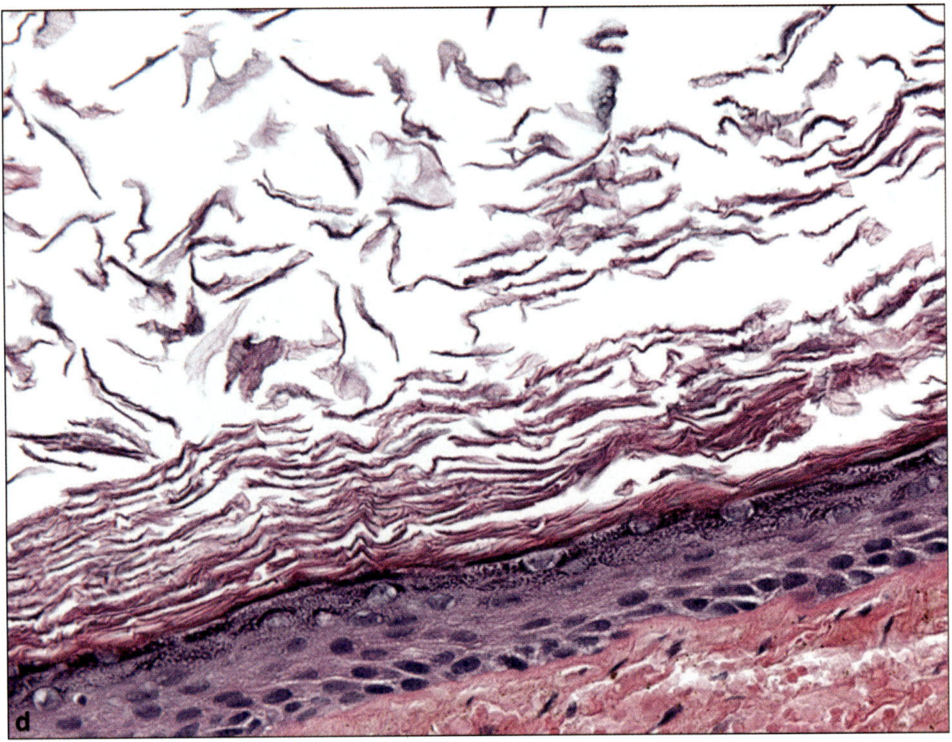

Pathology

The gross features of these cysts are identical to those encountered in other locations, with the flaky or pearly contents representing accumulated squamous material. Microscopically, sections of the wall demonstrate keratinizing squamous epithelium with subjacent adnexal glands (Figure 3.120d). Some of these lesions will have undergone rupture and thus have elicited a prominent foreign body giant cell reaction.

Neuroenteric (Enterogenous) Cysts

Clinical and Radiological Features

These are most commonly located in the spinal cord region and may occur at all ages. Solitary lesions occur most commonly in the cervical spinal canal and those with associated malformations occur most frequently in the lumbosacral region. They produce symptoms related to mass effect depending on the level of brainstem or spinal cord affected. MRI demonstrates a hypodense lesion on T1-weighted images with iso- to hypointense signal as compared with CSF (Figure 3.121a).

Pathology

The cyst wall is composed of variable amounts of columnar, ciliated or nonciliated epithelium, most commonly resembling gastrointestinal and less commonly respiratory epithelium with approximately one-third showing mixed differentiation (Figure 3.121b). These cells form a single or pseudostratified layer over basement membrane. Some cysts may show mucus or serous glands, smooth muscle, lymphoid elements, and others may show ependymal and other glial components.

Neuroepithelial Cysts

Ependymal Cyst

These may occur in diverse extraventricular locations including over the convexities, within the brain parenchyma, or near the midbrain, and may also occur in the intramedullary spinal cord, most commonly in the thoracic segments. They are lined by benign ciliated GFAP-positive ependymal cells, which may be used to distinguish these from neurenteric cysts.

Pineal Cyst

These are usually found incidentally and are usually asymptomatic unless they achieve an unusually large size in the range of 1–2 cm (Figure 3.122a). Symptomatic examples usually occur in early adulthood with the usual features of a pineal mass, including headache, signs and symptoms of obstructive hydrocephalus, or hypothalamic dysfunction.

These cysts have no well-defined lining but exist as a large cystic space surrounded by fibrillary glial tissue, often including Rosenthal fibers (Figure 3.122b).

Figure 3.121. Neuroenteric (enterogenous) cyst. (a) An axial T1 contrast-enhanced MR image shows a mass slightly inferior to the right cerebellar pontine angle at the pontomedullary junction. This neuroenteric cyst was isointense to CSF on T2 and T1 sequences. Often, neuroenteric cysts, which contain mucin-secreting goblet cells, will be hyperintense to CSF on T2 and T1 sequences, thereby allowing them to be distinguished from arachnoid cysts. Intracranial neuroenteric cysts are very rare; the vast majority occur in the posterior fossa, often at the pontomedullary junction. Arachnoid cysts and cystic schwannomas could appear similar to neuroenteric cysts on MR imaging. (b) Both ciliated and nonciliated columnar epithelium including a possible goblet cell, lining an enterogenous cyst.

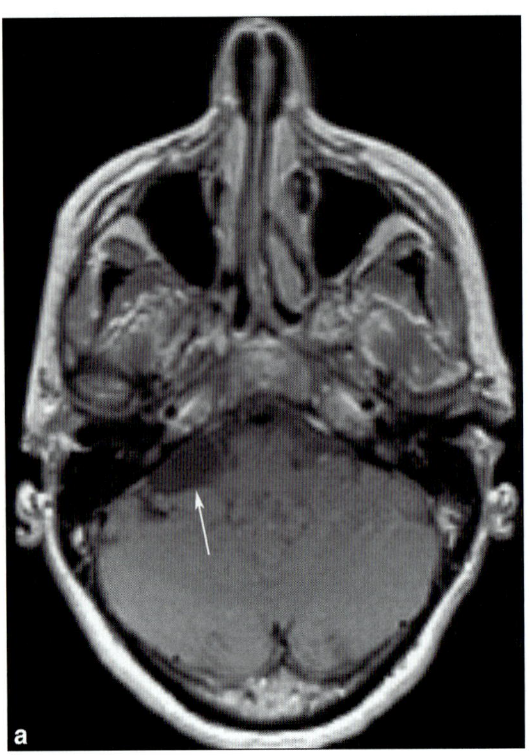

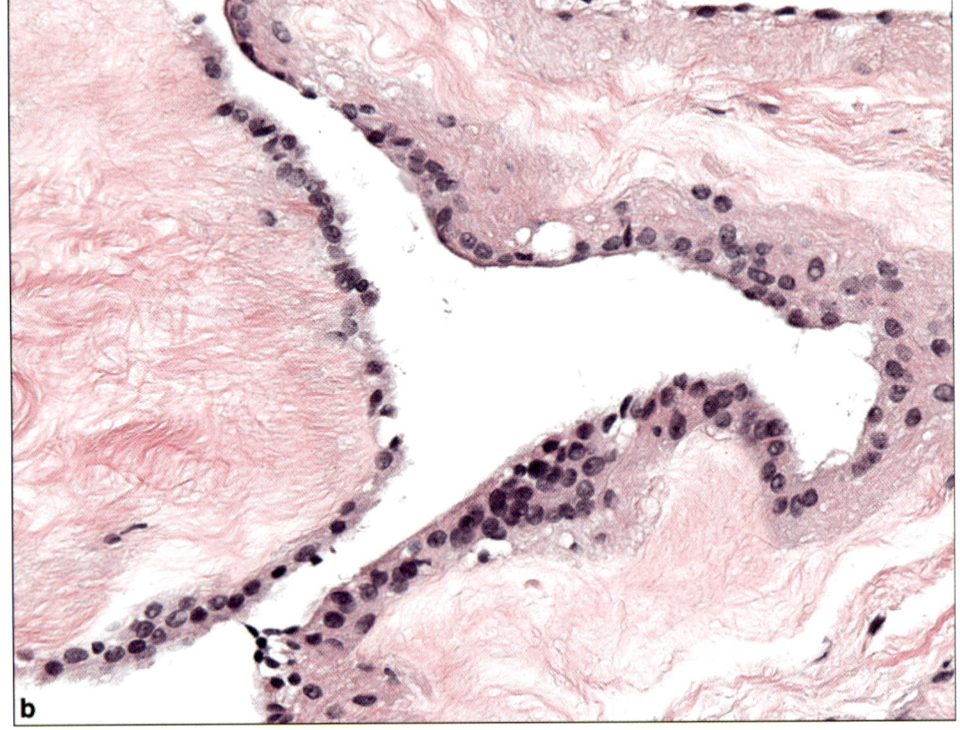

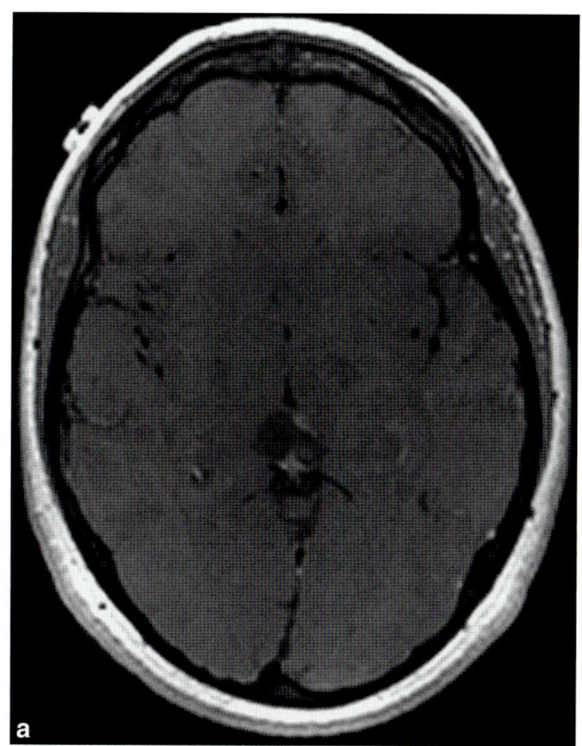

Figure 3.122. Pineal cyst. (a) An axial T1 contrast-enhanced MR image shows a bilobed pineal region cystic mass with a peripheral rim of enhancement. This pineal cyst deviates the tectum and narrows the Sylvian aqueduct. Typically, pineal cysts are isointense or slightly hyperintense relative to CSF on T1 and T2 imaging. Occasionally, pineal cysts are complicated by internal hemorrhage, which drastically alters the signal characteristics of the cyst. Some arachnoid cysts and pineocytomas can appear very similar to pineal cysts by MR imaging.

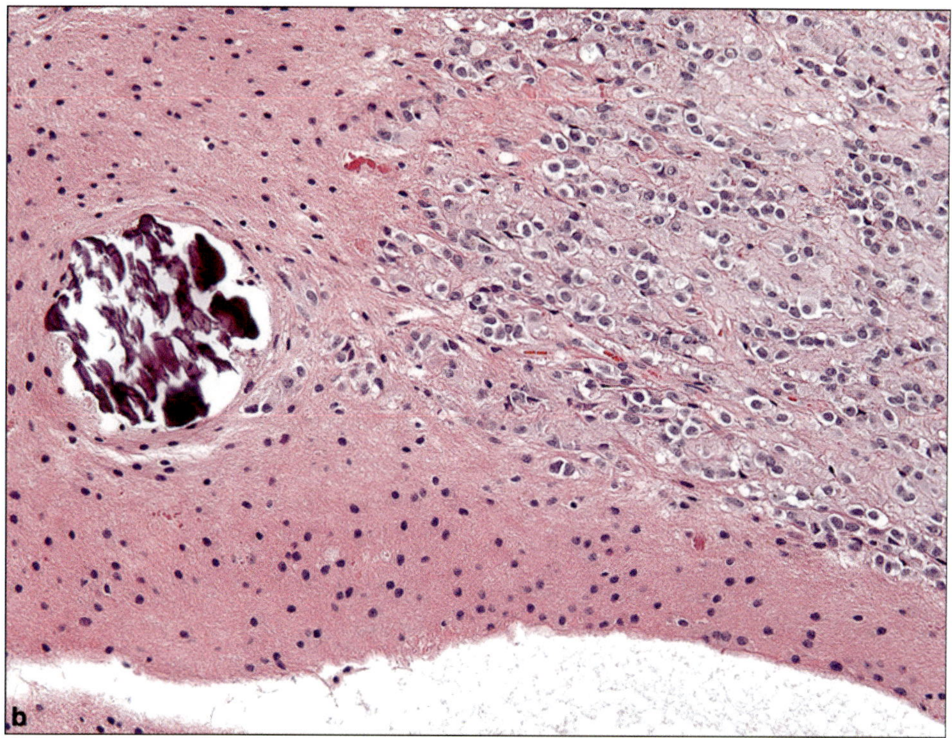

REFERENCES

Cannon TC, Bane BL, Kistler D, Schoenhals GW, Hahn M, Leech RW, et al. Primary intracerebellar osteosarcoma arising within an epidermoid cyst. *Arch Pathol Lab Med* 1998; 122: 737–9.

Cohen M, Lanska D, Roessmann U, Karaman B, Ganz E, Whitehouse P, et al. Amyloidoma of the CNS.I. Clinical and pathologic study. *Neurology* 1992; 42: 2019–23.

Coons SW, Rekate HL, Prenger EC, Wang N, Drees C, Ng YT, et al. The histopathology of hypothalamic hamartomas: study of 57 cases. *J Neuropathol Exp Neurol* 2007; 66: 131–41.

Gandhi D, Wee R, Goyal M. CT and MR imaging of intracerebral amyloidoma: case report and review of the literature. *AJNR Am J Neuroradiol* 2003; 24: 519–22.

Gluszcz A. A cancer arising in a dermoid of the brain. A case report. *J Neuropathol Exp Neurol* 1962; 21: 383–7.

Goldman SA, Gandy SE. Squamous cell carcinoma as a late complication of intracerebroventricular epidermoid cyst. Case report. *J Neurosurg* 1987; 66: 618–20.

Maixner W. Hypothalamic hamartomas – clinical, neuropathological and surgical aspects. *Childs Nerv Syst* 2006; 22: 867–73.

Passero S, Filosomi G, Cioni R, Venturi C, Volpini B. Arachnoid cysts of the middle cranial fossa: a clinical, radiological and follow-up study. *Acta Neurol Scand* 1990; 82: 94–100.

Penner CR, Thompson L. Nasal glial heterotopia: a clinicopathologic and immunophenotypic analysis of 10 cases with a review of the literature. *Ann Diagn Pathol* 2003; 7: 354–9.

Valdueza JM, Cristante L, Dammann O, Bentele K, Vortmeyer A, Saeger W, et al. Hypothalamic hamartomas: with special reference to gelastic epilepsy and surgery. *Neurosurgery* 1994; 34: 949–58; discussion 958.

Wester K. Peculiarities of intracranial arachnoid cysts: location, sidedness, and sex distribution in 126 consecutive patients. *Neurosurgery* 1999; 45: 775–9.

Younus M, Coode PE. Nasal glioma and encephalocele: two separate entities. Report of two cases. *J Neurosurg* 1986; 64: 516–19.

PATHOLOGY OF THE SELLAR REGION

Mohanpal Dulai and Hannes Vogel

The sellar region is a crowded and convergent crossroad of central and peripheral neural, meningeal, vascular, bone and soft tissue structures that predicts a wide diversity of primary or metastatic neoplasms arising from within any of these elements. The principle neoplasm of the sellar region is the anterior pituitary adenoma followed by neoplasms arising from the posterior pituitary. Knowledge of the surrounding anatomy predicts the types of symptoms that may arise from mass lesions in this region such as visual disturbances due to optic nerve compression; cranial neuropathies involving cranial nerves III, IV, V, and VI in the adjacent cavernous sinus; hypopituitarism or other more isolated endocrinopathies; and many others.

PITUITARY ADENOMAS

Benign pituitary adenomas account for the vast majority of tumors of the sellar region, and account for 10–15% of intracranial neoplasms. They are distinctly rare in children, only representing around 2% of all pituitary adenomas (Diamond, 2006; Kane et al., 1994). Pituitary adenomas were once classified along histochemical staining lines; however, this has been replaced by immunohistochemical profiling of adenomas and is an important adjunct to clinical care.

Pituitary adenomas cause clinical symptoms in one of two general ways: as a mass lesion or through abnormal hormone secretion. A large surgical series of pituitary adenomas indicates that the most common immunohistochemical subtypes of pituitary adenomas in decreasing frequency are prolactinomas, combined sparsely and densely granulated growth hormone–cell adenomas and null cell adenomas, followed by approximately equal frequencies of corticotroph cell adenomas and gonadotroph cell adenomas (Horvath et al., 2002). Although they are rare, the clinicopathologic identification of silent corticotroph adenomas subtypes 1, 2, and 3 is also important.

Pituitary adenomas are classified as either microadenomas, measuring less than or equal to 10 mm in greatest dimension or macroadenomas, measuring greater than 10 mm in diameter. When pituitary adenomas cause mass effect, the results include headache, visual field disturbances, and loss of normal anterior pituitary hormone production because of compression-induced atrophy of the remaining anterior pituitary gland. There is often a mild elevation in serum prolactin concentration, usually less than 200 ng/ml due to pituitary stalk compression, known as "stalk effect" (Lopes et al., 1997; Young et al., 1996). Invasion of cavernous sinus can result in cranial neuropathies involving cranial nerves III, IV, or VI, manifested as ophthalmoplegias. Gradual hypopituitarism may be clinically insidious. In the opposite sense, pituitary adenomas may produce acute hemorrhagic necrosis, or pituitary apoplexy, most commonly seen in the gonadotropin-producing adenomas.

Transsphenoidal resection of pituitary adenomas is the main form of therapy after a course of medical therapy, particularly in patients with hyperprolactinemia and some patients with growth hormone-producing adenomas (Pickett, 2005). This is important for the pathologist to remember since there is a characteristic histologic alteration of prolactin-producing cells under the influence of the dopamine agonist used to treat these adenomas. Radiation therapy may be used in cases of incompletely resected adenomas or recurrent tumors and in other situations in which surgical complete resection is not feasible, but this is generally avoided because of the risk of local side effects.

Most pituitary adenomas show typical features of a neuroendocrine neoplasm, consisting of monotonous cells with round nuclei, delicate chromatin, and inconspicuous nucleoli (Figure 3.123). Cells are often arranged around microvasculature, and separation artifact will yield a papillary appearance to many of these tumors. Nuclear pleomorphism may be seen as in all neuroendocrine tumors (Figure 3.124). Mitotic figures are rare, and unless apoplectic, necrosis is also not a usual feature.

One of the histological hallmarks of pituitary adenomas is the loss of the normal nesting pattern of anterior pituitary cells as highlighted by reticulin staining (Figure 3.125). Adenomas will stand apart from adjacent nonneoplastic

Figure 3.123. Pituitary adenomas show a proliferation of monotonous cells in various architectural arrangements. The small nested pattern seen in normal anterior pituitary is lost.

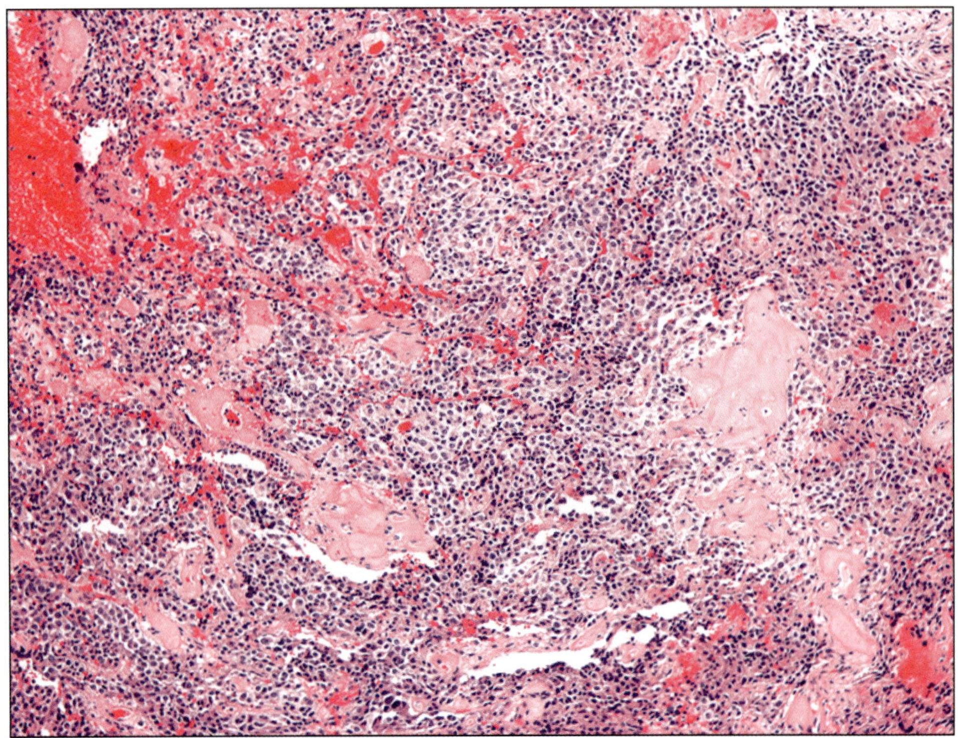

anterior pituitary tissue and this may be complemented by hormone immunostaining, particularly in instances of microadenomas.

The reticulin stain may be useful in identifying pituitary hyperplasia by highlighting enlarged acini of anterior pituitary cells, which still retain the surrounding reticulin network (Figure 3.126). However, highly fragmented specimens may show reticulin-free zones in the enlarged nests of hyperplastic pituitary, imitating the appearance of true adenomas. Pituitary hyperplasia may occur in a number of well-recognized circumstances. *Growth hormone cell hyperplasia* may accompany growth hormone–releasing hormone (GHRH), producing neuroendocrine tumors of other tissues. *Prolactin cell hyperplasia* is a normal feature of pregnancy and is also seen with estrogen treatment and long-standing primary hypothyroidism. Corticotropin-releasing hormone-producing tumors or otherwise undefined hypothalamic stimulation may cause *corticotroph cell hyperplasia*. *Thyrotroph cell hyperplasia* is associated with hypothyroidism. Both corticotroph hyperplasia and thyrotroph hyperplasia may precede the formation of true adenomas. *Gonadotroph hyperplasia* may be seen in cases of hypogonadism such as in Klinefelter's or Turner's syndrome (Al-Gahtany et al., 2003).

Pituitary adenomas are immunopositive for cytokeratin or chromogranin in 90% of cases and EMA in greater than 50%. Results of immunostaining for pituitary hormones are variable but require close inspection for focal or, at times, very weak expression. Dural invasion by tumor cells is not uncommon and often results in shrunken cells morphologically resembling lymphocytes (Figure 3.127). Immunohistochemistry may be useful in this setting for accurate diagnosis.

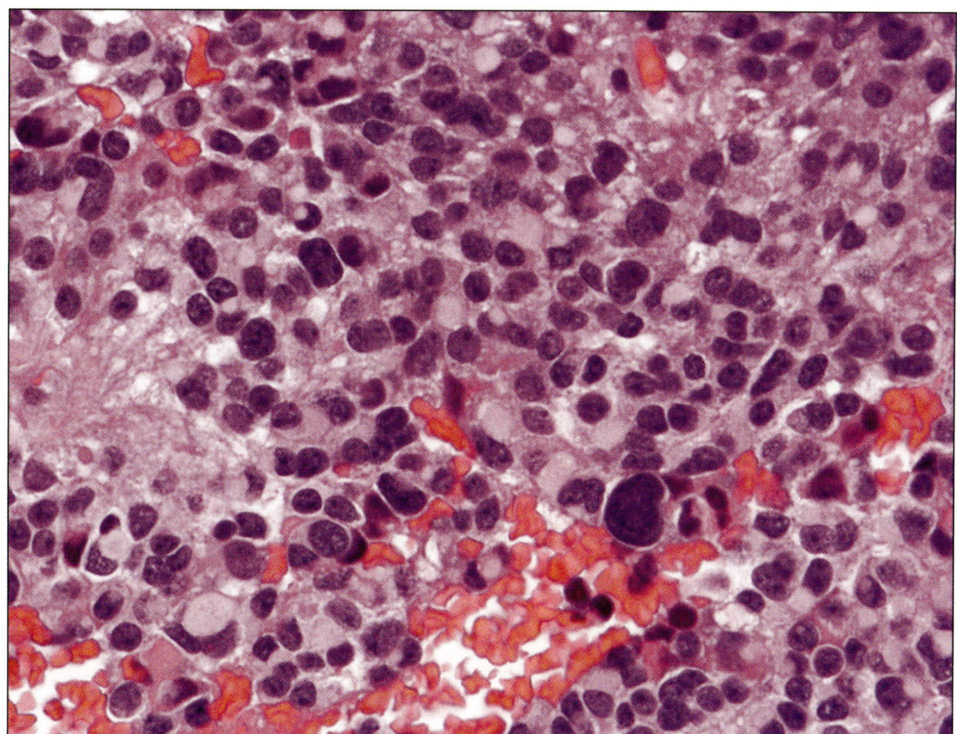

Figure 3.124. As in any neuroendocrine neoplasm, a significant amount of pleomorphism can be seen in pituitary adenomas.

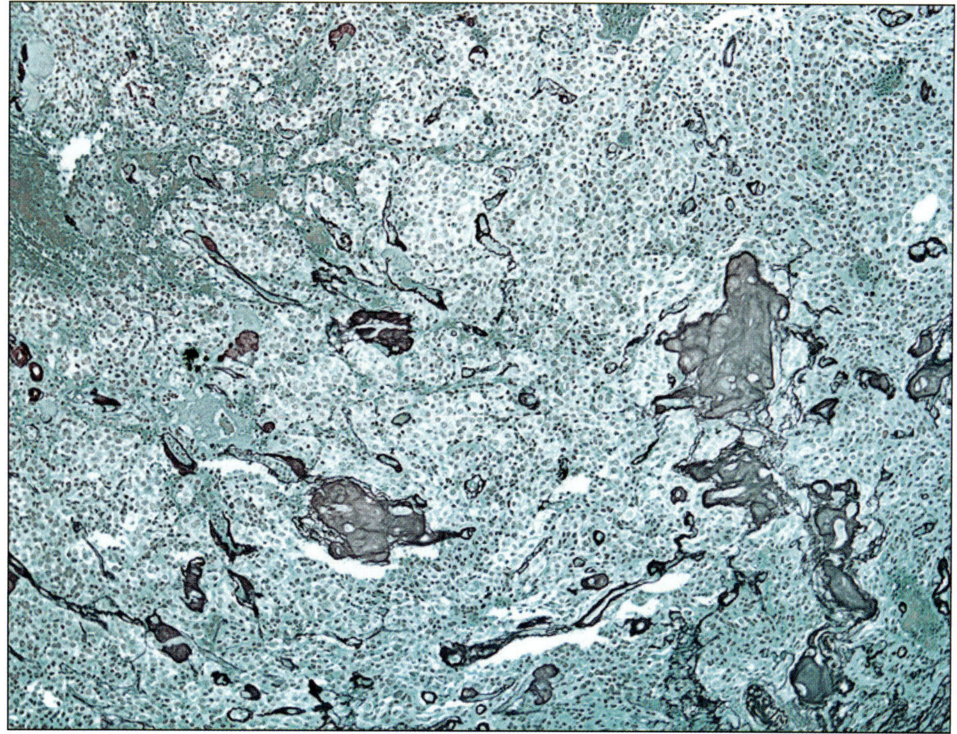

Figure 3.125. Reticulin staining in this adenoma demonstrates an absence of the reticulin around small nests of cells, which should be present in normal anterior pituitary.

Intraoperative Assessment of Pituitary Adenomas

This is the responsibility of the diagnostic pathologist when the neurosurgeon desires confirmation of adenoma versus nonneoplastic anterior pituitary tissue. In this situation, a cytological preparation made as a touch preparation is called

Figure 3.126. Pituitary hyperplasia is seen on the left with enlarged acini of cells, which retain the surrounding reticulin network. The tissue on the right side of the image retains the normal small nested pattern.

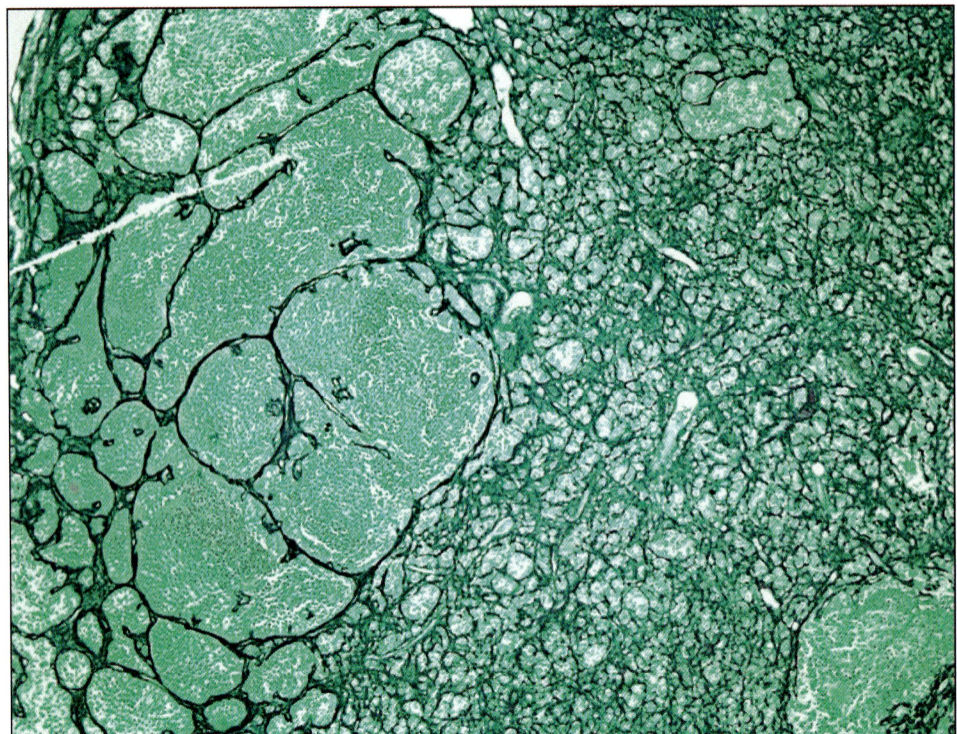

Figure 3.127. Dural invasion by pituitary adenomas is not uncommon. The cells often appear small with dense nuclei resembling lymphocytes.

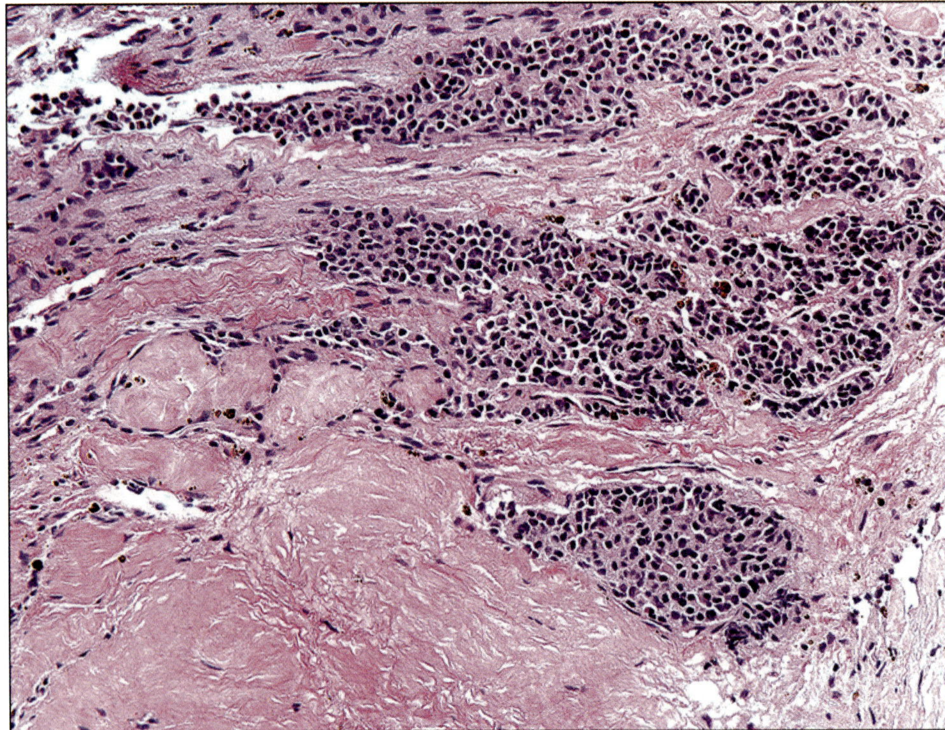

for, even preferentially over a frozen section or smear preparation. Pituitary adenoma cells typically exfoliate abundantly, yielding sheets of monotonous and discohesive cells onto the slide (Figures 3.128 and 3.129). When this does not occur, the diagnostician should revert to frozen section, in particular to exclude other neoplasms, which may mimic pituitary adenomas, such as meningiomas or metastatic tumors.

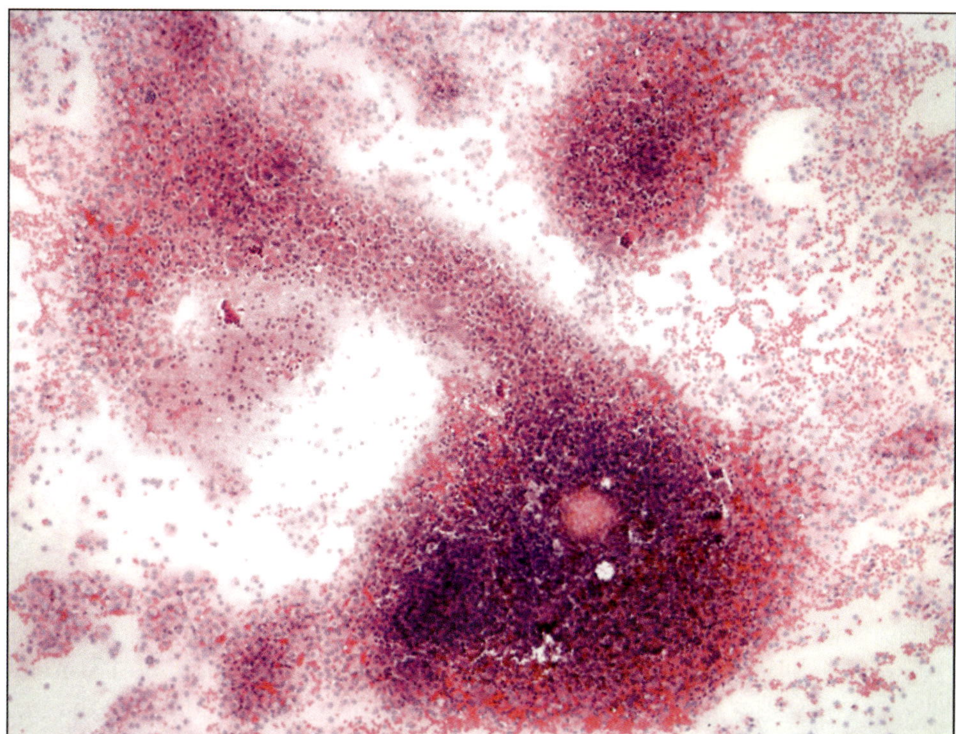

Figure 3.128. An intraoperative touch preparation from a pituitary adenoma shows exhuberant exfoliation of cells.

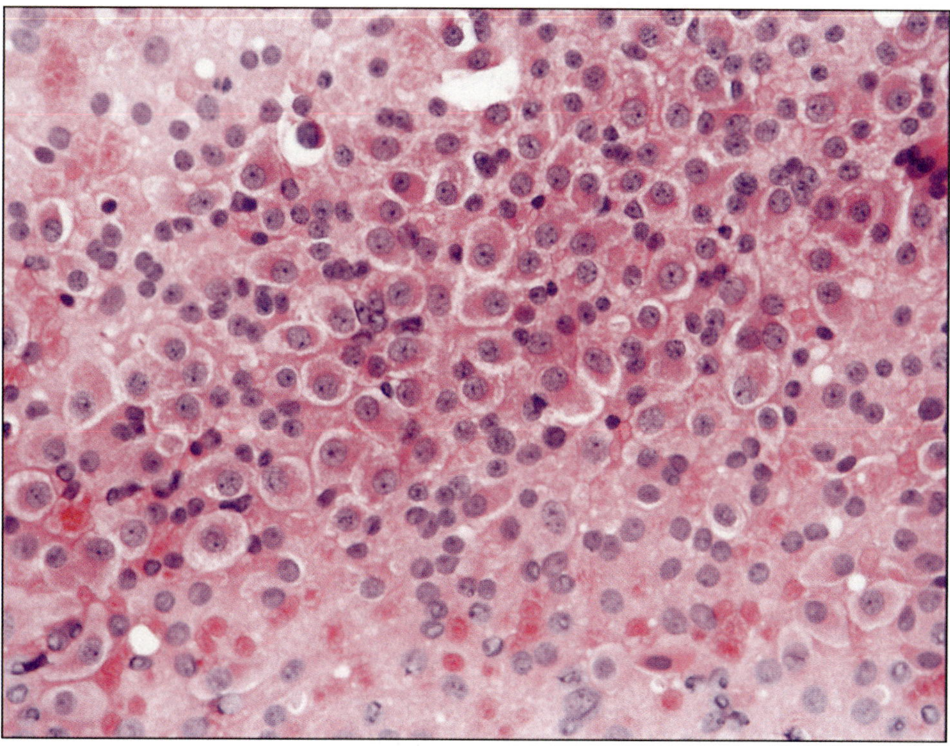

Figure 3.129. Monotonous sheets of discohesive neoplastic cells from an intraoperative touch preparation is diagnostic of pituitary adenoma.

The following descriptions will highlight individual features of the various subtypes of pituitary adenoma as defined by their hormone product. Further details and definitive descriptions may be found in the volume entitled World Health Organization Classification of Tumours: Pathology and Genetics of Tumours of Endocrine Organs (Lloyd et al., 2004).

Growth Hormone–Producing Adenoma

Clinical and Radiological Features

Approximately 10–20% of pituitary adenomas are growth hormone producing. These tumors may be associated with gigantism if onset is prepubertal before epiphyseal plates in long bones are closed, or acromegaly in adults, which may be insidious and continue for years before the diagnosis is established (Burger et al., 2002). When a tumor lacks significant hormonal effect, it may cause mass effect. Interestingly, relatively few adenomas associated with gigantism or acromegaly produce growth hormone alone, and an important subgroup includes adenomas that coproduce prolactin. Radiographically, these tumors will cause lateral expansion of the sella or grow upward.

Pathology

Growth hormone–producing adenomas are either densely granulated (acidophilic) (Figure 3.130) or sparsely granulated (chromophobic) lesions. The majority of adenomas associated with acromegaly produce prolactin, thyroid-stimulating hormone (TSH), and alpha-subunit in addition to growth hormone, and are, in turn, most often densely granulated adenomas. Immunohistochemically, they show strong and diffuse growth hormone immunoreactivity (Figure 3.131). These are defined ultrastructurally as containing large numbers of secretory granules in the 300- to 450-nm range (Figure 3.132).

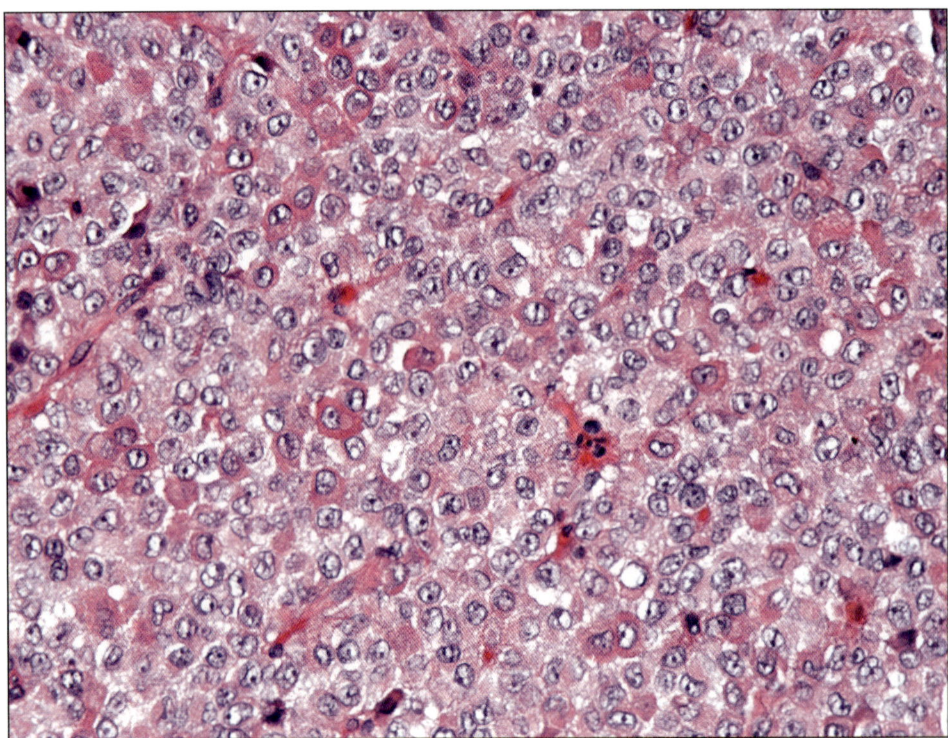

Figure 3.130. Densely granulated growth hormone adenoma with dense acidophilic cytoplasm.

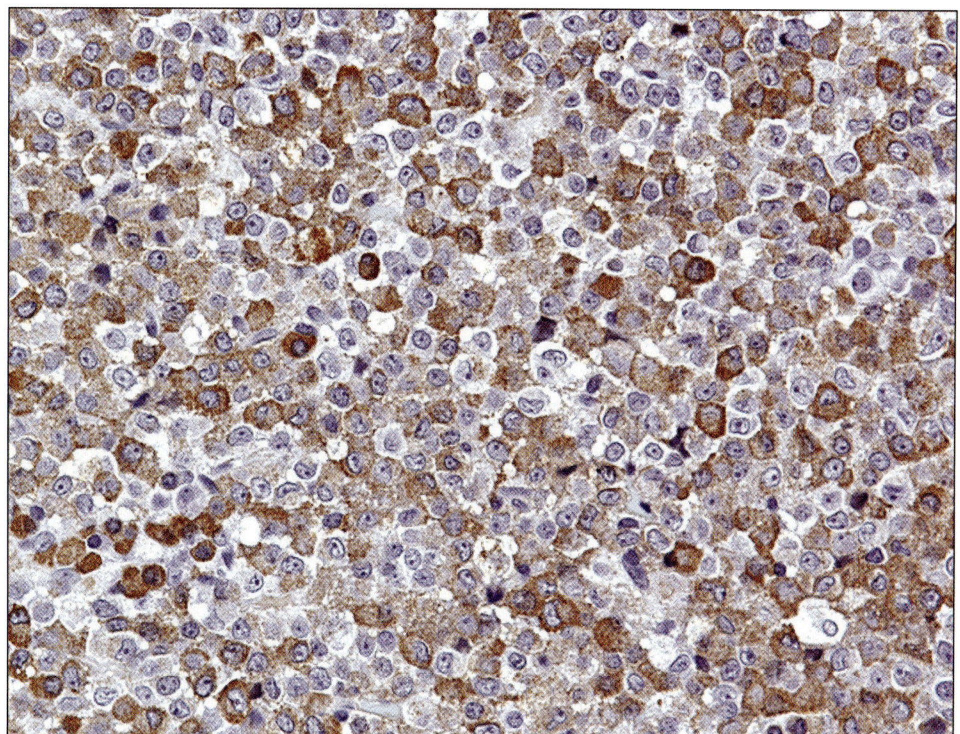

Figure 3.131. Growth hormone immunohistochemistry in a densely granulated growth hormone adenoma.

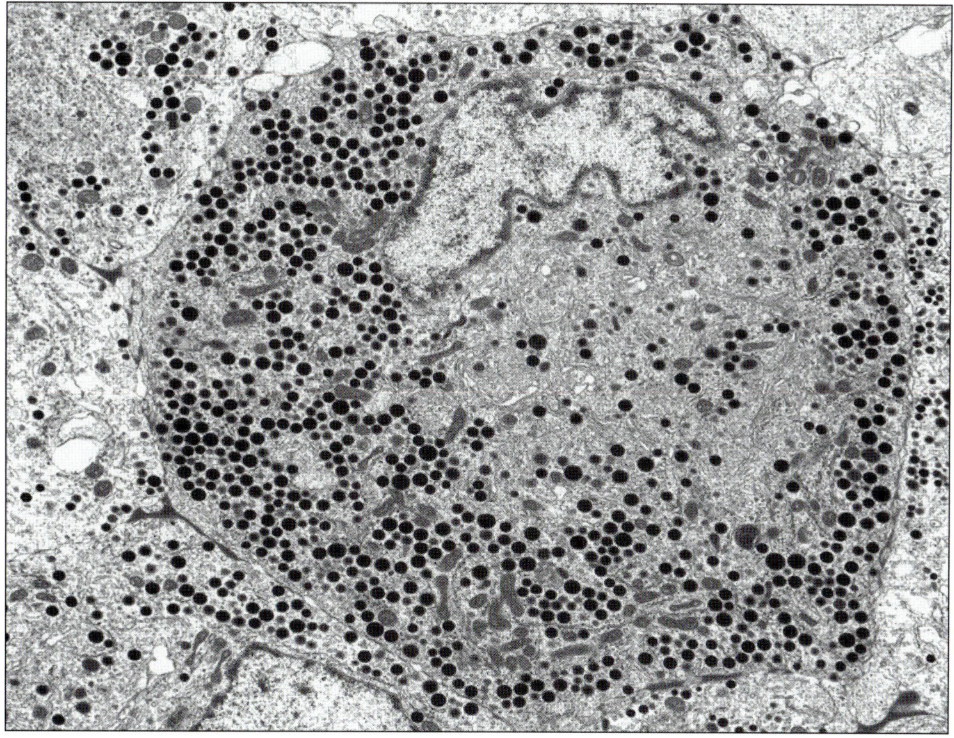

Figure 3.132. By electron microscopy, the cytoplasm in densely granulated growth hormone secreting adenomas is packed with neurosecretory granules measuring 300–450 nm.

By contrast, the sparsely granulated adenoma (Figure 3.133) shows weak or nearly absent staining for growth hormone (Figure 3.134) as well as the distinctive presence of fibrous bodies, round cytokeratin immunopositive structures seen as perinuclear masses (Figure 3.135). Electron microscopy

Figure 3.133. Sparsely granulated growth hormone adenoma with round eosinophilic fibrous bodies.

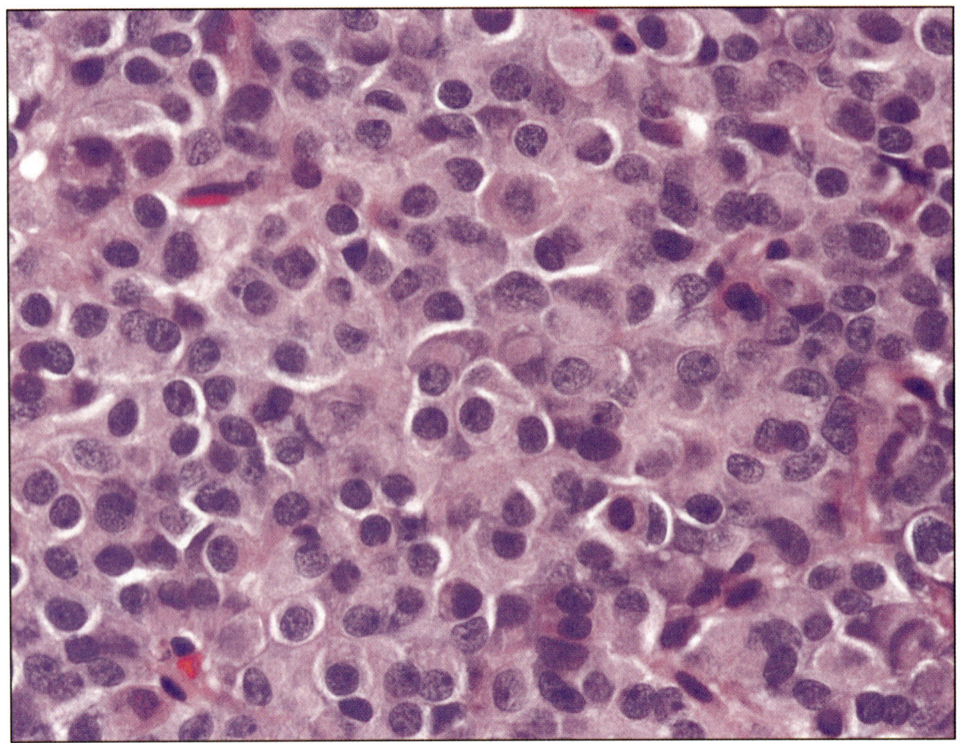

Figure 3.134. Weak immunoreactivity for growth hormone in a sparsely granulated growth hormone adenoma.

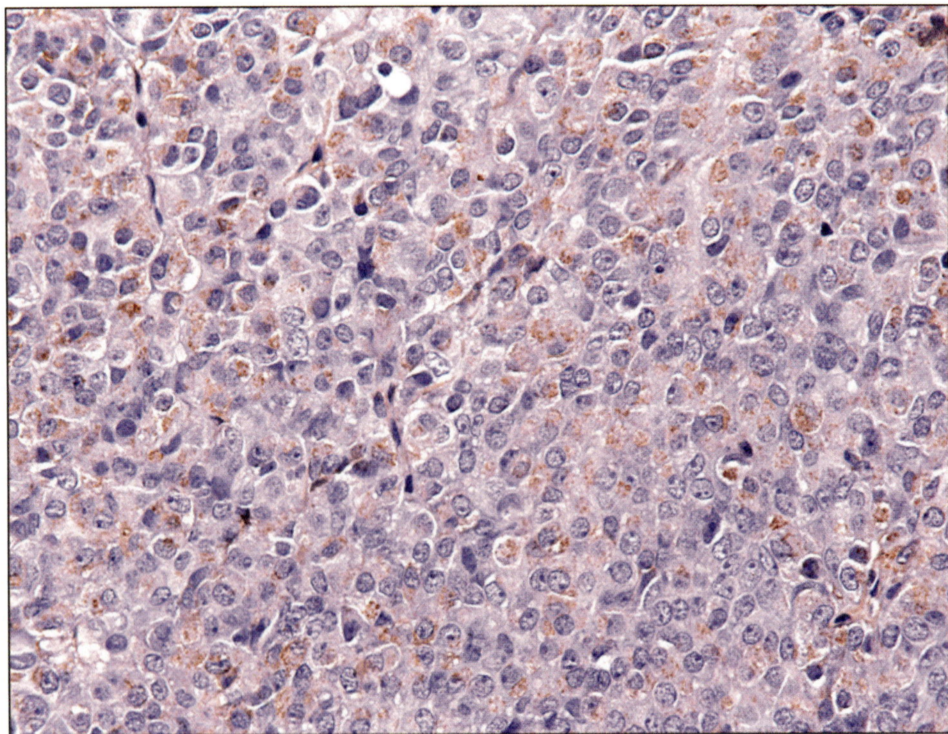

reveals a paucity of secretory granules, which are usually in the 100- to 250-nm range with occasional cytoplasmic fibrous bodies composed of concentric aggregates of intermediate filaments and smooth endoplasmic reticulum (Figure 3.136).

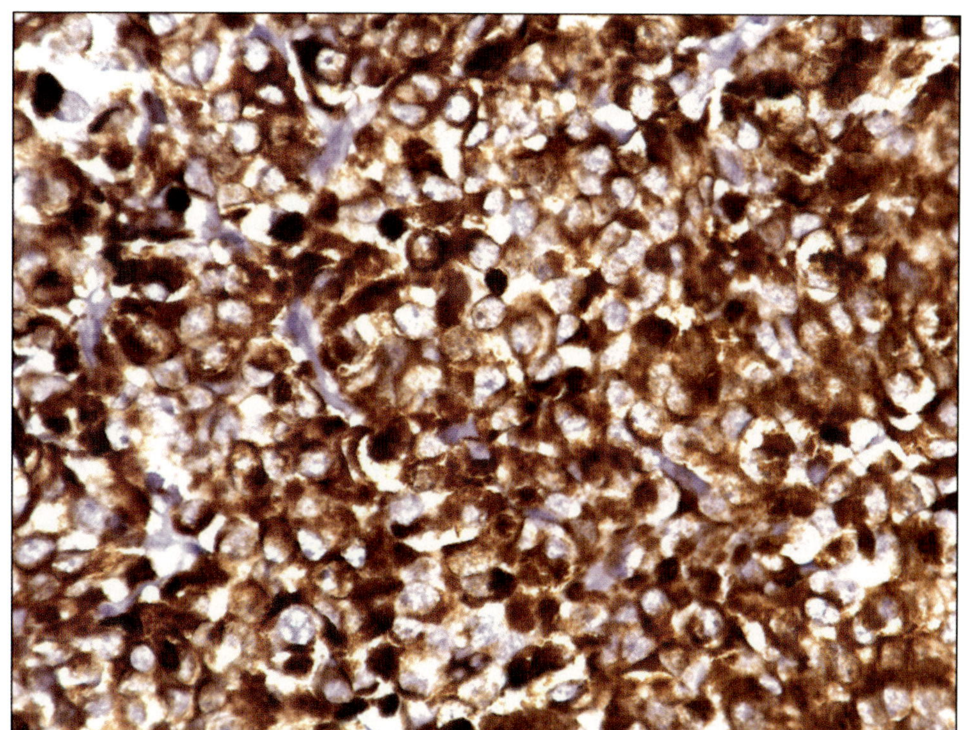

Figure 3.135. Fibrous bodies are dense round cytoplasmic structures highlighted with the low-molecular-weight cytokeratin CAM5.2.

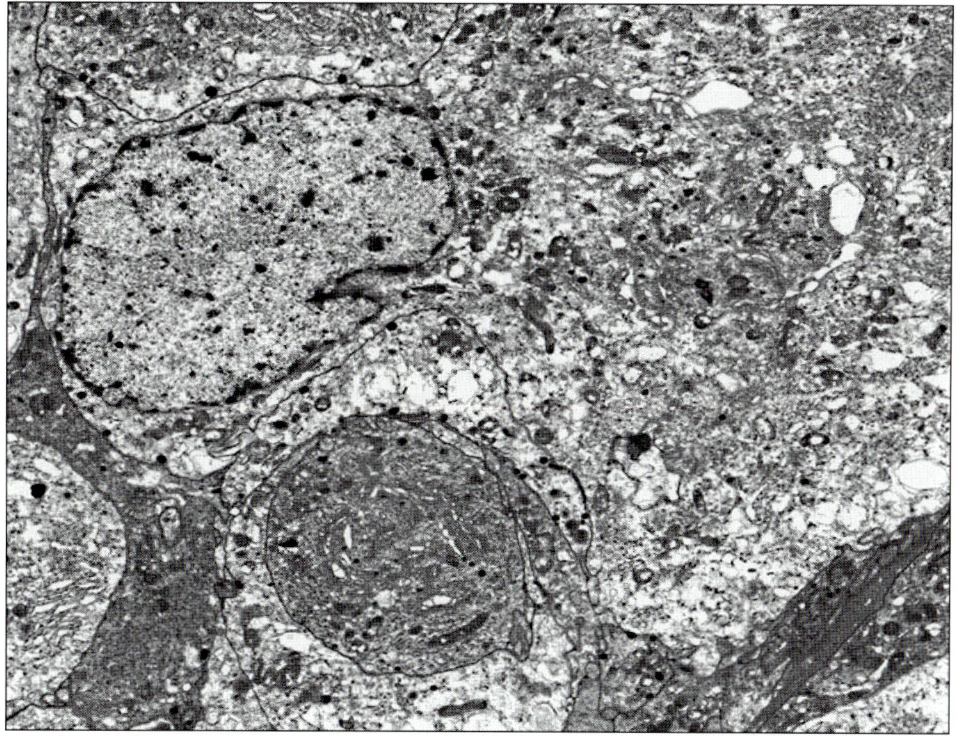

Figure 3.136. This electron micrograph depicts a sparsely granulated growth hormone secreting adenoma. Only a few scattered neurosecretory granules are seen, and a fibrous body is present in the lower half of the field.

Sparsely granulated growth hormone adenomas are associated with a distinctly poorer prognosis and a propensity for aggressive recurrence. This may be reflected in a higher proliferation index in comparison with the mammosomatotroph adenomas (Thapar et al., 1996).

Prolactin-Producing Adenoma

Clinical Features

Prolactinoma is one of the most common types of pituitary adenoma and the most common type of incidentally found pituitary adenoma at autopsy (McComb et al., 1983), and their incidence appears to be increasing (Randall et al., 1985). Clinical manifestations vary with the sex and age of the patient.

Hyperprolactinemia accounts for the endocrine symptoms, with the serum prolactin level usually paralleling the tumor size. Levels of prolactin over 200 ng/ml are usually indicative of a prolactin-producing adenoma (Randall et al., 1985). Elevations below this level may be seen in a variety of mass lesions that compress the pituitary stalk and thus impede the flow of prolactin inhibiting factor (dopamine) from the hypothalamus to the anterior pituitary. This results in the aforementioned stalk effect whereby there is disinhibition of release of prolactin by normal lactotrophs and symptoms of mild hyperprolactinemia. Young women more often become symptomatic when the adenoma is less than 1 cm in size (Delgrange et al., 1997) and develop amenorrhea and galactorrhea rather than symptoms of a mass lesion. In some men and postmenopausal women, large or even giant prolactinomas are more often functionally silent or produce reproductive and sexual dysfunction, including decreased libido and sexual impotence in men. In the absence of prolactin secretion, they produce symptoms due to mass effect related to compression of the optic nerves or invasion of local structures (Nishioka et al., 2002).

Pathology

These adenomas contain abundant rough endoplasmic reticulum and thus appear either chromophobic or basophilic (Figure 3.137). Analogous to growth hormone–producing adenomas, prolactin cell adenomas have sparsely and, much rarer, densely granulated variants. Immunostaining for prolactin will typically reveal a paranuclear localization coinciding with the Golgi apparatus (Figure 3.138). In approximately 10% of cases, the variable presence of psammomatous calcifications is noted, sometimes in great abundance, whereas calcification is rare in other forms of pituitary adenoma.

Prolactinomas are also rarely associated with massive amyloid deposition in the form of spherical concentrically laminated eosinophilic bodies (Figure 3.139), which are birefringent under polarized light when stained with Congo red (Figures 3.140 and 3.141). This finding is even more rarely associated with corticotroph cell adenomas.

An important morphologic feature of prolactinomas may be seen in the almost universal use of preoperative bromocriptine, a dopamine agonist used to treat prolactinomas. It causes dramatic tumor shrinkage and at the cytological level, cell atrophy resulting in a "small blue cell tumor"

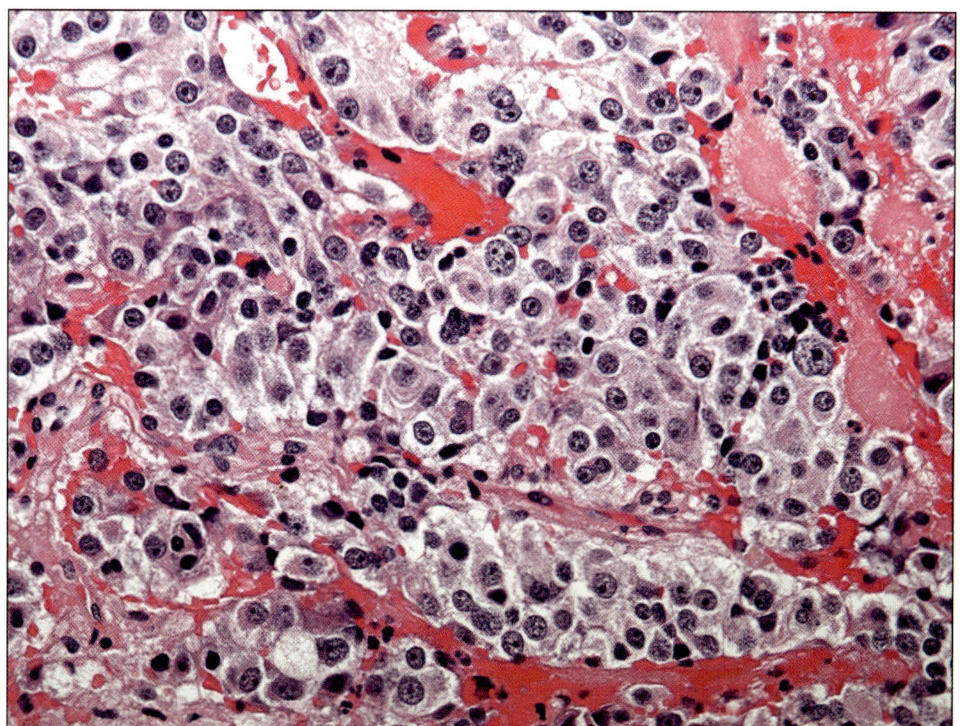

Figure 3.137. Prolactinoma cells are often chromophobic or amphophilic.

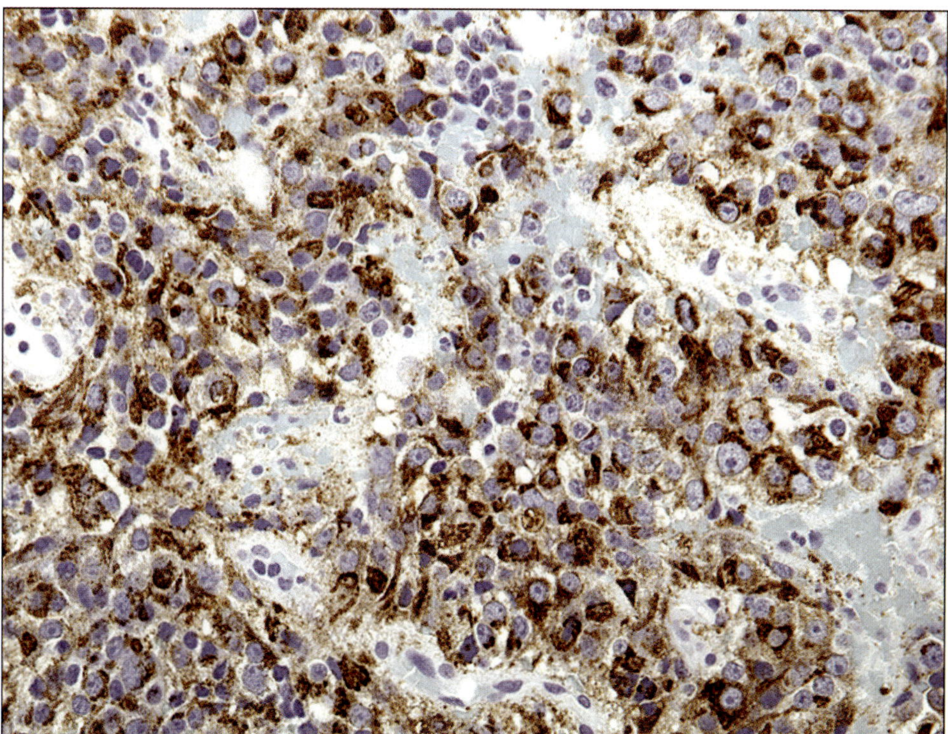

Figure 3.138. Immunohistochemical staining for prolactin is often concentrated adjacent to the nucleus on only one side of the cell, a term referred to as "Golgi pattern."

appearance, sometimes accompanied by extensive fibrosis after long-term treatment (Figure 3.142). Ultrastructural features include misplaced exocytosis, in which granules are excreted into intercellular positions instead of into the capillary border.

Figure 3.139. Prolactinomas often contain regions of amyloid deposition.

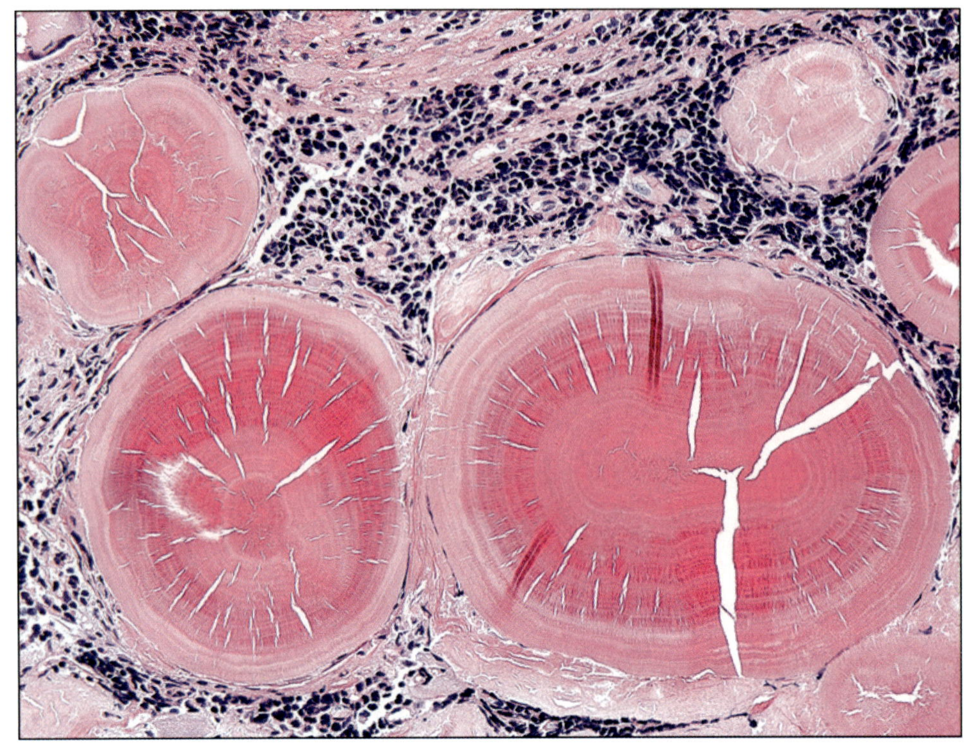

Figure 3.140. Congo red in a prolactinoma highlights the amyloid.

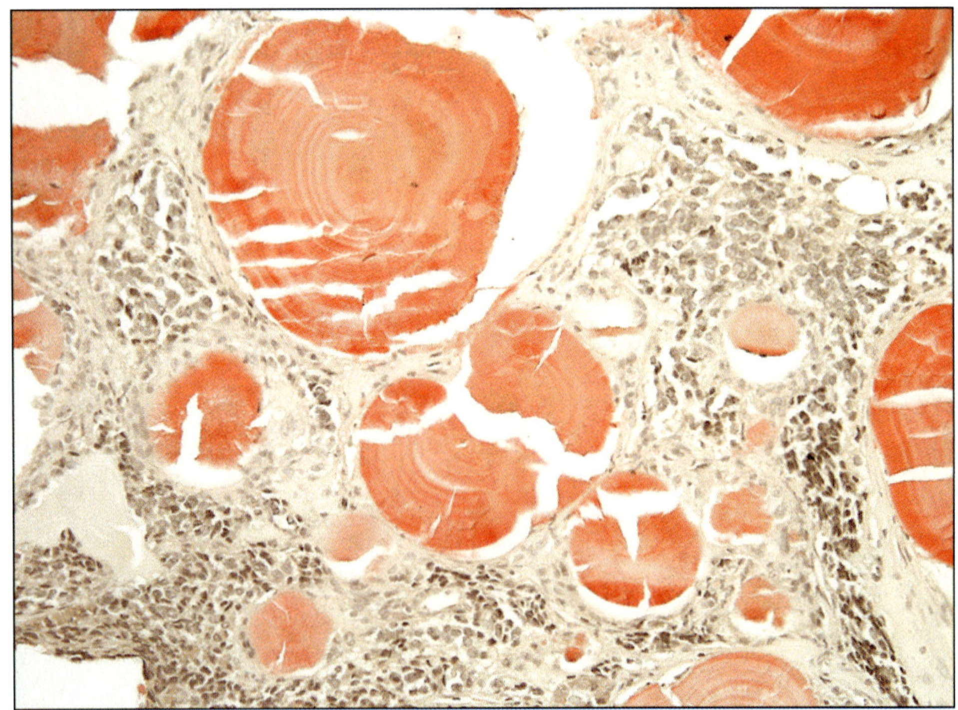

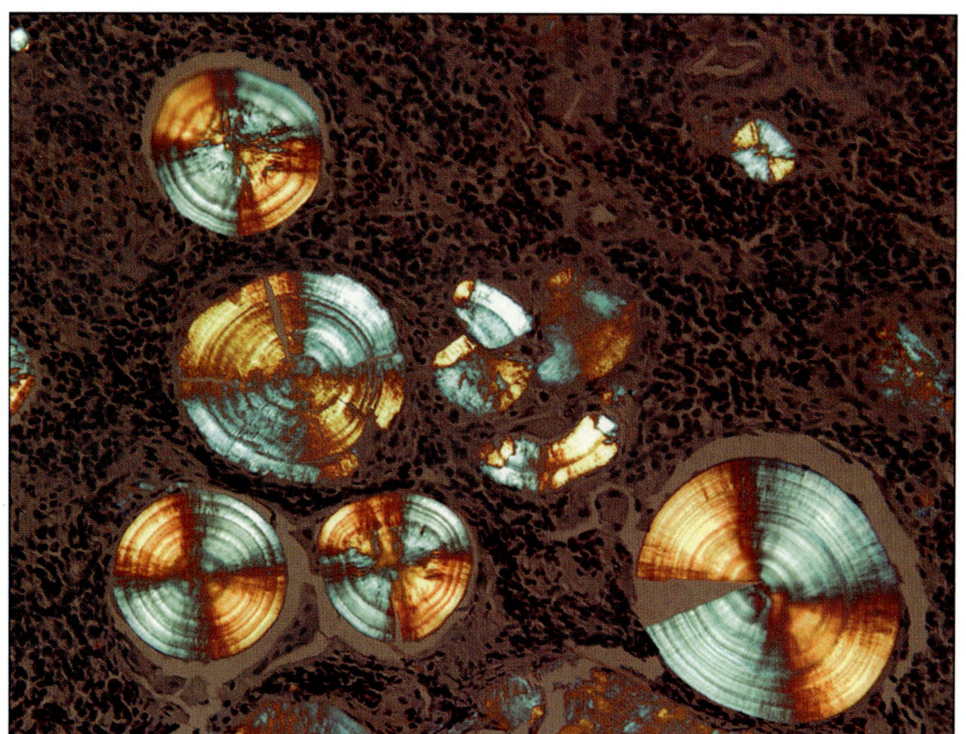

Figure 3.141. Under polarized light, the amyloid stained with Congo red shows bright apple-green birefringence.

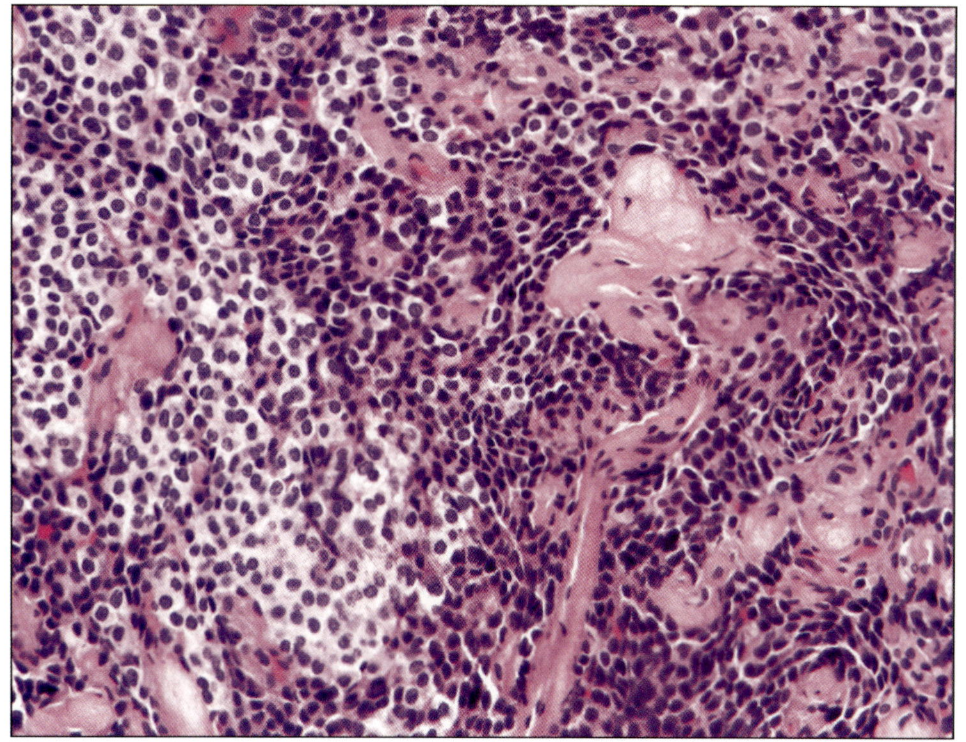

Figure 3.142. This prolactinoma suffered long-term treatment with a dopamine agonist prior to surgical resection. This causes shrinkage of the tumor cells with patchy fibrosis. Some unaffected portions of adenoma are still seen on the left.

Mixed Growth Hormone and Prolactin-Producing Adenomas

One example of this phenomenon, the *mixed growth hormone/prolactin cell adenoma*, is a generally indolent tumor associated with acromegaly, more so than the effects, if any, of hyperprolactinemia (Kontogeorgos et al., 2004). This tumor is recognizable in H&E-stained sections as a truly admixed tumor, composed of eosinophilic (densely granulated) growth hormone cells and chromophobic (sparsely granulated) prolactin cells, also reflected in their immunoreactivity for the respective hormones.

The second example, the *mammosomatotroph cell adenoma,* is a rare and unusual tumor associated with an indolent course and either gigantism or acromegaly. It is notable for both growth hormone and prolactin production within a single cell type, and corresponding immunoreactivity for both hormones in the same cells, which are acidophilic by H&E. Electron microscopy will reveal a unique presence of large (1000–1500 nm) ovoid or irregular secretory granules as well misplaced exocytosis (Felix et al., 1986; Kontogeorgos et al., 2004).

The third example is the *acidophil stem cell adenoma,* representing the growth hormone and prolactin cell line and accounting for approximately 2% of growth hormone-producing tumors. These are often rapidly growing and invasive macroadenomas without growth hormone effects because of usually normal growth hormone levels. It may be associated with hyperprolactinemia but with levels disproportionately low for the size of the corresponding tumor (Horvath et al., 1981; Kontogeorgos et al., 2004).

Microscopically, acidophil stem cell adenomas are usually chromophobic with immunopositivity for prolactin generally greater than that for

Figure 3.143. Acidophil stem cell adenoma demonstrating amphophilic and focally oncocytic cytoplasm with numerous cytoplasmic vacuoles.

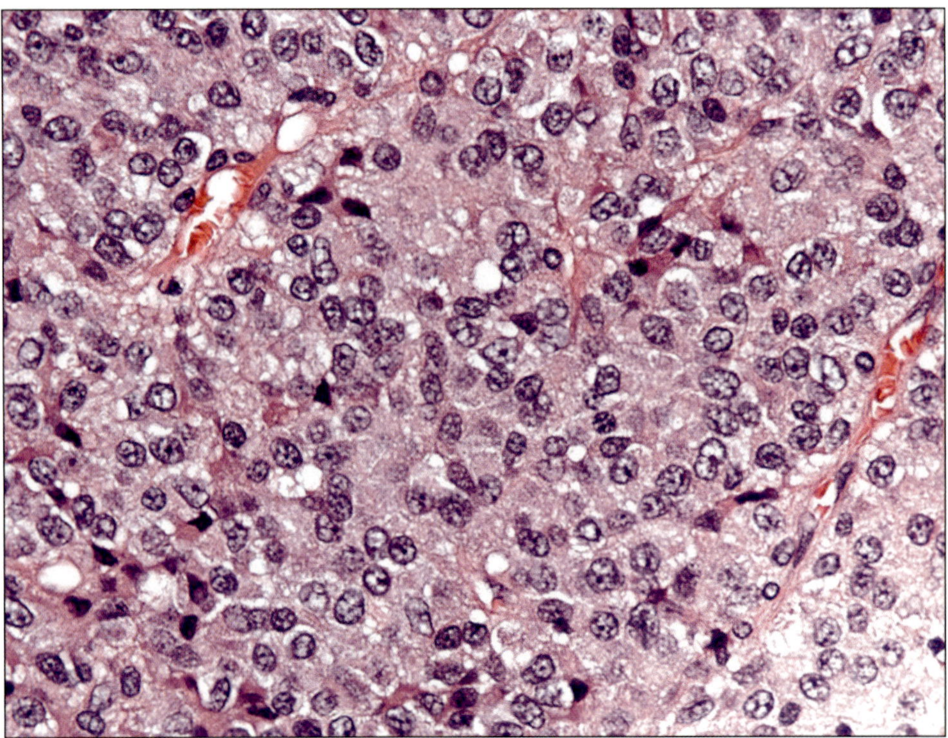

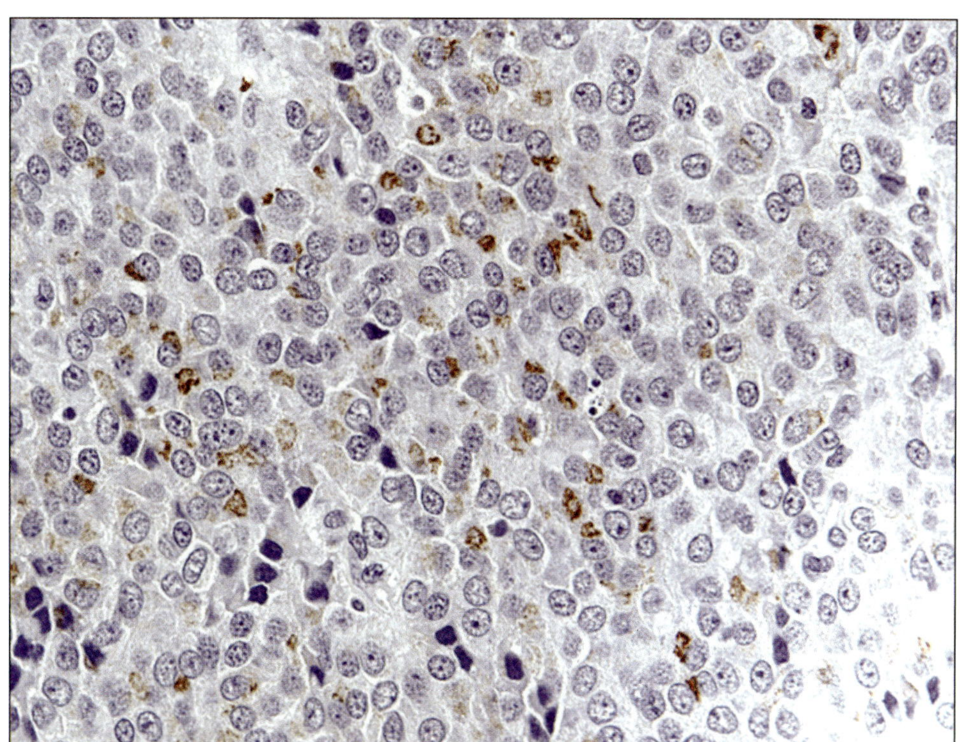

Figure 3.144. The acidophil stem cell adenoma from Figure 3.143 shows prominent Golgi staining for prolactin.

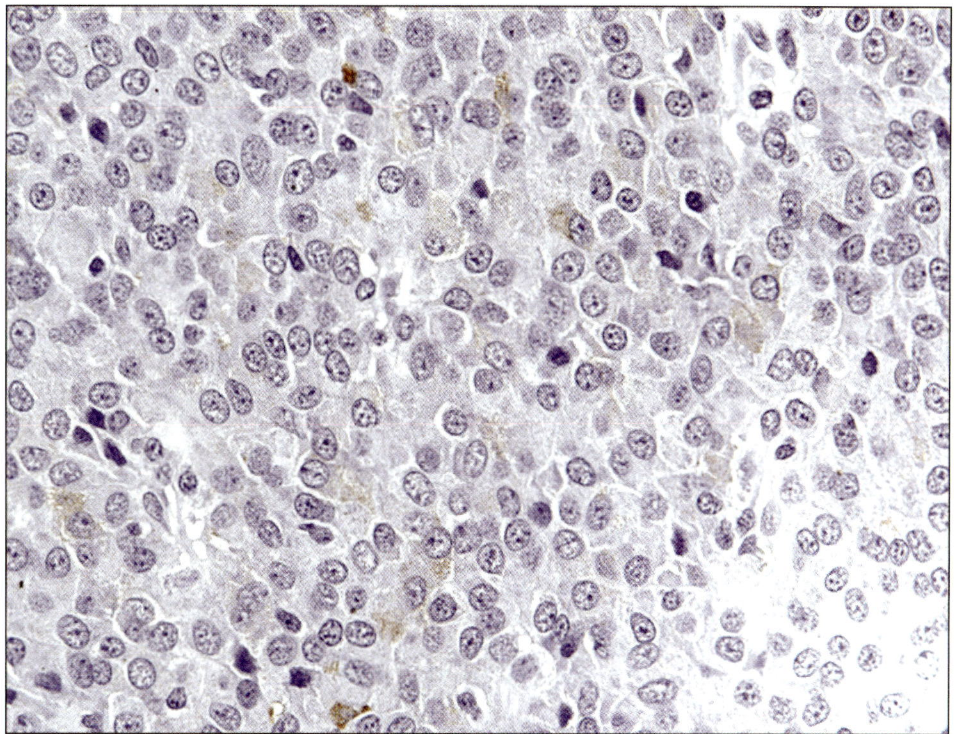

Figure 3.145. The same tumor from Figures 3.143 and 3.144 shows less immunoreactivity for growth hormone.

growth hormone. Oncocytic change and cytoplasmic vacuoles due to giant, swollen mitochondria may be seen (Figures 3.143–3.145). Fibrous bodies, which stain for low molecular weight cytokeratin (Figure 3.146), as well as misplaced exocytosis, may be noted by electron microscopy.

Figure 3.146. Fibrous bodies can be highlighted in acidophil stem cell adenomas by low molecular weight cytokeratin.

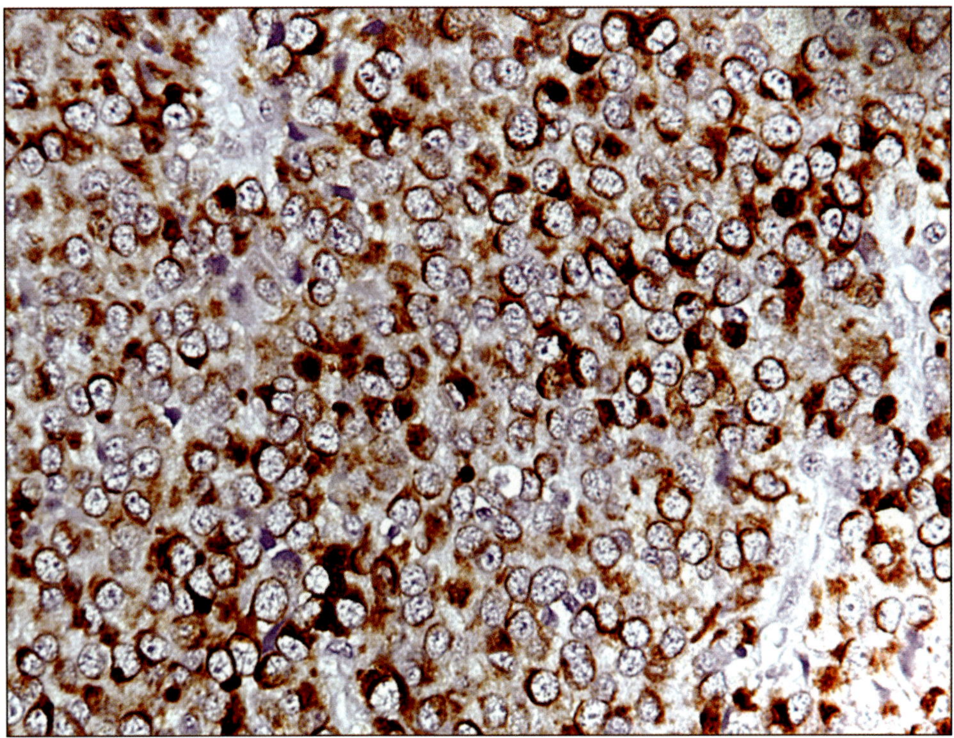

ACTH-Producing Adenoma

Clinical Features

Adrenocorticotropic hormone ACTH or corticotroph cell adenomas synthesize proopiomelanocortin (POMC) from which ACTH and other peptides are manufactured (Trouillas et al., 2004). These tumors are associated with several clinical syndromes with the common feature of cortisol excess and Cushing's disease. Classically, these are due to microadenomas and account for approximately 10–15% of all pituitary adenomas (Trouillas, 2002). They are five times more common in women and require intervention because of the potentially fatal consequences of cortisol excess. A second syndrome seen with progressive adenomas is Nelson syndrome in patients having undergone adrenalectomy in the presence of a pituitary corticotroph adenoma, which was initially unapparent radiographically (Thapar et al., 1992). Corticotroph cell adenomas also include subtypes 1 and 2 of the so-called silent adenomas, which are frequently invasive with a higher recurrence rate (Scheitauer et al., 2000; Psaras et al., 2007). Table 3.1 outlines the details of these silent corticotroph adenoma subtypes as well as silent subtype 3.

Pathology

As previously stated, these lesions are frequently microadenomas and, thus may represent only a small portion of the anterior pituitary resection specimen, a potential challenge, not only in interpreting permanent sections, but also in intraoperative evaluation. The reticulin stain may be invaluable in detecting the

Table 3.1. Silent Pituitary Adenoma Subtypes

Silent Adenoma	Gender Predilection	Clinical Characteristics	Light Microscopy	Electron Microscopy	Immuno / Special Stains
Subtype 1 (Corticotroph)	Female	Older individuals than normally seen for corticotroph adenomas; macroadenoma; high tendency for hemorrhage and apoplexy; often invasive; higher recurrence	Identical to functional corticotroph adenomas; Basophilic	Identical to functional corticotroph adenomas; numerous secretory granules (indented or heart shaped); presence of type I cytokeratin filaments (perinuclear)	Widespread ACTH; POMC
					Strong PAS positivity
Subtype 2 (Corticotroph)	Male	Macroadenoma; higher tendency for hemorrhage and apoplexy; often invasive; higher recurrence	Chromophobic, amphophilic or slightly basophilic cytoplasm; Resembles typical null-cell adenomas	Small cells; smaller and fewer secretory granules (drop-shaped); absence of type I cytokeratin filaments	Patchy uneven ACTH; POMC
					Weak to absent PAS positivity
Subtype 3 (Noncorticotroph)	Slight female predominance	More aggressive and often invasive; macroadenomas; radiosensitive	Spindled; May be large with variably pleomorphic nuclei and abundant cytoplasm; Chromophobic or slightly acidophilic; Sometimes blotchy acidophilia	Large polar cells with prominent nucleoli and intranuclear inclusions (spheridia >> filaments); smooth ER (in contrast to other adenoma types); numerous segments of Golgi membranes scattered over large cytoplasmic area; minute sparse granules	Plurihormonal: GH, TSH, prolactin, or α-SU in any combination

Sources: Horvath et al. (2005), Psaras et al. (2007), Scheithauer et al. (2000), Thodou et al. (2007).

Figure 3.147. ACTH immunoreactivity is seen in this corticotroph adenoma.

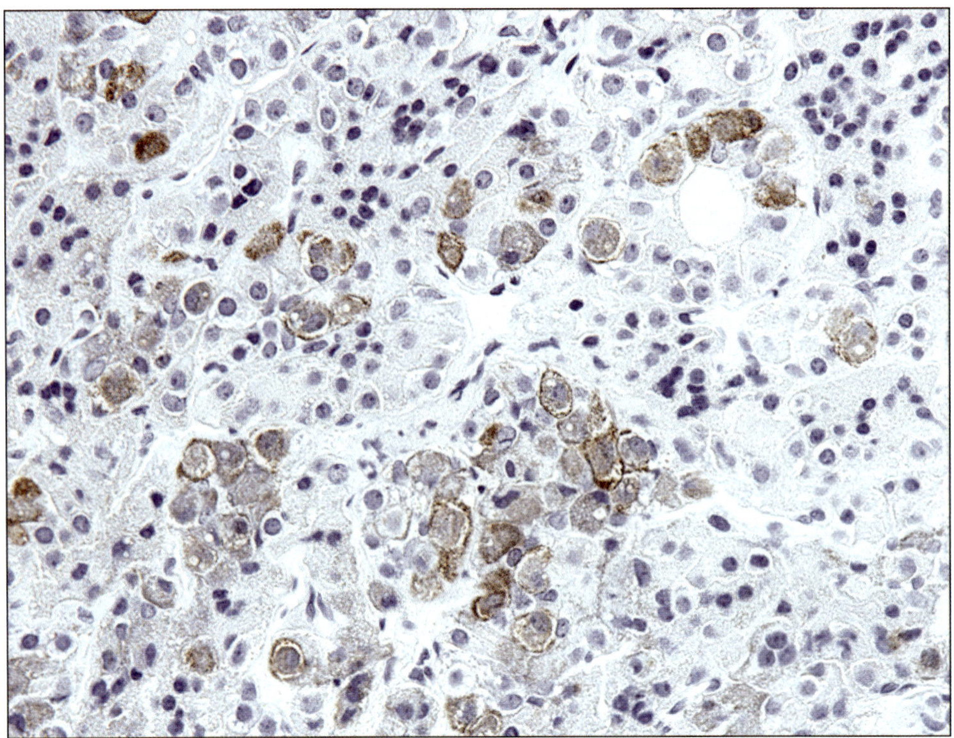

reticulin-free microadenoma. Corticotroph cell adenomas (Figure 3.147) are amphophilic to basophilic in H&E-stained sections and are strongly PAS positive. On rare occasions, amyloid deposition may be seen.

An interesting feature accompanying some ACTH-producing adenomas is the presence of prominent accumulations of keratin microfilaments imparting a hyaline appearance to the cytoplasm in nonneoplastic corticotrophs and rarely in corticotroph adenoma cells, known as *Crooke's hyaline change* (Figure 3.148). This feature occurs in response to glucocorticoid excess.

Corticotroph cell adenomas show immunoreactivity for ACTH. Mixed hormone patterns include concomitant gonadotropin or alpha-subunit production. Whereas galectin-3 positivity is seen in functioning adenomas, the silent corticotroph adenomas show infrequent immunoreactivity (Jin et al., 2005; Thodou et al., 2007). By electron microscopy, most corticotroph cell adenomas are densely granulated with somewhat pleomorphic, variably electron-dense, tear-shaped or heart-shaped granules.

Gonadotropin-Producing Adenoma

Clinical Features

Adenomas associated with follicle stimulating hormone (FSH) and luteinizing hormone (LH) production are part of a group of tumors known as glycoprotein adenomas that share production of the alpha-subunit common to FSH, LH, and TSH. Alpha-subunit elevations may be detectable in serum, even in the absence of

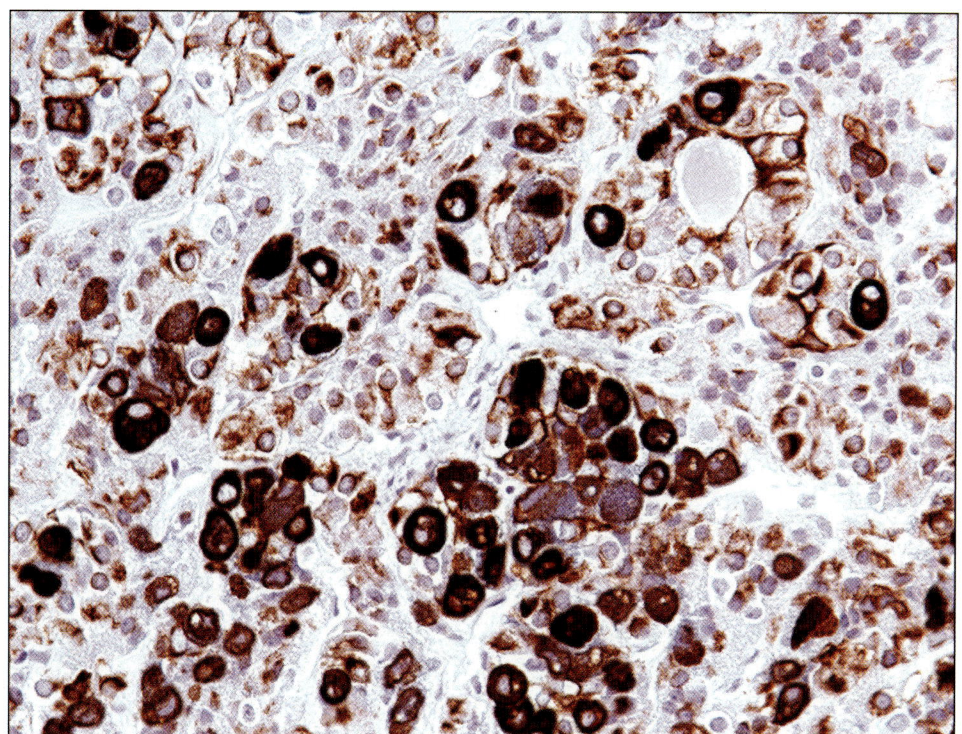

Figure 3.148. Crooke's hyaline change is identified here in nonneoplastic corticotroph cells as dense, homogeneous immunoreactivity for CAM5.2.

elevated hormone levels. These adenomas are less often associated with endocrine deficiencies, and rather present as macroadenomas with the usual results of headache, visual disturbances, and cranial nerve palsies (Snyder 1997; Asa et al., 2004). This type of pituitary adenoma is the one most commonly associated with pituitary apoplexy or hemorrhagic necrosis (Asa et al., 2004).

Pathology

These adenomas tend to be composed of sparsely granulated chromophobes (Figure 3.149) with a tendency for oncocytic change and a conspicuous perivascular arrangement. Immunopositivity for gonadotropins is often focal, with cells showing LH positivity (Figure 3.150) usually numbering fewer than those showing FSH positivity (Figure 3.151). Electron microscopy usually shows medium-sized secretory granules.

Thyrotropin-Producing Adenoma

Clinical Features

This least frequent form of pituitary adenoma is usually accompanied by elevated levels of TSH, but they may also arise in the setting of hypothyroidism in which there is preexisting thyrotroph hyperplasia. The majority of these tumors present as aggressive and invasive macroadenomas (Beck-Peccoz et al., 1996; Beck-Peccoz and Persani, 2008).

Figure 3.149.
Gonadotropin-producing
adenoma with chromophobic
cytoplasm and a prominent
perivascular arrangement.

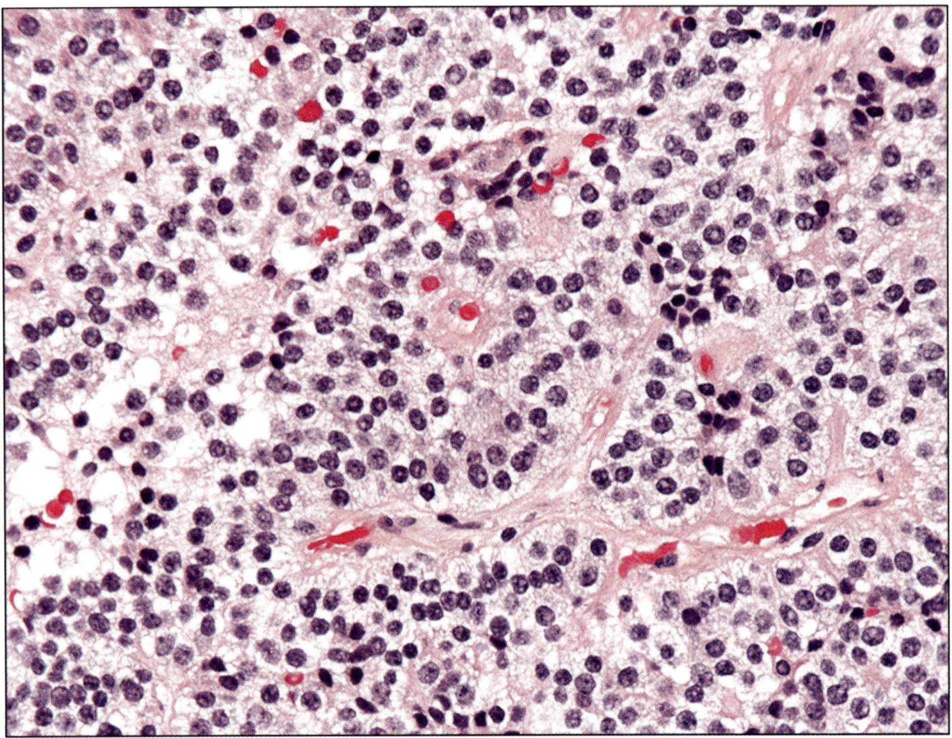

Figure 3.150.
Immunoreactivity for LH is
often weak and patchy in
gonadotropin-producing
adenomas.

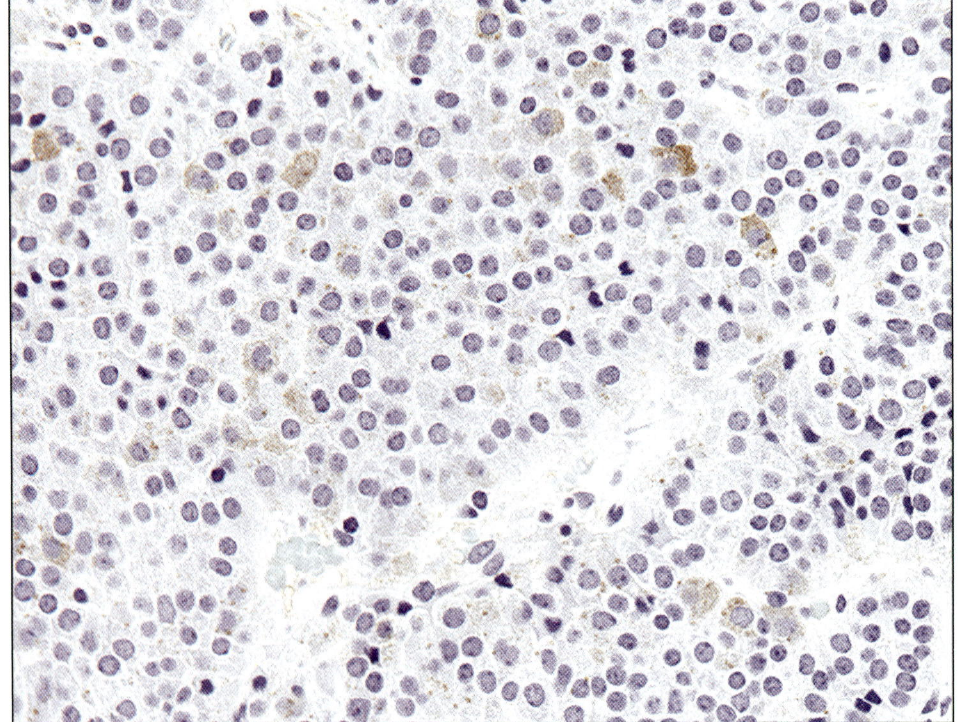

Pathology

Microscopy shows similar histologic features to gonadotroph cell adenomas, namely chromophobic with weak to no PAS positivity and arranged in
perivascular pseudorosettes. Solid tumor growth may also be observed.

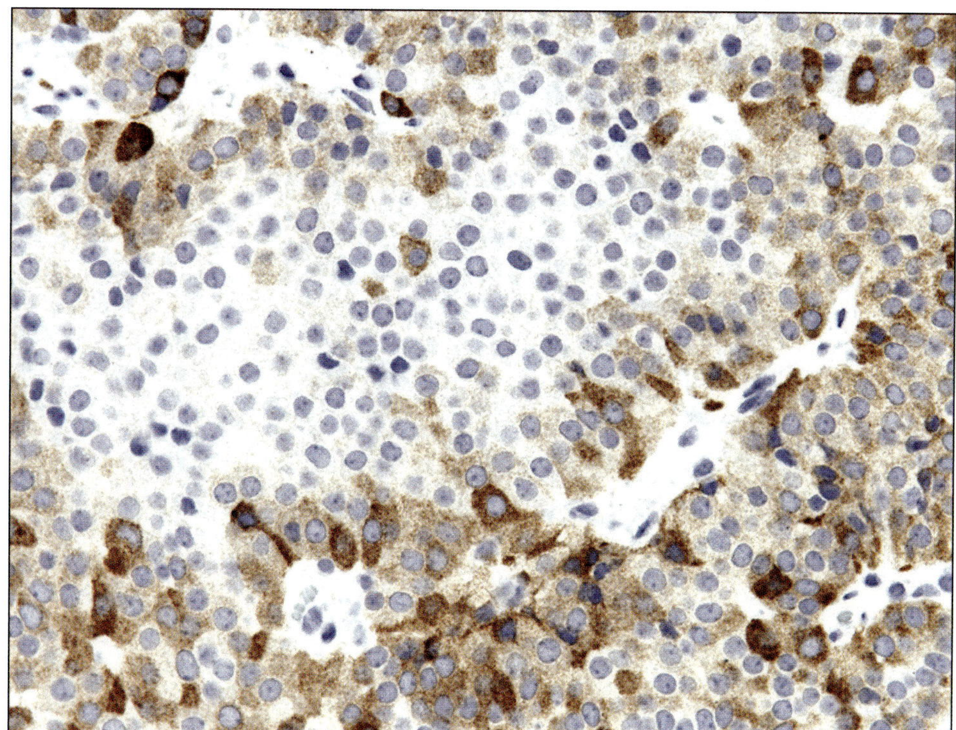

Figure 3.151. FSH often shows more prominent immunoreactivity than LH in gonadotroph adenomas.

Plurihormonal Adenoma

Clinical Features

These adenomas by definition produce hormones from both major classes of anterior pituitary cells: the amino acid hormones including growth hormone, prolactin and ACTH, and the glycoprotein hormones including LH, FSH, and TSH, which harbor the same alpha-subunit (Horvath et al., 2004). They tend to present as macroadenomas at the time of diagnosis with corresponding mass effect and hyperprolactinemia due to pituitary stalk effect. The *silent subtype 3* pituitary adenoma is a member of this category and is important to recognize because of its highly infiltrative behavior, rapid growth, and high recurrence rate (Al-Shraim et al., 2004; Horvath et al., 2005). These patients often have hyperprolactinemia and, when treated with a dopamine agonist, will show a fall in prolactin levels despite continued growth of the tumor. ACTH-producing adenomas, which show expression of alpha-subunit, comprise a rare plurihormonal subtype, characterized by aggressive behavior and higher recurrence (Berg et al., 1990).

Pathology

These are most often chromophobic adenomas or slightly acidophilic and are PAS negative. They may be monomorphous or plurimorphous with regard to cell type. By their nature, they show immunoreactivity for several hormones, the most common patterns being a combination of TSH, FSH, and growth hormone or a combination of prolactin and TSH. Excluded from this group designation are adenomas producing growth hormone, prolactin, and TSH as well as those with LH and FSH dual immunoreactivity (Horvath et al., 2004).

The silent adenoma subtype 3 (Table 3.1) usually expresses growth hormone, prolactin, TSH, and alpha-subunit in variable combinations. The cells are often spindled with chromophobic cytoplasm, which is rich with organelles. The nuclei may be large and sometimes pleomorphic.

Null Cell Adenoma

Clinical Features

Neither clinical nor immunohistochemical evidence of hormone production is seen in approximately 20% of pituitary adenomas. However, patients often present with hypopituitarism and mass effect, with the majority showing indolent progression (Kovacs et al., 1980).

Pathology

Most of these adenomas are chromophobic. They are perhaps most analogous to gonadotroph cell adenomas in showing occasional alpha-subunit or glycoprotein hormone immunopositivity (e.g., FSH and LH). Ultrastructurally, these typically show small poorly developed granules and sometimes mitochondrion-rich cytoplasm as is seen in some oncocytic tumors. *Oncocytic change* is not specific to null cell adenoma, being also associated with acidophil stem cell, silent corticotroph, and gonadotroph cell adenomas.

Atypical Pituitary Adenoma

Aside from the pituitary adenomas in which clinical behavior may be linked to the pathological and hormonal profile, an attempt has been made to define separate criteria that may be predictive of aggressive behavior and a higher likelihood of recurrence. Logically, these adenomas are associated with a higher mitotic rate (Figure 3.152). Accordingly, those with a MIB-1 labeling index exceeding 3% (Figure 3.153) along with extensive p53 immunoreactivity (Figure 3.154) may be considered atypical pituitary adenomas (Lloyd et al., 2004; Scheitauer et al., 2006). However, the predictive value in these determinations remains to be proven, considering the vagaries in defining p53 immunopositivity in these cases and the notion that immunoreactivity has not been shown to correlate with actual mutations in the *p53* tumor suppressor gene.

PITUITARY CARCINOMA

This is defined as a pituitary neoplasm, usually producing prolactin or ACTH, which has undergone craniospinal dissemination (e.g. subarachnoid or parenchymal) or systemic metastases such as to lymph nodes, liver, or bone

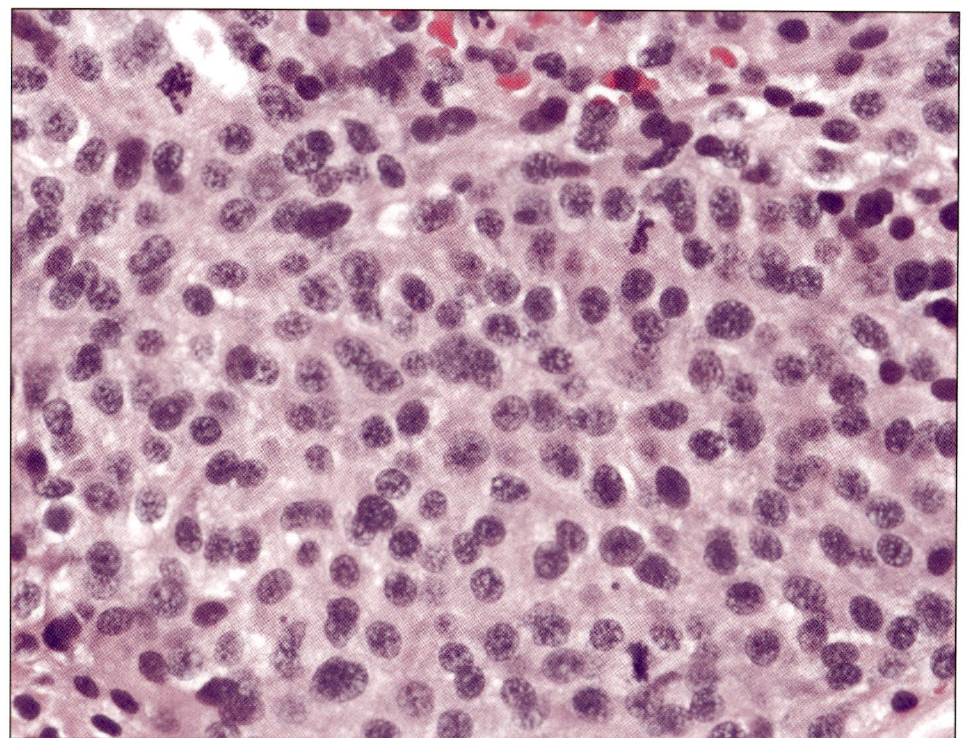

Figure 3.152. Several mitotic figures are seen in a single high-power field in this atypical adenoma, which otherwise looks cytologically bland.

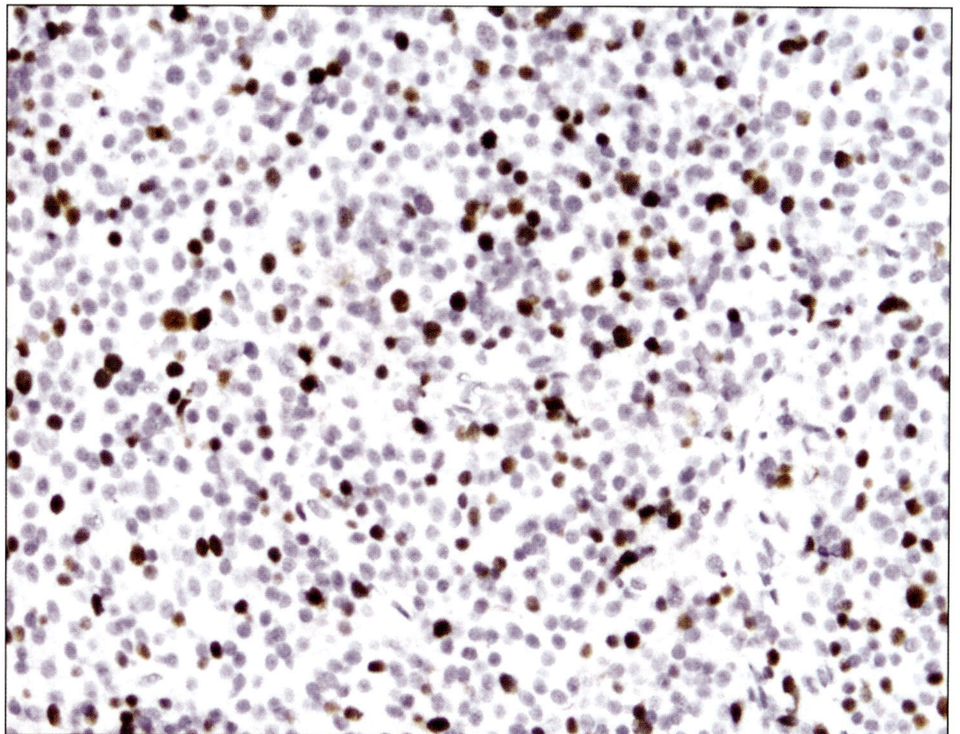

Figure 3.153. This atypical adenoma has a MIB-1 labelling index well above 3%.

(Scheithauer et al., 2004, 2006). The significance of direct brain invasion by an adenoma is controversial but currently does not fall under the rubric of carcinoma. Microscopically pituitary carcinoma may appear deceptively well-differentiated. However, a majority of these tumors have increased proliferation indices and overexpression of p53.

Figure 3.154. Atypical adenoma with extensive p53 immunoreactivity.

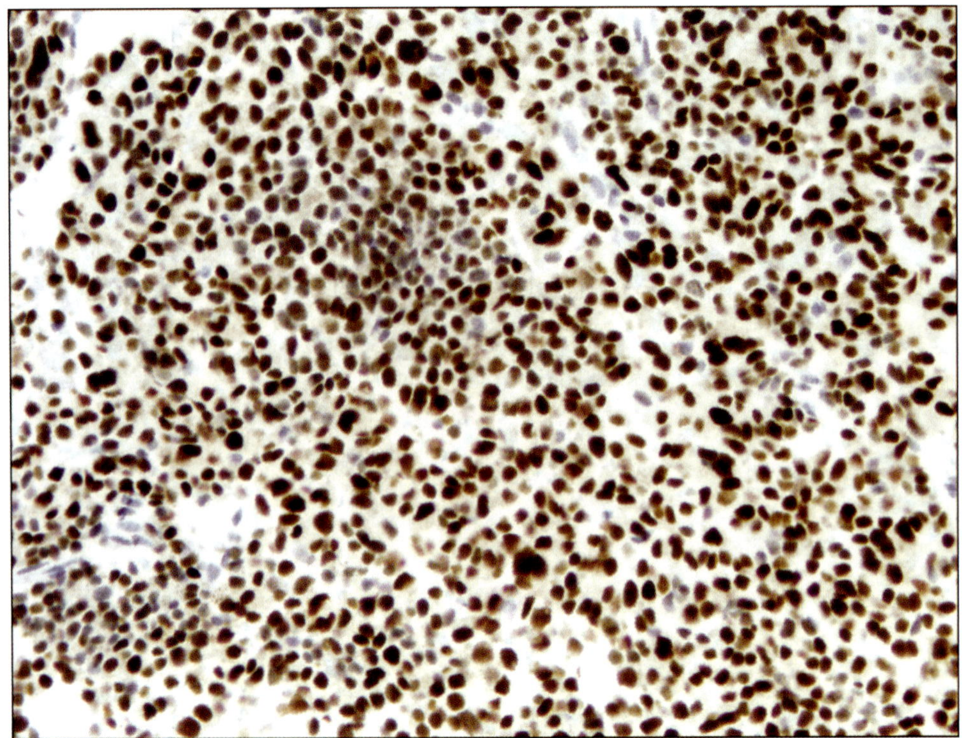

PITUITARY APOPLEXY

Apoplexy of the pituitary gland refers to hemorrhagic infarction of the gland, which can occur in a multitude of settings. Most commonly, this is seen in postpartum women as the result of hypotension. In the setting of pituitary adenoma, apoplexy is most often seen with gonadotropin-producing adenomas. However, silent corticotroph adenomas also have an increased tendency toward infarction. Clinical symptoms vary, but headache is by far the most common complaint (Glezer et al., 2008).

In the acute setting, CT or MRI with contrast administration is extremely helpful, demonstrating a high-intensity or heterogeneous pituitary gland sometimes accompanied by a sellar fluid level (Figure 3.155) or subarachnoid hemorrhage. Glucocorticoid therapy is required in these patients (Glezer et al., 2008).

GANGLIOCYTOMA

Clinical Features

The majority of these tumors appear to be associated with pituitary adenomas with evidence of hormone hypersecretion, especially growth hormone. As such, it seems reasonable that gangliocytic differentiation occurs as a metaplastic phenomenon, which is supported by the ultrastructure of cells showing intermediate differentiation between neurons and adenohypophysial cells (Geddes et al., 2000). Accordingly, the clinical features of these tumors may closely

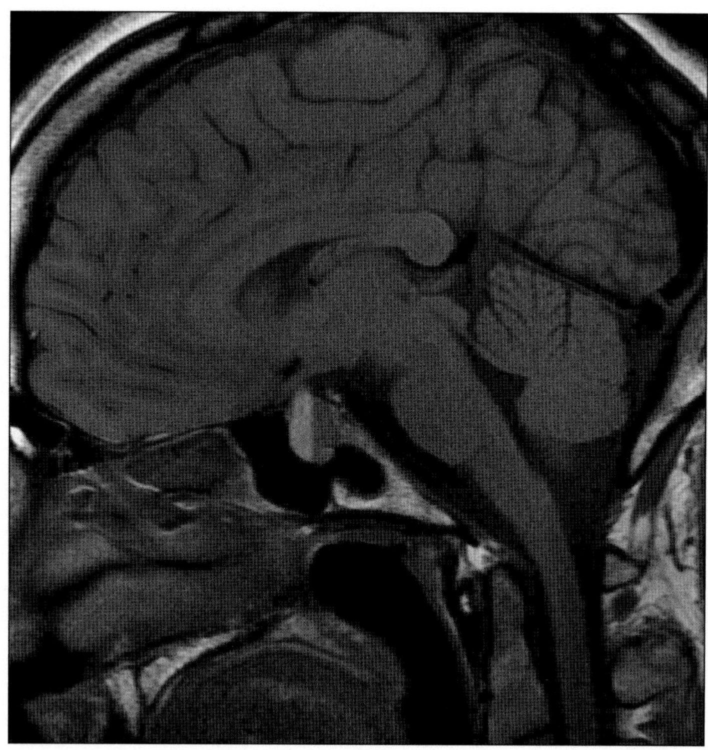

Figure 3.155. Pituitary apoplexy and hemorrhage. A sagittal T1-weighted MR image shows a fluid–fluid level within the sella turcica. The fluid–fluid level likely resulted from hemorrhage into a necrotic or cystic portion of this patient's growth hormone-secreting pituitary adenoma. The patient was undergoing treatment with somatostatin. The diploic space is slightly thickened, as can be seen in patients with acromegaly.

resemble those resulting from hormone hypersecretion of the corresponding adenoma. Interestingly, acromegaly due to hypothalamic gangliocytoma producing growth hormone releasing hormone (GHRH) has been reported (Asa et al., 1984).

Pathology

This is viewed as a true metaplastic phenomenon within a pituitary adenoma with cells of intermediate neuronal differentiation forming a spectrum with cells demonstrating complete gangliocytic differentiation, including neuronal cell processes and Nissl substance. The Nissl substance may be marginated, and multinucleated neuronal cells with prominent nucleoli are not uncommon (Figure 3.156). Immunoreactivity is present for neuronal markers, including neurofilament and synaptophysin. Although neuronal cells demonstrating immunoreactivity for hormonal markers of the associated pituitary adenoma have been reported, these cases are in the minority. Gangliocytomas without associated pituitary adenoma may also arise very infrequently in the sellar or hypothalamic regions (Geddes et al., 2000).

SPINDLE-CELL ONCOCYTOMA OF THE ADENOHYPOPHYSIS

Clinical and Radiological Features

This newly recognized and rare entity occurs as a tumor of adults with an apparently equal sex distribution and a wide age range, but a mean age of 56 years.

Figure 3.156. This pituitary adenoma contained foci of gangliocytic differentiation. These large cells, some of which are multinucleated, have abundant granular cytoplasm with Nissl substance and large nuclei with prominent nucleoli.

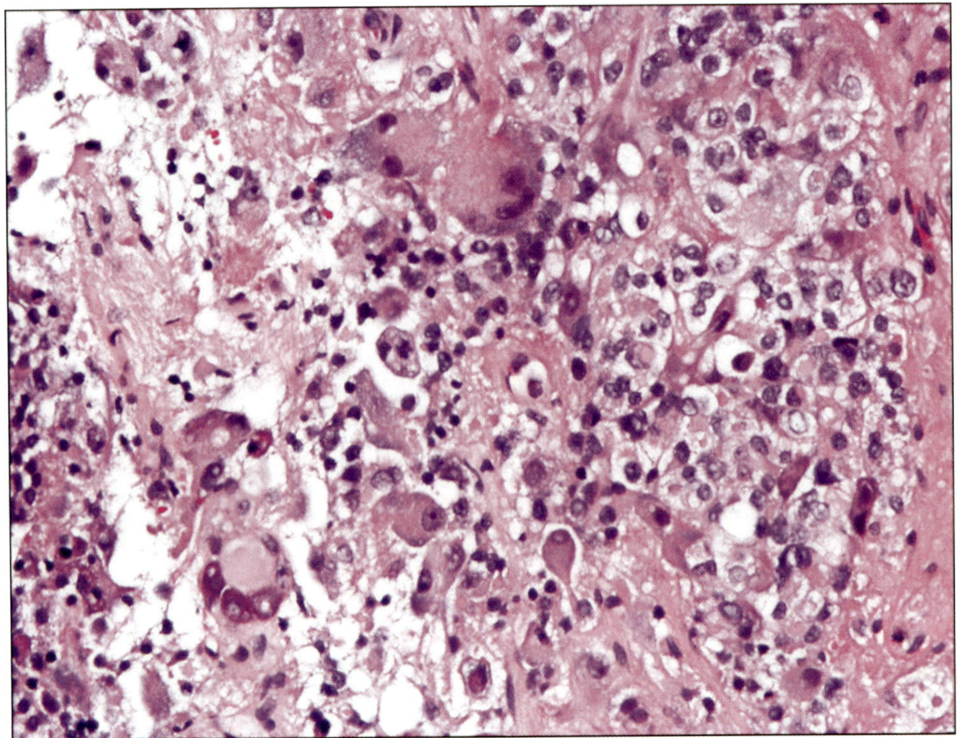

It originates in the adenohypophysis and the clinical presentation is generally identical to that of ordinary pituitary adenomas, producing hypopituitarism, visual field defects, and occasionally headache, nausea, and vomiting (Roncaroli and Scheithauer, 2007). The ultrastructural features along with its characteristic immunophenotype suggest a histogenetic origin in the folliculostellate cell of the anterior pituitary (Roncaroli et al., 2002). This entity has been classified as WHO Grade I.

Radiographic features include those of a sharply demarcated solid and contrast-enhancing sellar or suprasellar mass. Skull base destruction has been reported (Vajtai et al., 2006; Roncaroli and Scheithauer, 2007).

Pathology

These are grossly indistinguishable from pituitary adenomas. Histologically, spindle cell oncocytomas display spindled to epithelioid cells arranged in compact, interlacing fascicles. The cells typically have eosinophilic cytoplasm with variable degrees of oncocytic change (Figure 3.157). There may be mild to moderate nuclear atypia and pleomorphism. Patchy infiltrates of mature lymphocytes may be noted. Mitotic activity is typically low. Ultrastructural examination depicts well-formed desmosomes and cell junctions, numerous swollen mitochondria, and an absence of secretory granules, allowing its distinction from pituitary adenoma.

Spindle-cell oncocytomas are typically immunopositive for vimentin, EMA, and S-100 protein, as well as for galectin-3 (Figure 3.158). Immunoreactivity for GFAP, cytokeratins, synaptophysin, chromogranin, smooth muscle actin, desmin, and CD34 is generally absent (Kloub et al., 2005; Roncaroli and Scheithauer, 2007).

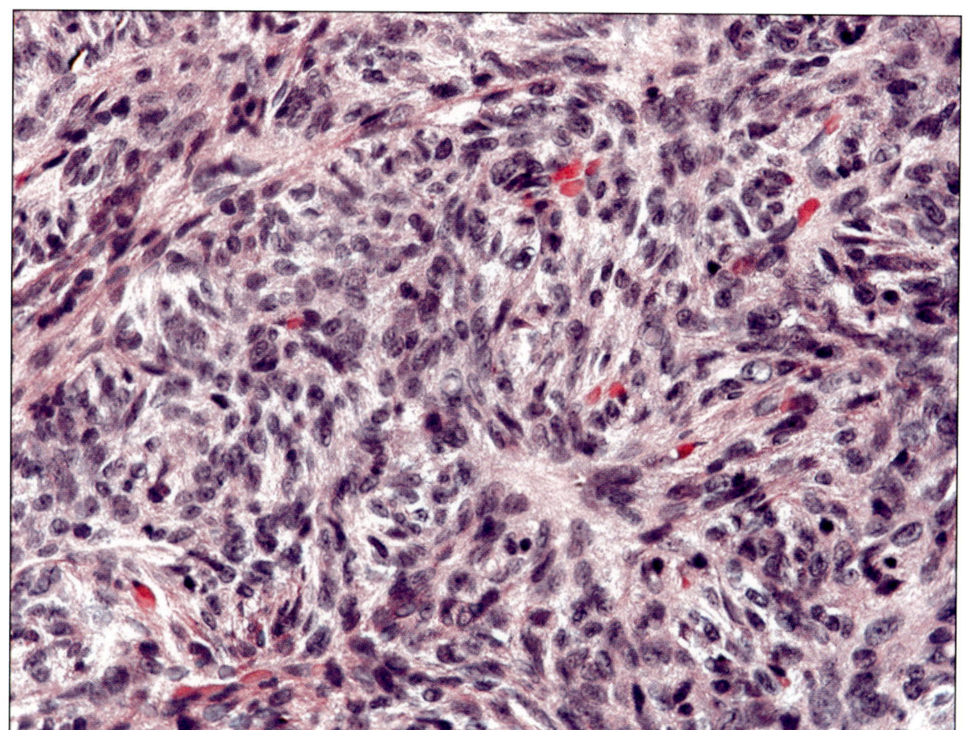

Figure 3.157. As the name implies, spindle-cell oncocytoma of the anterior pituitary is composed of spindled- cells arranged in fascicles with oncocytic cytoplasm.

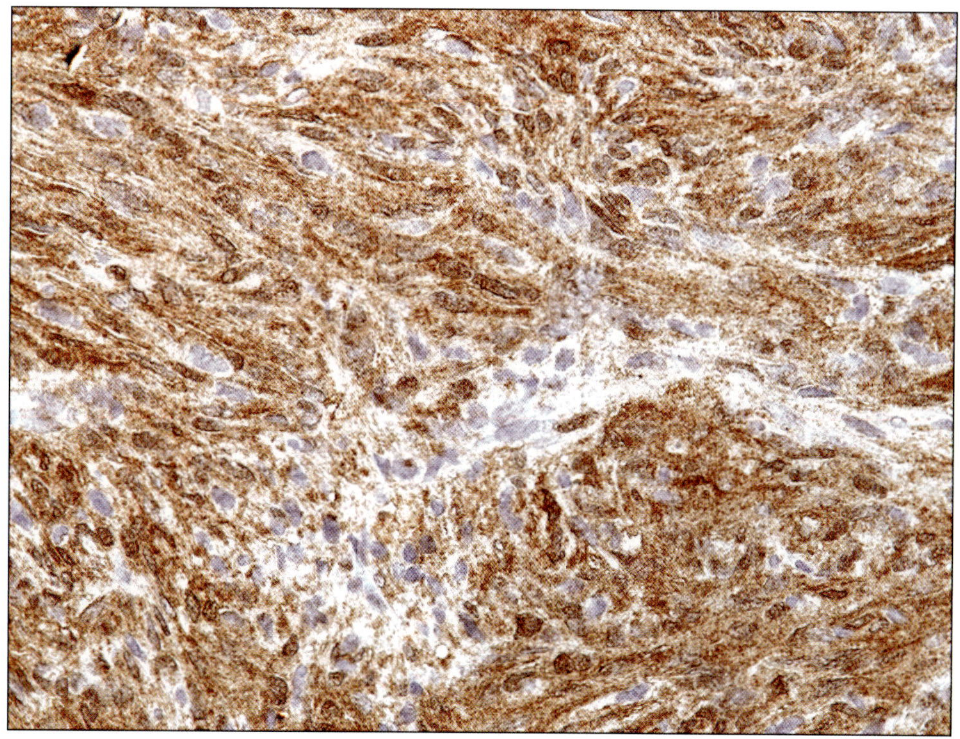

Figure 3.158. Galectin-3 stains the cytoplasm and some of the nuclei in spindle-cell oncocytoma.

PITUICYTOMA

Clinical and Radiological Features

The handful of cases in the known literature has been reported in adults and more commonly in males. The symptoms resemble those of other slow-growing

Figure 3.159. Pituicytomas have intersecting fascicles of spindled astrocytic cells, many of which have easily discernable cytoplasmic borders.

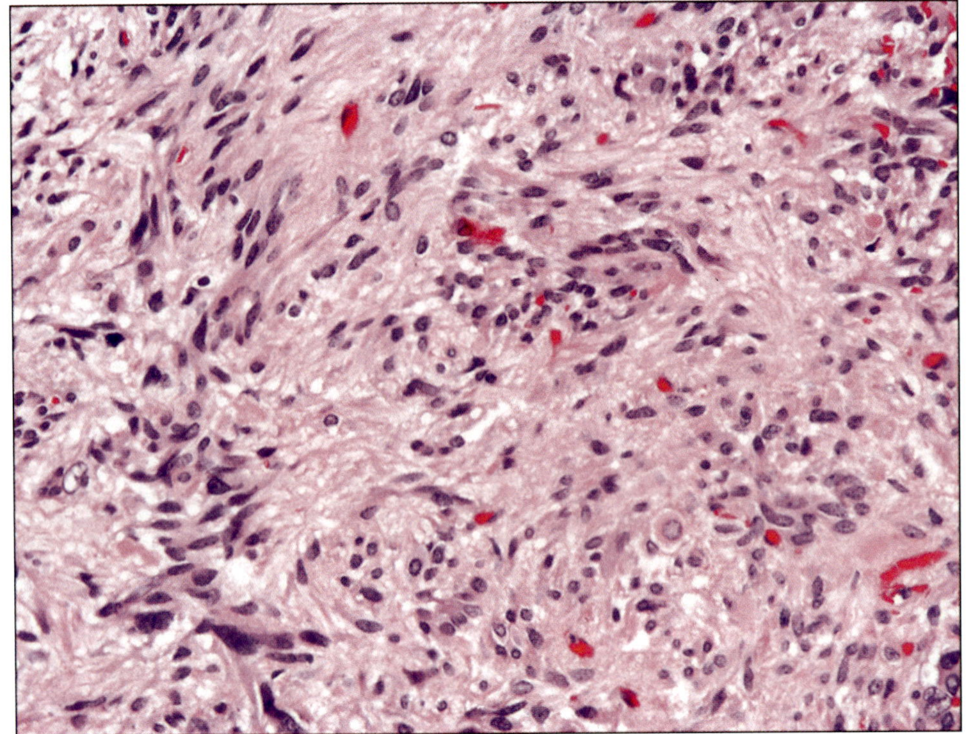

masses of the sellar or suprasellar region, with compression of the visual pathways or hypopituitarism and hyperprolactinemia due to pituitary stalk effect. These tumors are believed to originate in pituicytes, which are the specialized glial cells of the neurohypophysis, and their differences with granular cell tumors of the infundibulum may be explained by different subtypes of normal pituicytes in which these neoplasms originate (Takei et al., 1980). Their radiographic appearance is that of a solid circumscribed growth with diffuse contrast enhancement, rarely containing a cystic component (Brat et al., 2000).

Pathology

This WHO Grade I tumor is characterized by a compact arrangement of elongated bipolar spindle cells arranged in fascicles or a storiform pattern in which cell borders are discernable (Figure 3.159). The nuclei may be enlarged but show little atypia. Tumor cells often contain abundant eosinophilic cytoplasm, although obvious granular or oncocytic change is lacking.

Immunohistochemically, these may be distinguished from granular cell tumors by GFAP positivity (Figure 3.160), but they share S-100 protein expression (Brat et al., 2000). GFAP staining is sometimes only focal or even absent. Cytokeratin, neuronal, and neuroendocrine markers are negative.

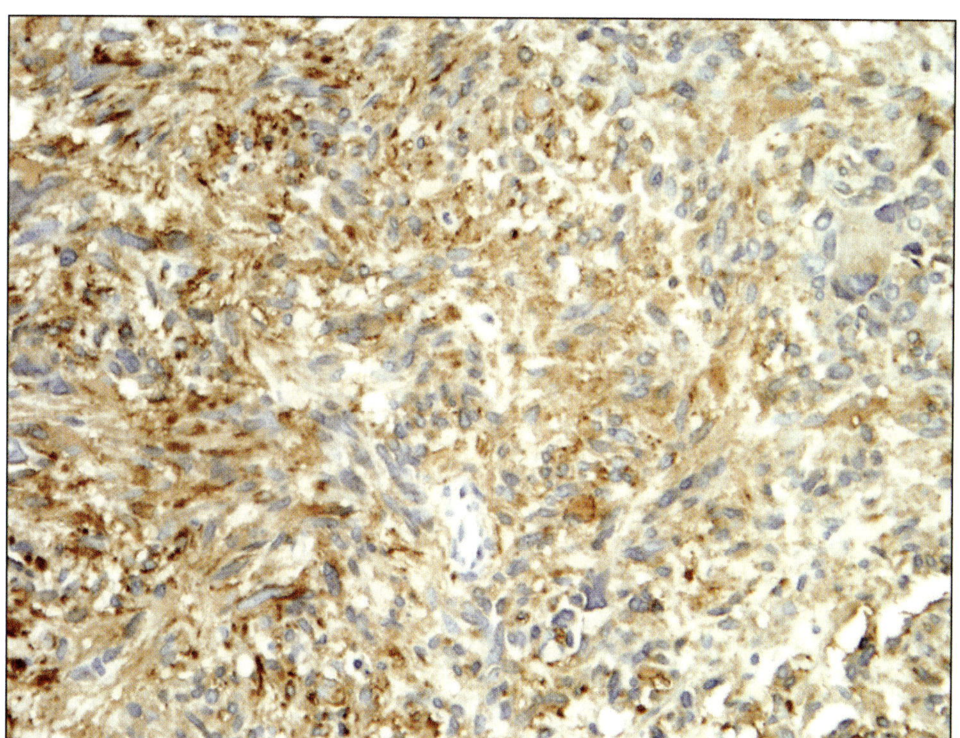

Figure 3.160. The tumor cells in pituicytoma show GFAP immunoreactivity.

GRANULAR CELL TUMOR OF THE NEUROHYPOPHYSIS

Clinical and Radiological Features

These WHO grade I tumors only rarely present as a mass lesion prompting surgical biopsy. They occur most frequently in females between the ages of 30 and 60 years and become symptomatic because of suprasellar extension and mass effect upon visual pathways. Hyperprolactinemia due to pituitary stalk effect may occur. They are believed to arise from the glia of the posterior pituitary, which undergo granular degeneration, thus nosologically linking these tumors with *pituicytoma* (Fuller et al., 2007). Granular cell tumors may arise from normally occurring nests or tumorlets of granular cells found with increasing frequency in old age. They can be multiple and are a relatively common incidental finding at autopsy. Cooccurrence with pituitary adenomas has been noted on occasion (Tomita and Gates, 1999); however, these tumors are not histogenetically linked. Radiographically, granular cell tumors are circumscribed solid masses with uniform contrast enhancement.

Pathology

These appear as hypocellular lesions composed of large polygonal cells with granular eosinophilic cytoplasm (Figure 3.161) containing PAS-positive and diastase-resistant cytoplasm (Figure 3.162). The nuclei are round with small nucleoli and are often eccentrically placed. Perivascular aggregates of lymphocytes may be noted.

Figure 3.161. Granular cell tumor of the neurohypophysis is composed of sheets of large polygonal cells with abundant granular cytoplasm due to lysosomal accumulation. The nuclei are bland and often eccentrically located.

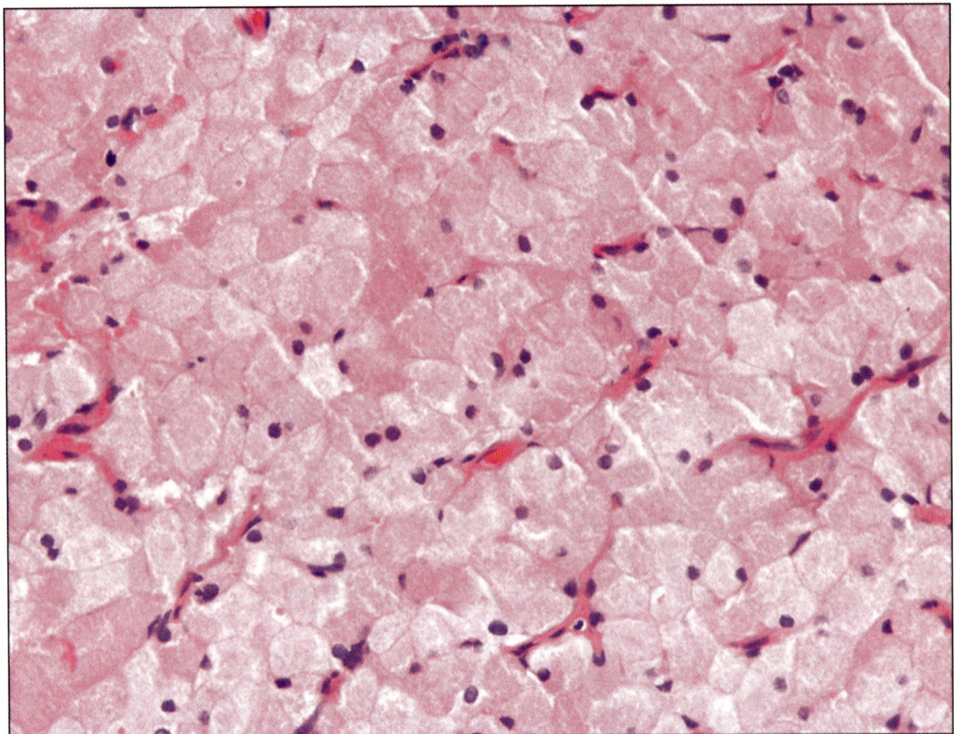

Figure 3.162. Granular cell tumors contain PAS-positive granules, which are resistant to diastase.

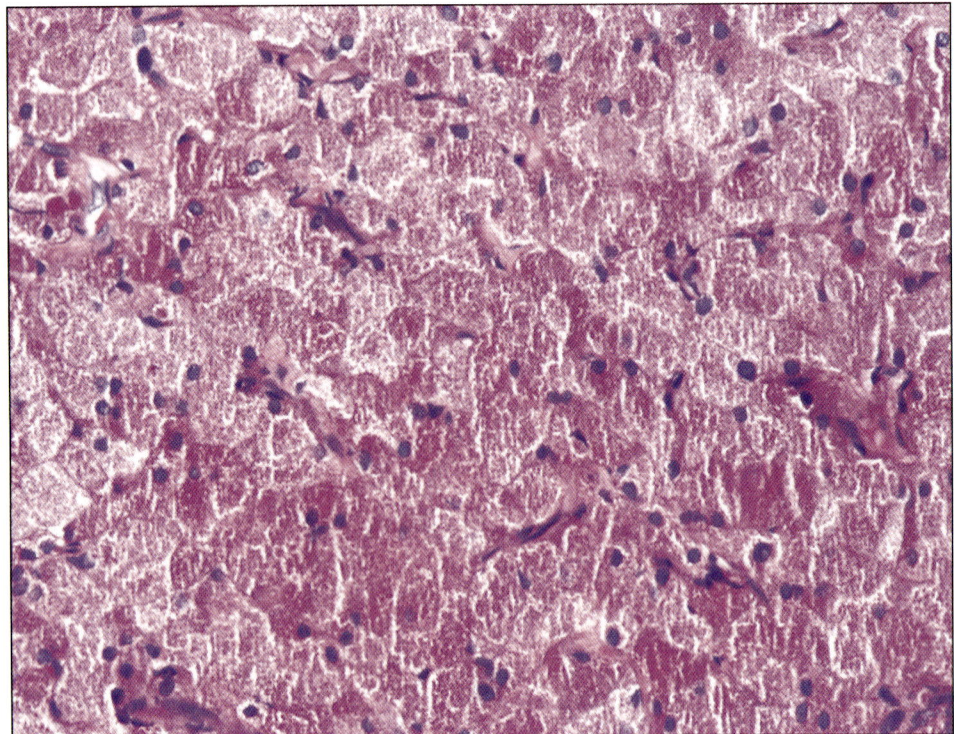

Electron microscopy reveals membrane-bound dense bodies, multivesicular bodies, lamellated membranous structures, and vacuoles, all thought to be derived from autophagic lysosomal bodies. Granular cell tumors of the neurohypophysis are immunopositive for S-100 protein and show rare positivity for GFAP, further supporting the hypothesis that they arise from pituicytes (Nishioka, 1993).

CRANIOPHARYNGIOMA

These tumors are usually intimately associated with the sellar or suprasellar region. However, they may be more akin to cysts and other mass lesions of maldevelopmental origin rather than neoplasms in the traditional sense. They account for between 2% and 5% of all primary intracranial neoplasms (Karavitaki and Wass, 2008). Both adamantinomatous and papillary types correspond to WHO Grade I.

Adamantinomatous Craniopharyngioma

Clinical and Radiological Features

This is the most common nonneuroepithelial intracerebral neoplasm in children and the most common sellar tumor in children, estimated to represent approximately 5–15% of all intracranial tumors in this age group (Karavitaki and Wass, 2008). They exhibit a bimodal age distribution, also with a second peak incidence in adults aged 45–60 years (Rushing et al., 2007).

Believed to arise from tooth primordia present in Rathke's pouch remnants, craniopharyngiomas are most commonly located in a suprasellar position with intrasellar extension (Prabhu and Brown, 2005). Unusual locations such as the sphenoid sinus or cerebellopontine angle have been reported. The most frequent neurologic symptom is related to compression of the visual pathways, more frequent in the adult setting, and endocrine deficiencies, which are conversely more frequent in children than in adults (Yaşargil et al., 1990). Diabetes insipidus may be seen in children but is more frequent in adults. Other nonspecific symptoms include cognitive impairment and personality changes. With compression of the third ventricle, obstructive hydrocephalus may be seen (Karavitaki and Wass, 2008).

Radiographic imaging may provide a high degree of accuracy in predicting the diagnosis of craniopharyngioma. CT scans show contrast enhancement of the solid portion and the typical calcifications. T1-weighted MRI studies show hyperintense cystic structures and isointense solid components, which also show contrast enhancement (Figure 3.163) (Rossi et al., 2006).

Pathology

The gross appearance of craniopharyngiomas is highly characteristic, being a lobulated mass with a spongy consistency because of the variably cystic component. Most frequently, the neurosurgeon will report the cyst contents as a greenish-brown thick liquid classically resembling motor oil. This derives from the lipid- and cholesterol-rich content of the keratinous portion of the cyst wall undergoing degeneration blended with the sequelae of microhemorrhage. Given the opportunity, microscopic inspection of the cyst fluid will show rectangular refractile cholesterol crystals with certain structural irregularities that have evoked the designation "state of Utah" crystals (Figure 3.164).

Figure 3.163. MRI with contrast of a craniopharyngioma showing a cystic mass with solid, heterogeneously enhancing components.

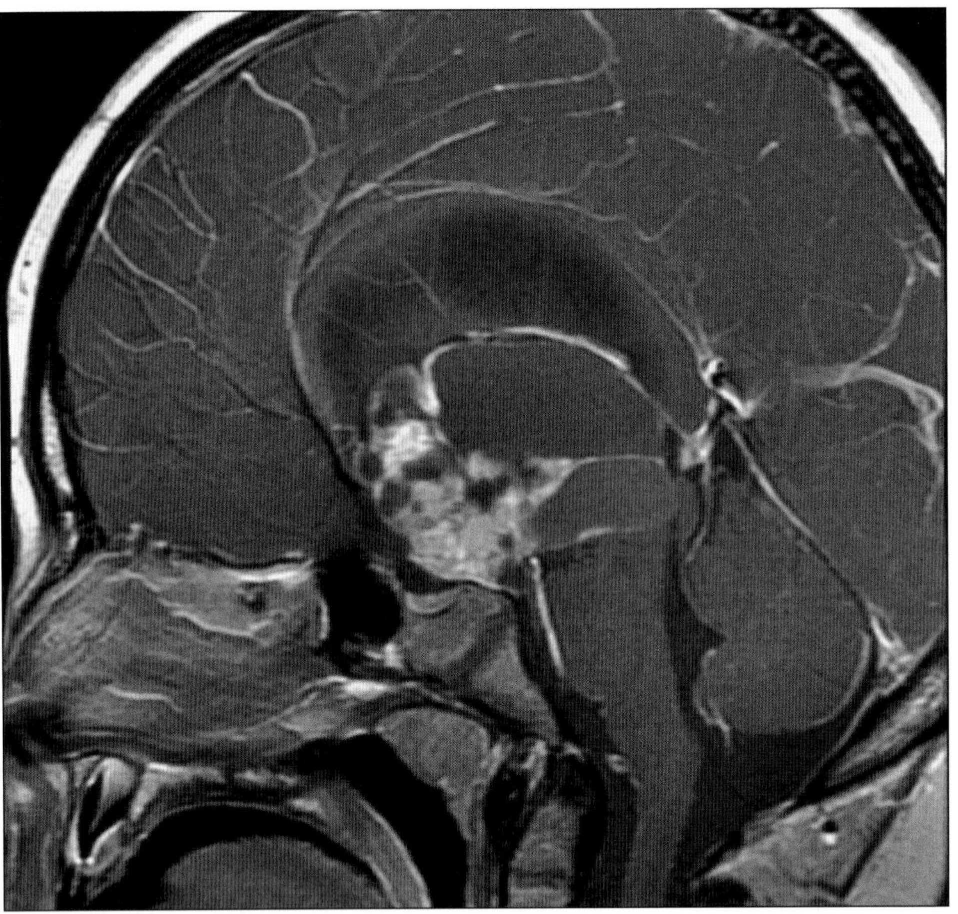

The histology of craniopharyngiomas and the designation adamantinomatous draws from the similarity with that of ameloblastomas or adamantinomas of the jaw. A variety of appearances may prevail but most often there is a layer of pallisading basaloid cells, forming anastomosing cords associated with keratinizing squamous epithelium. Looser sheets of squamous epithelium connected by tenuous cytoplasmic processes is referred to as stellate reticulum (Figure 3.165). There are usual intervening cystic spaces. Squamous elements may combine to form eosinophilic masses of keratinized material known as wet keratin (Figure 3.166). The wet keratin will often undergo mineralization, portions of which may undergo ossification. A granulomatous or foreign body giant cell reaction to foci of prior hemorrhage or calcific material may be seen. However, when predominantly associated with cholesterol clefts in the absence of an adamantinomatous epithelial component, *xanthogranuloma of the sella* should be considered.

When craniopharyngiomas impinge upon brain tissue, they evoke an intense gliotic reaction characterized by a proliferation of Rosenthal fibers (Figure 3.167). This provides the basis for a diagnostic pitfall whereby a biopsy of tissue surrounding a craniopharyngioma undergoing brain invasion may be misinterpreted as pilocytic astrocytoma, particularly when the fingers of infiltrating craniopharyngioma are not apparent and the biopsy is done in the context of a ring-enhancing suprasellar lesion in a child, which would

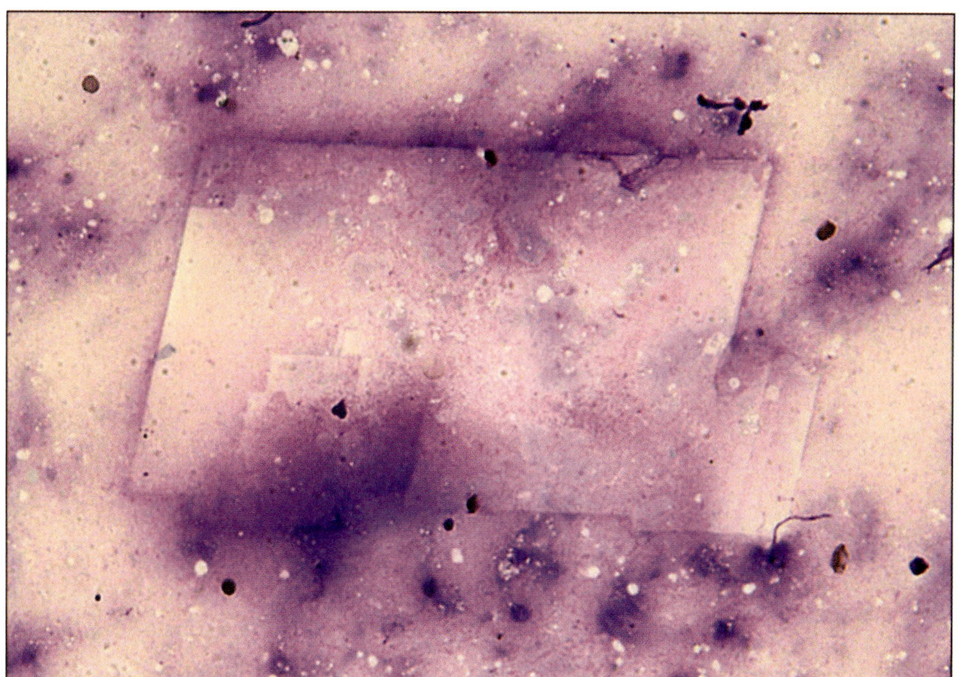

Figure 3.164. Cholesterol crystals seen in aspirates of craniopharyngiomas have rectangular shapes, sometimes resembling the shape of Utah.

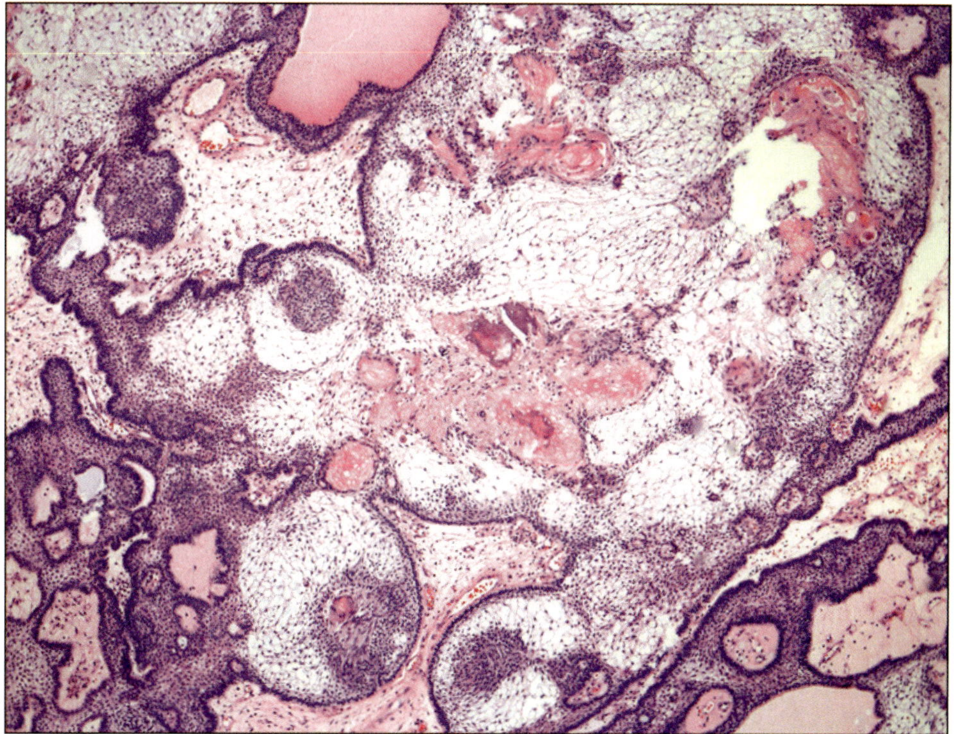

Figure 3.165. This adamantinomatous craniopharyngioma contains squamous epithelium, which is lined by pallisading basaloid cells. Hypocellular regions of stellate reticulum are seen, and wet keratin with mineralization is present in the center of the field.

otherwise be suspicious for pilocytic astrocytoma. The other diagnostic dilemma posed by craniopharyngiomas is in distinguishing them from Rathke's cleft cysts undergoing extensive squamous metaplasia, or with epidermoid cysts.

Epidermoid cysts tend to lack the oily fluid contents of craniopharyngiomas and are more likely to have flaky keratinized contents. The distinctive features of

Figure 3.166. Stellate reticulum of a craniopharyngioma with a focus of wet keratin on the right.

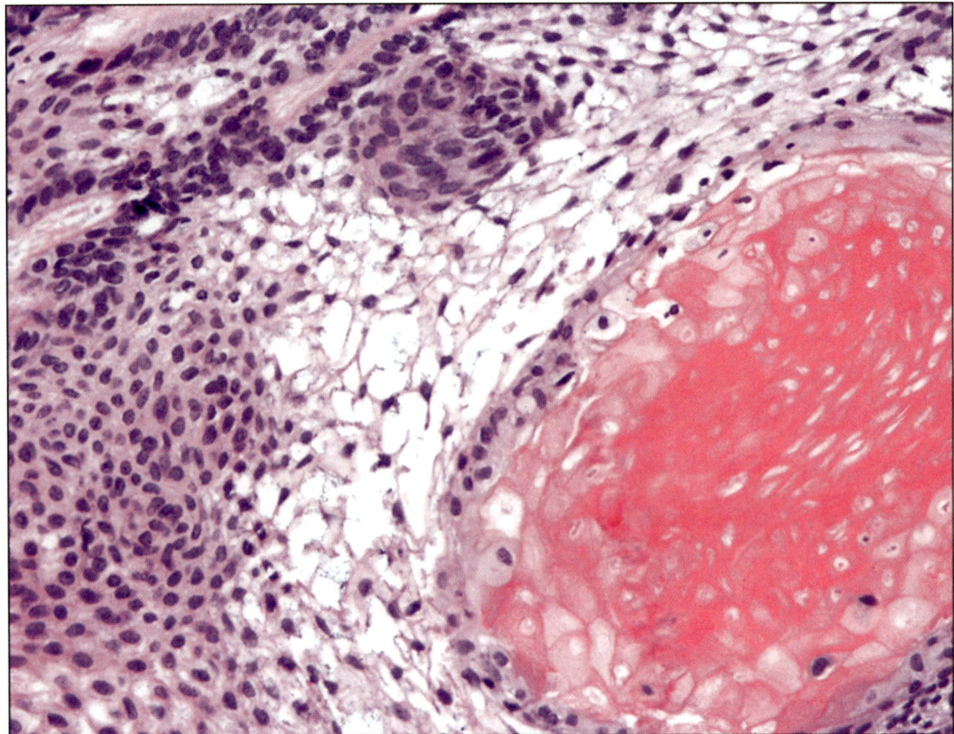

Figure 3.167. The squamous epithelium is delimited by pallisaded basaloid cells in adamantinomatous craniopharyngioma. Numerous Rosenthal fibers are often present in the adjacent glial tissue.

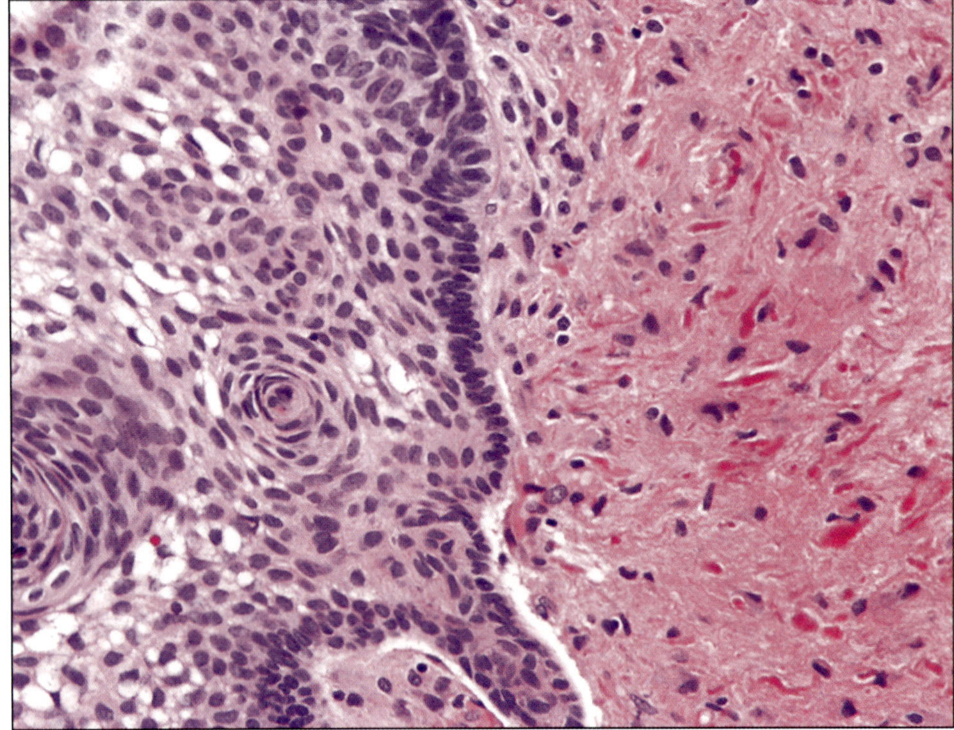

epithelium in craniopharyngiomas are also usually more varied and complex than that of the wall of an epidermoid cyst. In distinguishing a *Rathke's cleft cyst* undergoing squamous metaplasia, careful inspection will often reveal a thin layer of ciliated columnar epithelium undermined by the metaplastic squamous tissue, and frank keratinization is not usually seen.

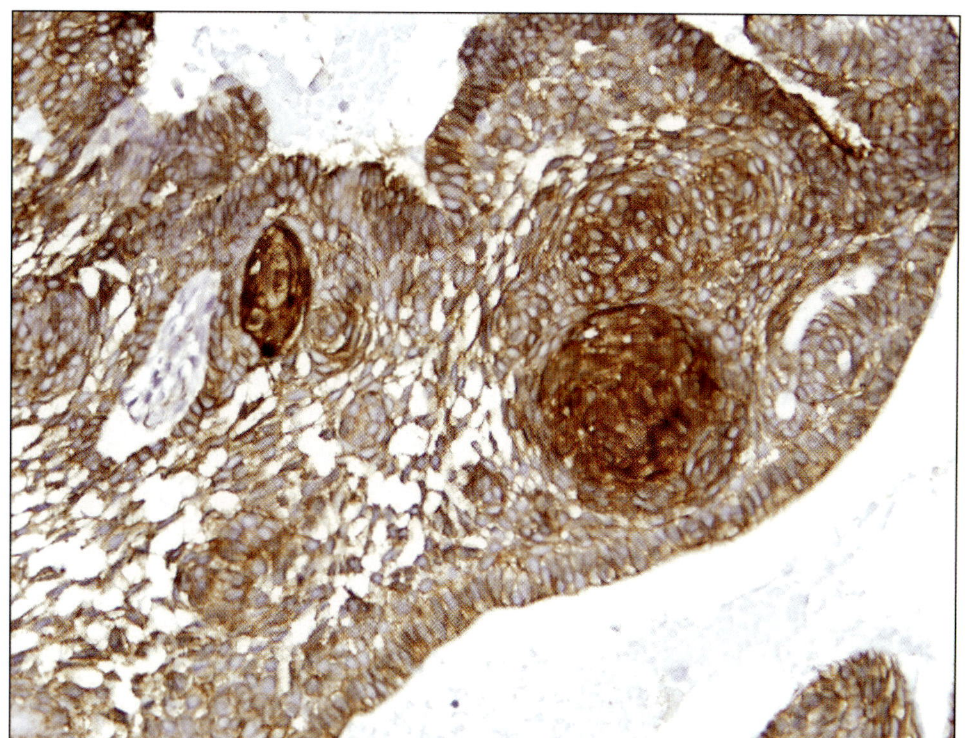

Figure 3.168. Beta-catenin demonstrates diffuse cytoplasmic immunoreactivity in adamantinomatous craniopharyngioma with scattered epithelial nodules exhibiting nuclear positivity as well.

Immunohistochemistry is not generally needed for the diagnosis of cranio-pharyngiomas. However, as expected, they are variably immunopositive for cytokeratins, with limited staining for epithelial membrane antigen and carcinoembryonic antigen. Although cytoplasmic beta-catenin immunoreactivity is present, nodules of squamous epithelium demonstrating nuclear positivity is seen in adamantinomatous craniopharyngiomas (Figure 3.168) but not in the papillary subtype (Buslei et al., 2005; Hofmann et al., 2006). Malignant transformation of craniopharyngioma after irradiation has been reported but is considered distinctly rare (Kristopaitis et al., 2000).

Papillary Craniopharyngioma

Clinical and Radiological Features

Believed to arise from the primordia of the buccal mucosa (Prabhu and Brown, 2005), this craniopharyngioma subtype seems to occur exclusively in adults with a mean age of 40–55 years (Adamson et al., 1990; Crotty et al., 1995). Although initial reports cited a lower incidence of recurrence compared to adamantinomatous craniopharyngiomas, more recent data have shown that recurrence and overall survival may be more directly related to extent of surgical resection and postsurgical therapies (Van Effenterre and Boch, 2002; Karavitaki and Wass, 2008).

Neuroimaging of the papillary craniopharyngioma shows a noncalcified and more homogeneous lesion in CT and MRI images as compared with the adamantinomatous type (Crotty et al., 1995; Sartoretti-Schefer et al., 1997).

Figure 3.169. Papillary craniopharyngiomas are formed by squamous epithelium surrounding fibrovascular cores. These do not have stellate reticulum or wet keratin.

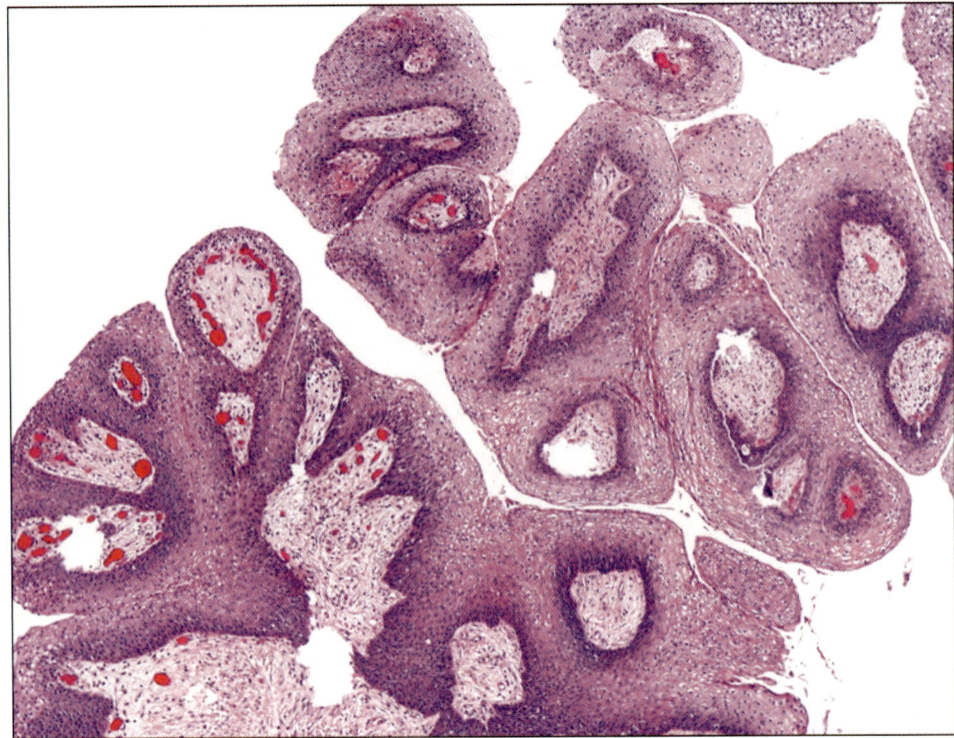

Figure 3.170. Pallisading of the basal cells is not seen in papillary craniopharyngioms, and there is a lack of surface epithelial maturation.

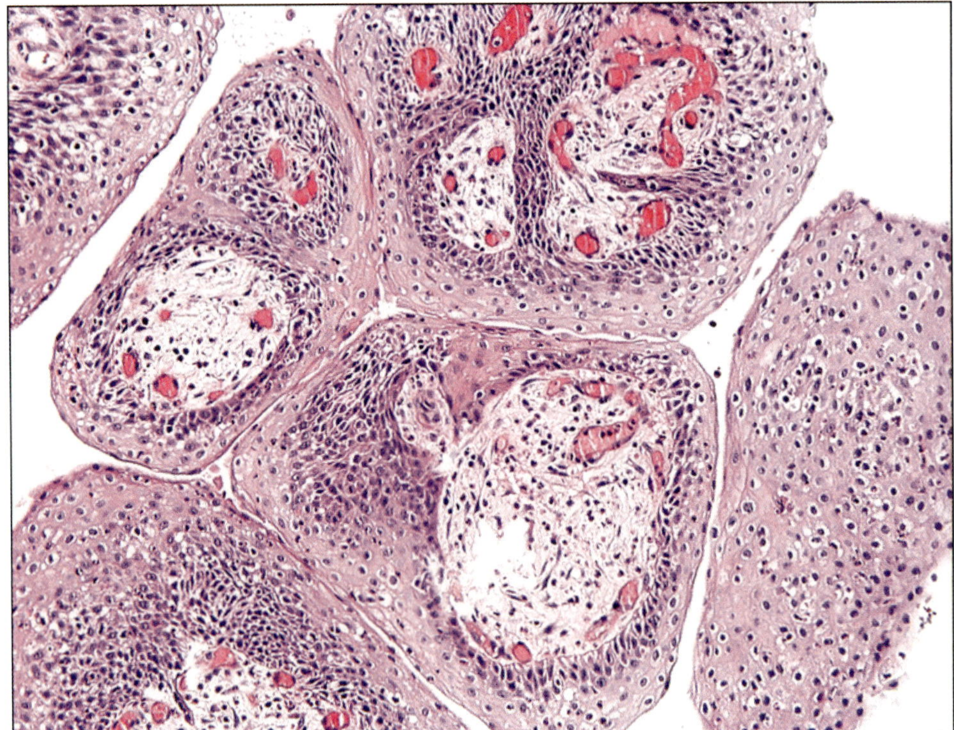

Pathology

Papillary craniopharyngiomas are identified by sheets of well-differentiated squamous epithelial cells without surface maturation, usually surrounding fibrovascular cores forming papillary-like structures (Figures 3.169 and 3.170). Generally, these tumors do not demonstrate surface maturation of the

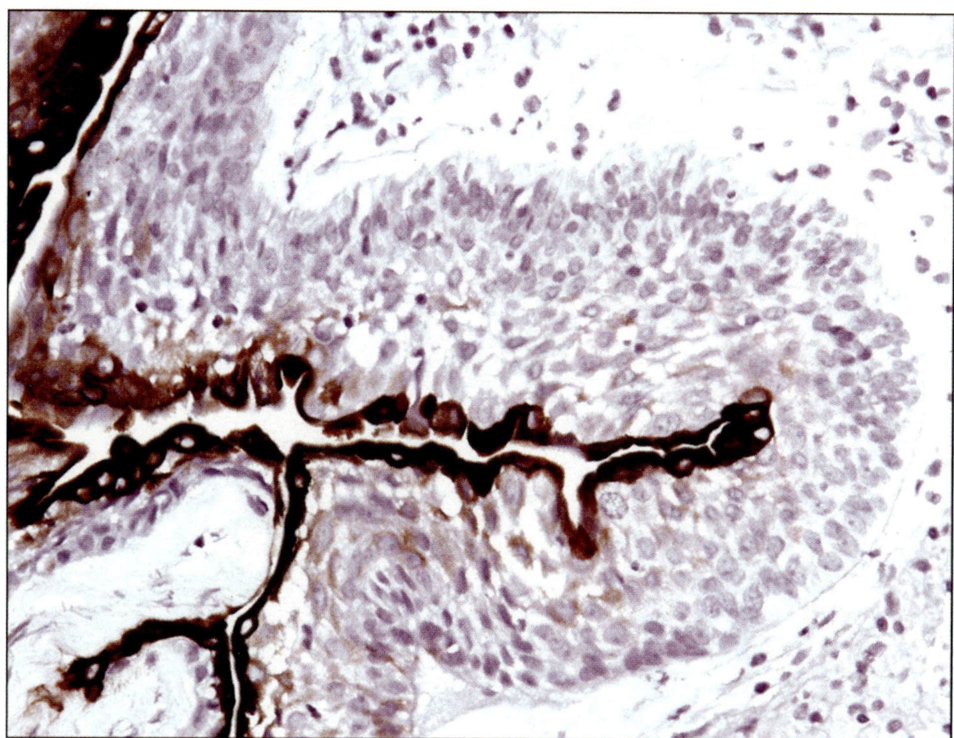

Figure 3.171. CK7 stains only the surface epithelium in papillary craniopharyngiomas, whereas full-thickness staining is seen in adamantinomatous craniopharyngiomas.

squamous epithelium, pallisading basal cells, wet keratin, or calcification. Ciliated epithelial or goblet cells may be noted (Rushing et al., 2007).

Immunohistochemistry utilizing CK7 may be helpful. In papillary craniopharyngiomas, immunoreactivity is seen only in the superficial layers (Figure 3.171). Diffuse CK7 positivity is seen in adamantinomatous craniopharyngiomas, but the basal layer may show weak or absent staining (Kurosaki et al., 2001; Tateyama et al., 2001).

RATHKE'S CLEFT CYST

Clinical and Radiological Features

Rathke's cleft cysts are believed to originate from small asymptomatic remnants of Rathke's pouch, an embryonic outpouching from the buccal cavity involved in the formation of the anterior pituitary gland. They are more common in females and are a common incidental finding in autopsies. There is a wide age of incidence ranging from the teens to late adulthood (Glezer et al., 2008). Larger symptomatic cysts are relatively rare by comparison, the majority being intrasellar lesions capable of suprasellar extension. Only rarely do they arise as a suprasellar cyst (Barrow et al., 1985). Symptoms are referable to regional mass effect indistinguishable from those of other sellar tumors.

Pathology

Symptomatic cysts usually range between 1 and 3 cm in maximum diameter. Unlike craniopharyngiomas, the cyst wall is usually thin and translucent,

Figure 3.172. Rathke's cleft cysts are lined by ciliated columnar cells with occasional goblet cells.

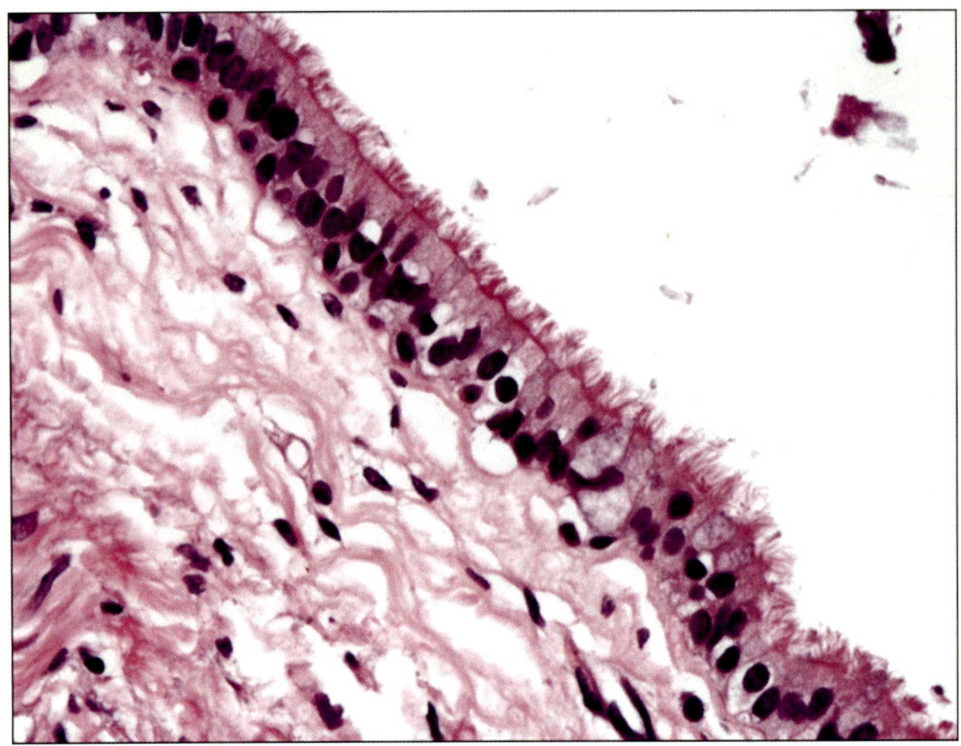

containing turbid mucus or clear fluid contents. Microscopy of the lining epithelium will show focally stratified columnar or cuboidal cells with cilia and occasional goblet cells (Figure 3.172). There is a subjacent thin connective tissue layer in which small glandlike structures may be seen. Nonkeratinizing squamous metaplasia may be extensive (Figure 3.173) (Burger et al., 2002; Rushing et al., 2007).

Distinguishing this lesion from craniopharyngiomas through the use of cytokeratin markers has shown mixed results to date. However, the nuclear beta-catenin positivity seen in adamantinomatous craniopharyngioma is not seen in Rathke's cleft cyst and can be a useful adjunct (Hofmann et al., 2006).

LYMPHOCYTIC HYPOPHYSITIS

Clinical and Radiological Features

Although rare cases have been reported in children, this idiopathic condition occurs most frequently in young women in the late stages of pregnancy or in the postpartum period, producing multiple but sometimes isolated endocrine deficiencies or clinical signs of hyperprolactinemia due to pituitary stalk effect. This carries the risk of the clinical misdiagnosis of prolactinoma. The pathogenesis is thought to be an autoimmune phenomenon (Gellner et al., 2008). The mass effect may be sufficient to cause a visual field disturbance. Treatment consists of surgical decompression, if necessary, and supplementation of endocrine deficiencies (Tashiro et al., 2002).

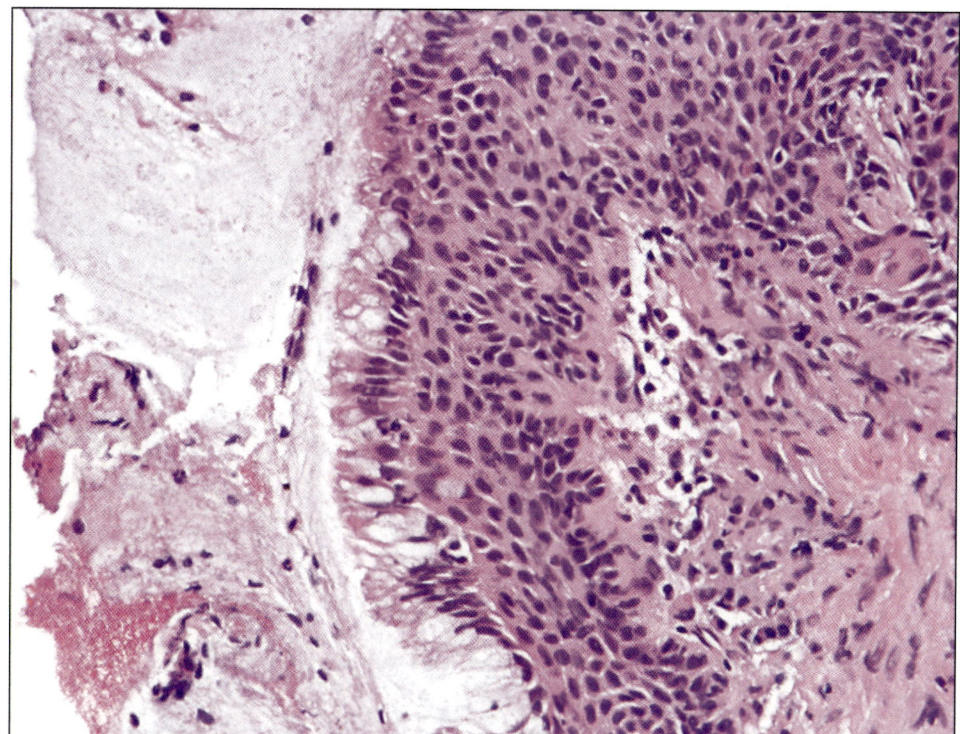

Figure 3.173. Rathe's cleft cysts may undergo extensive squamous metaplasia, but the surface may retain a columnar appearance with cilia and/or goblet cells.

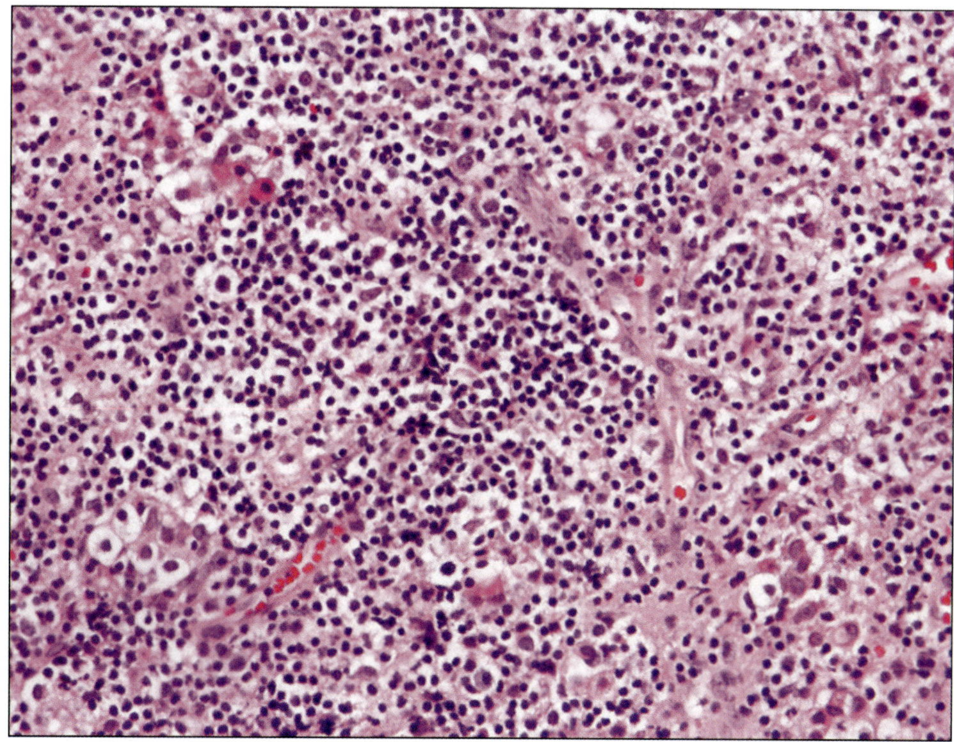

Figure 3.174. Lymphocytic hypophysitis manifests as small, mature-appearing lymphocytes infiltrating the anterior pituitary tissue. Plasma cells and eosinophils may also be seen.

Pathology

The biopsy will show anterior pituitary gland tissue overrun by B and T lymphocytes, plasma cells, and occasional eosinophils which distort the normal architecture (Figure 3.174). Lymphoid follicles with germinal centers may even be present. Although granulomas are not present, an infectious etiology such as fungal or tuberculous infection should nevertheless be considered and investigated by appropriate special stains. In late stages, the residual pituitary tissue is often fibrotic with atrophy of the parenchyma.

GIANT CELL GRANULOMATOUS HYPOPHYSITIS

Clinical and Radiological Features

This condition is presumably autoimmune and is sometimes accompanied by similar granulomatous infiltrates in other endocrine organs. Although there is no gender predilection, when women are affected, they are generally middle-aged and older, unlike the younger demographic seen with lymphocytic hypophysitis. Anterior pituitary failure and occasionally diabetes insipidus may occur (Honegger et al., 1997; Wilson et al., 2000). Diagnostic biopsy or decompression provides the rationale for surgical intervention.

Pathology

Although a lymphocytic infiltrate may be present, what distinguishes this entity from lymphocytic hypophysitis is the presence of epithelioid macrophages and prominent multinucleated giant cells with or without necrosis (Figure 3.175). Plasma cells and eosinophils may also be present (Figure 3.176).

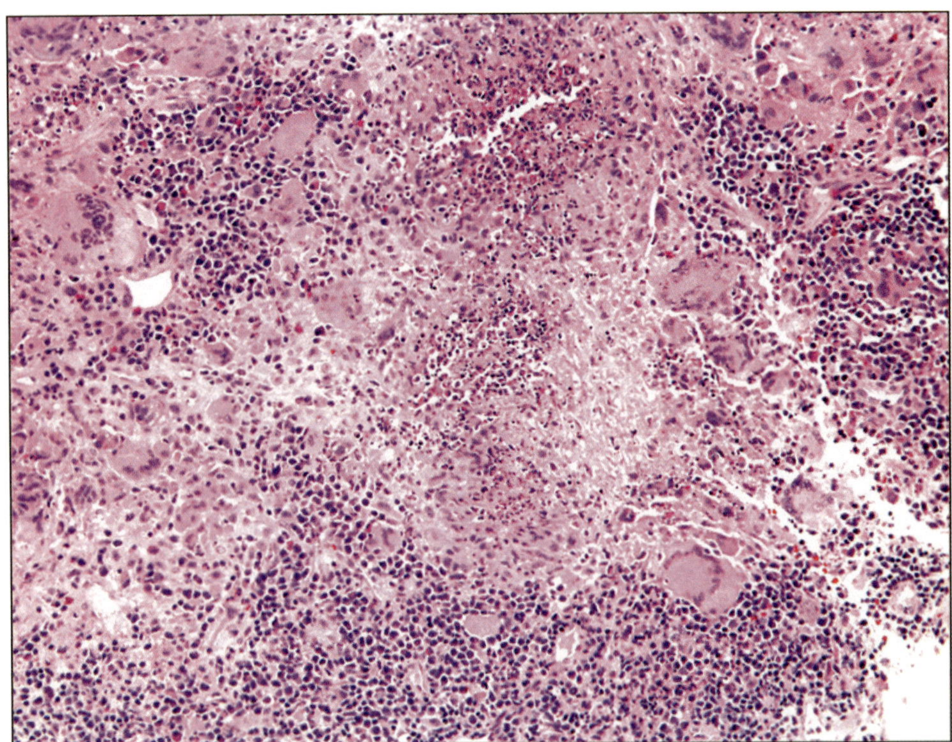

Figure 3.175. Giant cell granulomatous hypophysitis demonstrates foreign body giant cells with a variable mixture of inflammation and/or necrosis.

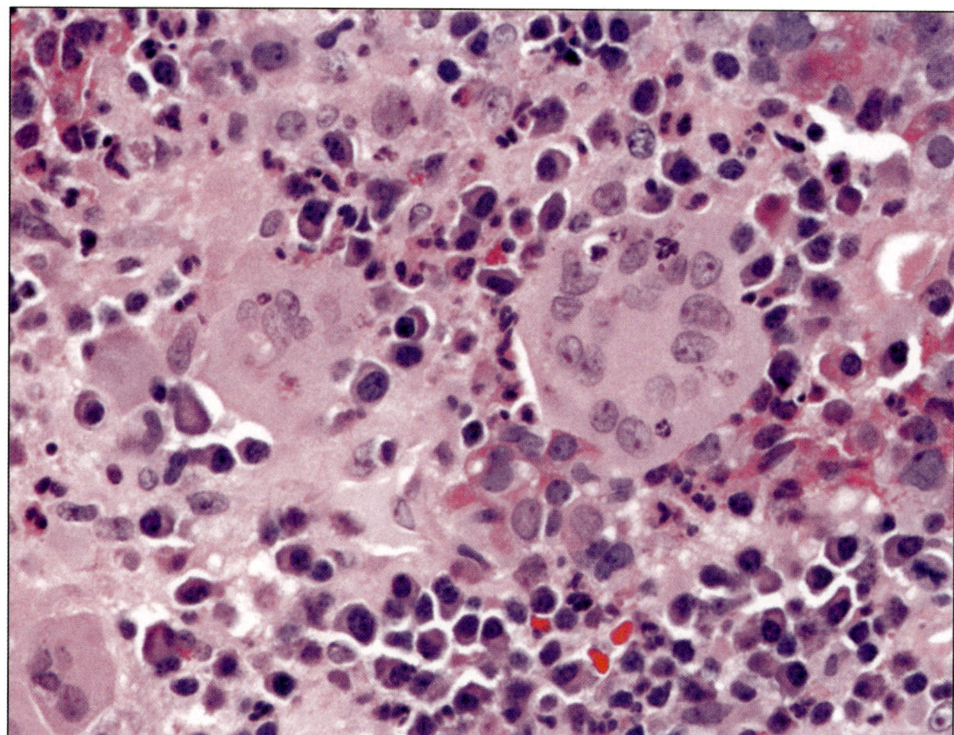

Figure 3.176. In addition to multinucleated giant cells and macrophages, the inflammatory infiltrate in a giant cell granuloma may contain a mixture of plasma cells, lymphocytes and eosinophils.

XANTHOGRANULOMA OF THE SELLAR REGION

Clinical and Radiological Features

These share some radiological and histologic features with craniopharyngioma; however, it has been noted that they tend to occur in adolescents and young adults with a long history of endocrine deficiencies and are usually not calcified. They are often well circumscribed and, hence, resectable lesions of the sella lacking significant suprasellar extension and carrying a more favorable outcome. Some authorities consider the xanthogranuloma of the sellar region to represent one end of the spectrum of degeneration in common cystic lesions of the region, namely Rathke's cleft cysts or colloid cysts, particularly those that have undergone rupture (Paulus et al., 1999; Yonezawa et al., 2003).

Pathology

These are composed of xanthomatous elements including cholesterol clefts, multinucleated giant cells, macrophages, chronic inflammatory cells, necrotic debris, and hemosiderin (Figure 3.177). A minority of cases may show cystlike epithelium, squamous, or cuboidal cells, but adamantinomatous epithelium is not seen.

MISCELLANEOUS LESIONS

The sellar region can be home to a multitude of less common neoplasms including *meningiomas*, *schwannomas* and *germ cell tumors*, of which the most

Figure 3.177.
Xanthogranuloma of the
sellar region with prominent
cholesterol clefts surrounded
by numerous giant cells,
chronic inflammation, and
hemosiderin.

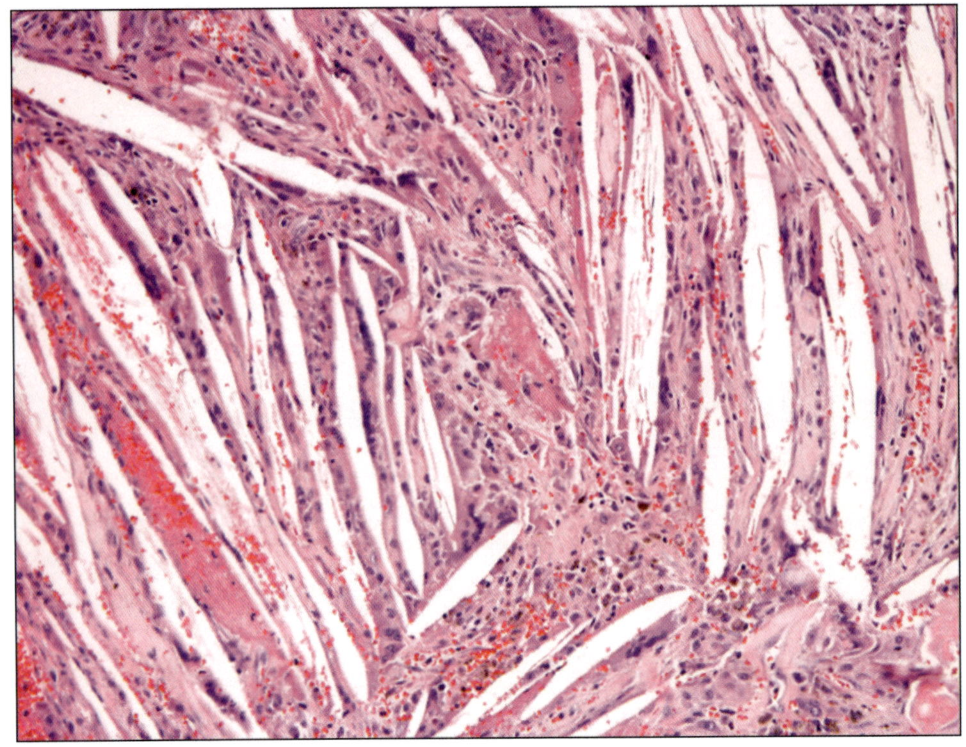

common are *germinoma* and *teratoma* (Glezer et al., 2008). *Plasmacytoma* is not uncommonly seen, and may mimic a *pituitary adenoma* (Dhanani et al., 1990). Other lesions including *Langerhans cell histiocytosis* and adult *acute lymphoblastic leukemia* may also be seen, the latter infiltrating in a peripituitary fashion in about half the cases (Masse et al., 1973). Systemic inflammatory disorders such as *sarcoidosis* and *Wegener granulomatosis* may manifest in the sella but typically have multiorgan involvement (Glezer et al., 2008). *Metastatic lesions* to the pituitary (breast and lung carcinoma being most common) are often silent, but when present, occur primarily in the neurohypophysis. Diabetes insipidus is the most common presenting symptom in this setting (Glezer et al., 2008; Sioutos et al., 1996).

REFERENCES

Adamson TE, Wiestler OD, Kleihues P, Yaşargil MG. Correlation of clinical and pathological features in surgically treated craniopharyngiomas. *J Neurosurg* 1990; 73: 12–17.

Al-Gahtany M, Horvath E, Kovacs K. Pituitary hyperplasia. *Hormones (Athens)* 2003; 2: 149–58.

Al-Shraim M, Asa SL. The 2004 World Health Organization classification of pituitary tumors: what is new? *Acta Neuropathol* 2006; 111: 1–7.

Asa SL, Scheithauer BW, Bilbao JM, Horvath E, Ryan N, Kovacs K, et al. A case for hypothalamic acromegaly: a clinicopathological study of six patients with hypothalamic gangliocytomas producing growth hormone-releasing factor. *J Clin Endocrinol Metab* 1984; 58: 796–803.

Asa SL, Ezzat S, Watson RE, Lindell EP, et al. Gonadotropin producing adenoma. In: Delellis RA, LLoyd RV, Heitz PU, Eng C, editors. *World Health Organization Classification of Tumours: Pathology and Genetics of Tumours of Endocrine Organs.* Lyon, IARC, 2004, 30–2.

Barrow DL, Spector RH, Takei Y, Tindall GT. Symptomatic Rathke's cleft cysts located entirely in the suprasellar region: review of diagnosis, management, and pathogenesis. *Neurosurgery* 1985; 16: 766–72.

Beck-Peccoz P, Brucker-Davis F, Persani L, Smallridge RC, Weintraub BD. Thyrotropin-secreting pituitary tumors. *Endocr Rev* 1996; 17: 610–38.

Beck-Peccoz P, Persani L. Thyrotropinomas. *Endocrinol Metab Clin North Am* 2008; 37: 123–34.

Berg KK, Scheithauer BW, Felix I, Kovacs K, Horvath E, Klee GG, Laws ER Jr. Pituitary adenomas that produce adrenocorticotropic hormone and alpha-subunit: clinicopathological, immunohistochemical, ultrastructural, and immunoelectron microscopic studies in nine cases. *Neurosurgery* 1990; 26: 397–403.

Brat DJ, Scheithauer BW, Staugaitis SM, Holtzman RN, Morgello S, Burger PC. Pituicytoma: a distinctive low-grade glioma of the neurohypophysis. *Am J Surg Pathol* 2000; 24: 362–8.

Burger PC, Scheithauer BW, Vogel FS. *Surgical Pathology of the Nervous System and Its Coverings.* New York: Churchill Livingstone, 2002.

Buslei R, Nolde M, Hofmann B, Meissner S, Eyupoglu IY, Siebzehnrubl F, et al. Common mutations of beta-catenin in adamantinomatous craniopharyngiomas but not in other tumours originating from the sellar region. *Acta Neuropathol* 2005; 109: 589–97.

Crotty TB, Scheithauer BW, Young WF Jr, Davis DH, Shaw EG, Miller GM, Burger PC. Papillary craniopharyngioma: a clinicopathological study of 48 cases. *J Neurosurg* 1995; 83: 206–14.

Delgrange E, Trouillas J, Maiter D, Donckier J, Tourniaire J. Sex-related difference in the growth of prolactinomas: a clinical and proliferation marker study. *J Clin Endocrinol Metab* 1997; 82: 2102–7.

Dhanani AN, Bilbao JM, Kovacs K. Multiple myeloma presenting as a sellar plasmacytoma mimicking a pituitary tumor. Report of a case and review of the literature. *Endocr Pathol* 1990; 1: 245–48.

Diamond FB, Jr. Pituitary adenomas in childhood: development and diagnosis. *Fetal Pediatr Pathol* 2006; 25: 339–56.

Felix IA, Horvath E, Kovacs K, Smyth HS, Killinger DW, Vale J. Mammosomatotroph adenoma of the pituitary associated with gigantism and hyperprolactinemia. A morphological study including immunoelectron microscopy. *Acta Neuropathol* 1986; 71: 76–82.

Fuller GN, Wesseling P. Granular cell tumor of the neurohypophysis. In: Louis DN, Ohgaki H, Wiestler OD, Cavenee WK, editors. *WHO Classification of Tumours of the Nervous System.* Lyon: IARC, 2007, 241–2.

Geddes JF, Jansen GH, Robinson SF, Gomori E, Holton JL, Monson JP, et al. 'Gangliocytomas' of the pituitary: a heterogeneous group of lesions with differing histogenesis. *Am J Surg Pathol* 2000; 24: 607–13.

Gellner V, Kurschel S, Scarpatetti M, Mokry M. Lymphocytic hypophysitis in the pediatric population. *Childs Nerv Syst* 2008; 24: 785–92.

Glezer A, Paraiba DB, Bronstein MD. Rare sellar lesions. *Endocrinol Metab Clin North Am* 2008; 37: 195–211.

Hofmann BM, Kreutzer J, Saeger W, Buchfelder M, Blümcke I, Fahlbusch R, Buslei R. Nuclear beta-catenin accumulation as reliable marker for the differentiation between cystic craniopharyngiomas and rathke cleft cysts: a clinico-pathologic approach. *Am J Surg Pathol* 2006; 30: 1595–603.

Honegger J, Fahlbusch R, Bornemann A, Hensen J, Buchfelder M, Müller M, Nomikos P. Lymphocytic and granulomatous hypophysitis: experience with nine cases. *Neurosurgery* 1997; 40: 713–22.

Horvath E, Kovacs K, Singer W, Smyth HS, Killinger DW, Erzin C, Weiss MH. Acidophil stem cell adenoma of the human pituitary: clinicopathologic analysis of 15 cases. *Cancer* 1981; 47: 761–71.

Horvath E, Scheitauer BW, Kovacs K, Lloyd RV. Hypothalamus and pituitary. In: Graham DI, Lantos PL, editors. *Greenfield's Neuropathology*, 7th edn. London: Edward Arnold, 2002, 983–1062.

Horvath E, Lloyd RV, Kovacs K, Sano T, et al. Plurihormonal adenoma. In: Delellis RA, LLoyd RV, Heitz PU, Eng C, editors. *World Health Organization Classification of Tumours: Pathology and Genetics of Tumours of Endocrine Organs*. Lyon: IARC, 2004, 35.

Horvath E, Kovacs K, Smyth HS, Cusimano M, Singer W. Silent adenoma subtype 3 of the pituitary – immunohistochemical and ultrastructural classification: a review of 29 cases. *Ultrastruct Pathol* 2005; 29: 511–24.

Jin L, Riss D, Ruebel K, Kajita S, Scheithauer BW, Horvath E, Kovacs K, Lloyd RV. Galectin-3 expression in functioning and silent ACTH-producing adenomas. *Endocr Pathol* 2005; 16: 107–14.

Kane LA, Leinung MC, Scheithauer BW, Bergstralh EJ, Laws ER, Jr., Groover RV, et al. Pituitary adenomas in childhood and adolescence. *J Clin Endocrinol Metab* 1994; 79: 1135–40.

Karavitaki N, Wass JA. Craniopharyngiomas. *Endocrinol Metab Clin North Am* 2008; 37: 173–93.

Kloub O, Perry A, Tu PH, Lipper M, Lopes MB. Spindle cell oncocytoma of the adenohypophysis: report of two recurrent cases. *Am J Surg Pathol* 2005; 29: 247–53.

Kontogeorgos G, Watson RE, Lindell EP, Barkan AL, et al. Growth hormone producing adenoma. In: Delellis RA, LLoyd RV, Heitz PU, Eng C, editors. *World Health Organization Classification of Tumours: Pathology and Genetics of Tumours of Endocrine Organs*. Lyon: IARC, 2004, 14–19.

Kovacs K, Horvath E, Ryan N, Ezrin C. Null cell adenoma of the human pituitary. *Virchows Arch A Pathol Anat Histol* 1980; 387: 165–74.

Kristopaitis T, Thomas C, Petruzzelli GJ, Lee JM. Malignant craniopharyngioma. *Arch Pathol Lab Med* 2000; 124: 1356–60.

Kurosaki M, Saeger W, Lüdecke DK. Immunohistochemical localisation of cytokeratins in craniopharyngioma. *Acta Neurochir (Wien)* 2001; 143: 147–51.

Lloyd RV, Kovacs K, Young WF Jr. Pituitary tumours. In: Delellis RA, LLoyd RV, Heitz PU, Eng C, editors. *World Health Organization Classification of Tumours: Pathology and Genetics of Tumours of Endocrine Organs*. Lyon: IARC, 2004, 10–13.

Lopes MB, Salmon I, Nagy N, Decaestecker C, Pasteels JL, Laws ER Jr, Kiss R. Computer-assisted microscope analysis of feulgen-stained nuclei in gonadotroph adenomas and null-cell adenomas of the pituitary gland. *Endocr Pathol* 1997; 8: 109–20.

Masse SR, Wolk RW, Conklin RH. Peripituitary gland involvement in acute leukemia in adults. *Arch Pathol* 1973; 96: 141–2.

McComb DJ, Ryan N, Horvath E, Kovacs K. Subclinical adenomas of the human pituitary. New light on old problems. *Arch Pathol Lab Med* 1983; 107: 488–91.

Nishioka H, Immunohistochemical study of granular cell tumors and granular pituicytes of the neurohypophysis. *Endocr Pathol* 1993; 4: 140–45.

Nishioka H, Haraoka J, Akada K, Azuma S. Gender-related differences in prolactin secretion in pituitary prolactinomas. *Neuroradiology* 2002; 44: 407–10.

Paulus W, Honegger J, Keyvani K, Fahlbusch R. Xanthogranuloma of the sellar region: a clinicopathological entity different from adamantinomatous craniopharyngioma. *Acta Neuropathol* 1999; 97: 377–82.

Pickett CA. Update on the medical management of pituitary adenomas. *Curr Neurol Neurosci Rep* 2005; 5: 178–85.

Prabhu VC, Brown HG. The pathogenesis of craniopharyngiomas. *Childs Nerv Syst* 2005; 21: 622–7.

Psaras T, Honegger J, Buslei R, Saeger W, Klein D, Capper D, et al. Atypical type II silent corticotrophic adenoma developing into Cushing's disease upon second recurrence. *Exp Clin Endocrinol Diabetes* 2007; 115: 610–15.

Randall RV, Scheithauer BW, Laws ER, Jr., Abbound CF, Ebersold MJ, Kao PC. Pituitary adenomas associated with hyperprolactinemia: a clinical and immunohistochemical study of 97 patients operated on transsphenoidally. *Mayo Clin Proc* 1985; 60: 753–62.

Roncaroli F, Scheithauer BW, Cenacchi G, Horvath E, Kovacs K, Lloyd RV, Abell-Aleff P, Santi M, Yates AJ. 'Spindle cell oncocytoma' of the adenohypophysis: a tumor of folliculostellate cells? *Am J Surg Pathol* 2002; 26: 1048–55.

Roncaroli F, Scheithauer BW. Papillary tumor of the pineal region and spindle cell oncocytoma of the pituitary: new tumor entities in the 2007 WHO classification. *Brain Pathol* 2007; 17: 314–8.

Rossi A, Cama A, Consales A, Gandolfo C, Garrè ML, Milanaccio C, Pavanello M, Piatelli G, Ravegnani M, Tortori-Donati P. Neuroimaging of pediatric craniopharyngiomas: a pictorial essay. *J Pediatr Endocrinol Metab* 2006; 19: 299–319.

Rushing EJ, Giangaspero F, Paulus W, Burger PC. Craniopharyngioma. In: Louis DN, Ohgaki H, Wiestler OD, Cavenee WK, editors. *WHO Classification of Tumours of the Nervous System*. IARC, Lyon, 2007, pp. 238–40.

Sartoretti-Schefer S, Wichmann W, Aguzzi A, Valavanis A. MR differentiation of adamantinous and squamous-papillary craniopharyngiomas. *AJNR Am J Neuroradiol* 1997; 18: 77–87.

Scheithauer BW, Jaap AJ, Horvath E, Kovacs K, Lloyd RV, Meyer FB, et al. Clinically silent corticotroph tumors of the pituitary gland. *Neurosurgery* 2000; 47: 723–9.

Scheithauer BW, Kovacs K, Horvath E, Roncaroli F, et al. Pituitary carcinoma. In: Delellis RA, LLoyd RV, Heitz PU, Eng C, editors. *World Health Organization Classification of Tumours: Pathology and Genetics of Tumours of Endocrine Organs*. IARC, Lyon, 2004, pp. 36–39.

Scheithauer BW, Gaffey TA, Lloyd RV, Sebo TJ, Kovacs KT, Horvath E, Yapicier O, Young WF Jr, Meyer FB, Kuroki T, Riehle DL, Laws ER Jr. Pathobiology of pituitary adenomas and carcinomas. *Neurosurgery* 2006; 59: 341–53.

Sioutos P, Yen V, Arbit E. Pituitary gland metastases. *Ann Surg Oncol* 1996; 3: 94–9.

Snyder PJ. Gonadotroph and other clinically nonfunctioning pituitary adenomas. *Cancer Treat Res* 1997; 89: 57–72.

Takei Y, Seyama S, Pearl GS, Tindall GT. Ultrastructural study of the human neuro-hypophysis II. Cellular elements of neural parenchyma, the pituicytes. *Cell Tissue Res* 1980; 205: 273–87.

Tashiro T, Sano T, Xu B, Wakatsuki S, Kagawa N, Nishioka H, Yamada S, Kovacs K. Spectrum of different types of hypophysitis: a clinicopathologic study of hypophysitis in 31 cases. *Endocr Pathol* 2002; 13: 183–95.

Tateyama H, Tada T, Okabe M, Takahashi E, Eimoto T. Different keratin profiles in craniopharyngioma subtypes and ameloblastomas. *Pathol Res Pract* 2001; 197: 735–42.

Thapar K, Smith MV, Elliot E, Kovacs K, Laws E. Corticotroph adenomas of the pituitary. Long term results of operative treatment. *Endocr Pathol* 1992; 3: S51–53.

Thapar K, Kovacs K, Scheithauer BW, Stefaneanu L, Horvath E, Pernicone PJ, Murray D, Laws ER Jr. Proliferative activity and invasiveness among pituitary adenomas and carcinomas: an analysis using the MIB-1 antibody. *Neurosurgery* 1996; 38: 99–106.

Thodou E, Argyrakos T, Kontogeorgos G. Galectin-3 as a marker distinguishing functioning from silent corticotroph adenomas. *Hormones (Athens)* 2007; 6: 227–32.

Tomita T, Gates E. Pituitary adenomas and granular cell tumors. Incidence, cell type, and location of tumor in 100 pituitary glands at autopsy. *Am J Clin Pathol* 1999; 111: 817–25.

Trouillas J. [Pathology and pathogenesis of pituitary corticotroph adenoma]. *Neurochirurgie* 2002; 48: 149–62.

Trouillas J, Barkan AL, Watson RE, Lindell EP, et al. ACTH producing adenoma. In: Delellis RA, LLoyd RV, Heitz PU, Eng C, editors. *World Health Organization Classification of Tumours: Pathology and Genetics of Tumours of Endocrine Organs.* IARC, Lyon, 2004, pp. 26–9.

Vajtai I, Sahli R, Kappeler A. Spindle cell oncocytoma of the adenohypophysis: report of a case with a 16-year follow-up. *Pathol Res Pract* 2006; 202: 745–50.

Van Effenterre R, Boch AL. Craniopharyngioma in adults and children: a study of 122 surgical cases. *J Neurosurg* 2002; 97: 3–11.

Wilson JD, Jacobs M, Shuer L, Atlas S, Horoupian DS. Idiopathic giant-cell granulomatous hypophysitis. Report of a case with autopsy follow-up. *Clin Neuropathol* 2000; 19: 300–4.

Yaşargil MG, Curcic M, Kis M, Siegenthaler G, Teddy PJ, Roth P. Total removal of craniopharyngiomas. Approaches and long-term results in 144 patients. *J Neurosurg* 1990; 73: 3–11.

Yonezawa K, Shirataki K, Sakagami Y, Kohmura E. Panhypopituitarism induced by cholesterol granuloma in the sellar region – case report. *Neurol Med Chir* 2003; 43: 259–62.

Young WF Jr, Scheithauer BW, Kovacs KT, Horvath E, Davis DH, Randall RV. Gonadotroph adenoma of the pituitary gland: a clinicopathologic analysis of 100 cases. *Mayo Clin Proc* 1996; 71: 649–56.

METASTATIC NEOPLASMS OF THE CENTRAL NERVOUS SYSTEM

Gregory Moes and Hannes Vogel

Neuropathologists as well as surgical pathologists routinely evaluate CNS lesions from patients undergoing resection of a known metastasis for therapeutic reasons or from a patient with no known prior history of malignancy. The most common intracranial and intraspinal tumors are metastases (about 20%) and the incidence increases with age (Klos and O' Neill, 2004). The frequency of metastatic disease depends on the primary site, with lung, breast, skin (malignant melanoma), renal cell carcinoma, carcinoma of the gastrointestinal (GI) tract, particularly colon, and choriocarcinoma being the more common malignancies to involve the CNS in order of decreasing frequency. Four of these, lung, melanoma, renal cell and choriocarcinoma, are malignancies that tend to produce "hemorrhagic" foci (Mandybur, 1977). Hemorrhagic lesions should not automatically be considered more likely to be a metastasis, since some primary glial neoplasms can be abundantly hemorrhagic (Ragland et al., 1990).

In accordance with the most common types of systemic neoplasms in adults, the most common type of metastatic brain tumors are those that arise from lung cancers, the most common CNS metastases in men, and breast carcinoma, the most common metastases in women (Evans et al., 2004). Breast carcinomas, and others such as lung carcinoma in men, are particularly prone to metastasize to the sella turcica and thereby become symptomatic by causing diabetes insipidus (Bobilev et al., 2005; Teears and Silverman, 1975; Yap et al., 1979).

Particular tendencies of less common tumors should be kept in mind, such as the propensity of choriocarcinoma to spread to the CNS and occurrence of latent metastatic disease of melanoma (Cohn-Cedermark et al., 1998) and renal carcinoma. Solitary posterior fossa metastases originate from the prostate, uterus, or gastrointestinal tract 50% of the time (Delattre et al., 1988). One highly unusual but well-documented occurrence is metastatic carcinoma, most often breast or lung carcinoma, into preexisting meningiomas (Baratelli et al., 2004; Benedetto et al., 2007).

Soft tissue sarcomas and bone malignancies infrequently present as metastatic CNS disease. However, as patient survival increases because of chemotherapy, so does the likelihood of encountering these uncommon malignancies. These include malignant fibrous histiocytoma (Mandal and Mandal, 2007), Ewing sarcoma, rhabdomyosarcoma (Parasuraman et al., 1999), alveolar soft part sarcoma (Postovsky et al., 2003; Reichardt et al., 2003), osteosarcoma, and mesenchymal chondrosarcoma as well as others (Postovsky et al., 2003). CNS involvement by hematopoietic malignancies such as non-Hodgkin lymphoma may occur as multiple foci unlike Hodgkin disease, which uncommonly involves only the meninges (Jellinger and Radiaszkiewicz, 1976).

Figure 3.178. Metastatic tumors are multiple in half of cases with neuroimaging and often appear to arise in gray matter or the gray–white junction (arrows).

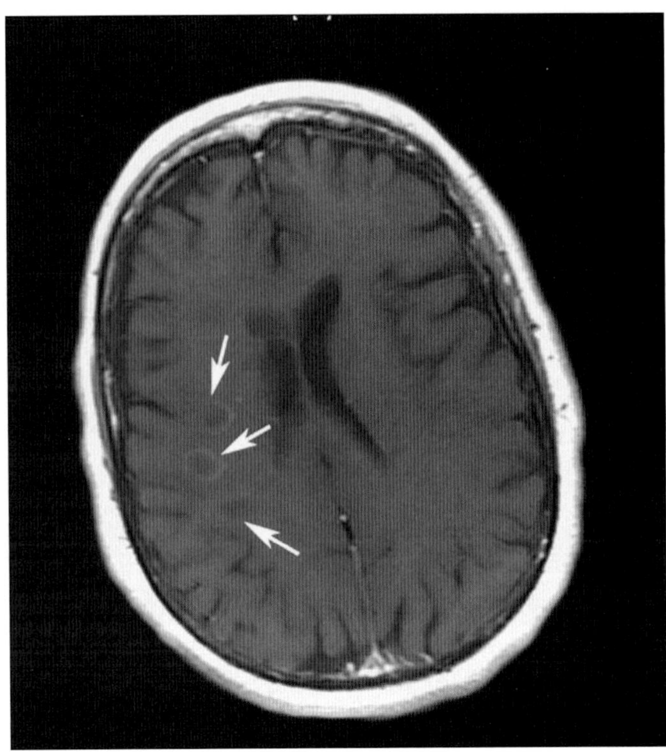

Clinical Features

The clinical symptoms of metastatic lesions are nonspecific and similar to those caused by any expanding mass lesion. These symptoms include seizures, headaches, mental changes, and or motor deficits. Sudden expansion of a lesion is usually secondary to intratumoral hemorrhage, a phenomenon more often noted in metastatic lesions prone to hemorrhage. Patients with head and neck carcinomas, such as squamous cell carcinoma and adenoid cystic carcinoma, are more likely to present with pain because of the proclivity of these carcinomas for perineural invasion and subsequent invasion of nerves at the base of the brain (Dumas and Perusse, 1999).

NEUROIMAGING

The lesions appear as spherical contrast ring enhancing lesions, sometimes with necrotic centers. They are often located in gray matter, with the epicenter near the gray–white junction (Figure 3.178). Since approximately 50% of patients will present with solitary metastasis, the presence and location additional lesions is an indicator of metastatic rather than primary disease. Additionally, solitary lesions identified in the deep white matter or the corpus callosum tend to be primary rather than metastatic disease. As metastatic disease spreads primarily as a hematogenous event, those arteries supplying the largest amount of blood, that is, middle cerebral artery and angulated branches of the arterial border zones are preferentially affected. The presence of calcifications, an uncommon finding in metastatic disease (Pedersen et al., 1989), should suggest a primary process, while a component of the metastasis can be characterized radiographically suggesting the primary source, such as melanin in metastatic melanoma (Isiklar et al., 1995).

Leptomeningeal, dural, or vertebral involvement by metastasis is best detected by MRI examination. Contrast-enhanced MR imaging will reveal diffuse thickening or nodular enhancement of the leptomeninges or dura in carcinomatosis.

Macroscopic Features

As a general rule, the lesions of metastatic disease are well-demarcated masses, with a firm consistency and the soft surrounding nonneoplastic rim of reactive brain parenchyma. Necrosis and hemorrhage will impart a variegated yellow–tan–hemorrhagic soft surface. Lesions of metastatic melanoma, when containing melanin deposits, as seen in 50% of melanomas, will appear black or dark brown.

Microscopic Features

The microscopic appearance of metastatic lesions follows their macroscopic and radiographically discrete nature from the surrounding nonneoplastic brain parenchyma (Figure 3.179). However, some metastatic lesions, particularly melanoma, small cell carcinoma of lung, and lymphoma will have a tendency to produce less defined boundaries from the nonneoplastic brain parenchyma at the microscopic level. Necrosis is usually abundant within the tumors and characteristically displays an abrupt transition between necrotic tumor and a rim of viable tumor parallel to blood vessels.

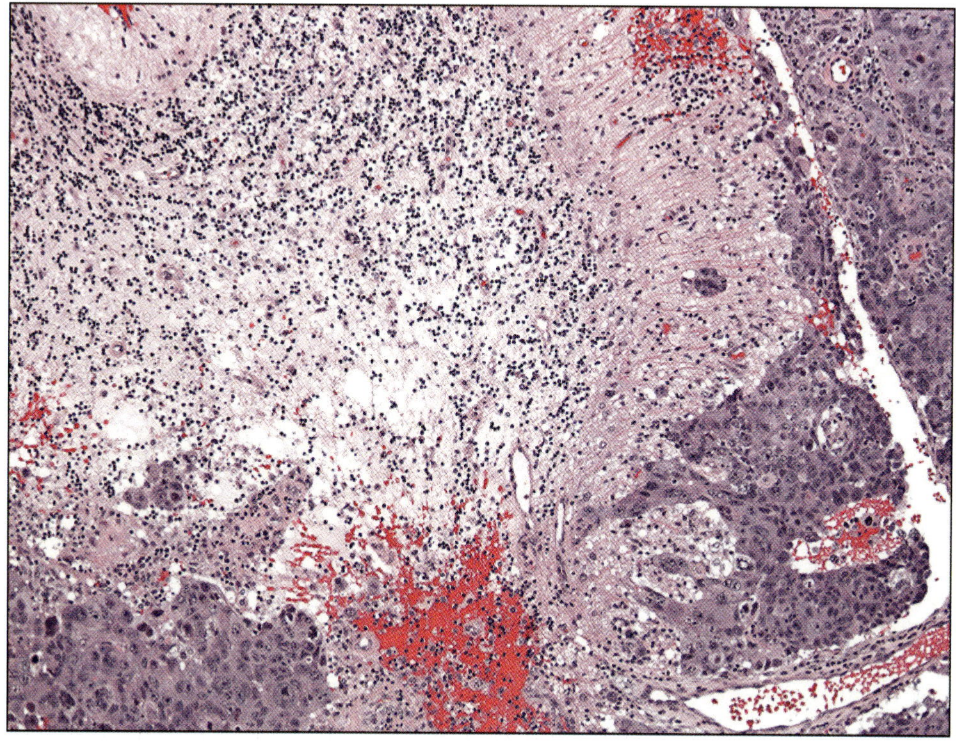

Figure 3.179. Most metastatic neoplasms to the brain grow with a pushing and non-infiltrating border as is seen in this example of carcinoma metastatic to the cerebellar parenchyme and subarachnoid space.

Figure 3.180. Metastatic colon adenocarcinoma retaining a histological appearance essentially the identical to that of the primary lesion.

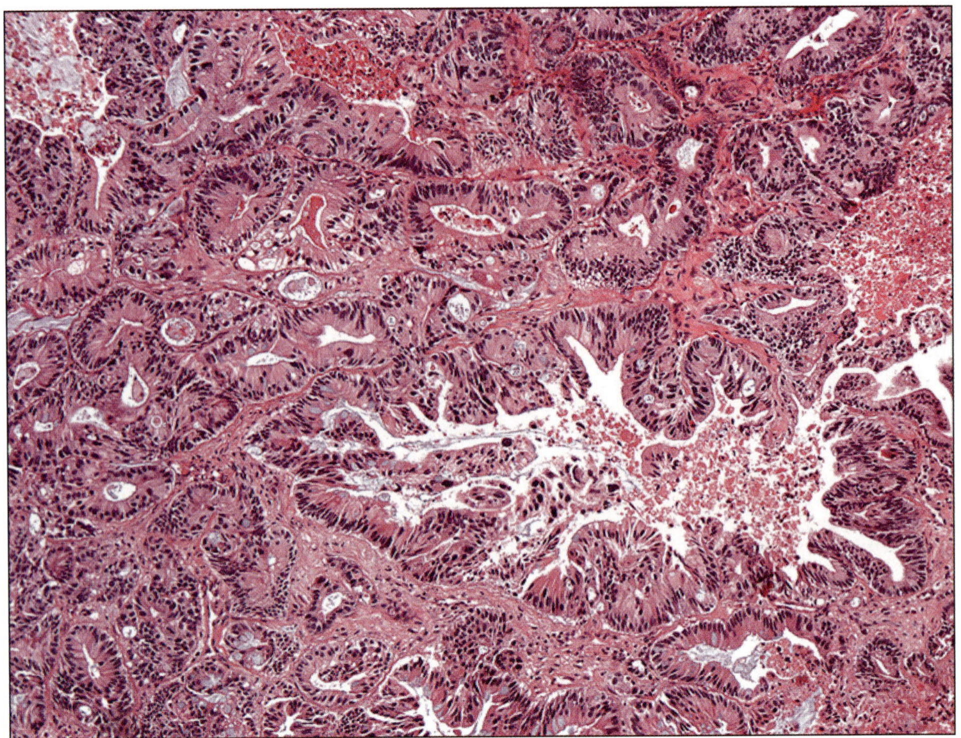

Histologically, metastatic lesions usually do not pose a diagnostic dilemma as the neoplasms attempt to recapitulate the histology of the primary site, which in cases of well-differentiated tumors may show specialized epithelium such as intestinal epithelium from metastatic GI tumors (Figure 3.180) and squamous epithelium of head and neck carcinomas. Occasionally, however, extensive necrosis or poorly differentiated tumors can lead to difficulty in the determination of metastatic versus primary brain lesions. In such cases, immunohistochemical, molecular, or ultrastructural analysis may be required.

Some metastatic lesions particular to areas less commonly involved by metastatic disease may trick the unwary. These include papillary carcinoma of the lung or thyroid mimicking a choroid plexus neoplasm or metastatic neuroendocrine carcinoma to the sella mimicking pituitary adenoma (Figure 3.181) (Chandra et al., 1984). Metastatic clear cell renal cell carcinoma to the dura or posterior fossa can pose diagnostic issues with hemangioblastoma because both lesions may exhibit abundant clear cytoplasm with uniform, round cell nuclei present in solid sheets or tubules within a prominent background vasculature (Weinbreck et al., 2008).

Metastatic melanoma, the "great mimicker", occasionally poses a problem as a result its myriad histologic patterns. Melanomas may vary from those composed of exclusively spindled or epithelioid cells to a mixture both morphologies and lack of melanin production in 50% of metastases. For these reasons, melanoma is typically on the short diagnostic differential list for lesions that do not show an extensive defining histologic pattern. Furthermore, metastatic melanoma is known for its proclivity to hemorrhage and one may overlook the scant diagnostic tissue admixed with abundant blood.

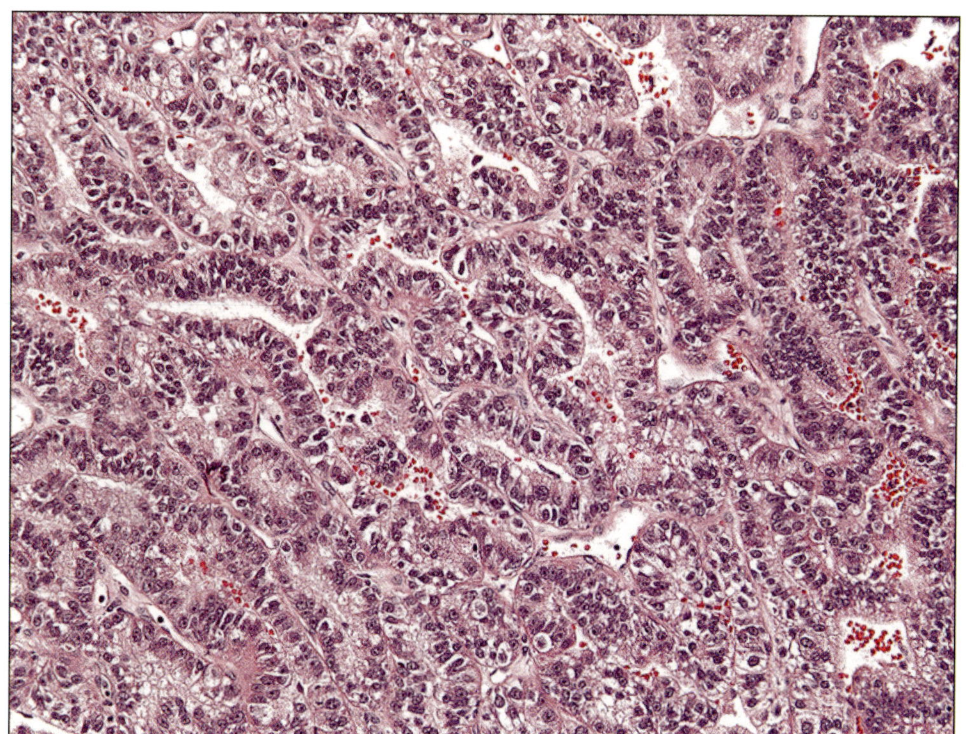

Figure 3.181. Example of metastatic well-differentiated renal cell carcinoma to the sella, mimicking pituitary adenoma.

Frozen Section and Cytological Features

Cytological smears reveal important clues to metastatic versus primary disease. Carcinoma tends to cluster in a nonfibrillary background while glial tumors will reveal a dispersed cell pattern within a fibrillar background. Both metastases and high-grade glial tumor may show necrosis or microvascular proliferation. Nuclear morphology, always superior in the cytological preparation, will typically reveal round pleomorphic nuclei with prominent nucleoli and well-defined cytoplasm characteristic of metastatic carcinoma. Glial tumors, on the other hand, typically reveal dispersed cells with elongate angular nuclei with indistinct or fibrillar cytoplasm (Savargaonkar and Farmer, 2001).

Immunohistochemistry

Immunohistochemistry is often useful to distinguish metastatic disease from primary neoplasms, to confirm the origin of a suspected metastasis, or as a tool in identifying the origin of a poorly differentiated malignancy.

- Cytokeratins and EMA are useful in distinguishing carcinoma from melanoma, sarcoma, and glioblastoma.
- A differentiating cytokeratin panel of CK7 and CK20 along with thyroid transcription factor 1 and CDX2 is useful in identifying the origin of a metastasis from more common metastatic lesions (Moskaluk et al., 2003; Rubin et al., 2001). For example, CK7+, TTF-1+ and CK20− neoplasm supports metastatic lung carcinoma,

while CK7−, CK20+, TTF-1− and CDX2+ supports metastatic colorectal carcinoma.

- Melanomas are positive for S-100 protein, HMB45, melan A, and MITF, although it must be kept in mind that a subset of melanomas can display cytokeratin positivity (Liu et al., 2004).
- Antibodies to such tissue specific antibodies as thyroglobulin, calcitonin, and prostate-specific antigen can be used to identify metastases from thyroid or prostate, respectively.
- Hep Par-1 and alpha-fetoprotein are useful markers for metastatic hepatocellular carcinoma (Leong et al., 1998).
- Metastatic germ cell tumors are distinguished not only by histologic features but by marker-specific subtypes of germ cell tumors and include OCT4, PLAP, and CD117 for germinoma (Hattab et al., 2005; Sever et al., 2005), βHCG for choriocarcinoma, AFP for yolk sac tumor, and CD30 for embryonal carcinoma.
- Differentiating conventional renal cell carcinoma from hemangioblastoma can be clarified by analysis for CD10, RCC, and EMA, which are usually positive in renal cell carcinoma while inhibin and epidermal growth factor receptor (EGFR) positively supports a diagnosis of hemangioblastoma (Bakshi et al., 2007; Bohling et al., 1996; Jung and Kuo, 2005).

MET	CK7	CK20	P63	CDX2	TTF-1	S-100	HMB45	MITF	SYNAP	OCT4	RCC	CD56	CD30	CK	EMA	AFP	βHCG
LAC	+	−	−	−	+	−	−	−	−	−	−	−	−	+	+/−	−	−
LSCCA	−	−	+	−	−	−	−	−	−	−	−	−	−	+	+/−	−	−
LSC	+/−	−	−	−	+	−	−	−	−	−	−	−	−	+	+/−	−	−
MM	−	−	−	−	−	+	+	+	−	−	−	−	−	−	+/−	−	−
GERM	−	−	−	−	−	+/−	−	−	−	+	−	−	−	−	+/−	−	+/−
EMB	−	−	−	−	−	−	−	−	−	−	−	−	+	+	+/−	−	−
YS	−	−	−	−	−	−	−	−	−	−	−	−	−	+	+	+	−
CHOR	−	−	−	−	−	−	−	−	−	−	−	−	−	+	+	−	+
RCCA	−	−	−	−	−	−	−	−	−	−	+	−	−	+	+	−	−

LAC, lung adenocarcinoma; LSCCA, lung squamous cell carcinoma; LSC, lung small cell carcinoma; MM, malignant melanoma; GERM, germinoma; EMB, embryonal carcinoma; YS, yolk sac tumor; CHOR, choriocarcinoma; RCCA, renal cell carcinoma.

DIFFERENTIAL DIAGNOSIS

The differential diagnosis of metastatic disease must always include the possibility of malignant glioma, primary CNS lymphoma, or hemangioblastoma. A thorough histologic examination will usually reveal clues to the identity of the malignancy. Differentiating lung small cell carcinoma from anaplastic oligodendroglioma, small cell glioblastoma, or primitive neuroectodermal tumor may be problematic given that all of the neoplasms may be comprised of small cells that may occasionally reveal discrete cytoplasmic borders, hyperchromatic nuclei, occasional nuclear molding, and abundant necrosis. Anaplastic oligodendroglioma will display fairly monotonous nuclei with perinuclear halos, an exaggerated hexagonally arrayed background vasculature and occasional foci of calcification. Close scrutiny of the interface will usually reveal a distinct and robust reactive parenchymal interface in metastatic disease than in primary tumors, a feature highlighted by GFAP immunohistochemical analysis.

Additionally, pronounced parenchymal infiltration and an absence of collagen within and surrounding the lesion are features of primary rather than metastatic disease. Carcinoma, as a general rule, will infiltrate predominantly as cohesive clusters of malignant cells and the individual neoplastic cells display their epithelial nature of round to polygonal-shaped cells with distinct cytoplasmic borders. Although glioblastoma may exhibit epithelial structures, that is, adenoid glioblastoma glioblastoma, these foci are a minor component of the overall histologic pattern.

Metastatic tumors that have the ability to produce spindle cell morphology and stimulate a high-grade glioma, that is, sarcomatoid renal cell carcinoma or spindle cell melanoma, may only be correctly identified by immunohistochemical analysis or by comparison to the primary tumor, if known.

Important histologic features ascribed to glioblastoma include random distribution of serpentine pseudopalisading necrosis, typically partially rimmed by blood vessels with microvascular proliferation. Metastatic tumors, on the other hand, tend to outgrow their blood supply and are prone to geographical necrosis with foci of viable neoplastic cells surrounding a central blood supply. When vascular proliferation is encountered in metastatic carcinomas (Ito et al., 1993), it is usually within the confines of the tumor and rarely approaches the exuberance of that seen in glioblastoma or anaplastic oligodendroglioma.

Systemic lymphoma, particularly large cell forms, may cause confusion with metastatic carcinoma or high-grade glioma. Radiographic findings of white matter, periventricular or corpus callosum lesions are features usually seen in lymphoma and in combination with the characteristic "onion skinning" infiltration around blood vessels, highlighted by reticulin staining, helps to distinguish lymphomas from epithelial or glial neoplasms. The diagnosis is confirmed by immunohistochemical analysis for B-cell and T-cell markers and immunoglobulin light stain monotypism. Clinical and radiographic correlation is then essential to determine whether the lymphoma is primary or a result of CNS involvement by a systemic lymphoma.

Specific problems areas include distinguishing metastatic small cell carcinoma from medulloblastoma of the cerebellum that occur in older patients, metastatic renal cell carcinoma from hemangioblastoma, and metastatic papillary carcinoma from choroid plexus carcinoma. Medulloblastoma forming neuroblastic (Homer Wright rosettes) or spongioblastic features, characterized by neoplastic cell nuclei arranged with their long axis in parallel arrangements, are important distinguishing features from small cell carcinoma, but unfortunately are not seen in the majority of medulloblastomas. In addition, large cell or anaplastic medulloblastoma can be very difficult on histologic grounds alone to exclude metastatic neuroendocrine carcinomas such as small cell carcinoma. Confounding the issue is that immunohistochemical analysis of both tumors may overlap, but generally, perinuclear cytokeratin staining and TTF-1 immunoreactivity seen in small cell carcinoma is not typically associated with medulloblastoma. In cases of large cell medulloblastoma, analysis for MYC amplification may add prognostic as well as diagnostic information, considering that some large cell medulloblastomas have MYC amplification (Leonard et al., 2001). Nevertheless, some cases may not be resolved and small cell carcinoma will have to be considered even with a negative imaging studies of the chest.

The differentiation between metastatic clear cell carcinoma from hemangioblastoma can be an issue due to their histological similarities. Immunohistochemical analysis is often required to demonstrate epithelial membrane antigen, CD10 and RCC positivity in renal cell carcinoma versus inhibin immunoreactivity in hemangioblastoma.

Differentiating metastatic well papillary adenocarcinoma from choroid plexus papilloma is another potential pitfall, particularly in patients with no preexisting history of carcinoma. Immunohistochemical analysis for BerEP4 can be useful since it labels 95% of metastatic carcinomas compared to choroid plexus tumors (10%) (Gottschalk et al., 1993). Most choroid plexus tumors have a CK7-positive/CK20-negative immunophenotype, a pattern of immunoreactivity that may be useful in differentiating these lesions from metastatic carcinomas that have a differing CK7/CK20 profile (Gyure and Morrison, 2000).

REFERENCES

Bakshi N, Kunju LP, Giordano T, Shah RB. Expression of renal cell carcinoma antigen (RCC) in renal epithelial and nonrenal tumors: diagnostic Implications. *Appl Immunohistochem Mol Morphol* 2007; 15: 310–15.

Baratelli GM, Ciccaglioni B, Dainese E, Arnaboldi L. Metastasis of breast carcinoma to intracranial meningioma. *J Neurosurg Sci* 2004; 48: 71–3.

Benedetto N, Perrini P, Scollato A, Buccoliero AM, Di Lorenzo N. Intracranial meningioma containing metastatic colon carcinoma. *Acta Neurochir (Wien)* 2007; 149: 799–803; discussion 803.

Bobilev D, Shelef I, Lavrenkov K, Tokar M, Man S, Baumgarten A, et al. Diabetes insipidus caused by isolated intracranial metatstases in patient with breast cancer. *J Neurooncol* 2005; 73: 39–42.

Bohling T, Hatva E, Kujala M, Claesson-Welsh L, Alitalo K, Haltia M. Expression of growth factors and growth factor receptors in capillary hemangioblastoma. *J Neuropathol Exp Neurol* 1996; 55: 522–7.

Chandra V, McDonald LW, Anderson RJ. Metastatic small cell carcinoma of the lung presenting as pituitary apoplexy and Cushing's syndrome. *J Neurooncol* 1984; 2: 59–66.

Cohn-Cedermark G, Mansson-Brahme E, Rutqvist LE, Larsson O, Johansson H, Ringborg U. Central nervous system metastases of cutaneous malignant melanoma – a population-based study. *Acta Oncol* 1998; 37: 463–70.

Delattre JY, Krol G, Thaler HT, Posner JB. Distribution of brain metastases. *Arch Neurol* 1988; 45: 741–4.

Dumas M, Perusse R. Trigeminal sensory neuropathy: a study of 35 cases. *Oral Surg Oral Med Oral Pathol Oral Radiol Endod* 1999; 87: 577–82.

Evans AJ, James JJ, Cornford EJ, Chan SY, Burrell HC, Pinder SE, et al. Brain metastases from breast cancer: identification of a high-risk group. *Clin Oncol (R Coll Radiol)* 2004; 16: 345–9.

Gottschalk J, Jautzke G, Paulus W, Goebel S, Cervos-Navarro J. The use of immuno-morphology to differentiate choroid plexus tumors from metastatic carcinomas. *Cancer* 1993; 72: 1343–9.

Gyure KA, Morrison AL. Cytokeratin 7 and 20 expression in choroid plexus tumors: utility in differentiating these neoplasms from metastatic carcinomas. *Mod Pathol* 2000; 13: 638–43.

Hattab EM, Tu PH, Wilson JD, Cheng L. OCT4 immunohistochemistry is superior to placental alkaline phosphatase (PLAP) in the diagnosis of central nervous system germinoma. *Am J Surg Pathol* 2005; 29: 368–71.

Isiklar I, Leeds NE, Fuller GN, Kumar AJ. Intracranial metastatic melanoma: correlation between MR imaging characteristics and melanin content. *AJR Am J Roentgenol* 1995; 165: 1503–12.

Ito T, Kitamura H, Nakamura N, Kameda Y, Kanisawa M. A comparative study of vascular proliferation in brain metastasis of lung carcinomas. *Virchows Arch A Pathol Anat Histopathol* 1993; 423: 13–17.

Jellinger K, Radiaszkiewicz T. Involvement of the central nervous system in malignant lymphomas. *Virchows Arch A Pathol Anat Histol* 1976; 370: 345–62.

Jung SM, Kuo TT. Immunoreactivity of CD10 and inhibin alpha in differentiating hemangioblastoma of central nervous system from metastatic clear cell renal cell carcinoma. *Mod Pathol* 2005; 18: 788–94.

Klos KJ, O'Neill BP. Brain metastases. *Neurologist* 2004; 10: 31–46.

Leonard JR, Cai DX, Rivet DJ, Kaufman BA, Park TS, Levy BK, et al. Large cell/anaplastic medulloblastomas and medullomyoblastomas: clinicopathological and genetic features. *J Neurosurg* 2001; 95: 82–8.

Leong AS, Sormunen RT, Tsui WM, Liew CT. Hep Par 1 and selected antibodies in the immunohistological distinction of hepatocellular carcinoma from cholangiocarcinoma, combined tumours and metastatic carcinoma. *Histopathology* 1998; 33: 318–24.

Liu Y, Sturgis CD, Bunker M, Saad RS, Tung M, Raab SS, et al. Expression of cytokeratin by malignant meningiomas: diagnostic pitfall of cytokeratin to separate malignant meningiomas from metastatic carcinoma. *Mod Pathol* 2004; 17: 1129–33.

Mandal S, Mandal AK. Malignant fibrous histiocytoma following radiation therapy and chemotherapy for Hodgkin's lymphoma. *Int J Clin Oncol* 2007; 12: 52–5.

Mandybur TI. Intracranial hemorrhage caused by metastatic tumors. *Neurology* 1977; 27: 650–5.

Moskaluk CA, Zhang H, Powell SM, Cerilli LA, Hampton GM, Frierson HF, Jr. Cdx2 protein expression in normal and malignant human tissues: an immunohisto-chemical survey using tissue microarrays. *Mod Pathol* 2003; 16: 913–19.

Parasuraman S, Langston J, Rao BN, Poquette CA, Jenkins JJ, Merchant T, et al. Brain metastases in pediatric Ewing sarcoma and rhabdomyosarcoma: the St. Jude Children's Research Hospital experience. *J Pediatr Hematol Oncol* 1999; 21: 370–7.

Pedersen H, McConnell J, Harwood-Nash DC, Fitz CR, Chuang SH. Computed tomography in intracranial, supratentorial metastases in children. *Neuroradiology* 1989; 31: 19–23.

Postovsky S, Ash S, Ramu IN, Yaniv Y, Zaizov R, Futerman B, et al. Central nervous system involvement in children with sarcoma. *Oncology* 2003; 65: 118–24.

Ragland RL, Wagner LD, Huang YP, Som PM, Teal JS, Handler MS. Streaming hypo-intensity in hemorrhagic glioblastoma multiforme. An illustrative case. *Neuroradiology* 1990; 32: 241–3.

Reichardt P, Lindner T, Pink D, Thuss-Patience PC, Kretzschmar A, Dorken B. Chemotherapy in alveolar soft part sarcomas. What do we know? *Eur J Cancer* 2003; 39: 1511–16.

Rubin BP, Skarin AT, Pisick E, Rizk M, Salgia R. Use of cytokeratins 7 and 20 in determining the origin of metastatic carcinoma of unknown primary, with special emphasis on lung cancer. *Eur J Cancer Prev* 2001; 10: 77–82.

Savargaonkar P, Farmer PM. Utility of intra-operative consultations for the diagnosis of central nervous system lesions. *Ann Clin Lab Sci* 2001; 31: 133–9.

Sever M, Jones TD, Roth LM, Karim FW, Zheng W, Michael H, et al. Expression of CD117 (c-kit) receptor in dysgerminoma of the ovary: diagnostic and therapeutic implications. *Mod Pathol* 2005; 18: 1411–16.

Teears RJ, Silverman EM. Clinicopathologic review of 88 cases of carcinoma metastatic to the putuitary gland. *Cancer* 1975; 36: 216–20.

Weinbreck N, Marie B, Bressenot A, Montagne K, Joud A, Baumann C, et al. Immunohistochemical markers to distinguish between hemangioblastoma and metastatic clear-cell renal cell carcinoma in the brain: utility of aquaporin1 combined with cytokeratin AE1/AE3 immunostaining. *Am J Surg Pathol* 2008; 32: 1051–9.

Yap HY, Tashima CK, Blumenschein GR, Eckles N. Diabetes insipidus and breast cancer. *Arch Intern Med* 1979; 139: 1009–11.

SKULL AND PARASPINAL NEOPLASMS, NONNEOPLASTIC MASSES, AND MALFORMATIONS

A surprising number of cases come to the attention of the surgical neuropathologist that represent extraneural masses originating in the bone or other soft tissues, simply because these are within the spectrum of practice in neurosurgery. These represent a wide gamut of etiologies including primary and metastatic neoplasms, infections, malformations, and others. Just as in the proper evaluation of any CNS lesion, knowledge of the radiographic features and overall clinical circumstances is of paramount importance in making a correct diagnosis. Many of the entities listed below may be seen in association with either the skull or spinal column even though they all have distinct sites of predilection.

Among the following, the most common benign entities to involve the skull are fibrous dysplasia, Langerhans cell histiocytosis, osteoma, dermoid cysts, and hemangiomas.

Neoplasms of the skull and skull base may be best conceptualized as arising in one of the following compartments:

- Pituitary region (Chapter 3G)
- Nasal and paranasal sinus region, including olfactory neuroblastoma, olfactory neuroepithelioma, neuroendocrine carcinoma, nasopharyngeal carcinoma, juvenile angiofibroma, and mucocele
- Orbital region, including meningioma, lymphoma, rhabdomyosarcoma, and malignant melanoma
- Middle ear compartment, including paraganglioma, cholesteatoma, squamous cell carcinoma, and endolymphatic sac tumor
- Skull base tumors, including chondroma, chondrosarcoma, chordoma, meningioma, and schwannoma

MALIGNANT NEOPLASMS

Chordoma

Clinical and Radiological Features

Almost all chordomas occur in the midline of the skull and vertebral axis with 40% of all cases arising in the clivus and are derived from notochordal remnants. A related entity is a nonneoplastic extraosseous nodule of nonneoplastic notochordal tissue in the spinal canal or posterior fossa in the prepontine cistern, known as *ecchordosis physaliphora* (Mehnert et al., 2004; Rotondo et al., 2007). Some "giant" examples may pose a semantic issue in distinguishing these from true chordomas, although the latter usually involve bone (Wolfe and Scheithauer, 1987).

Chordomas occur most commonly from adolescents through the seventh decade with a more common occurrence in men. They typically present with pain or other neurological deficits related to compression. The considerable difficulty in achieving surgical resection in most cases results in high incidence of recurrence. Radiation therapy may be of some therapeutic utility.

Radiologically, they are typically lytic lesions of bone and which are occasionally calcified. They show irregular contrast enhancement and are hyperintense on T2-weighted MR images (Figure 3.182a,b).

Pathology

Low-power microscopy shows a lobular tumor with intervening septa. The cells are arranged in irregular clusters or cords separated by variable amounts of mucin (Figure 3.182c–f). A subset of cells might show clear cytoplasmic expansion by small vacuoles, resulting in physaliphorous (Greek: "φυσαλλίς φέρειν") cells. Some examples may show nuclear pleomorphism or even occasional mitotic figures. There may also be cartilaginous or osseous differentiation although any significant chondroid differentiation should raise the possibility of a low-grade chondrosarcoma. Chordomas may also show frank malignant transformation, resulting in a mostly solid sarcomatous appearance. The hallmark immunohistochemical profile in chordomas consists of combined immunoreactivities for S-100 and cytokeratins or EMA.

Figure 3.182. Chordoma. (a) An axial T1-weighted contrast-enhanced MR image shows a multilobulated, enhancing mass arising from the spheno-occipital synchondrosis, deforming the pons and contacting the basilar artery. (b) On T2-weighted images the mass demonstrates high signal. Chordomas, like chondrosarcomas, often demonstrate high signal on T2-weighted images. However, skull base chordomas typically originate at the midline spheno-occipital synchondrosis, whereas chondrosarcomas most often arise off the midline at the petro-occipital fissure.

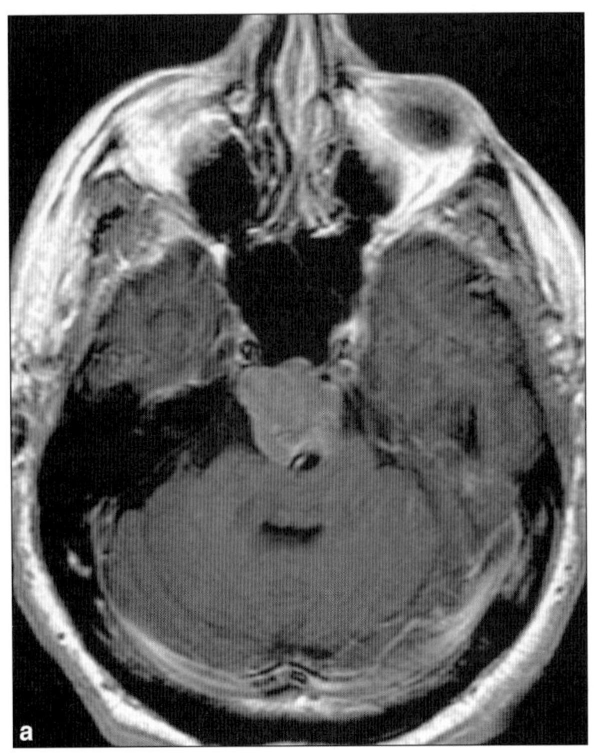

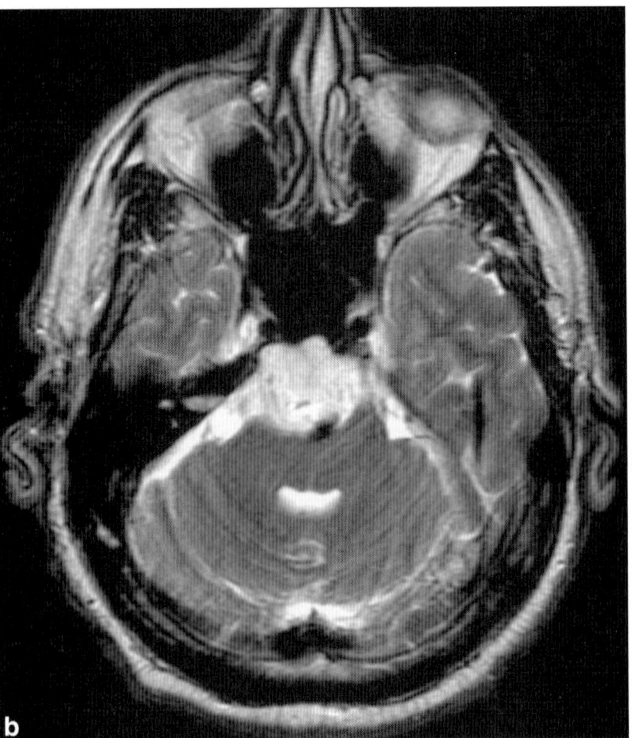

Olfactory Neuroblastoma (Esthesioneuroblastoma)

Clinical and Radiological Features

This distinctive neoplasm arises in the region of the cribriform plate with the potential for intracranial extension. They occur in a bimodal fashion in the

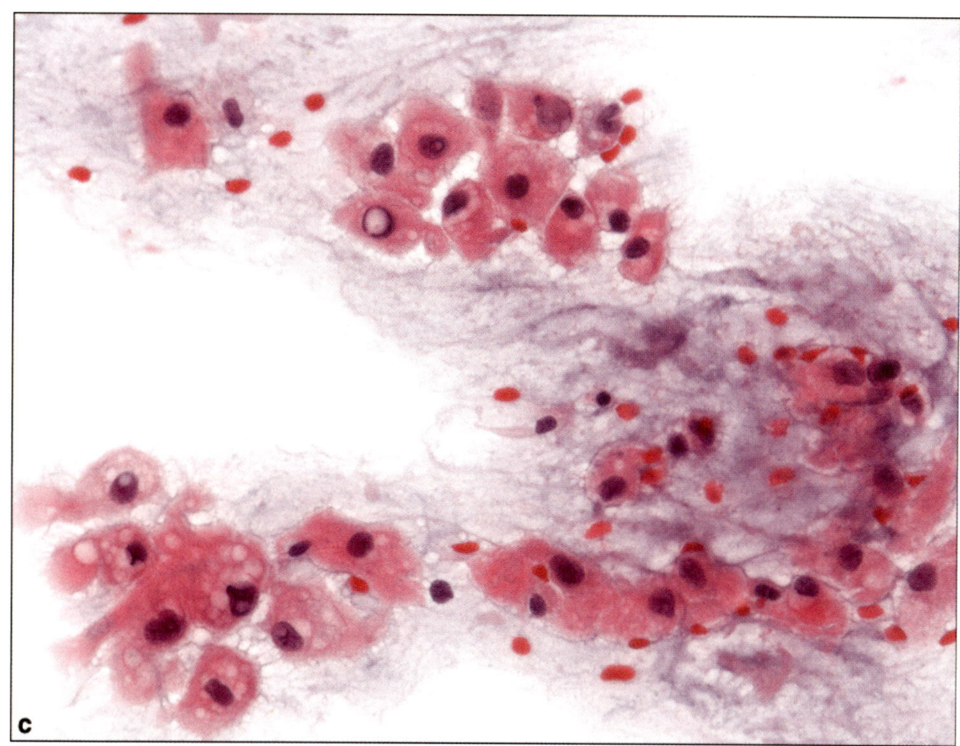

Figure 3.182. *continued*
(c) Squash cytological preparation, showing discrete cells in small clusters in a myxoid background. Note the vacuolated "physaliferous" cells seen well in these preparations.
(d) Characteristic H&E appearance with rows of epithelioid cells with a myxoid background. Many cells have clear cytoplasm and some are physaliphorous (Gr. "bubble-bearing"). Almost unique immunophenotype pairs
(e) S-100 and (f) cytokeratin reactivity.

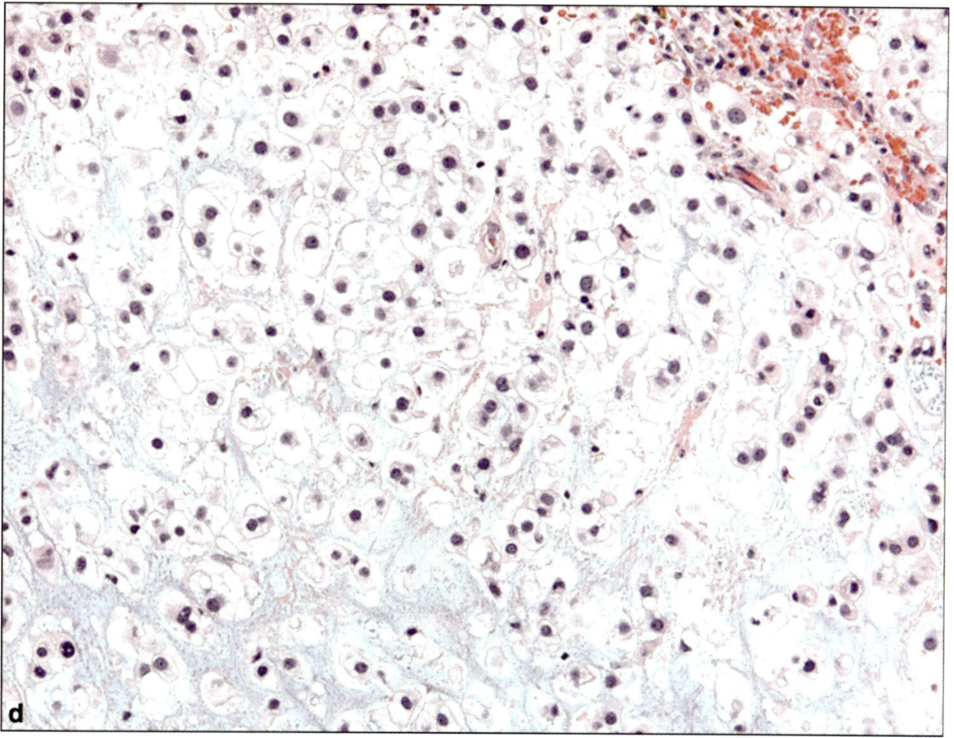

second and fifth decades. Presenting symptoms depend on the location of the mass, with intranasal examples causing nasal obstruction or epistaxis of sometimes surprisingly long duration, and intracranial lesions producing focal neurologic deficits. Radiologic features are those of an invasive mass involving regional soft tissues with variable signal and enhancement patterns.

Figure 3.182. *continued.*

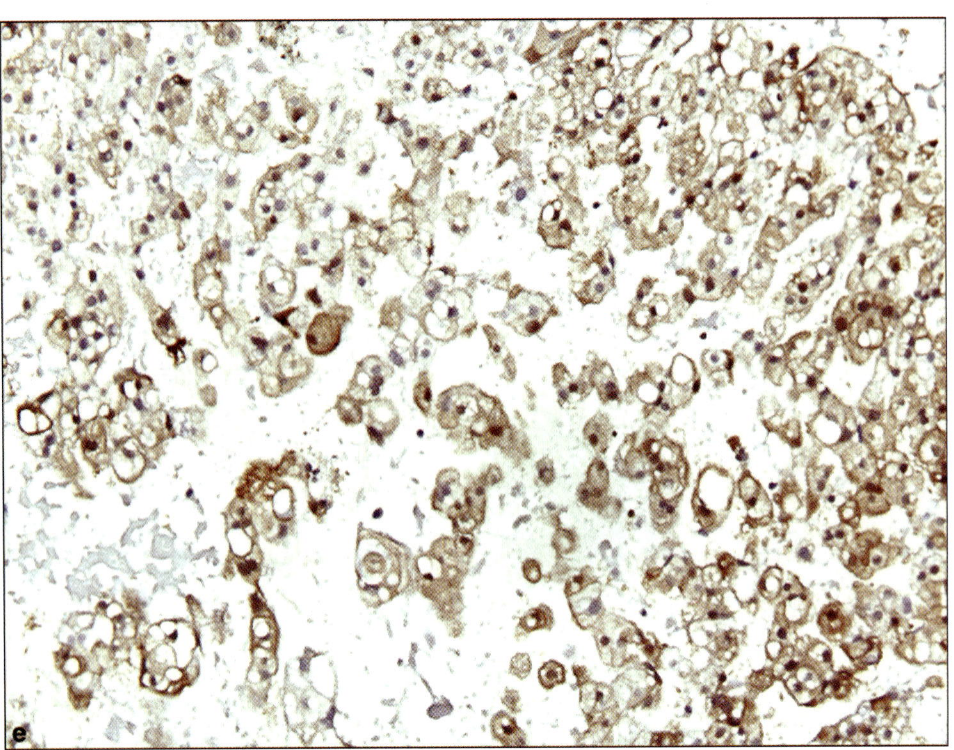

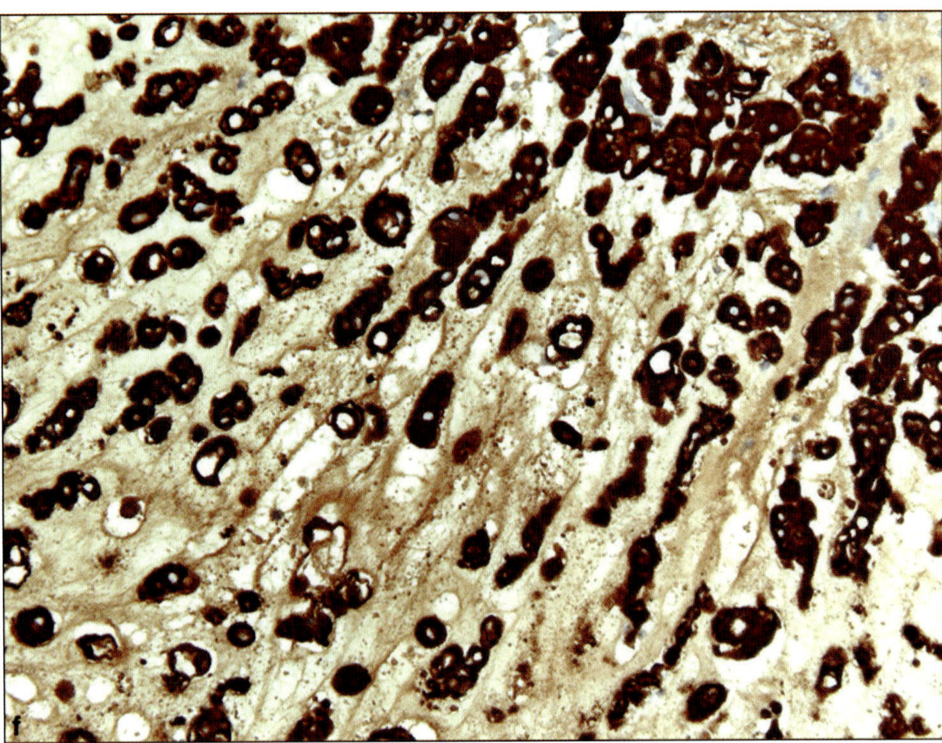

Pathology

The low-power appearance of olfactory neuroblastoma includes two main growth patterns: cellular nests and lobules with intervening vascular stroma is the most common pattern and less frequently diffuse patternless growth

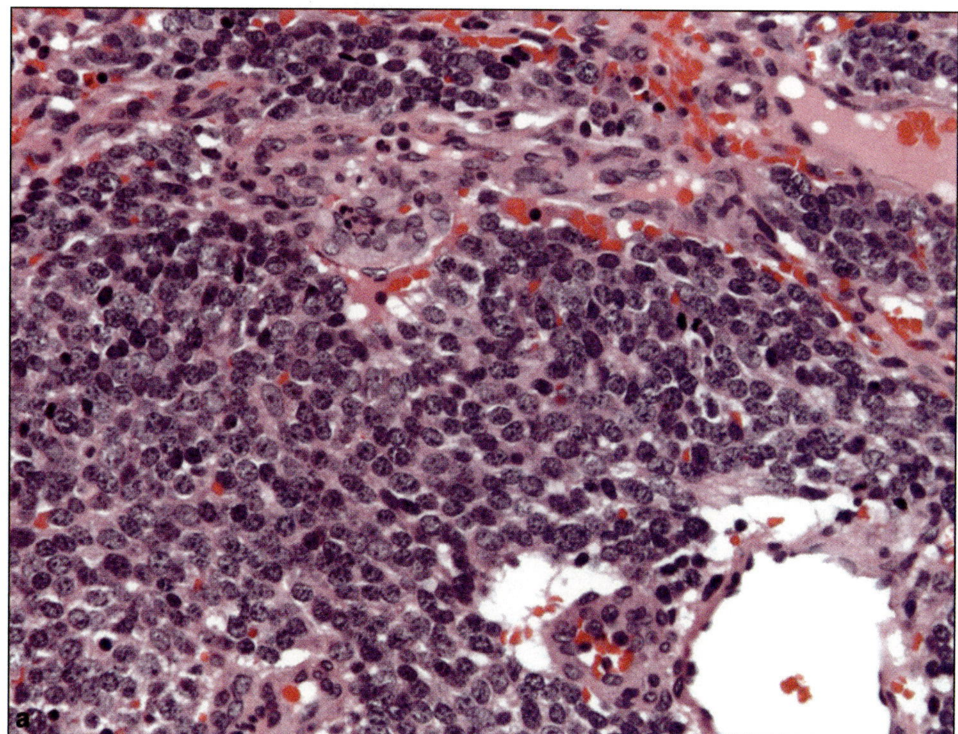

Figure 3.183. Esthesioneuroblastoma (olfactory neuroblastoma). (a) Usual features of a relatively undifferentiated neuroectodermal tumor, with large lobules of monotonous cells, that are (b) synaptophysin immunopositive, with (c) anti-S-100 labelling the bordering sustentacular cells.

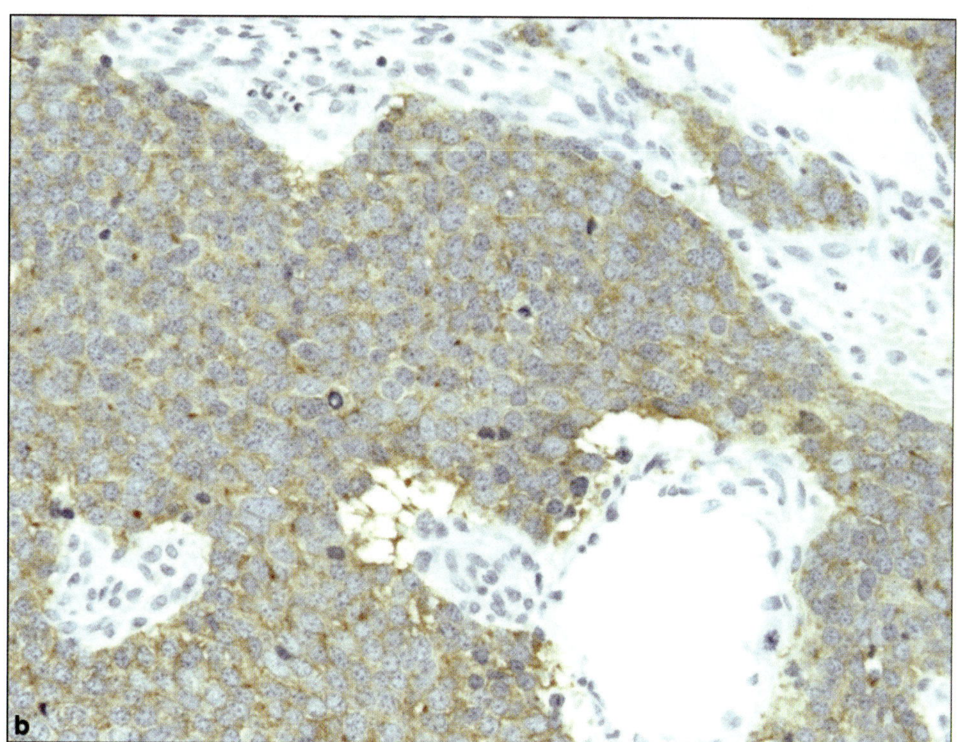

(Figure 3.183). Cytological features include monomorphous compact cells in a delicate neurofibrillary background, with occasional Homer Wright rosettes in a minority of lesions.

Immunohistochemistry is of great importance in confirming neuronal differentiation such as by the identification of synaptophysin, neurofilaments,

Figure 3.183. *continued.*

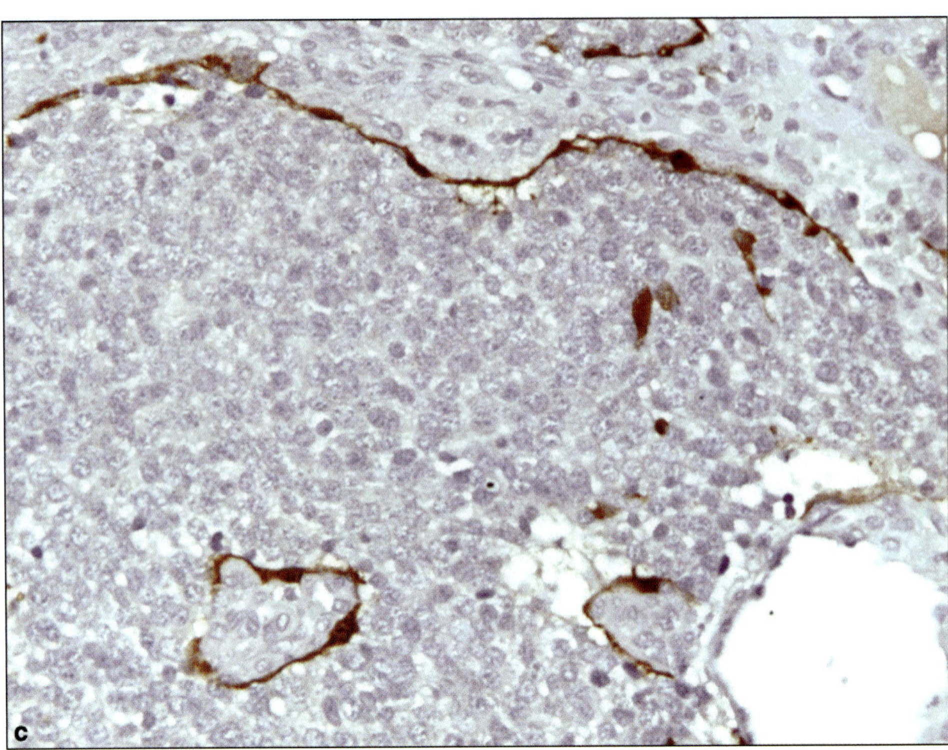

or microtubule associated protein. S-100 may be detected in the sustentacular cells at the edges of lobules or may also exist as scattered immunopositive cells within lobules. Immunohistochemistry is also important in excluding other cellular neoplasms that may occur in the region, such as melanoma, neuroendocrine carcinoma, sinonasal pituitary adenomas, and sinonasal undifferentiated carcinoma (SNUC) (Cohen et al., 2002; Luk et al., 1996).

Endolymphatic Sac Tumor

Clinical Features

These low-grade but locally invasive carcinomas occur in the temporal bone in the region of the inner ear and may extend into the posterior fossa and the cerebellopontine angle (Joseph et al., 2002). They generally occur in adults, but childhood examples have been reported. There is an association with Hippel–Lindau syndrome (Devaney et al., 2003; Horiguchi et al., 2001; Muzumdar et al., 2006).

Pathology

These tumors are characterized by papillary or solid growth of well-differentiated epithelium, or a follicular pattern resembling thyroid parenchyma (Figure 3.184). They are immunoreactive for cytokeratins, EMA, and sometimes S-100 protein.

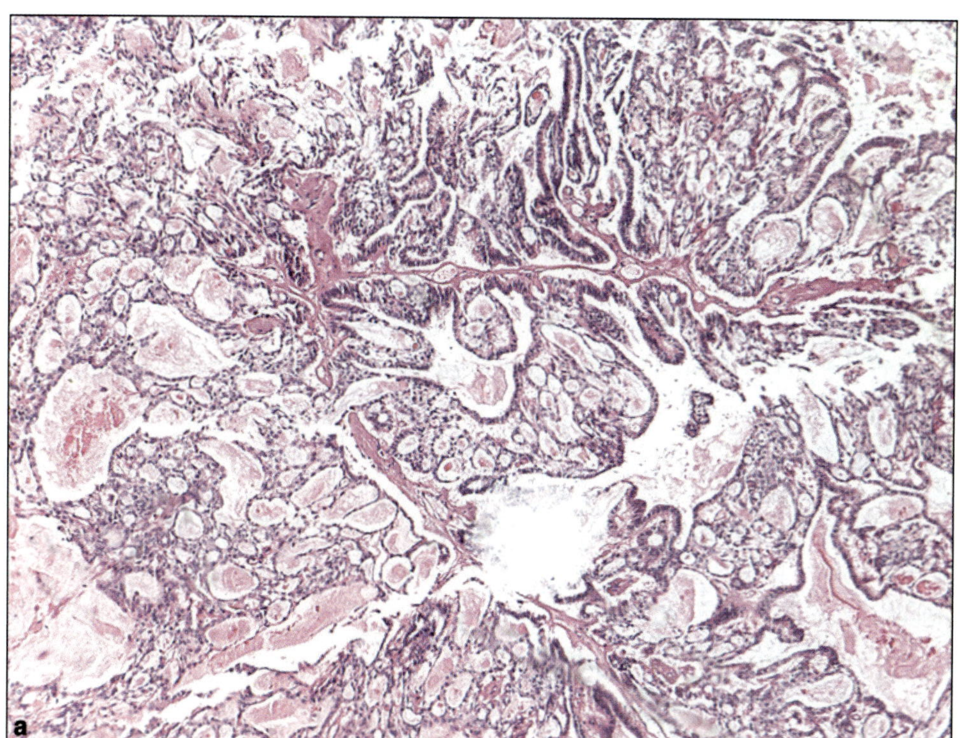

Figure 3.184. Endolymphatic sac tumor. (a,b) Vaguely papillary and cystic neoplasm with space lined by well-differentiated columnar epithelium.

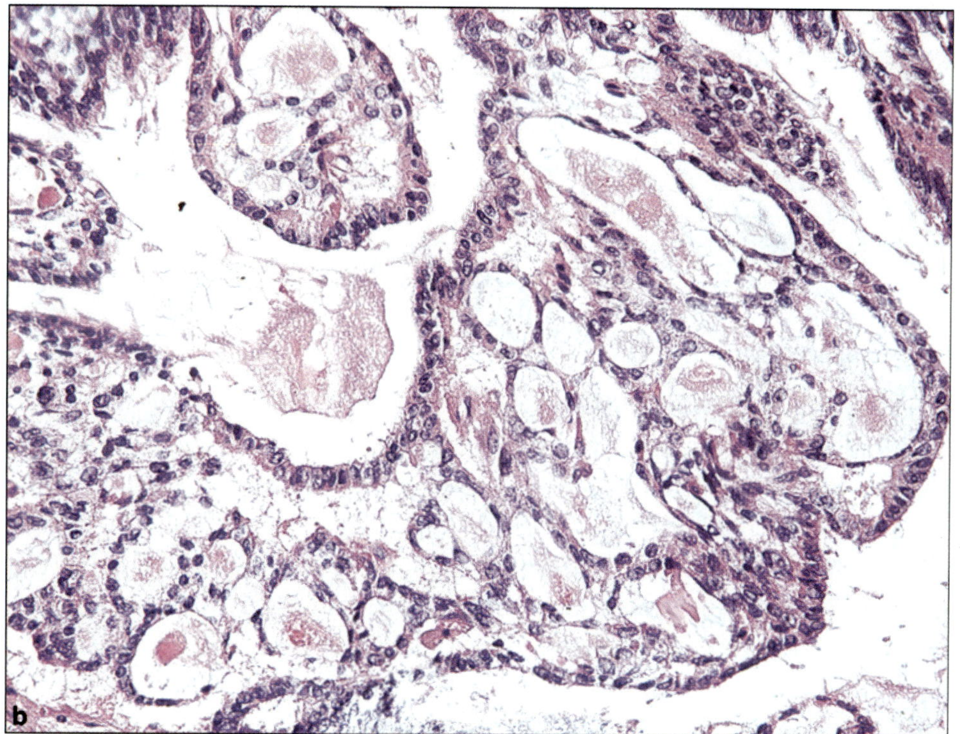

BENIGN MASSES

Fibrous Dysplasia

Clinical and Radiological Features

Fibrous dysplasia is a monostotic or polyostotic condition of unknown etiology characterized by benign but abnormal fibro-osseous proliferation.

Children and young adults are most frequently affected. It occurs most frequently in long bones of the extremities, ribs, or skull. Spinal or vertebral involvement is a rarity such that a biopsy is usually required for diagnosis when occurring in these lactiona (Gogia et al., 2007). There is an association of polyostotic disease with pigmented skin lesions and precocious sexual development, particularly in females, exemplifying the McCune Albright syndrome.

When involving the skull, fibrous dysplasia tends to involve anterior bone such as the facial, frontal, ethmoid, and sphenoid bones with decreasing incidence proceeding posteriorly (Figure 3.185a,b). Symptoms are referable to either mass effect causing asymmetry, proptosis, or because of compression of the optic nerve or other cranial neuropathies.

Plain films show a focal, well-defined area of rarefaction surrounded by a narrow rim of sclerotic bone with some known variations from the classic pattern. Examples of more extensive diffuse involvement may be seen in McCune Albright syndrome.

Pathology

Gross examination of the excision specimen usually displays an expansile lesion of bone, which contains a variably gritty or fibrous texture upon cross-section. The microscopic hallmark of fibrous dysplasia, although nonspecific, is the presence of plump spindle cells in a storiform pattern without cytological atypia (Figure 3.185c,d). Some tumors are myxoid. Spicules of metaplastic woven bone may be seen. The trabeculae of bone may form the so-called Chinese figure structures in a background of dense fibrous tissue with few osteocytes or osteoblasts.

Aneurysmal Bone Cyst

Clinical and Radiological Features

Aneurysmal bone cysts (ABCs) are an uncommon neurosurgical problem that may present as a rapidly growing mass mimicking a true neoplasm. They occur primarily in the first two decades of life (Saccomanni, 2007). Although ABCs usually involve the metaphysis of long bones, approximately 16% involve the spine and 4% involve the skull or mandible. When seen in the spine, they preferentially involve dorsal elements. The cause is unknown, however, some have been associated with prior fractures. They may also be seen as secondary lesions in various neoplastic and nonneoplastic conditions of bone, including giant cell tumor, chondroblastoma, chondromyxoid fibroma, nonossifying fibroma, osteoblastoma, fibrosarcoma, fibrous histiocytoma, osteosarcoma, and fibrous dysplasia (Martinez and Sissons, 1988). Curettage is the treatment of choice. However, there is a reported 20% recurrence rate.

Radiographic imaging suggests that these arise in the medullary cavity of bone, with the combination of features suggesting both osteolysis and

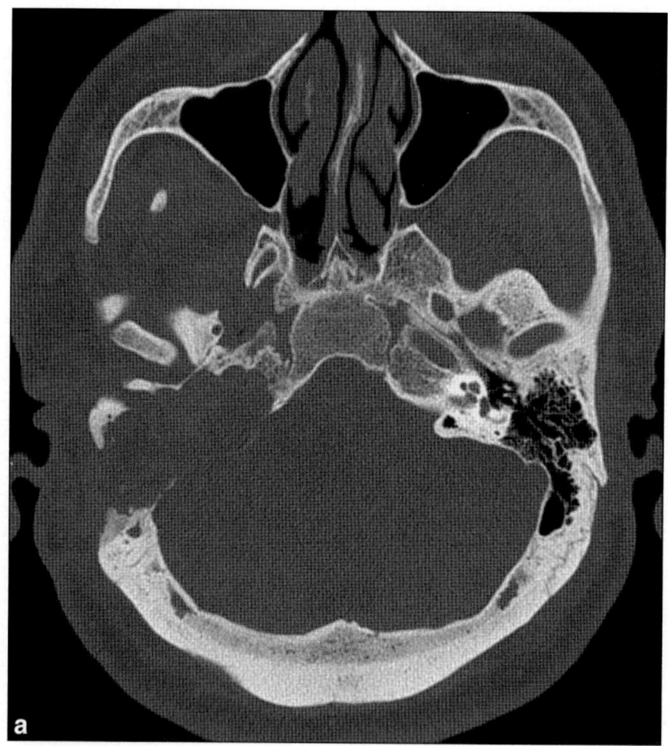

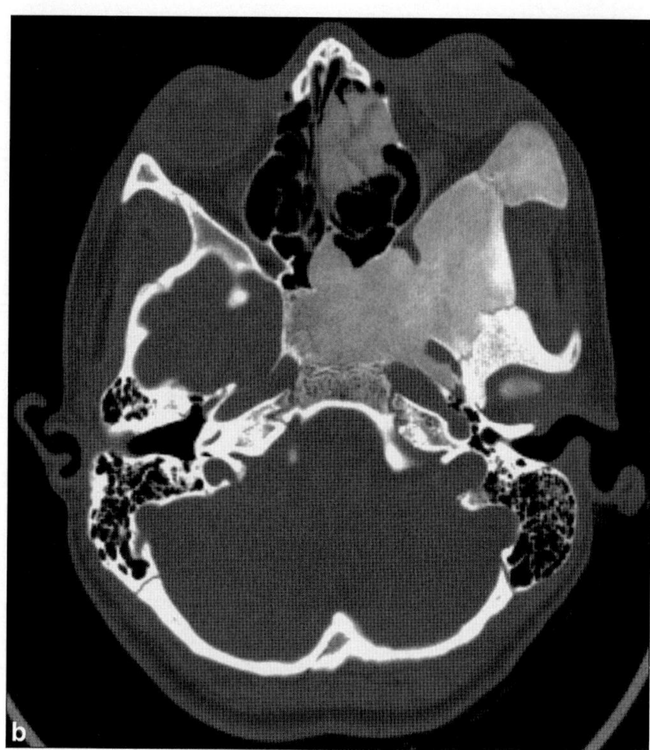

Figure 3.185. Fibrous dysplasia. (a) An axial CT image shows a lytic lesion centered within the petrous portion of the temporal bone. (b) In most cases, the CT appearance of fibrous dysplasia combined with the patient's clinical history is sufficient to permit a confident diagnosis and biopsy is avoided. Histopathology may be dominated by either the (c) spindle-cell parenchymal component, or (d) woven bone.

generation of new bone in the cyst wall (Figure 3.186a). A thin rim of residual subperiosteal bone may be noted. The expanded region of the cyst has a bubbly appearance and blood fluid levels may be noted. Internal septations may be noted by CT and MR imaging.

Figure 3.185. *continued.*

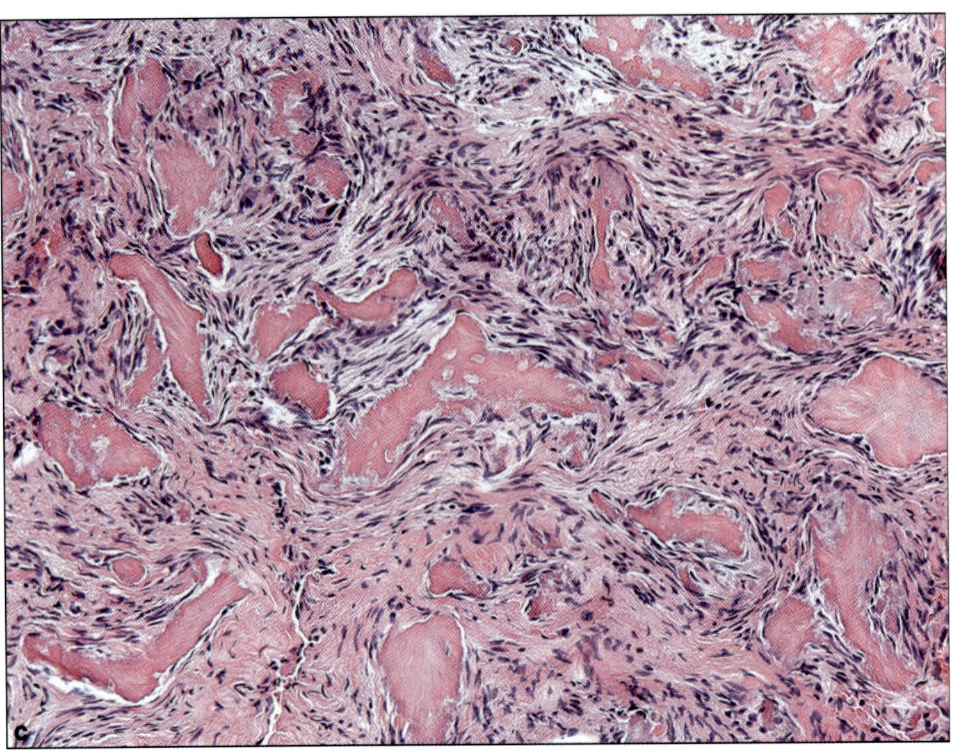

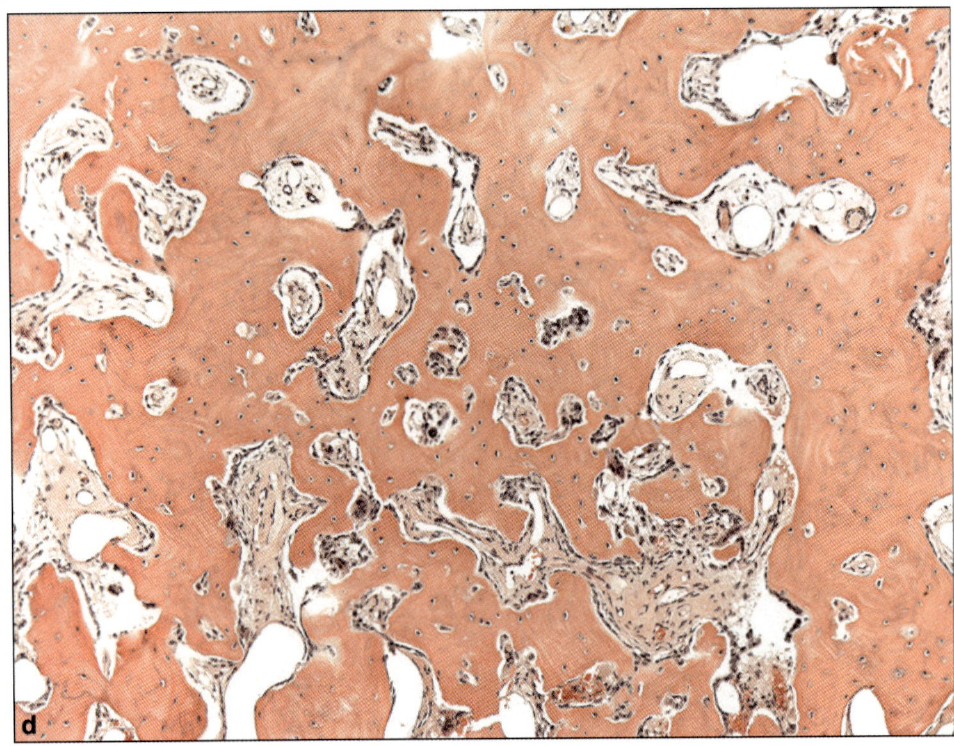

Pathology

ABCs are composed of blood or serum-filled cystic spaces separated by septae in which loosely arranged spindle cells are interspersed with benign giant cells (Figure 3.186b). A fine line of osteoid tissue may typically be found beneath

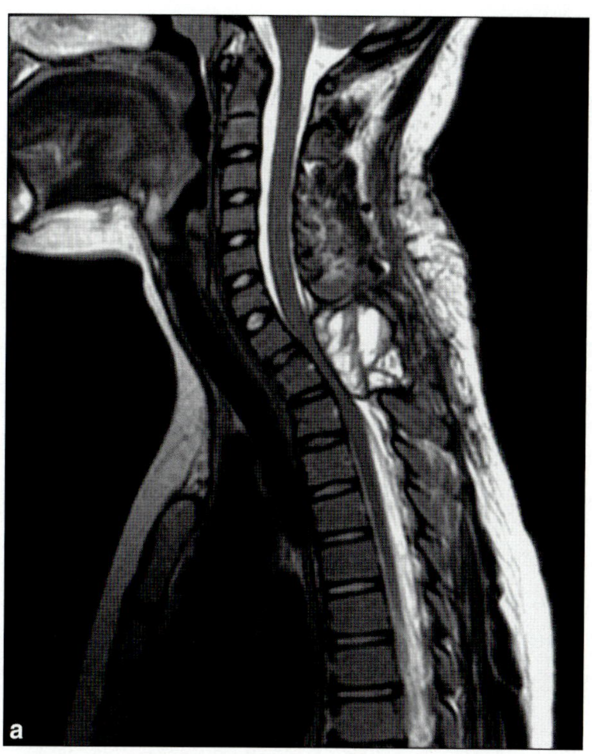

Figure 3.186. Aneurysmal bone cyst ABC. (a) Sagittal T2 MR image of the spine shows an expansile, fluid–fluid level containing mass with a narrow zone of transition in the neural arch of the first thoracic vertebra. There is cord compression. The fluid–fluid levels are the result of blood products and characteristic of an aneurysmal bone cyst. By MR, a telangiectatic osteogenic sarcoma could have a similar appearance. (b) Hemorrhagic lesion with focal organization and scattered giant cells.

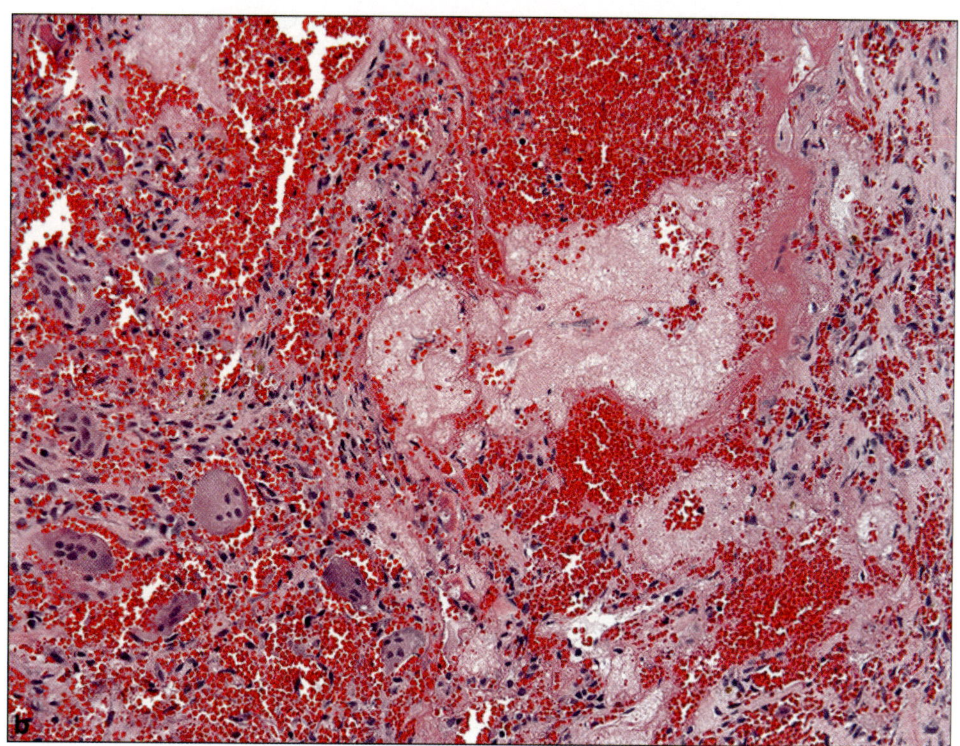

the lining of the septum. The cells lining the cysts are not endothelial. Solid areas are composed of spindle cells with prominent mitotic activity but no atypia. A noncystic type of ABC has been described (solid ABC) with solid areas composed of admixed spindle cells, giant cells, and osteoid.

Calcifying Pseudoneoplasm of the Neuraxis

Clinical and Radiological Features

This rare and enigmatic entity has been reported in several locations, apparently arising from the craniospinal meninges or spinal bones (Bertoni et al., 1990). The alternative and wholly nonspecific term of fibro-osseous lesion has also been applied to this entity. They are considered sporadic. Symptoms are referable to the compressive effect on the adjacent structures, including cranial nerves when occurring at the base of the skull. Excision is curative. Radiologically, these lesions are discrete densely calcified and exceedingly dense masses of the leptomeninges by CT imaging.

Pathology

These are discrete and friable masses, which may contain rock-hard elements. Microscopically they show a mixture of granular or fibrillar material with radial striations, dense calcification, and ossification, and a variable coating by meningothelial-like cells. A foreign body giant cell reaction may also be noted.

Crystal Arthropathy

Clinical and Radiological Features

Gout is a relatively common metabolic disorder usually affecting the distal joints of the appendicular skeleton, more common in males and usually associated with hyperuricemia. Tophaceous gout of the vertebra, particularly the facet joints and posterior column of the spine may mimic a diverse array of other pathological entities including infectious spondylodiscitis and epidural abscess on magnetic resonance imaging (Suk et al., 2007; Yen et al., 2005), or another destructive metastatic process (Cabot et al., 2005) The condition is only rarely responsible for cord compression.

Radiographic imaging shows homogeneous or heterogeneous peripheral enhancement gadolinium enhancement in MR imaging studies. Diffuse stippled calcifications may be found in the tophi by CT imaging (Hsu et al., 2002).

Pseudogout, a term applied to patients with calcium pyrophosphate crystal deposition disease, may also rarely affect the paraspinal joints (Fidler et al., 1996; Kinoshita et al., 1998).

Pathology

The continued deposition of monosodium urate crystals eventually results in tophaceous gout. Histologically, the resected tophi consist of large crystalline deposits surrounded by fibrous tissue and rimmed by histiocytes and giant cells (Figure 3.187). Routine processing will result in dissolving of the crystals, which are water soluble. However, examination of unstained sections by polarized

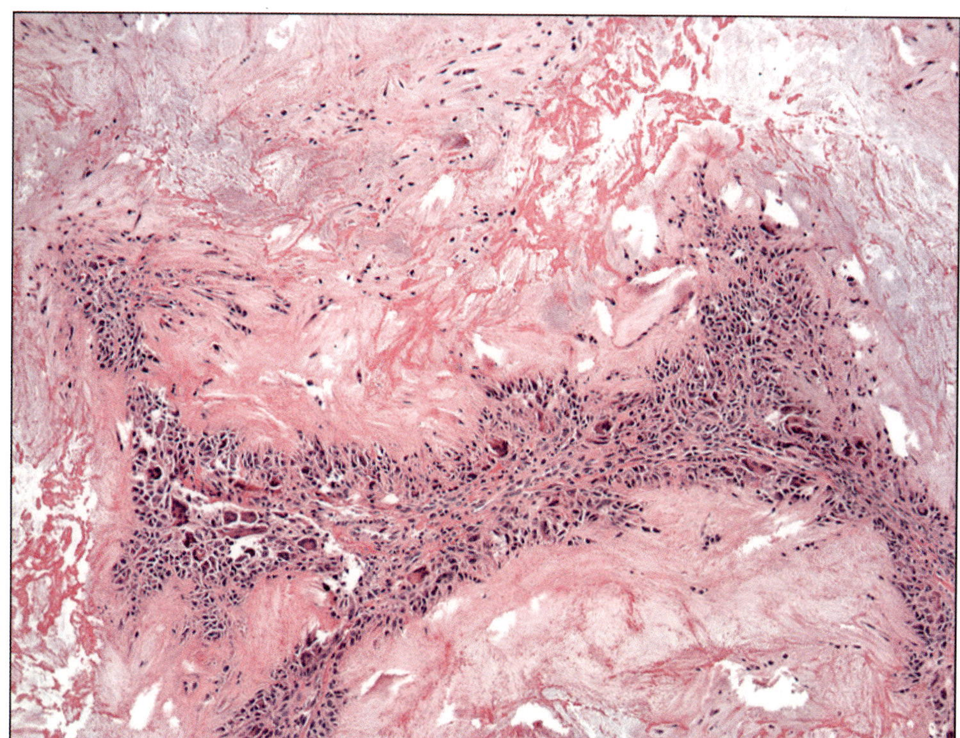

Figure 3.187. Gouty tophus, with acellular masses of amorphous material representing partically dissolved crystals surrounded by histiocytes and foreign body giant cells.

light will generally demonstrate crystalline nature of the deposits. In cases of *pseudogout*, chalky white deposits may be noted grossly, which upon microscopic examination show typical small rhomboidal crystals that are weakly birefringent.

HEMATOMA

Clinical Features

Spinal epidural hematomas may result from trauma, particularly following lumbar puncture for diagnostic or therapeutic purposes, rarely vascular malformations, and are potentiated by anticoagulation therapy. They are more common in adults and rare in children. Spinal epidural hematomas may have an acute compressive effect on the spinal cord and poor neurological outcome if not recognized and treated in a timely fashion. Any level of the spinal cord may be involved, depending upon the etiology. Spontaneous epidural spinal hematomas are believed to be more common in the dorsal space.

Pathology

The histology of hematomas is nonspecific regardless of the location, and findings depend upon the length of time the hematoma has undergone organization. Given appropriate clinical suspicion, an evacuated specimen may require close microscopic examination for elements of a vascular malformation.

Figure 3.188. Herniated nucleus pulposus, with characteristic myxoid degeneration of fibrocartilage and clusters of chondrocytes, sometimes called "chondrocyte cloning."

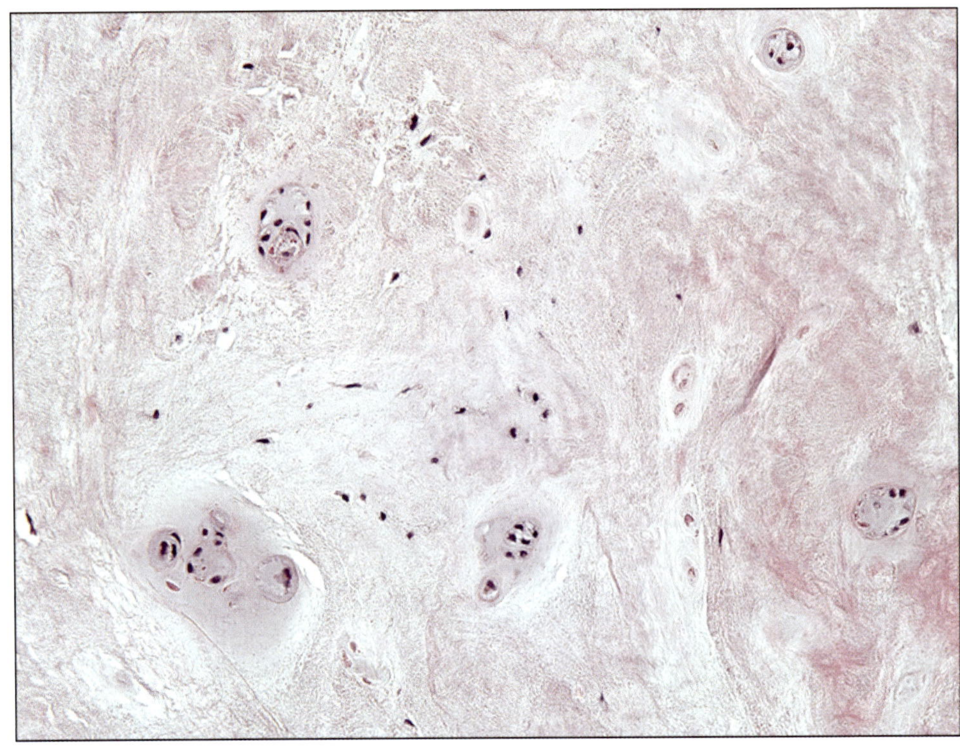

HERNIATED NUCLEUS PULPOSUS

Clinical Features

This is invariably a manifestation of aging and loss of structural and chemical integrity in intervertebral disks. Lumbar lesions far exceed those at other levels, followed by the cervical and lastly the thoracic spine.

Pathology

The typical surgical specimen displays a mixture of degenerating fibrocartilage and annulus fibrosus with focal microvascular proliferation, chondrocyte proliferation or "cloning," and necrosis (Figure 3.188).

LIGAMENTUM FLAVUM CYSTS

Clinical Features

These are a rare and distinctive type of benign cysts capable of spinal compression. A series of four cases in older adults showed exclusive occurrence in the lower lumbar region, with favorable outcomes after surgical intervention (DiMaio et al., 2005). Long-standing deterioration of the associated joint is considered to be the etiology.

Pathology

Histological sections may reveal ligamentum flavum with associated cystic degeneration and fibrosis, necrosis, and calcification in more advanced cases.

SPINAL DURAL ARTERIOVENOUS FISTULA

Clinical Features

Spinal dural arteriovenous fistulas are the commonest type of spinal vascular malformation. These arteriovenous shunts are located entirely outside the spinal cord, and cause chronic a progressive myelopathy believed to stem from the effects of increased venous pressure and impaired venous drainage on the spinal cord.

Pathology

A surgical biopsy of this entity would be exceedingly rare. However, a report of the spinal cord biopsy in a documented case of spinal dural arteriovenous fistula showed thickened and hyalinized blood vessels and degenerative changes of white matter attributed to the ischemic consequences of chronic focal venous congestion (Hurst et al., 1995).

SYNOVIAL CYST

Clinical Features

Synovial cysts are viewed as a degenerative phenomenon, thus the condition more frequently affects older adults. Symptoms most commonly include radicular pain and focal neurological deficits. It is believed that synovial cysts are associated with facet joint osteoarthritis but not with degenerative disk disease. The lumbar region is most commonly affected, followed by the cervical region, then the thoracic region, in which synovial cysts are distinctly rare.

Pathology

Recognizable synovium is not always readily apparent in histologic sections. A fibrous wall may predominate but the collapsed and furthermore, the fragmented nature of the specimen, may not suggest a cystic lesion. When synovium is present, it is often hyperplastic and sometimes inflamed (Figure 3.189).

MALFORMATIONS

Meningocele and Myelomeningocele

Clinical Features

Meningocele refers to herniation of meningeal tissue, with the additional component of spinal cord tissue in myelomeningocele, through a vertebral defect. These are immediately apparent at birth or may have been diagnosed prenatally through the detection of elevated serum or amniotic fluid alpha-fetoprotein, the hallmark albeit not specific, of a neural tube defect, followed by imaging in utero.

Myelomeningocele may occur at any level, but lumbosacral lesions are the most frequent and are almost always associated with a Chiari type II malformation and hydrocephalus. Lesions above the 12th thoracic vertebra may

Figure 3.189. Synovial cyst. Many surgical specimens may not include any recognizable synovial lining, and when present may show the effects of chronic inflammation.

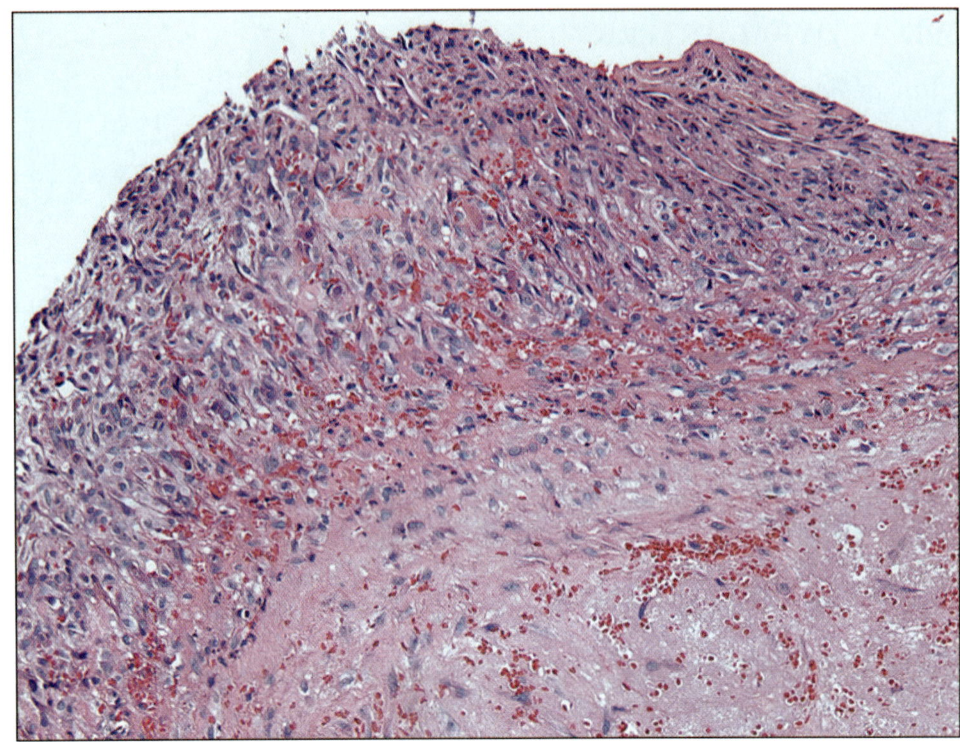

Figure 3.190. Meningocele specimen with central defect, which prior to resection and closure of the defect, had surrounded exposed lumbosacral neural tissue.

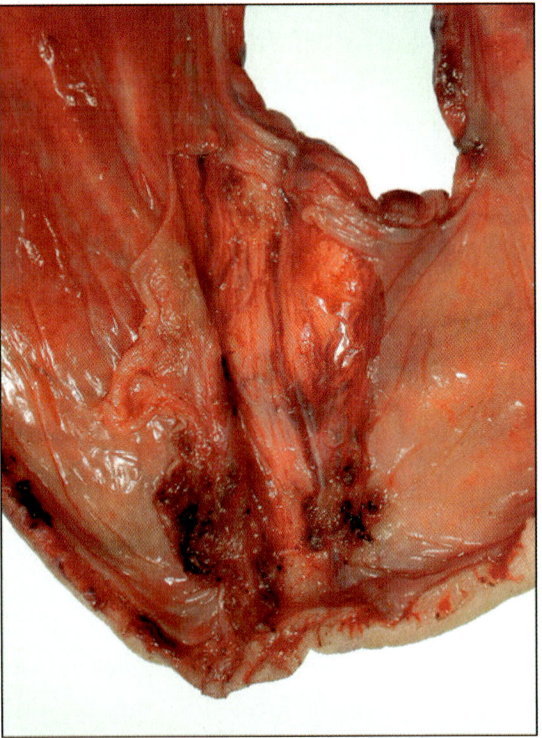

be associated with malformations in other systems, more severe neurological deficits, and are more common in females (Ellison and Love, 2004). Meningoceles do not have protrusion of spinal cord, however, it may bear abnormalities such as hydromyelia, splitting, or tethering.

Pathology

The surgical specimen will often show the macroscopic features of the lesion before excision, mainly an ovoid hyperemic lesion covered by a delicate membrane (Figure 3.190). Sectioning of the central lesion may display elements of the myelocele, namely disorganized neural tissue accompanied by islands of glial and ependymal tissue, and ectatic irregular vascular connective tissue. The surrounding skin lacks rete pegs and skin appendages.

Tethered Spinal Cord

Clinical and Radiological Features

This entity is represented by progressive neurological dysfunction such as urinary incontinence, mixed motor and sensory deficits, orthopedic abnormalities of the lower extremities including foot deformities, gait difficulty, and spasticity. It is often suspected when a sacral cutaneous abnormality such as hypertrichosis, cutaneous hemangioma, or lipoma is detected. Tethered cord may escape detection until well into adulthood.

Imaging abnormalities include laminar defects and malformations, a scoliotic or lordotic deformity, and others (Bui et al., 2007). Spinal cord motion studies may reveal the absence of the characteristic pulsatile movement of the spinal cord with heart beats.

Pathology

The neurosurgical specimen consists of a small fragment of fibrous tissue representing the excision of the distal filum terminale. Microscopy will show a predominance of fibrous tissue with possible nerve twigs and ependymal cell aggregates (Figure 3.191).

Encephalocele

Clinical and Radiological Features

Encephalocele is defined as the herniation of brain tissue through a skull defect, most commonly in the occipital region and less frequently in the parietal or frontoethmoidal areas. Some occipital encephaloceles are a component of Meckel syndrome, which also includes polydactyly and polycystic kidneys. The herniated mass is totally or partially covered by normal skin and hair and is attached to one hemisphere by and narrow pedicle.

MR imaging is considered the procedure of choice in radiographically demonstrating protrusion of brain tissue or at least the opening associated with an encephalocele, thus distinguishing them from completely extracranial masses such as a dermoid cysts (Lusk and Lee, 1986) or an anterior nasal glioma.

Figure 3.191. Tethered spinal cord. A typical surgical resection consists of a band of tissue with an admixture of fibroadipose tissues, possibly ependymal elements and some nerve twigs.

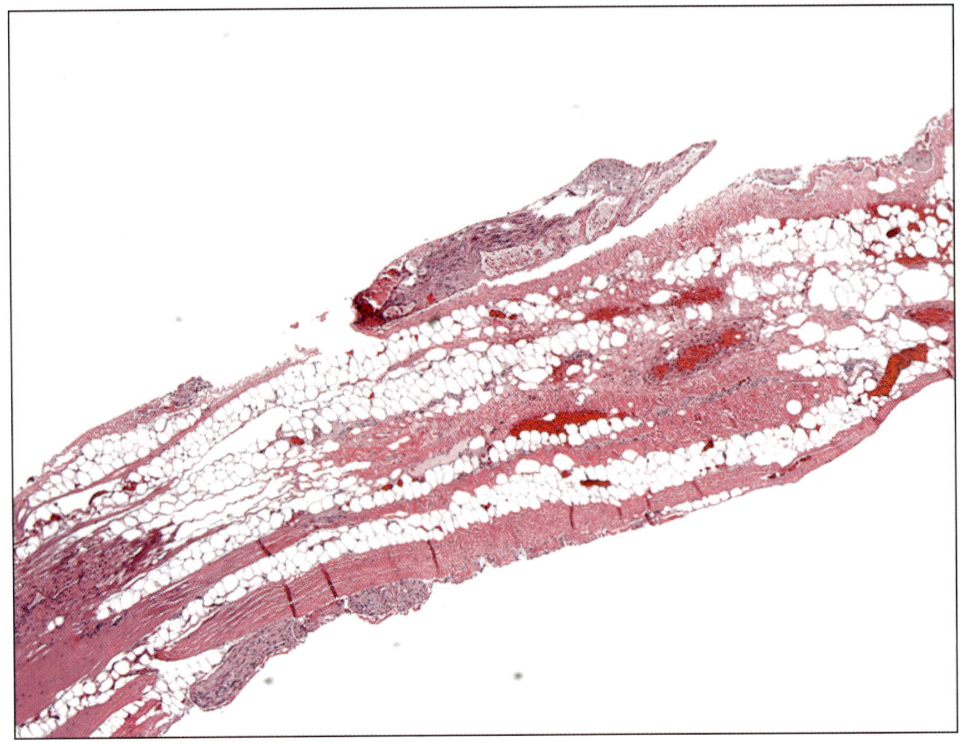

Pathology

The tissue components of an encephalocele may range from disorganized fibrous meningeal and vascular tissue to brain tissue with a disordered laminar pattern and even a ventricular space that connects with an intracranial ventricle.

REFERENCES

Bertoni F, Unni KK, Dahlin DC, Beabout JW, Onofrio BM. Calcifying pseudoneo-plasms of the neural axis. *J Neurosurg* 1990; 72: 42–8.

Bui CJ, Tubbs RS, Oakes WJ. Tethered cord syndrome in children: a review. *Neurosurg Focus* 2007; 23: 1–9.

Cabot J, Mosel L, Kong A, Hayward M. Tophaceous gout in the cervical spine. *Skeletal Radiol* 2005; 34: 803–6.

Cohen ZR, Marmor E, Fuller GN, DeMonte F. Misdiagnosis of olfactory neuroblas-toma. *Neurosurg Focus* 2002; 12: e3.

Devaney KO, Ferlito A, Rinaldo A. Endolymphatic sac tumor (low-grade papillary adenocarcinoma) of the temporal bone. *Acta Otolaryngol* 2003; 123: 1022–6.

DiMaio S, Marmor E, Albrecht S, Mohr G. Ligamentum flavum cysts causing incapa-citating lumbar spinal stenosis. *Can J Neurol Sci* 2005; 32: 237–42.

Ellison D, Love S. *Neuropathology: A Reference Text of CNS Pathology*. Edinburgh, New York: Mosby, 2004.

Fidler WK, Dewar CL, Fenton PV. Cervical spine pseudogout with myelopathy and Charcot joints. *J Rheumatol* 1996; 23: 1445–8.

Gogia N, Marwaha V, Atri S, Gulati M, Gupta R. Fibrous dysplasia localized to spine: a diagnostic dilemma. *Skeletal Radiol* 2007; 36 Suppl. 1: S19–23.

Horiguchi H, Sano T, Toi H, Kageji T, Hirokawa M, Nagahiro S. Endolymphatic sac tumor associated with a von Hippel–Lindau disease patient: an immunohistochemical study. *Mod Pathol* 2001; 14: 727–32.

Hsu CY, Shih TT, Huang KM, Chen PQ, Sheu JJ, Li YW. Tophaceous gout of the spine: MR imaging features. *Clin Radiol* 2002; 57: 919–25.

Hurst RW, Kenyon LC, Lavi E, Raps EC, Marcotte P. Spinal dural arteriovenous fistula: the pathology of venous hypertensive myelopathy. *Neurology* 1995; 45: 1309–13.

Joseph BV, Chacko G, Raghuram L, Rajshekhar V. Endolymphatic sac tumor: a rare cerebellopontine angle tumor. *Neurol India* 2002; 50: 476–9.

Kinoshita T, Maruoka S, Yamazaki T, Sakamoto K. Tophaceous pseudogout of the cervical spine: MR imaging and bone scintigraphy findings. *Eur J Radiol* 1998; 27: 271–3.

Luk IS, Chan JK, Chow SM, Leung S. Pituitary adenoma presenting as sinonasal tumor: pitfalls in diagnosis. *Hum Pathol* 1996; 27: 605–9.

Lusk RP, Lee PC. Magnetic resonance imaging of congenital midline nasal masses. *Otolaryngol Head Neck Surg* 1986; 95: 303–6.

Martinez V, Sissons HA. Aneurysmal bone cyst. A review of 123 cases including primary lesions and those secondary to other bone pathology. *Cancer* 1988; 61: 2291–304.

Mehnert F, Beschorner R, Kuker W, Hahn U, Nagele T. Retroclival ecchordosis physaliphora: MR imaging and review of the literature. *AJNR Am J Neuroradiol* 2004; 25: 1851–5.

Muzumdar DP, Goel A, Fattepurkar S, Goel N. Endolymphatic sac carcinoma of the right petrous bone in Von Hippel-Lindau disease. *J Clin Neurosci* 2006; 13: 471–4.

Rotondo M, Natale M, Mirone G, Cirillo M, Conforti R, Scuotto A. A rare symptomatic presentation of ecchordosis physaliphora: neuroradiological and surgical management. *J Neurol Neurosurg Psychiatry* 2007; 78: 647–9.

Saccomanni B. Aneurysmal bone cyst of spine: a review of literature. *Arch Orthop Trauma Surg* 2008; 128: 1145–7.

Suk KS, Kim KT, Lee SH, Park SW, Park YK. Tophaceous gout of the lumbar spine mimicking pyogenic discitis. *Spine J* 2007; 7: 94–9.

Wolfe JT, 3rd, Scheithauer BW. "Intradural chordoma" or "giant ecchordosis physaliphora"? Report of two cases. *Clin Neuropathol* 1987; 6: 98–103.

Yen PS, Lin JF, Chen SY, Lin SZ. Tophaceous gout of the lumbar spine mimicking infectious spondylodiscitis and epidural abscess: MR imaging findings. *J Clin Neurosci* 2005; 12: 44–6.

CNS-RELATED SOFT TISSUE TUMORS

Josef Záměčník and Hannes Vogel

ADIPOSE TUMORS

Intracranial and Spinal Lipomas

Clinical Features

Intracranial lipomas carry an incidence ranging from 0.1% to 0.5% of all brain tumors and generally occur at midline sites such as the anterior corpus callosum, choroid plexus, quadrigeminal plate, and base of the brain (Eghwrudjakpor et al., 1991), clinically manifesting as epilepsy in some cases (Loddenkemper et al.,

Figure 3.192. Classic lipoma of the corpus callosum. A sagittal T1-weighted MR image shows a curvilinear, high signal intensity mass in the interhemispheric fissure, consistent with a lipoma. The splenium of the corpus callosum is focally hypoplastic. Other lipid-containing intracranial masses, such as dermoids and teratomas, occur; however, the characteristic location and commonly associated dysgenisis of the corpus callosum almost always permits a confident imaging-based diagnosis of a corpus callosum lipoma.

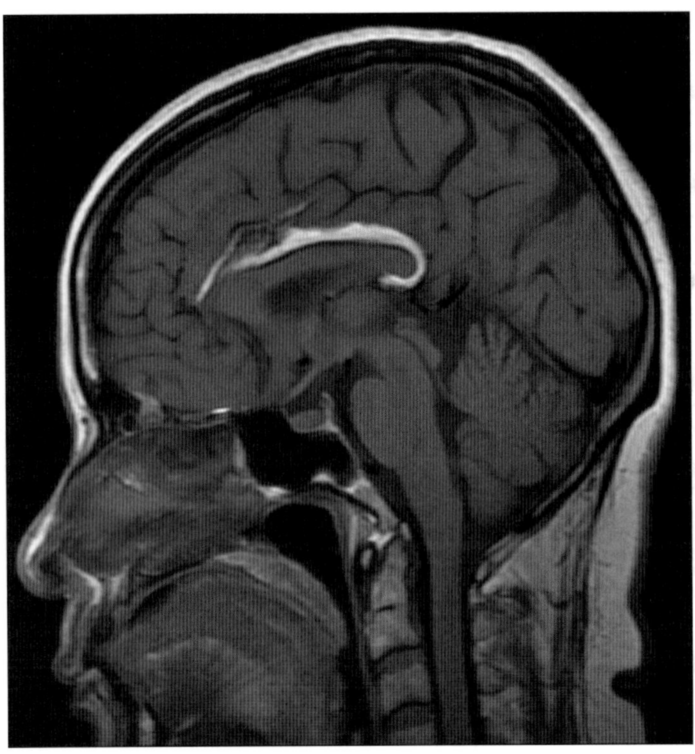

2006). Intracranial lipomas can also be associated with a wide spectrum of brain malformations, the most important being corpus callosum agenesis or dysgenesis (Donati et al., 1992) (Figure 3.192). A separate distinct entity is the lipoma of the internal auditory canal, which manifests due to focal mass effect. Intracranial lipomas usually do not require surgical resection.

Spinal lipomas are also commonly found in the lumbosacral region and are frequently associated with caudal dysraphic neural tube defects and thus may be termed lipomeningocele or similar appropriate designation. They are sometimes associated with the clinical entity of tethered spinal cord or a sacral sinus tract connecting the midline subcutis with the caudal spinal region. Surgical resection of caudal lipomas occurs as part of reparative surgical procedures such as untethering of the filum terminale.

Pathology

Lipomas are characterized by the presence of mature adipose tissue, often lobulated in appearance with delicate but prominent microvasculature (Budka, 1974; Harrison et al., 1990; Truwit and Barkovich, 1990). Spinal examples are often encapsulated.

Angiolipoma

Clinical Features

Angiolipomas are extremely rare intracranial tumors, have a female predominance, and are associated with seizures or progressive neurological deficits due to mass effect, or rarely with subarachnoid hemorrhage (Pirotte et al., 1998; Vilela et al., 2005). They appear to have a predilection for the sellar area (Lach and Lesiuk, 1994). Spinal extradural angiolipomas are also distinctly rare, generally occurring as a localized lesion causing progressive neurological impairment and back pain, sometimes also with subarachnoid hemorrhage (Raghavendra et al., 2007). As such, angiolipomas are generally either dorsolateral or ventrolateral to the spinal dura, sometimes with bony involvement or spinal root compression.

Angiolipomas are considered either noninfiltrating or infiltrating. Both types are considered benign but can be locally destructive of bone, muscle, neural, and connective tissues.

Pathology

Grossly, angiolipomas are typically white to yellow in appearance with a red tinge. Angiolipomas are composed of mature adipocytes and vascular channels. The vascular component often contains fibrin thrombi, which are absent in typical epidural lipomas. Infiltrating examples can be distinguished from noninfiltrating lesions by the absence of a well-circumscribed capsule. Angiomyolipomas are a variant of angiolipoma characterized by vascular smooth muscle proliferation.

Liposarcoma

Clinical Features

Liposarcoma has been described as either a dural or a leptomeningeal lesion (Kothandaram, 1970; Sima et al., 1976). As with all sarcomatous lesions of the brain or dura, a metastatic process must be carefully excluded.

Pathology

A histological spectrum exists for liposarcoma ranging from well differentiated to dedifferentiated, myxoid, and pleomorphic liposarcomas. The pathology of the most reported cases appears to be that of well-differentiated liposarcoma. Intracranial examples should be considered part of liposarcomatous differentiation in a glioblastoma or a metastatic lesion until proven otherwise.

Hibernoma

Clinical Features

This entity is exceedingly rare within the central nervous system having only been reported in the intradural extraaxial spinal cord.

Pathology

This tumor is composed of adipose tissue cells resembling brown fat, and thus appear as sheets or lobules of finely microvacuolated cells (Figure 3.193) (Chitoku et al., 1998).

Figure 3.193. Hibernoma.

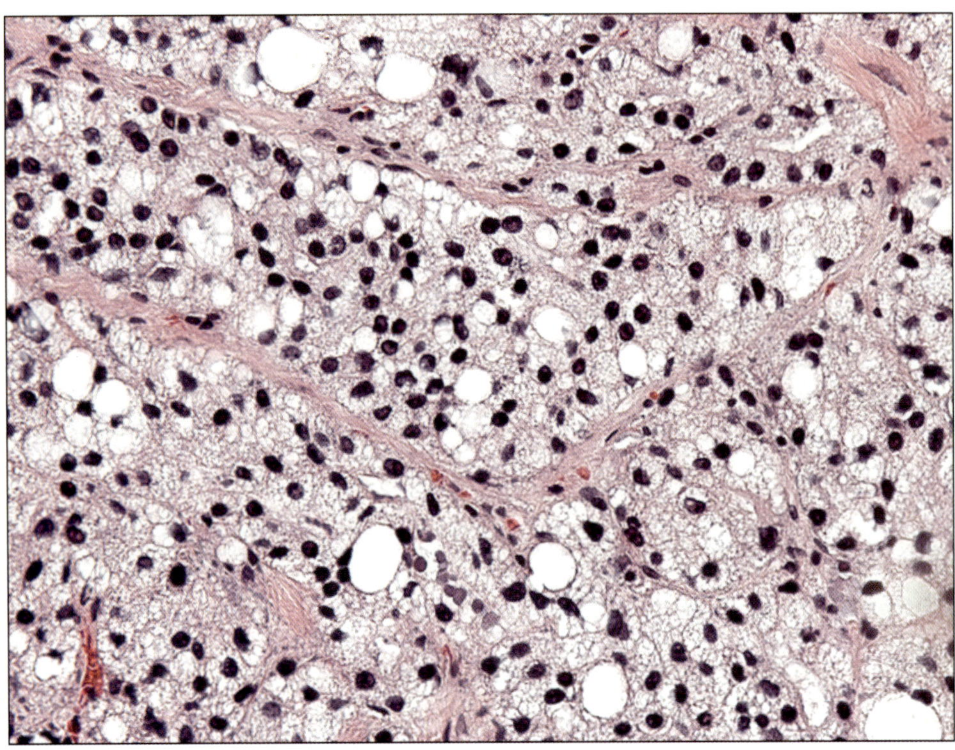

Figure 3.194. Epidural lipomatosis. A sagittal T1-weighted MR image of the lumbar spine shows abundant adipose tissue in the epidural space (arrow). Epidural lipomatosis usually occurs in the midthoracic and lower lumbar spine and can contribute to spinal stenosis.

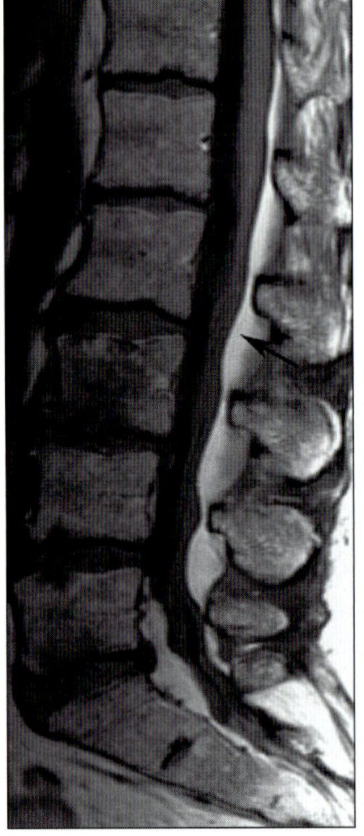

Epidural Lipomatosis

Clinical and Radiological Features

This condition is seen as a diffuse hypertrophy or enlargement of spinal epidural adipose tissue (Figure 3.194) and is a rare complication of steroid therapy (Quint et al., 1988), obesity, or endogenous steroid excess (Fogel et al., 2005) but has also been reported as idiopathic (Akhaddar et al., 2008; Fan et al., 2004; Shah et al., 2005). The condition reportedly occurs most frequently in the thoracic cord and causes compressive myelopathic or radiculopathic symptoms. Surgical decompression is occasionally required and the condition may partially abate with lessening of steroid dosage.

Pathology

The histological appearance of this lesion would be indistinguishable from that of benign adipose tissue.

FIBROUS TUMORS

Fibromatosis

Clinical Features

Fibromatosis, sometimes referred to as desmoid tumor, is a rare cause of an intracranial mass or spinal cord compression (Friede and Pollak, 1979; Mitchell et al., 1991; Rutigliano et al., 1994). They occur more often in adolescents or adults. They probably occur as a subset of head and neck fibromatosis, which accounts for almost one-fourth of extraabdominal fibromatosis. This exceedingly rare condition has only been described as a circumferential epidural mass extending from the cervical to thoracic levels with a poorly circumscribed mass in the left side of the neck, and as a rapidly growing cervical paraspinous mass in a 19-month-old female (Kriss and Warf, 1994).

Pathology

Grossly, these occur as an infiltrative lesion involving fascia, periosteum, or muscles. The cut surface is gritty with a course trabeculated appearance. Microscopy shows broad, elongated fascicles of pale eosinophilic fibroblasts and myofibroblasts with collagenous, focally hyalinized, or myxoid stroma. Muscle infiltration is common. The cellularity and mitotic activity varies. The tumor cells show variable actin and desmin immunopositivity.

Cranial Fasciitis

Clinical Features and Radiological Features

Cranial fasciitis is a rare, self-limiting fibroblastic process of the superficial and deep fascia. This occurs most commonly in children as a cranial or extracranial mass that manifests as a rapidly growing nodule in the head and neck region (Figure 3.195) (Hussein, 2008; Sarangarajan and Dehner, 1999). Accompanying

Figure 3.195. Cranial fasciitis. A coronal T1-weighted image shows a heterogeneously enhancing, well-demarcated mass centered within the left epidural space and displacing the cerebellum medially. Laterally, the mass extends into the subcutaneous tissues.

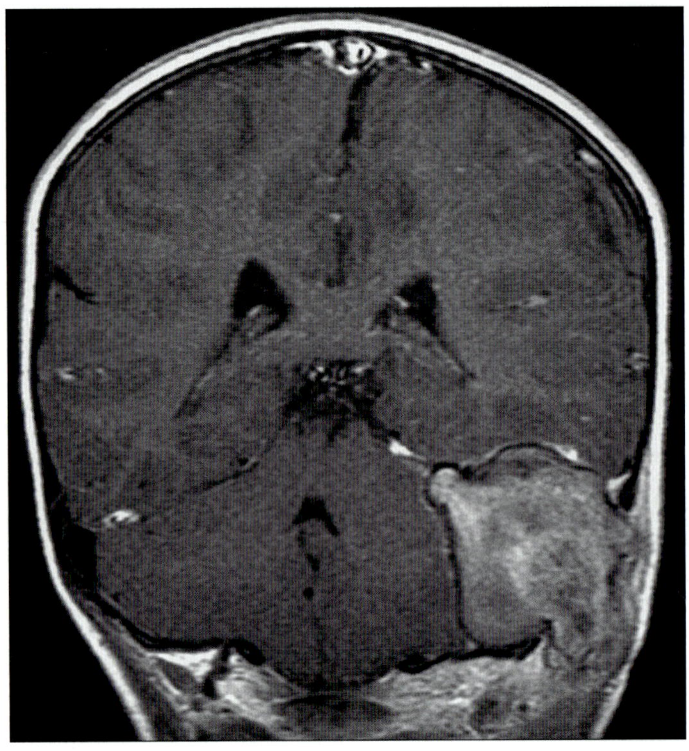

Figure 3.196. (a) Cranial fasciitis, composed of spindle cells in a fibromyxoid matrix, (b) in which mitotic activity may be readily apparent. (c) Cells may be immunoreactive for smooth muscle actin.

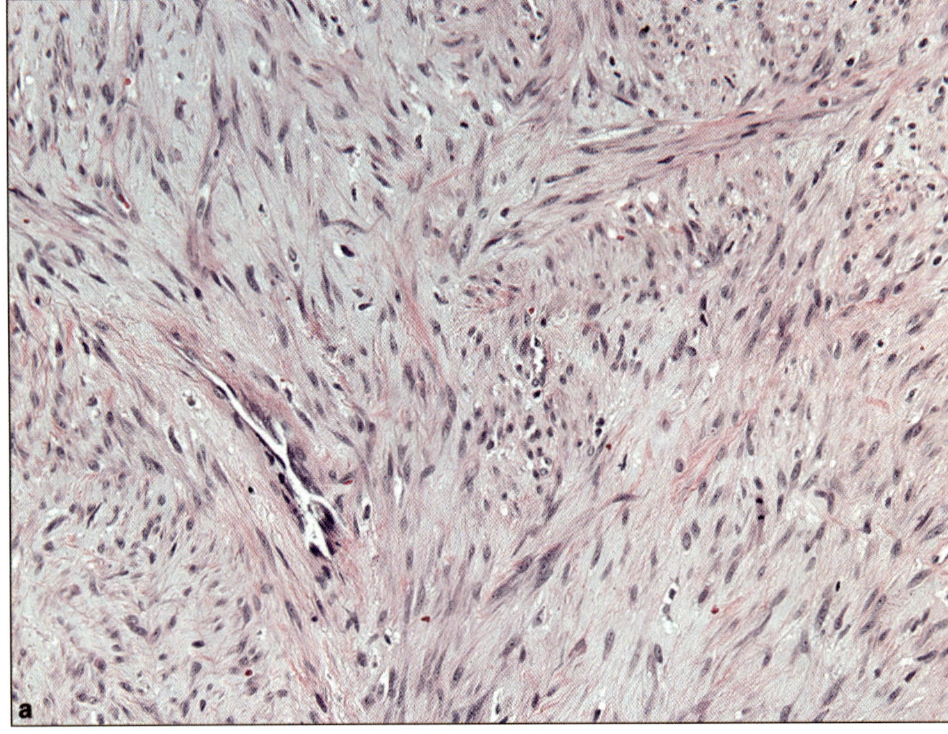

bony erosion is commonly noted. Although most cases of cranial fasciitis are reported to occur spontaneously in the very young, some cases involved older patients as lesions that developed at prior craniotomy sites in a delayed fashion (Summers et al., 2007).

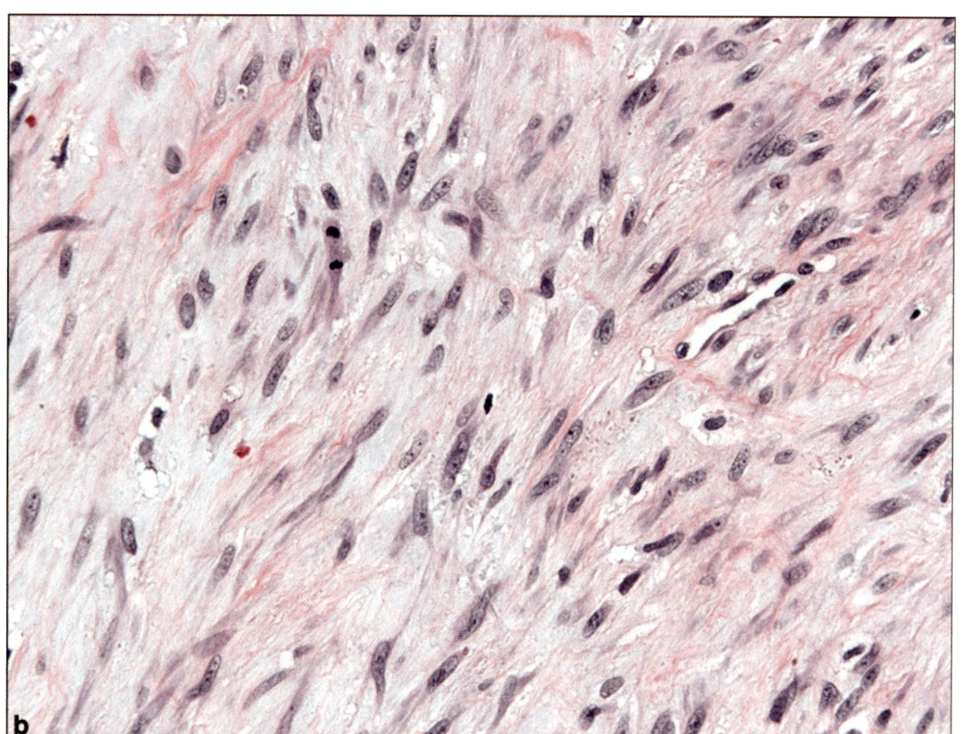

Figure 3.196. *continued.*

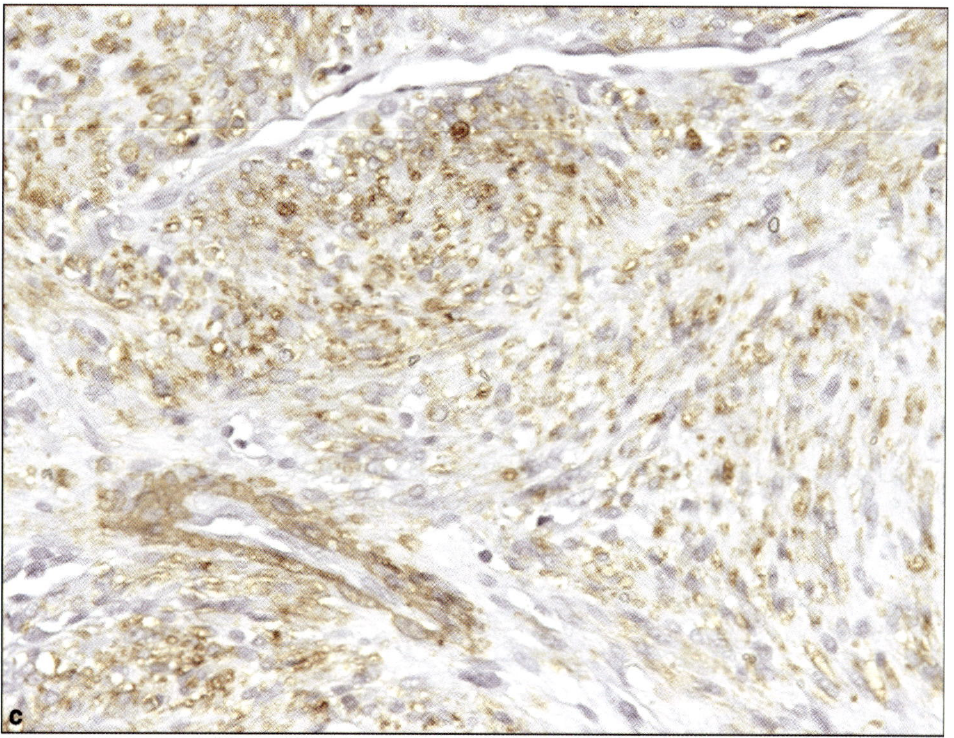

Pathology

The pathologic features are considered to be identical to those of nodular fasciitis – mitotically active spindle-shaped cells embedded in a myxoid matrix with occasionally extravasated erythrocytes (Figure 3.196). The lesional cells may be immunoreactive for smooth muscle actin.

Solitary Fibrous Tumor

Clinical Features

This entity is a well-known mimic of meningiomas of both the spinal and intracranial meninges. It occurs between the teens and seventh decade, most frequently in the fifth decade with a slight predominance in females. MRI shows uniform contrast enhancement with peritumoral edema, therefore is of essentially no use in distinguishing these from meningiomas by neuroradiology.

Some solitary fibrous tumors were probably previously recognized as fibrous meningiomas. Contemporary classification of this tumor (Fletcher et al., 2002) includes cases previously diagnosed as hemangiopericytoma, a well-recognized tumor by that name of the dura although they are clearly fibroblastic, rather than pericytic in nature (Gengler and Guillou, 2006) and lipomatous hemangiopericytoma, more rarely recognized as an intracranial tumor.

Pathology

Typical solitary fibrous tumors show a patternless architecture of variable cellularity separated by thick bands of hyalinized collagen (Figure 3.197). The branching or "staghorn" blood vessels commonly associated with hemangiopericytomas may be seen. The cells are round to spindle-shaped, monotonous without atypical features and in a syncytial background, thus providing occasional difficulty in distinguishing these from fibrous meningiomas (see page 205). Necrosis is usually absent. Mitotic figures are sparse except in malignant examples containing greater than four mitoses per ten high-power fields, along with infiltrative margins and cytological atypia (Gold et al., 2002).

Valuable diagnostic support lies in immunohistochemistry, demonstrating almost invariable positivity for CD34 and CD99, but negativity for S-100, actin, and desmin. However, immunohistochemical analysis can be frustrating in that a minority may show weak expression of EMA. Although CD34 immunopositivity was noted in some meningiomas, it is not as strong and diffuse as in solitary fibrous tumors.

Inflammatory Myofibroblastic Tumor

Clinical Features

This neoplasm was once considered either synonymous with inflammatory pseudotumor or plasma cell granuloma but is now recognized as a true neoplasm (Coffin et al., 1998) because of the demonstration of associated anaplastic lymphoma kinase (ALK) fusion genes. One series shows a male predominance with a wide age range (Coffin et al., 1995). They may appear in imaging studies as either a plaquelike lesion or discrete mass of the dura.

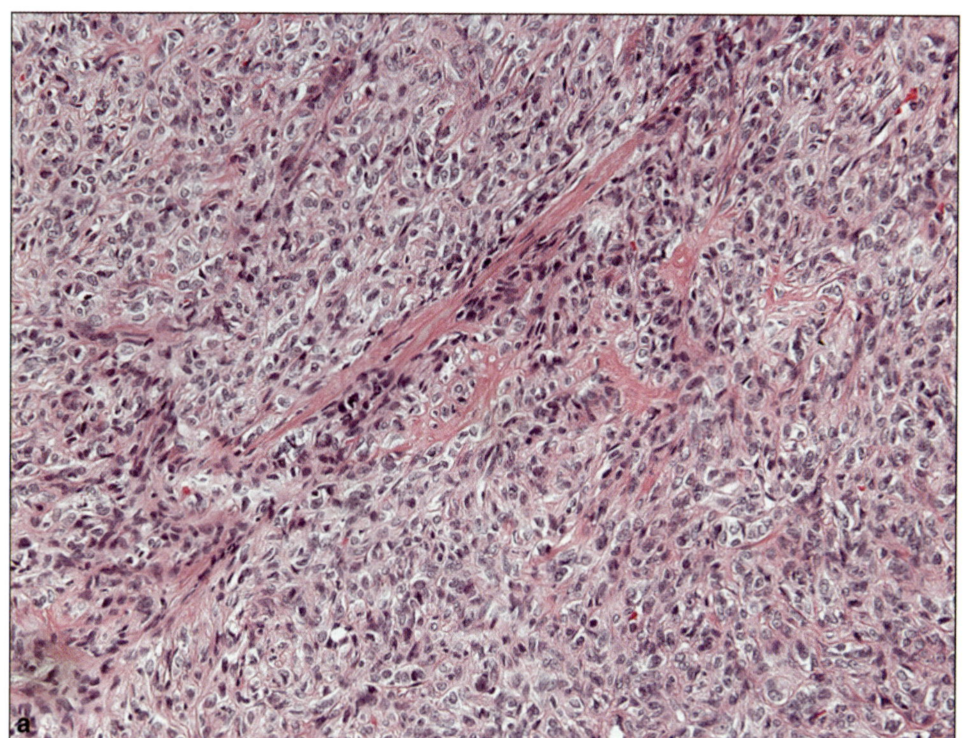

Figure 3.197. (a) Aggregates of ovoid and spindle cells of solitary fibrous tumor. (b) Immunostaining for CD34 may show tumor cell positivity as well as outline the distinctive blood vessels.

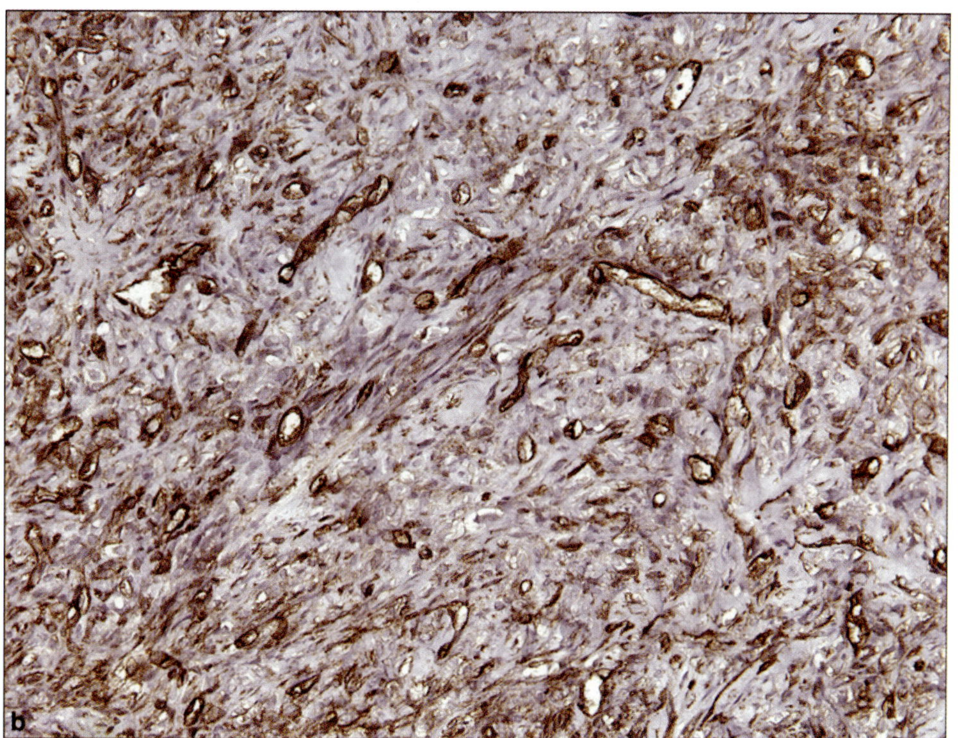

Late recurrence may occur in a minority of cases. There is small risk of metastasis, which is however difficult to predict based on histopathological features. Proliferative and apoptotic immunohistochemical markers do not correlate well with morphology or outcome. ALK reactivity is associated with local recurrence; on the other hand, absent ALK expression is associated with

Figure 3.198. Inflammatory myofibroblastic tumor, demonstrating elements predominated by (a) inflammatory cells, (b) admixed fibroblasts, and (c) myofibroblasts.

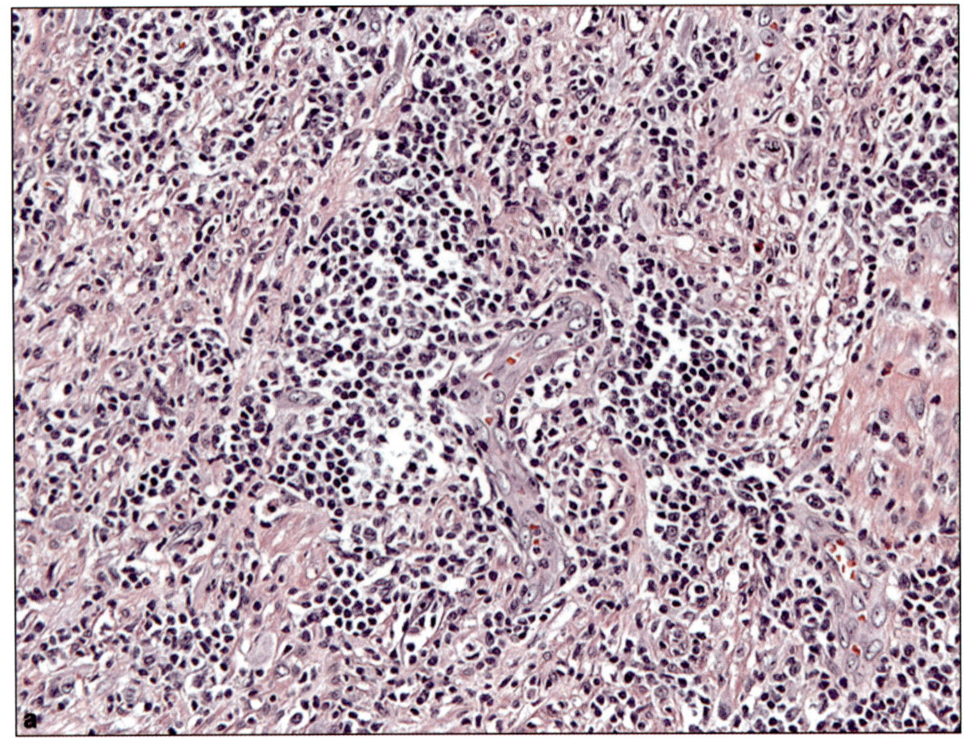

distant metastases in younger patients. Thus, ALK reactivity may be considered a favorable prognostic indicator (Coffin et al., 2007).

Pathology

Three basic histological patterns are seen in this tumor depending upon the relative contribution of the three respective cytological components of inflammatory myofibroblastic tumors: spindled myofibroblasts, admixed fibroblasts, and inflammatory cells (Figure 3.198). An edematous myxoid background may exist with abundant blood vessels and an infiltrate dominated by plasma cells, but containing also lymphocytes and eosinophils resembling granulation tissue or other reactive processes. A compact spindle-cell proliferation may be seen, resembling fibromatosis or smooth muscle neoplasm and the third pattern resembles a scar or desmoid-like fibromatosis with sparse inflammation. ALK immunopositivity occurs in less than 50% of inflammatory myofibroblastic tumors, which may be complemented by fluorescence in situ hybridization for ALK rearrangements, believed to occur mainly in children (Jeon et al., 2005).

Fibrosarcoma

Clinical Features

This rare tumor reported as an intracranial tumor apparently arising from the leptomeninges is nonetheless the second most common type of intracranial primary sarcoma (Oliveira et al., 2002) with a distribution similar to that of meningioma. Some may occur in childhood but the majority have been

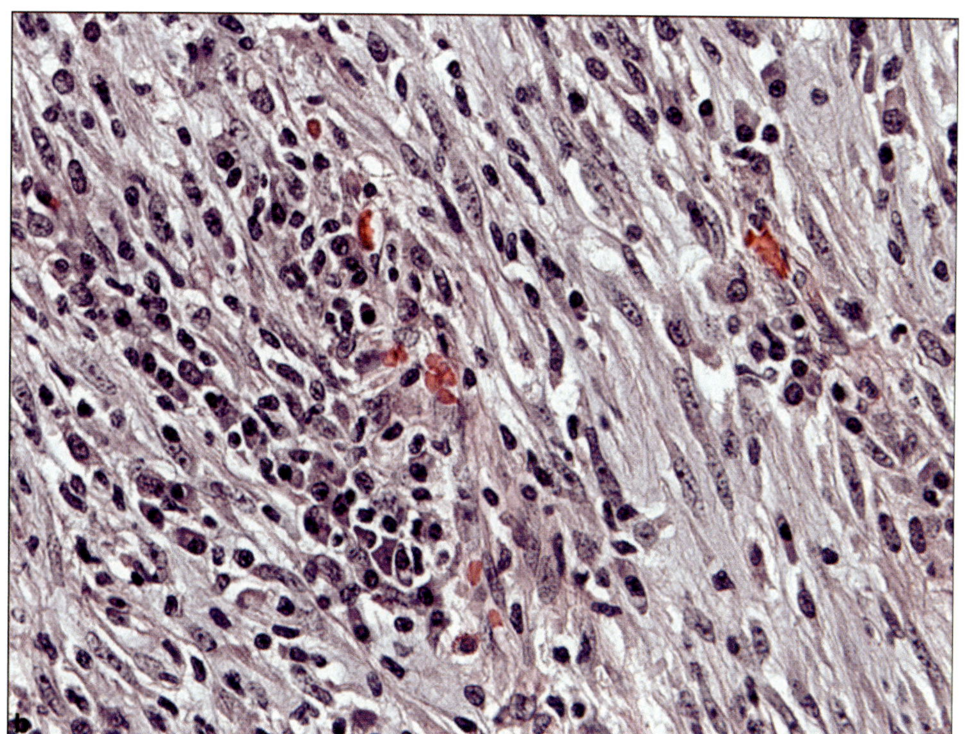

Figure 3.198. *continued.*

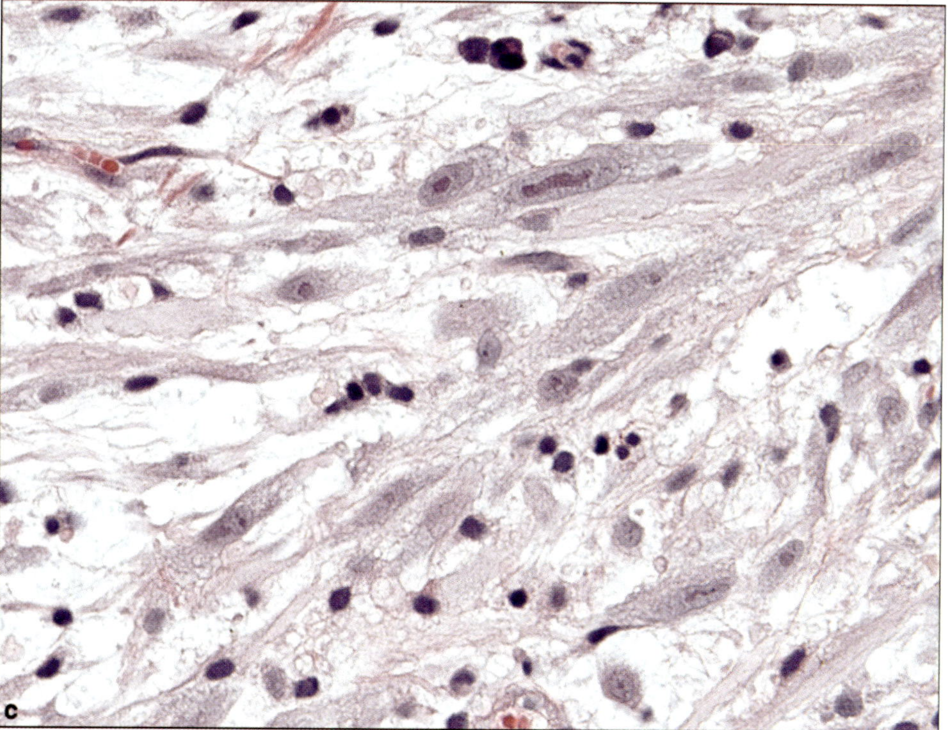

reported in adults (Cai and Kahn, 2004). There is a distinct tendency for local recurrence, or even metastasis and meningeal seeding (Gaspar et al., 1993).

Pathology

Fibrosarcoma typically shows a herringbone pattern of spindle cells in long bundles, with marked cellularity and mitotic activity, often with areas of

Figure 3.199. Fibrosarcoma, a malignant spindle cell neoplasm that may arise in the CNS-associated soft tissues but must be distinguished from malignant solitary fibrous tumor or metastatic fibrosarcoma.

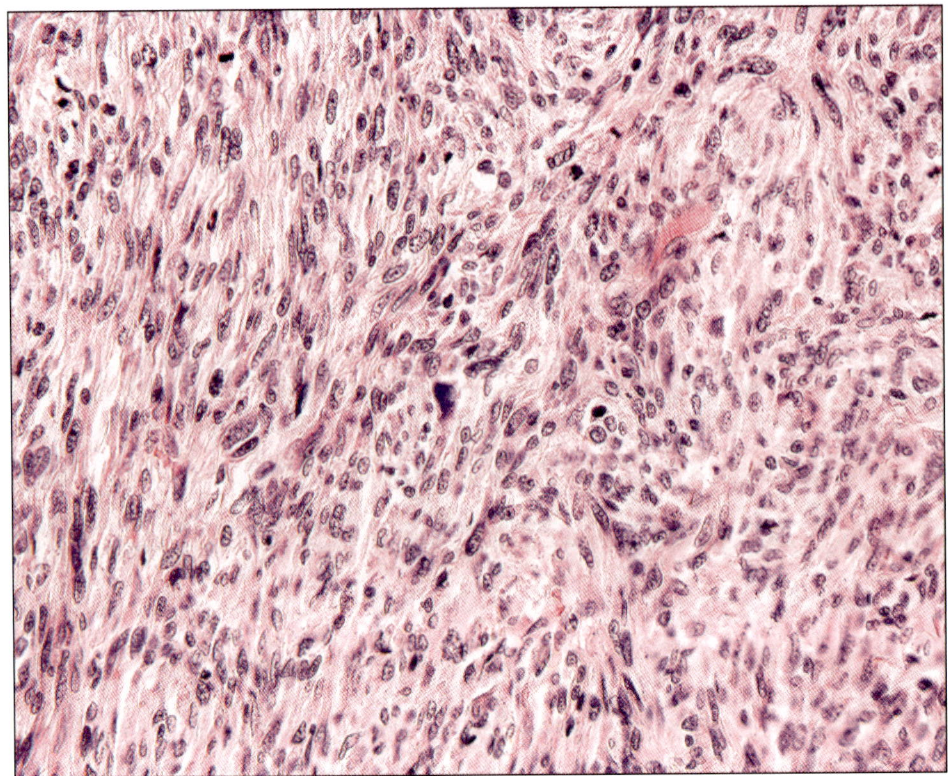

intralesional necrosis (Figure 3.199). The histological assessment of this lesion should be one of excluding other spindle cell neoplasms, which are more common in these locations such as malignant solitary fibrous tumor or metastatic fibrosarcoma. These tumors are immunopositive for vimentin and focally for smooth muscle actin, representing myofibroblastic differentiation (Fletcher et al., 2002).

FIBROHISTIOCYTIC TUMORS

The so-called fibrohistiocytic tumors represent a poorly defined group of tumors composed of cells that suggest both fibroblastic and histiocytic differentiation. However, classification has been controversial since virtually none of the lesions show histiocytic differentiation (Fletcher et al., 2002). Many malignant examples are now classified as sarcomas and the tumors described below should be considered diagnoses of exclusion or a matter of careful histological description without known histogenetic significance. Some tumors previously diagnosed as fibroxanthomas have been subsequently diagnosed as pleomorphic xanthoastrocytoma after the discovery of GFAP immunopositivity in these putative examples (Zimmerman, 1979).

Malignant Fibrous Histiocytoma

Clinical Features

This tumor has been rarely reported as an intracerebral neoplasm, although more commonly than other sarcomas of exceeding rarity (Oliveira et al., 2002).

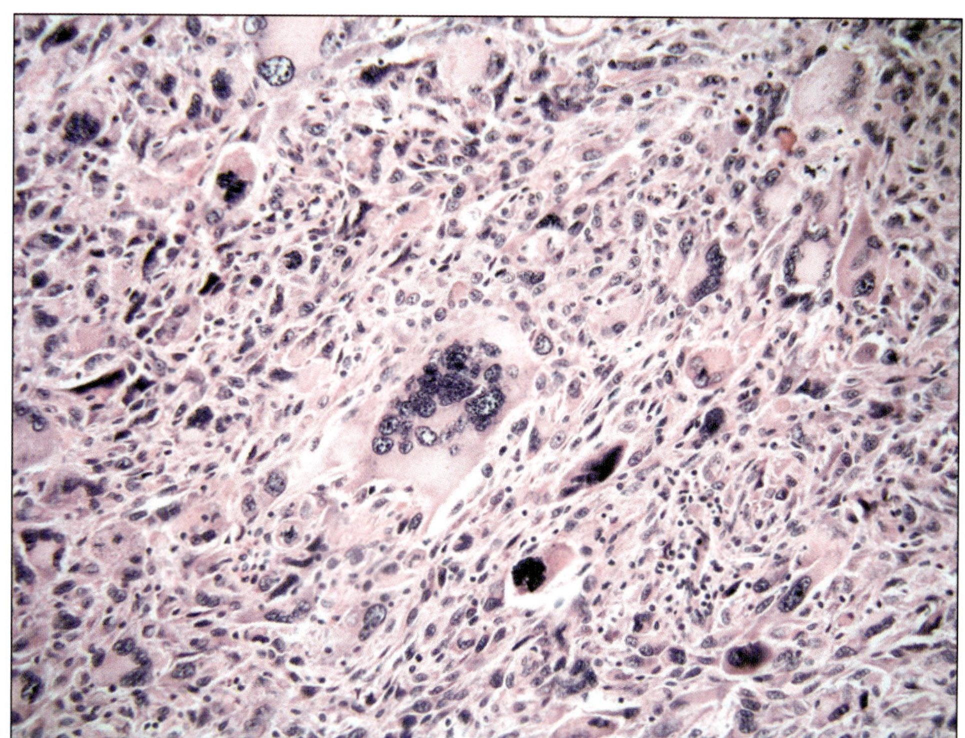

Figure 3.200. Malignant fibrous histiocytoma of the pleomorphic type.

It is also been recognized as a posttreatment tumor, occurring after treatment for childhood brain tumors (Broniscer et al., 2004; Martinez-Salazar et al., 1997). They occur as intraparenchymal hemispheric tumors.

Pathology

Both the pleomorphic and myxoid variants of malignant fibrous histiocytoma (MFH) have been described in the CNS. Myxoid MFH is considered to represent a myxoid liposarcoma. Pleomorphic malignant fibrous histiocytoma is a term considered synonymous with undifferentiated pleomorphic sarcoma and either term may be used (Fletcher et al., 2002). Accordingly, they are very heterogeneous in appearance and cellularity, sometimes including extensively fibrous stroma. There is marked cytological and nuclear pleomorphism with bizarre giant cells, admixed spindle cells, and rounded histiocyte-like cells, which may have foamy cytoplasm (Figure 3.200). Metaplastic change including carcinomatous, melanocytic, leiomyomatous, and rhabdomyosarcomatous differentiation has been described.

MYOGENIC TUMORS

Leiomyoma

Clinical Features

Intracranial leiomyomas have been rarely described, including those with a dural association (Ali et al., 2006), and in the sellar (Kroe et al., 1968) and suprasellar regions (Kleinschmidt-DeMasters et al., 1998), or from the orbital apex (Kulkarni et al., 2000). This seemingly sporadic occurrence has been superseded by the well-documented development of EBV-associated dural as well as other soft tissue smooth muscle tumors: either leiomyomas or relatively well-differentiated leiomyosarcomas in acquired immunodeficiency syndrome AIDS (Bargiela et al., 1999) or in other congenital or acquired forms of immunodeficiency (Kleinschmidt-DeMasters et al., 1998). An intraparenchymal parietal lobe pleomorphic angioleiomyoma has also been described (Lach et al., 1994).

The diagnostician must be aware of the possibility of the so-called benign metastasizing leiomyoma in which metastatic but otherwise well-differentiated smooth muscle tumors may affect the nervous system (Alessi et al., 2003; de Ruiter et al., 2006).

Pathology

Leiomyomas are spindle-cell neoplasms, characterized by monotonous waves of elongated cells with brightly eosinophilic cytoplasm and cigar-shaped nuclei forming intersecting fascicles. They lack mitotic activity as compared with sarcomatous counterparts. The lesions most likely to be confused with leiomyomas are fibrous meningioma or schwannoma; the strong immunoreactivity for both smooth muscle actin and S-100 with EMA negativity allows for the separation of these entities.

Leiomyosarcoma

Clinical Features

These have been reported as rare tumors of young adults, usually attached to the dura and mimicking meningioma, and in the sella (Kroe et al., 1968). As with leiomyomas, an association between EBV and these tumors occurring in individuals affected with AIDS has been well documented (Deyrup et al., 2006).

Pathology

Leiomyosarcomas show intersecting fascicles of eosinophilic spindle cells, occasionally presenting a hemangiopericytoma-like vascular pattern (Figure 3.201). They are usually highly cellular; however, fibrous and myxoid variants have been described. Mitotic activity is readily identifiable although variable.

Rhabdomyosarcoma

Clinical Features

Rhabdomyosarcomas occur predominately as parenchymal tumors in young patients both within the hemispheres or the posterior fossa (Celli et al., 1998; Taratuto et al., 1985). They behave aggressively and are rarely curable. The

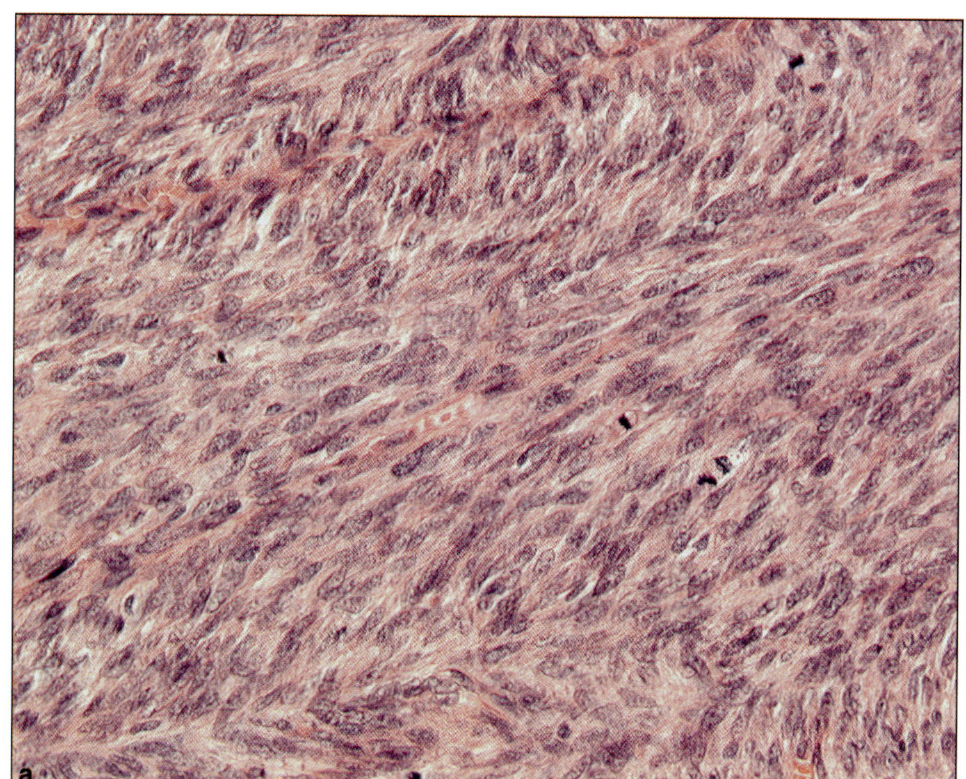

Figure 3.201.
Leiomyosarcoma.
(a) Aggressive spindle-cell
neoplasm, which is
immunopositive for
(b) smooth muscle actin and
(c) desmin.

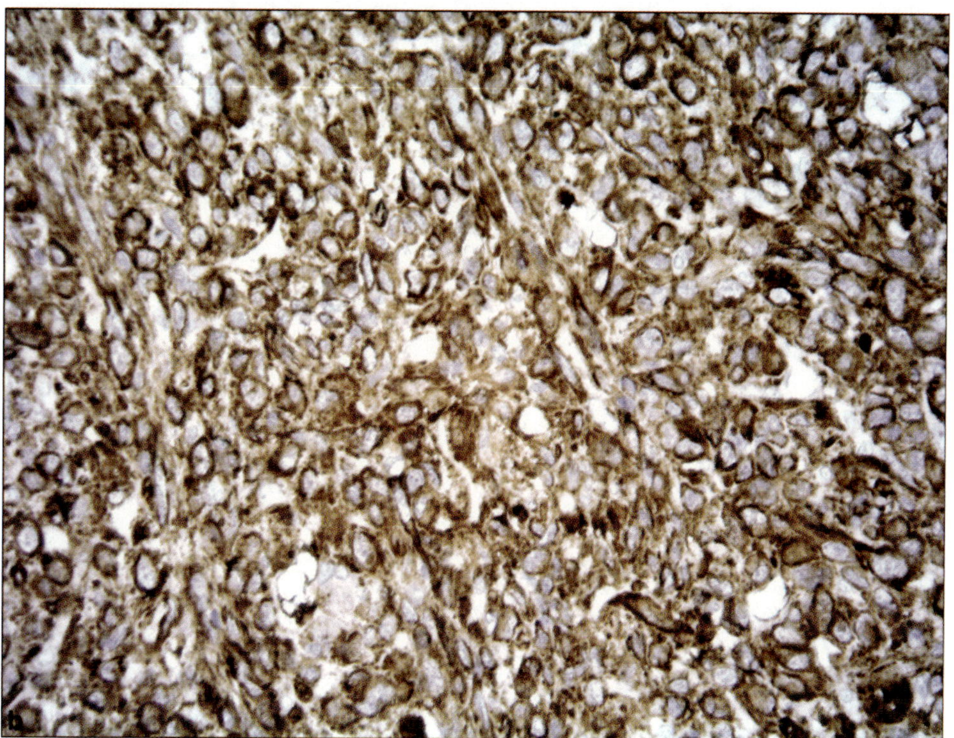

medical literature describes more instances of metastatic rhabdomyosarcoma to the brain than of primary examples. There is no intracranial intraparenchymal example of the benign counterpart except in a single report of rhabdomyoma of the seventh cranial nerve (Vandewalle et al., 1995).

Figure 3.201. *continued.*

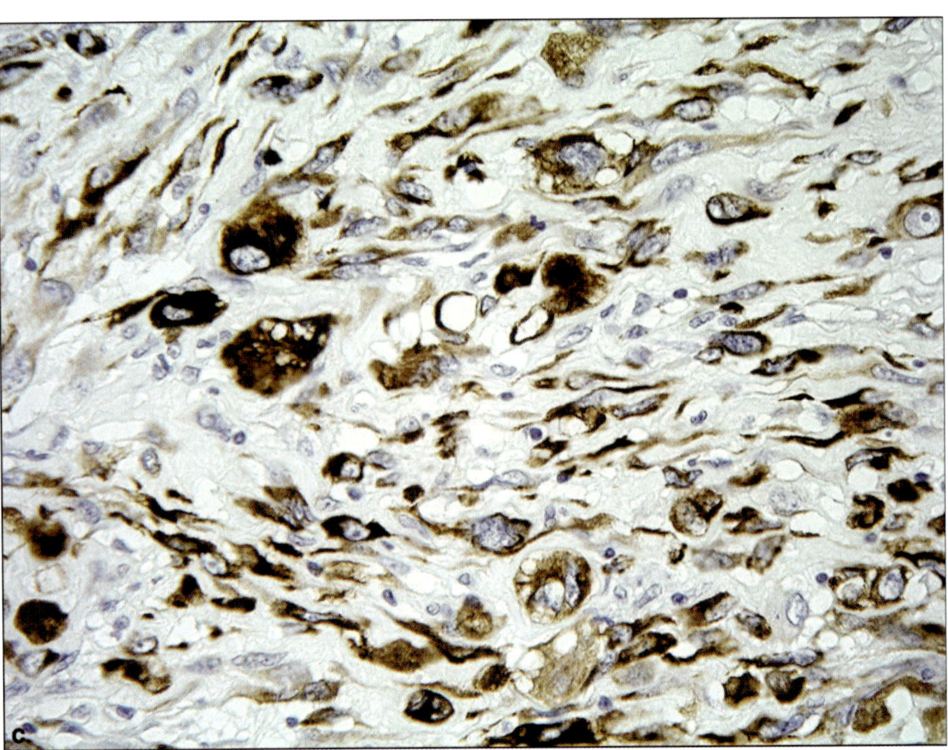

Figure 3.202.
(a) Rhabdomyosarcoma, a poorly differentiated example of the embryonal type, the most common to arise in the CNS. These are typically immunopositive for
(b) MyoD1 and (c) desmin.

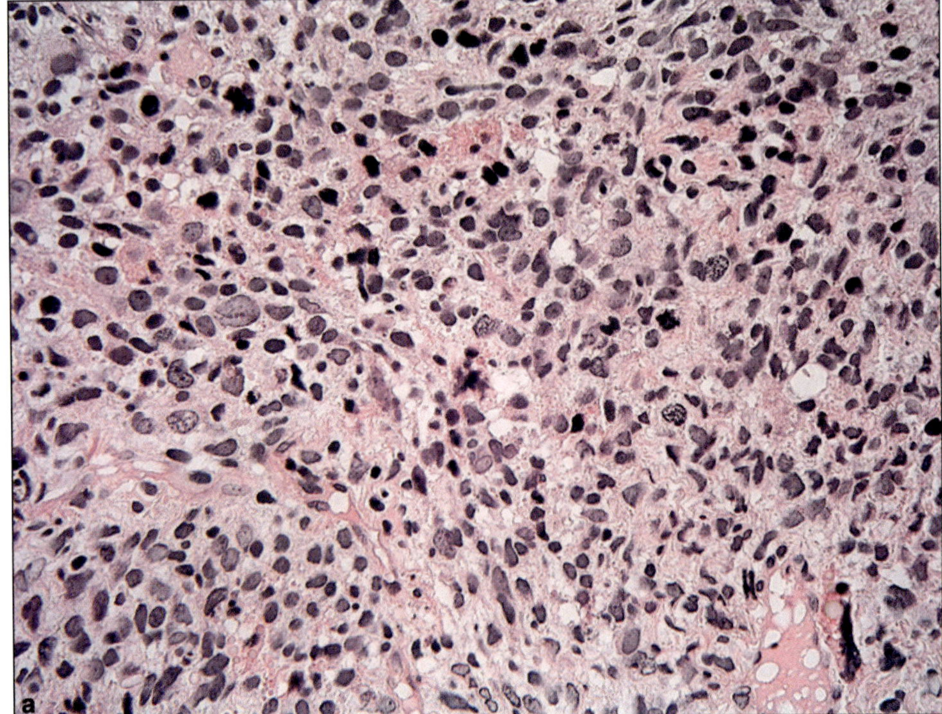

Pathology

The most common subtype of CNS rhabdomyosarcoma is embryonal; the pleomorphic subtype has been reported (Oliveira et al., 2002) and only metastatic alveolar rhabdomyosarcoma has been reported in the brain. Histological features

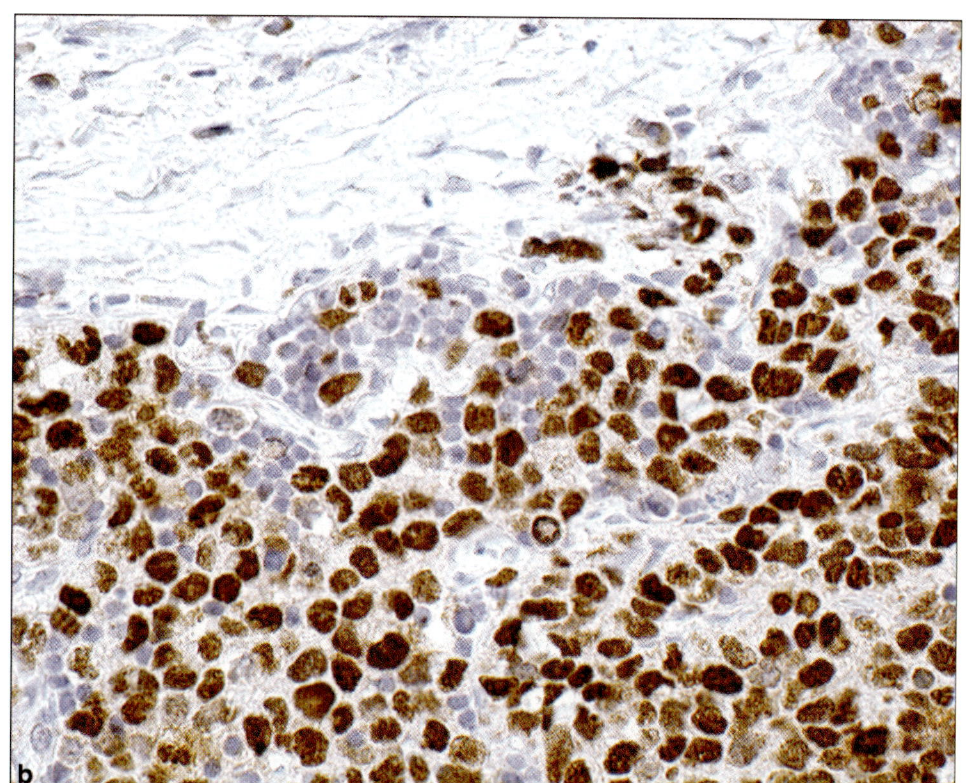

Figure 3.202. *continued.*

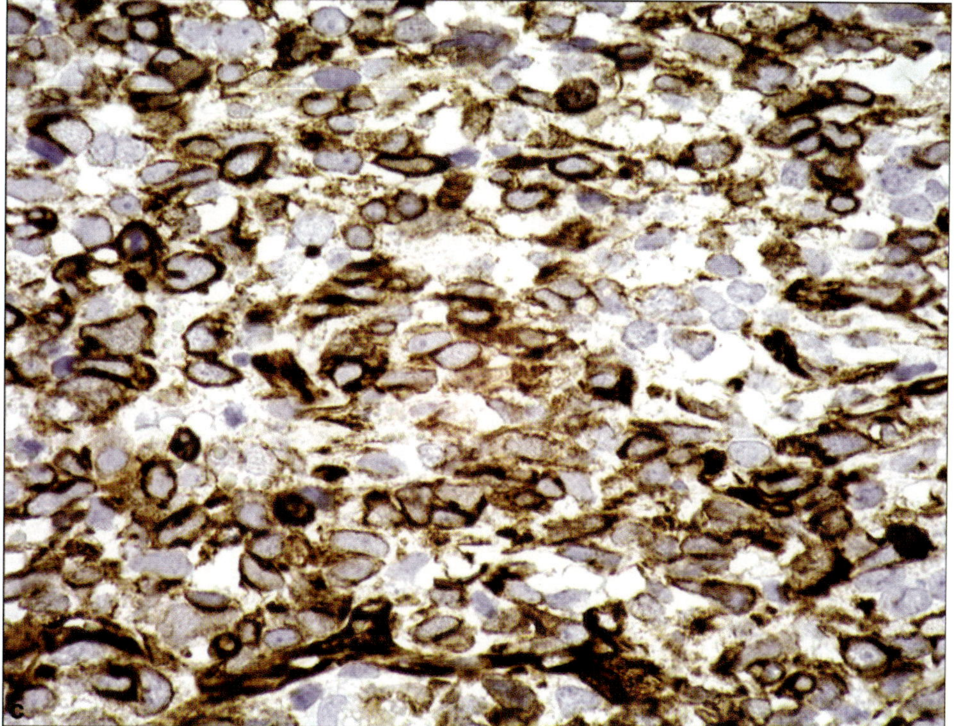

are analogous to embryonic skeletal muscle, composed of primitive cells displaying various stages of early myogenesis (Figure 3.202). Stellate cells with varying amounts of elongation and cytoplasmic eosinophilia are seen. Terminal differentiation can be seen as strap cells containing cross striations and myotubes with centrally placed nuclei. Immunohistochemical results tend to reflect the degree of differentiation, with only vimentin detectable in the most primitive cells, then acquiring desmin, actin, and myosin. Nuclear MyoD1 and myogenin reactivity are highly specific for rhabdomyosarcoma (Cessna et al., 2001).

CARTILAGINOUS TUMORS

Chondroma

Clinical Features

Chondromas are a rare occurrence at the skull base (Higashida et al., 2007; Rathore et al., 2005) where they produce symptoms depending on which structures are affected by compression.

Pathology

Chondromas are expansile and noninvasive benign tumors of cartilage, which may rarely show endochondral ossification (Figure 3.203). They are hypocellular and almost avascular, and lack the mitotic activity, cellularity, and atypia of their sarcomatous counterparts. Malignant transformation of chondroma to chondrosarcoma has been described (Miyamori et al., 1990).

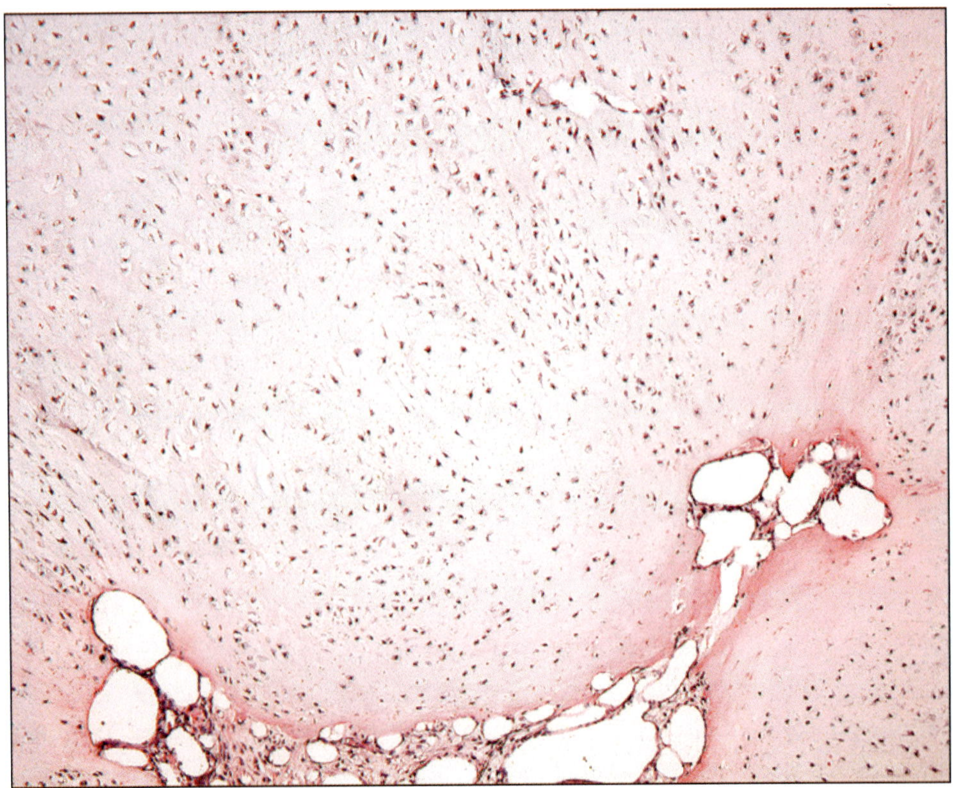

Figure 3.203. Chondroma with the typical benign and relatively hypocellular microscopic appearance.

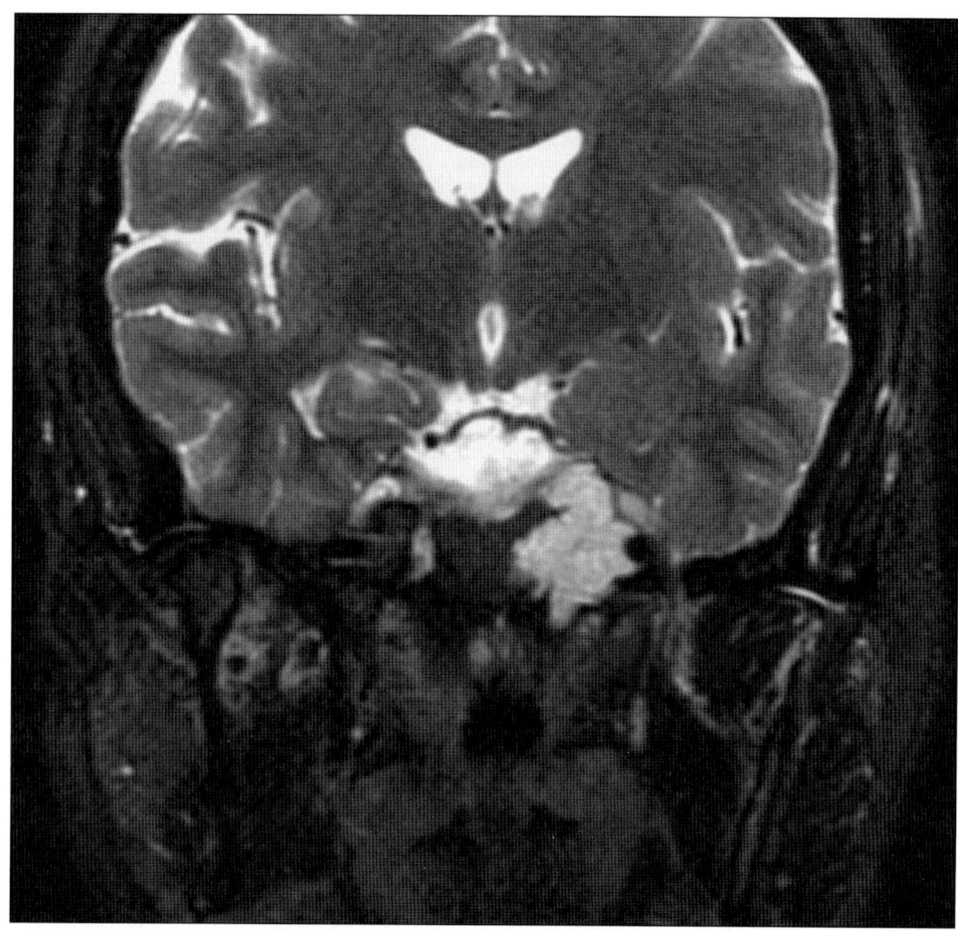

Figure 3.204. Chondrosarcoma. On STIR images, this multilobulated enhancing mass centered at the left petro-occipital fissure demonstrates high signal. Chondrosarcomas, like chordomas, often demonstrate high signal on T2-weighted images. However, skull base chondrosarcomas most often arise off the midline at the petro-occipital fissure, whereas chordomas typically originate at the midline spheno-occipital synchondrosis. On CT imaging, approximately half of chondrosarcomas display chondroid calcifications.

Chondrosarcoma

Clinical and Radiological Features

Chondrosarcomas are encountered either in the skull base or arising from the meninges (Lee et al., 1988; Oruckaptan et al., 2001) (Figure 3.204). They are generally tumors of adulthood.

Pathology

Chondrosarcomas are hypercellular as compared with their benign counterparts (Figure 3.205). The chondrocytes are atypical, vary in size and shape and contain enlarged hyperchromatic nuclei. Mitotic activity and binucleation may be seen. Larger lesions may show necrosis, hemorrhage, and cystic degeneration.

The greatest challenge in diagnosing these lesions is distinguishing them from chordoma or mesenchymal chondrosarcoma. Chordomas are acknowledged to sometimes exhibit chondroid differentiation and thus constitute a subtype known as chondroid chordoma, now believed to more closely approximate true low-grade chondrosarcomas.

Immunohistochemistry is usually unambiguous in distinguishing the two, with both chondrosarcomas and chordomas expressing S-100 protein but only chordomas expressing cytokeratins.

Figure 3.205. (a, b) Low-grade chondrosarcoma showing greater cellularity and cellular pleomorphism than in chondromas, (c) which may progress to lesions of more aggressive features including mitotic activity and necrosis.

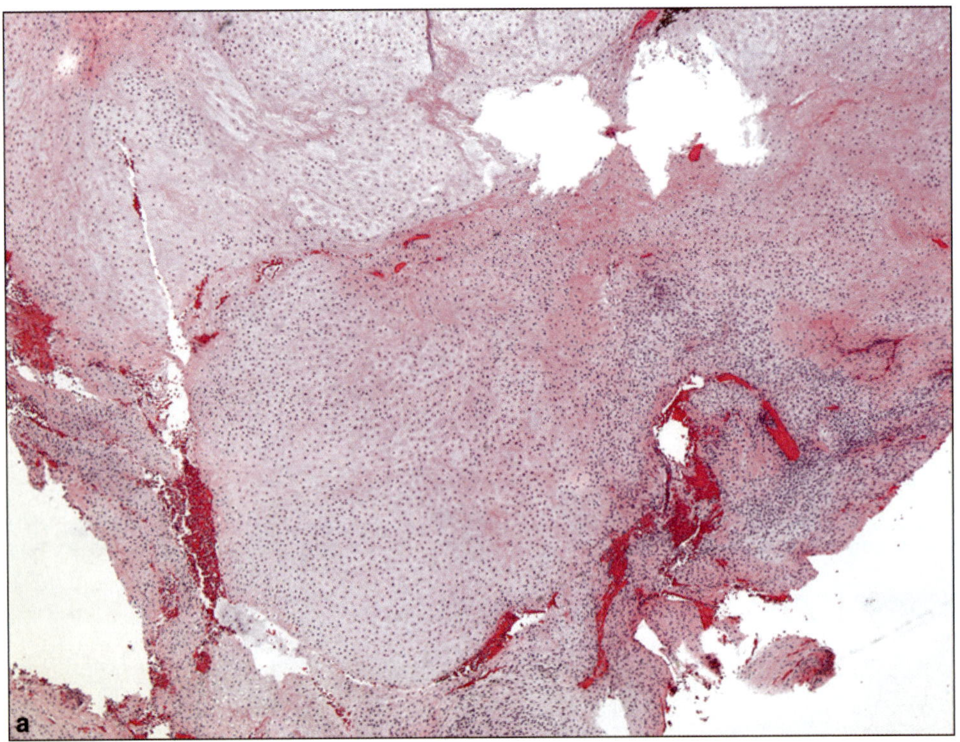

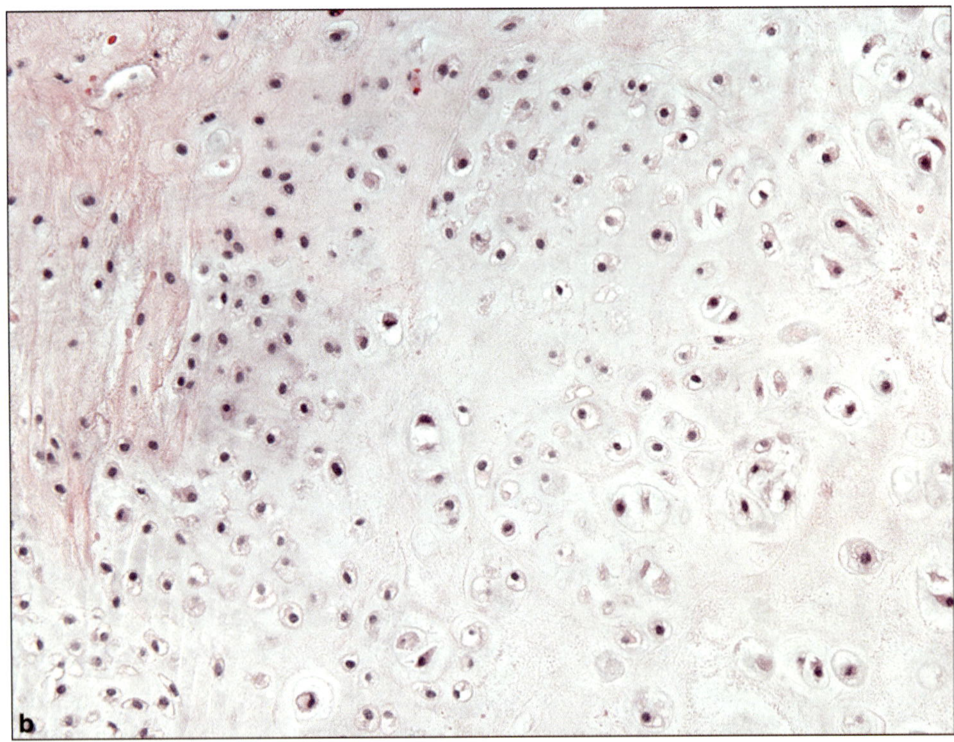

Mesenchymal Chondrosarcoma

Clinical Features

The CNS is the most common site of occurrence for mesenchymal chondrosarcoma (Bingaman et al., 2000; Rushing et al., 1996); however, extraaxial osseous examples may affect the skull or spine. They generally occur in children and young

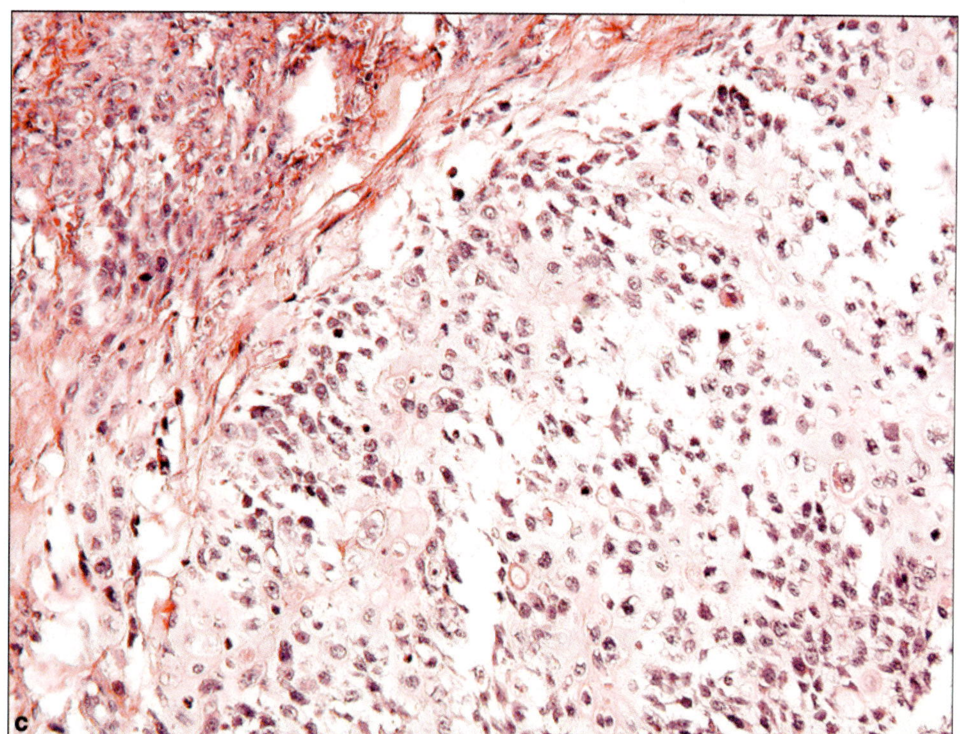

Figure 3.205. *continued.*

adults. Radiographically they are most likely to be confused with cranial or spinal meningiomas. The prognosis remains unpredictable (Nakashima et al., 1986).

Pathology

These tumors show a characteristic mosaic pattern of pale staining well-differentiated chondroid tissue with more compact cellular aggregates of poorly differentiated round or rarely spindled small cells with hyperchromatic nuclei, combined with a palisading architecture and prominent blood vessels (Figure 3.206). Mesenchymal chondrosarcomas are typically CD99 positive (Granter et al., 1996), which indicates the potential diagnostic overlap with Ewing sarcoma. The presence of cartilaginous component, however, rules out not only Ewing sarcoma, but also other "small blue cell" neoplasms including malignant lymphomas.

OSSEOUS TUMORS

Osteoma and Osteoid Osteoma

Clinical and Radiographic Features

This lesion most commonly affects the skull as a solitary lesion involving the frontal bone or frontal sinus, but any other skull bone may be involved (Larrea-Oyarbide et al., 2008). There is usually a male predominance and occurrence in early adulthood. They may also present with facial asymmetry.

Osteomas may be seen as part of the triad in Gardner syndrome of osteomas, familial polyposis coli, and soft tissue tumors (Bilkay et al., 2004). Skull osteomas may also be seen in response to an invading meningioma. They have

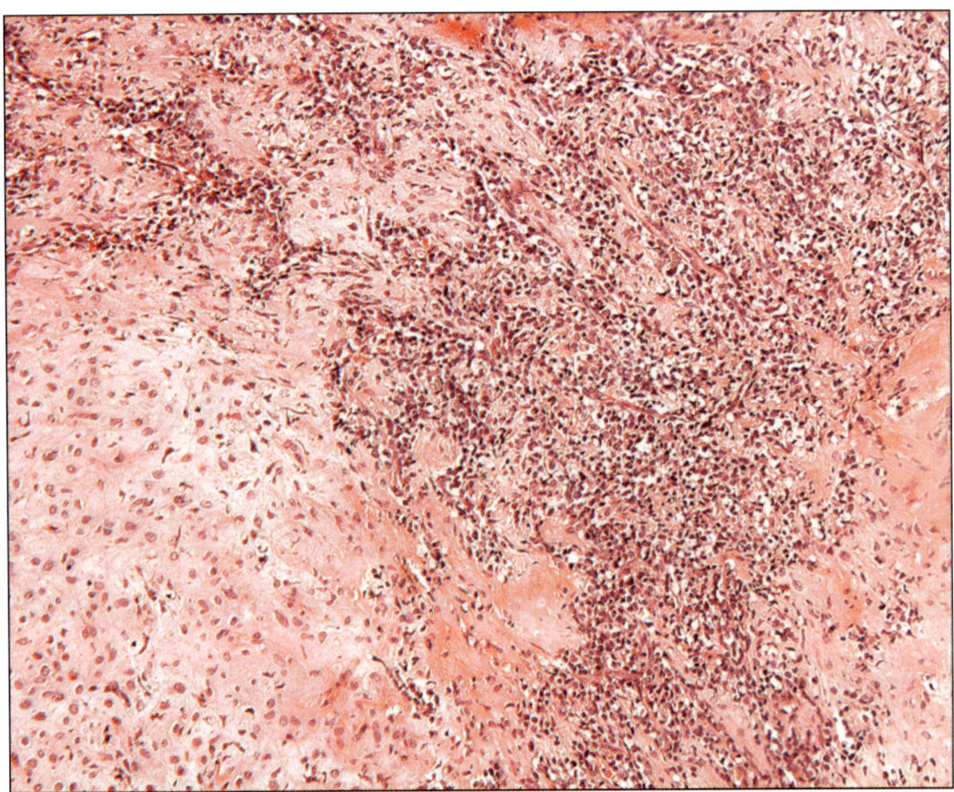

Figure 3.206. Variable degrees of differentiation in mesenchymal chondrosarcoma.

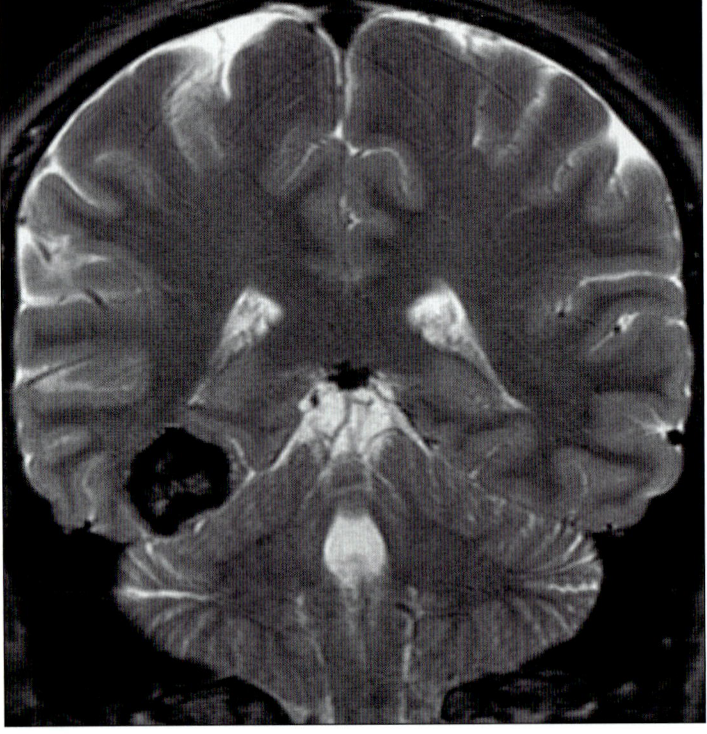

Figure 3.207. A rare example of an intracranial osteoma. A coronal STIR MR image shows a strikingly low signal mass with some central intermediate intensity centered within the right medial temporal lobe. There is no surrounding vasogenic edema. This osteoma did not enhance, and it paralleled the signal intensity of bone in other sequences.

also rarely been described within the brain parenchyma (Figure 3.207) or as dural based. Surgical excision is curative.

This lesion is to be distinguished from osteoid osteoma, a tumor of children or adolescents, seen most commonly in long bones but sometimes in the

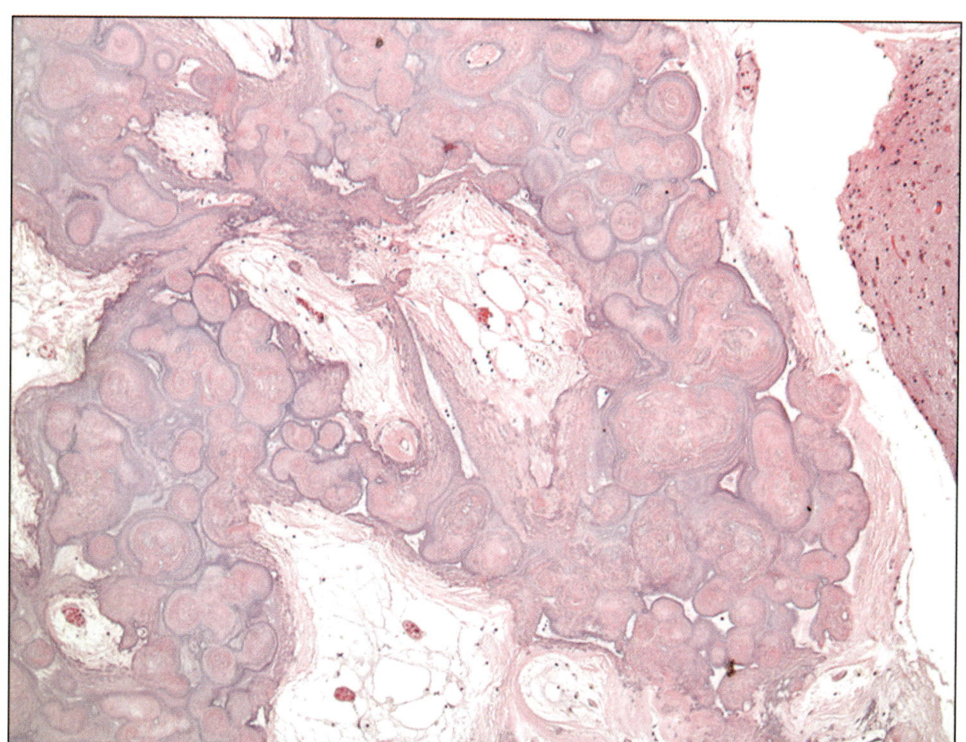

Figure 3.208. Low power appearance of a rare intracerebral osteoma.

vertebral bodies (Kan and Schmidt, 2008), and causing pain relieved by salicylates and nonsteroidal anti-inflammatory drugs.

Pathology

Osteomas are grossly rock hard, which require extensive decalcification prior to sectioning and paraffin embedding. Microscopy shows broad trabeculae of lamellar bone, often with true marrow spaces, as distinguished from fibrous dysplasia (Figure 3.208). *Osteoid osteoma* is a benign bone tumor, consisting of the nidus from osteoid and woven bone surrounded by a halo of reactive sclerotic bone (Figure 3.209).

Osteosarcoma

When osteosarcoma affects the CNS, it is most often due to primary skull or spine involvement. However, it has rarely been described to arise from the meninges (Lam et al., 1981) or brain parenchyma (Bauman et al., 1997; Sipos et al., 1997). In the latter circumstance, osteosarcomatous differentiation within gliosarcoma, or metastatic disease should both be excluded. Osteosarcoma is also a well-known late complication of Paget's disease (Jattiot et al., 1999).

Pathology

Osteosarcoma is a malignant neoplasm with an osteoid or bony matrix. There are many forms; however, most display features of a spindle-cell tumor with anaplasia, pleomorphism, and a wealth of other diverse forms of differentiation (Figure 3.210).

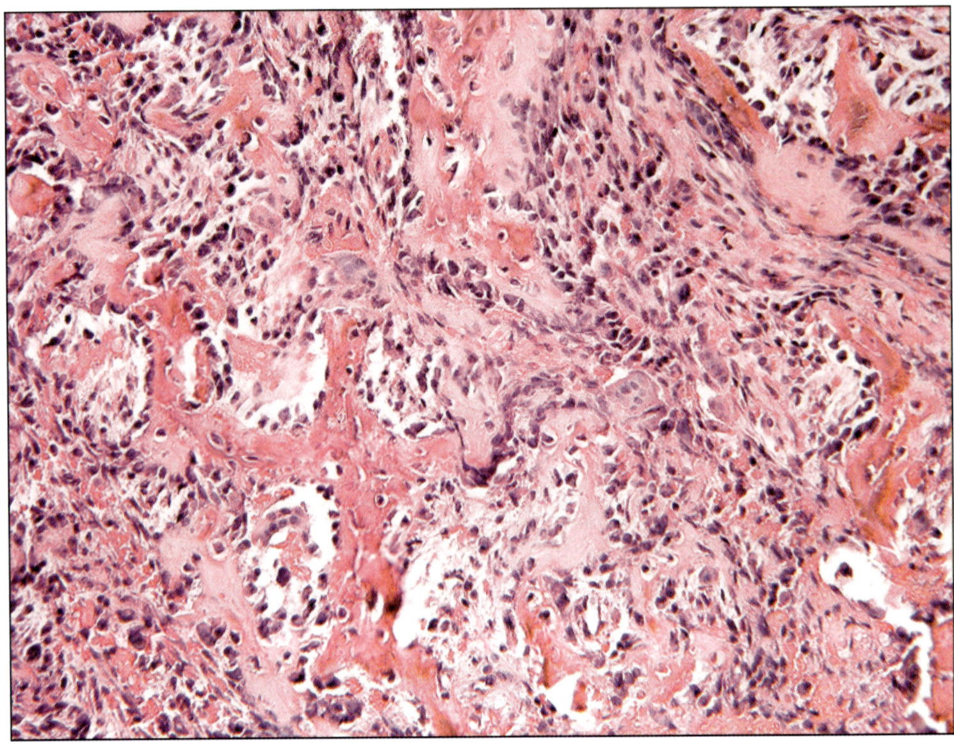

Figure 3.209. Osteoid osteomas are composed of mixed osteoid and woven bone.

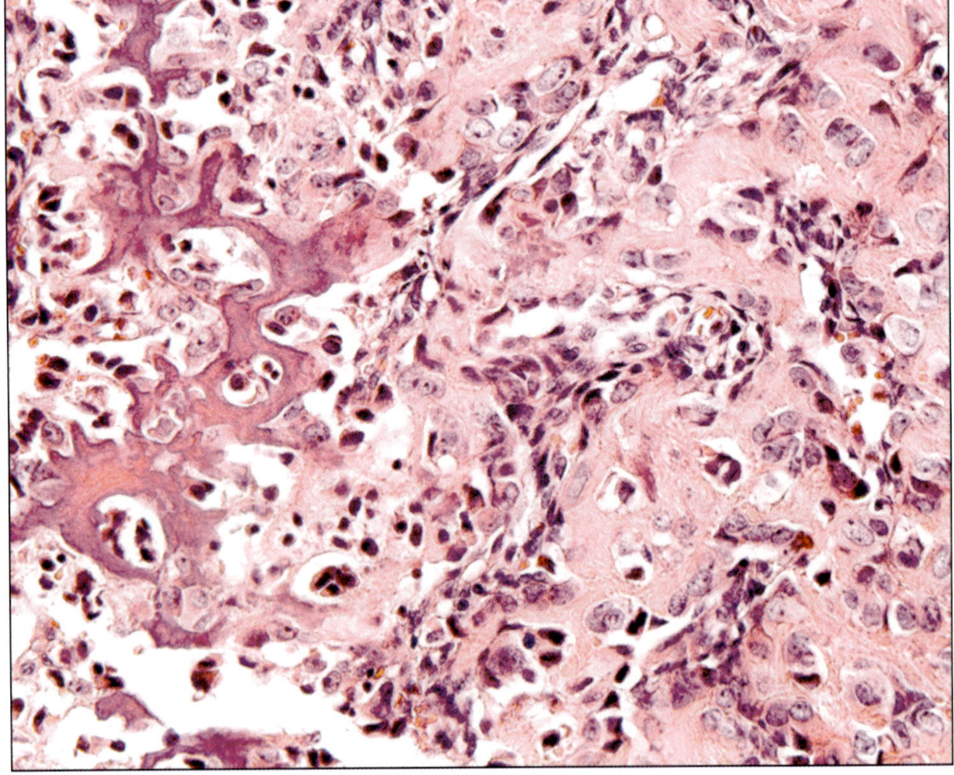

Figure 3.210. Osteosarcomas show a variety of appearances representing a malignant neoplasm with osteoid differentiation that must be distinguished from a gliosarcoma with osteosarcoma as a component.

VASCULAR TUMORS

Hemangioma

Clinical Features

These most commonly impinge upon the CNS as a primary process of bone, particularly within the parietal bone (Paradowski et al., 2007) or vertebral bodies (Lee et al., 2007), sometimes presenting as a process causing acute spinal cord compression (Dickerman and Bennett, 2005; Templin et al., 2004). Hemangiomas vary considerably in size.

Radiographic imaging shows a honeycomb pattern of radiating spicules, which allow their distinction from aneurysmal bone cysts. Epidural and parenchymal, including spinal cord and cranial nerve, examples have been noted (Kim et al., 2006; Templin et al., 2004).

Aggressive hemangiomas typically occur in the thoracic spine and their imaging appearance can mimic malignancy (Figure 3.211). MR imaging is generally diagnostic in the evaluation of the more common nonaggressive hemangiomas, because of their characteristic high signal on T1-weighted

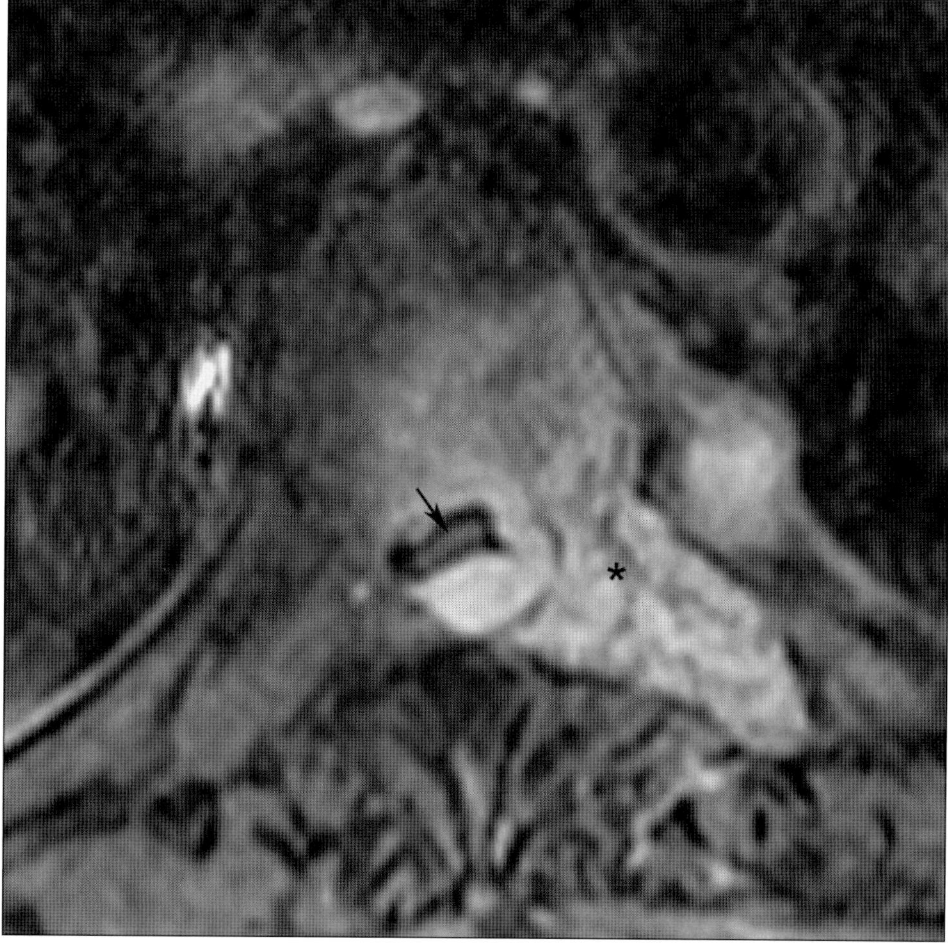

Figure 3.211. Aggressive vertebral hemangioma. Axial T1-weighted contrast-enhanced MR image with fat saturation shows an intensely enhancing midthoracic mass centered within the left pedicle (asterisk), extending into the epidural space and causing spinal cord compression (arrow).

Figure 3.212. (a) Low power microscopic appearance of cavernous hemangioma of bone. (b) Endothelial-lined spaces may be seen at higher power.

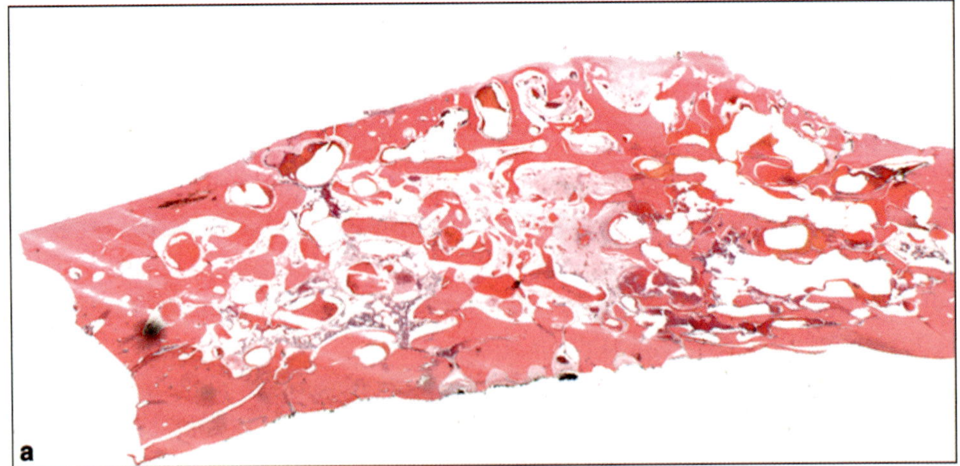

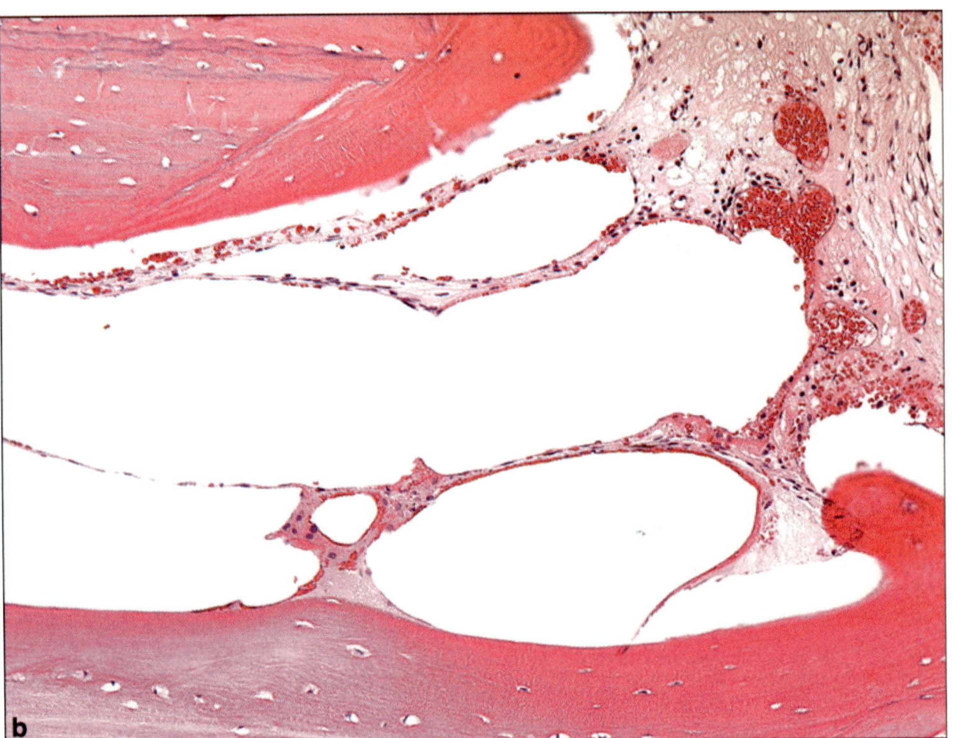

images. The high T1 signal is thought to be absent in the aggressive variety of hemangioma because of a lower ratio of fat to vascular stroma.

Pathology

Hemangiomas are classified as either capillary or cavernous. Hemangiomas of bone are usually of the cavernous type. They consist of endothelial lined vascular spaces with variable amounts of fibrous septation (Figure 3.212). Some examples may show the same evidence of involution or maturation with age as may be noted in soft tissue examples.

Intravascular Papillary Endothelial Hyperplasia (Masson's Tumor)

Clinical Features

This entity does not represent a neoplasm; however, intracranial examples, just as in other tissues, may be confused with true malignancy, particularly angiosarcoma. The condition has also been referred to as pseudoangiosarcoma or intravascular angiomatosis. The process is presumed to begin within arterial thromboemboli and venous thrombi. Cases have been most frequently reported to originate in the cavernous sinus with extension into the sella and thereby producing cranial neuropathies (Kristof et al., 1997). Another has been reported to arise in a cerebral hemisphere (Cagli et al., 2004) and rarely within the vertebral canal (Porter et al., 1995; Taricco et al., 1999).

Pathology

Microscopically, the lesion shows conspicuous intravascular papillary structures lined with plump endothelial cells, sometimes showing heaping, pleomorphism, and occasional mitotic figures, thus the potential for misdiagnosing this lesion as angiosarcoma (Figure 3.213). The key to recognition is in identifying

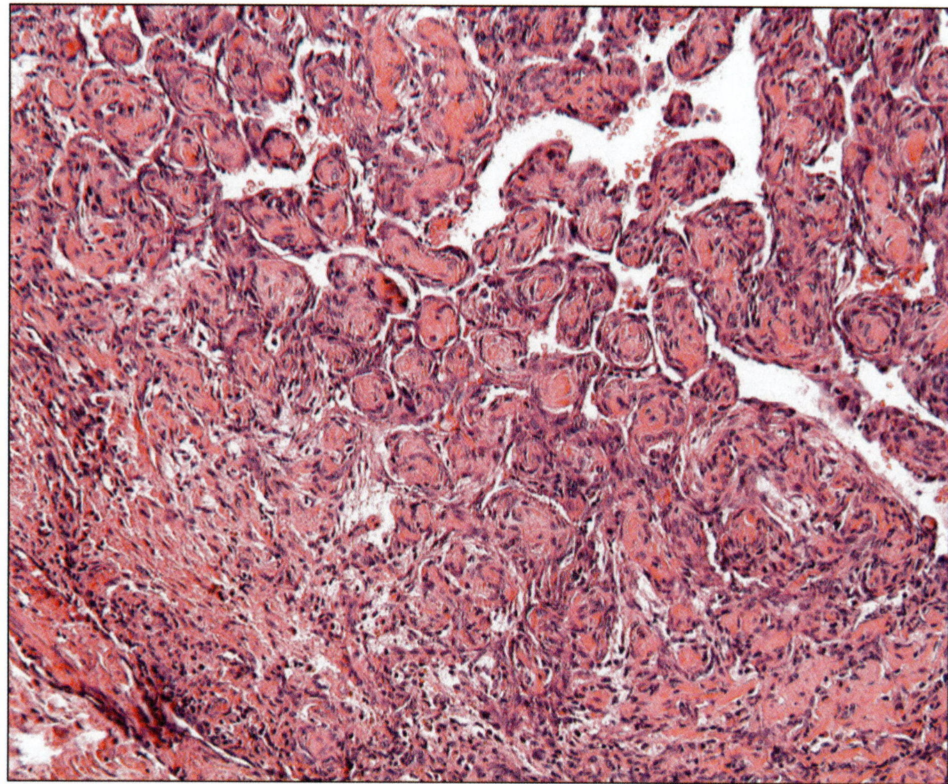

Figure 3.213. Intravascular papillary endothelial hyperplasia (Masson's tumor).

an underlying thrombotic matrix, apparently undergoing organization by the proliferative vascular process.

Epithelioid Hemangioendothelioma

Clinical Features

Aside from its usual location in the lungs, liver, or bone, this tumor may occur in intracranial locations and appears to preferentially affect middle-aged adults (Fernandes et al., 2006; Nora and Scheithauer, 1996). Other locations include the suprasellar region (Baehring et al., 2004; Hamlat et al., 2004), the cerebellopontine angle (Tammam et al., 1997), and as a metastatic malignancy (Diaz et al., 2004; Endo et al., 2004). Radiographic features include those of a relatively well-demarcated tumor, sometimes with a cystic component and peritumoral edema. It is normally of intermediate-grade malignancy and relatively favorable prognosis.

Pathology

A vaguely nodular architecture with limited necrosis is usually present. Tumor cells are round or polygonal, arranged in trabecules or small nests within a chondroid or myxoid stroma. Cytological features include cells with abundant eosinophilic cytoplasm, with vacuolation and sometimes intracytoplasmic vascular lumens sometimes containing erythrocytes (Figure 3.214). Nuclei are round or indented, with minor atypia and relatively few mitotic figures. Immunomarkers of vascular differentiation including CD34 and CD31 and factor VIII–related antigen may be weak or variable but will confirm the endothelial nature of the tumor, although the variable cytokeratin positivity in a proportion of cases might be misleading (Gray et al., 1990).

Angiosarcoma

Clinical Features

These may rarely arise in the intracranial compartment, sometimes even within schwannomas (Ito et al., 2007) and malignant peripheral nerve sheath tumors (Mentzel and Katenkamp, 1999) as has been documented in other locations and in association with neurofibromatosis-1. An epithelioid angiosarcoma has also been reported as a primary brain tumor (Fuse et al., 1995). Its more frequent occurrence in the scalp, sometimes as a diffusely infiltrating neoplasm, may give rise to intracranial metastases (Ellegala et al., 2002).

Pathology

These tumors display profuse vascularity with anastomosing vascular channels lined by mitotically active, cytologically atypical endothelial cells. Some less

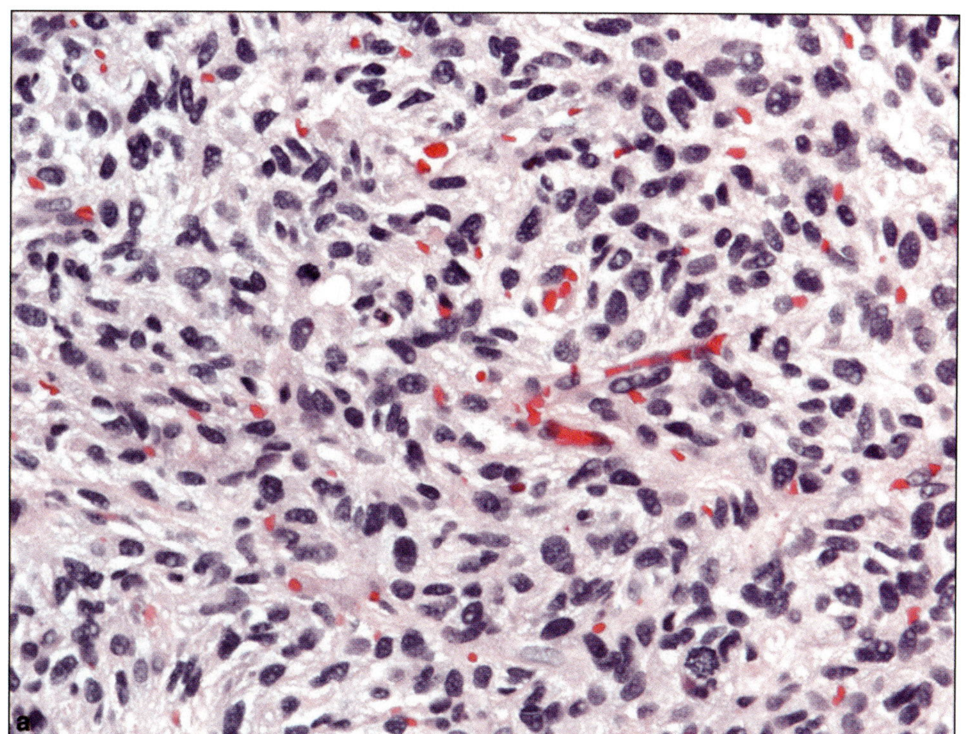

Figure 3.214. Epithelioid hemangioendothelioma. (a) Round to polygonal cells with scattered intracytoplasmic erythrocytes. (b) CD34 immunopositivity may be variable.

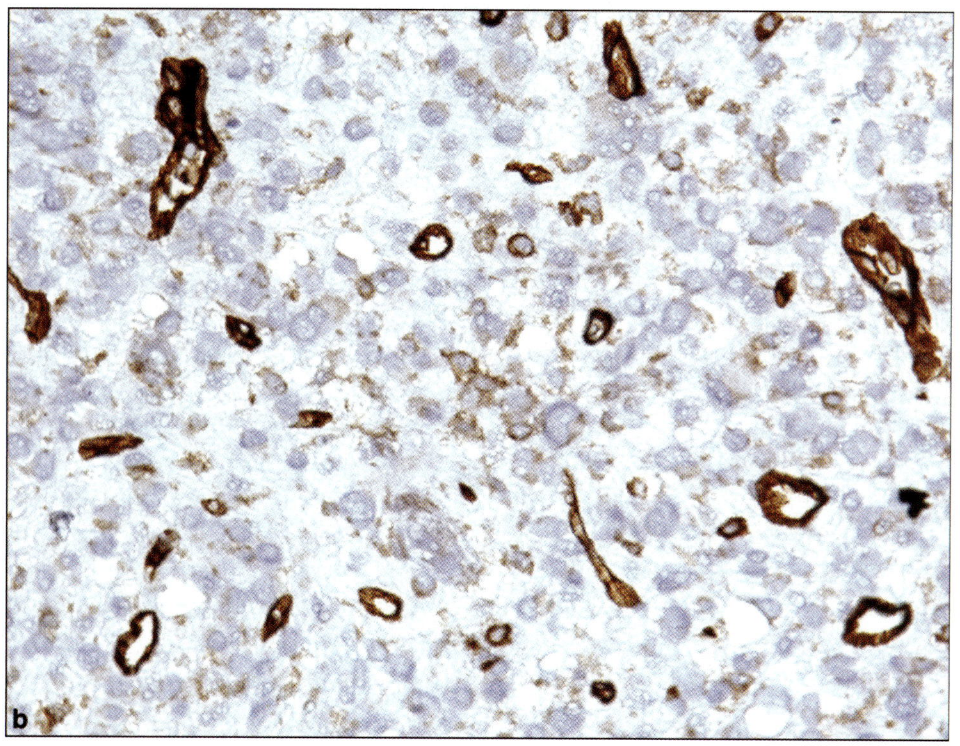

differentiated, often nodular epithelioid lesions with little lumen formation are less obvious and would prompt the use of immunohistochemical or ultrastructural studies in order to distinguish them from metastatic carcinoma (Figure 3.215). This dilemma is complicated by occasional focal reactivity for

Figure 3.214. *continued*
(c) Electron microscopy may
also reveal intracytoplasmic
erythrocytes.

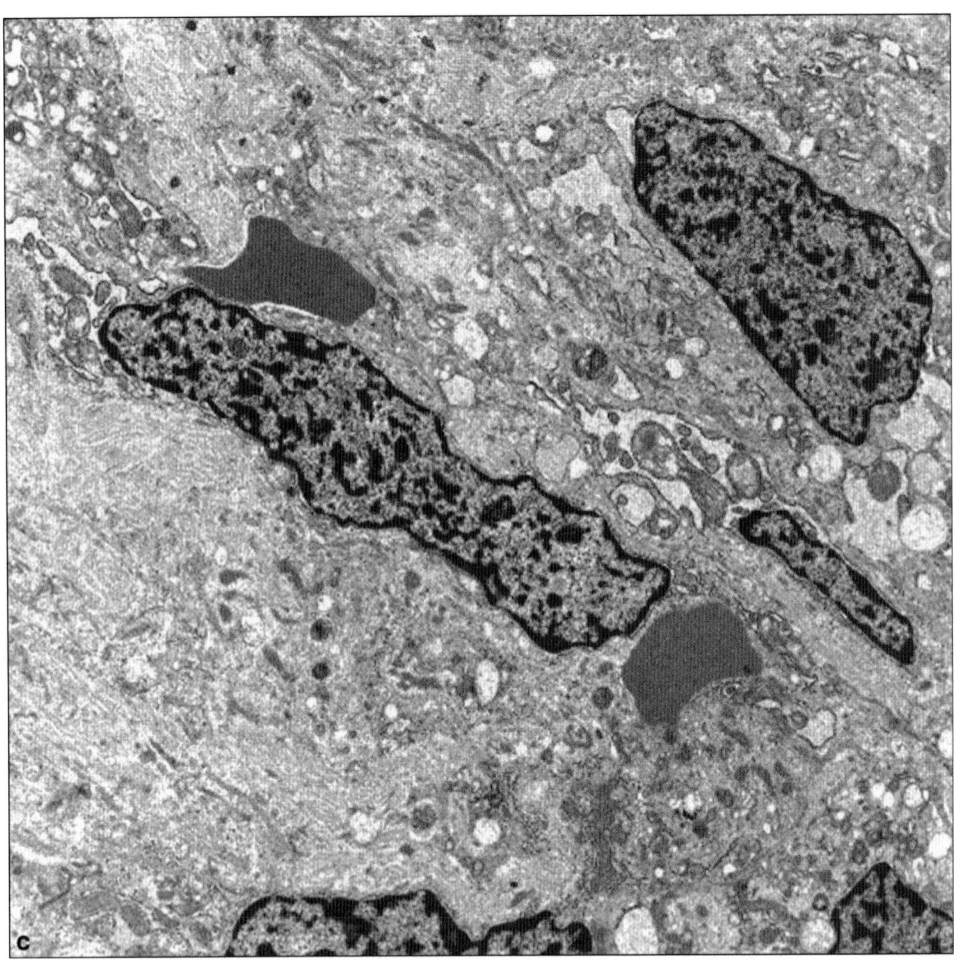

cytokeratin in angiosarcoma. Otherwise, immunohistochemistry may show positivity in the endothelial cells as well is sarcomatous cells outside the vessels for markers such as Ulex europeus agglutinin 1, CD31, and factor VIII–related antigen. It is of critical importance that gliosarcoma with an angiosarcomatous element be excluded.

Hemangioblastoma

Clinical and Radiological Features

This tumor is considered one the predominant vascular neoplasms of the CNS, although it is unclear that it is strictly derived from vascular tissues. It may be most accurate to say that hemangioblastoma is a vascularized neoplasm with stromal cells of uncertain histogenesis. Nonetheless, the hemangioblastoma is usually diagnosed with the descriptor of "capillary" because of the profusion of capillary-like spaces within the tumor. The name is otherwise confusing in the sense that "hemangioblast" refers to nondocumented cell type, and "-blastoma" usually connotes a primitive neoplasm, while in fact the morbidity and local tumor recurrence rate in solitary hemangioblastomas is low.

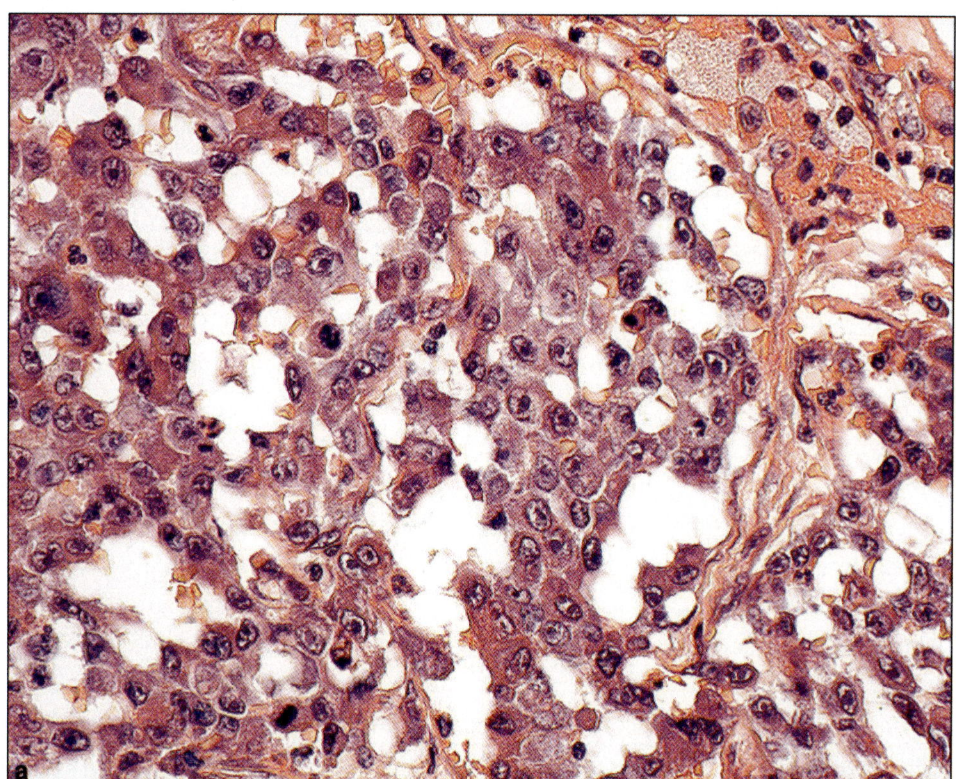

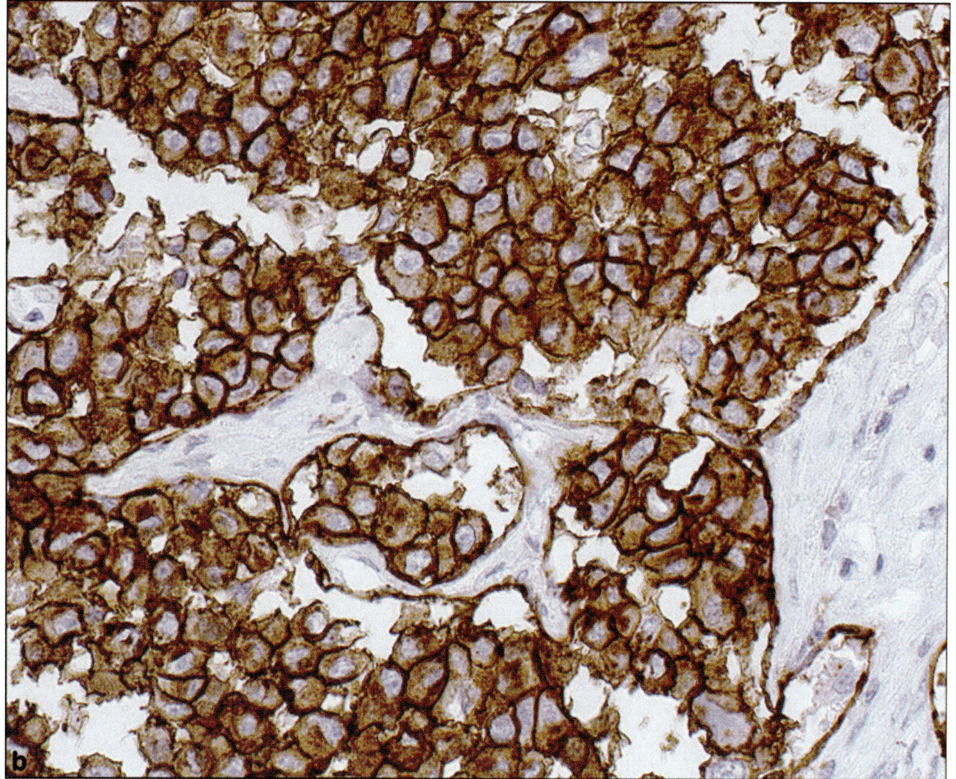

Figure 3.215. (a) Epithelioid variant of angiosarcoma, without obvious endothelial differentiation, but supported by (b) positive immunoreactivity for CD31.

They usually occur in adults and at a younger age and in a proportion of cases are associated with von Hippel–Lindau (VHL) disease. The prognosis is different in hemangioblastomas occurring in familial form associated with VHL disease because of the seemingly inevitable development of multiple CNS hemangioblastomas as well as renal cell carcinoma. This lowers the average life expectancy in this disease to between 40 and 50 years (Karsdorp et al., 1994). It is currently recommended that every patient with CNS hemangioblastoma, particularly those of younger age with multiple lesions, undergo analysis for germline mutations of the VHL gene. Yearly lifetime MRI screening of VHL patients should begin at the age of 10 years along with the family screening and counseling.

Hemangioblastomas may occur at any location in the nervous system; however, 80% occur in the posterior fossa, mostly in the cerebellar hemispheres with 13–14% in the vermis (Neumann et al., 1989). They may also occur at the caudal end of the fourth ventricle. Less than 5% of cases occur in the supratentorial compartment, involving the pituitary stalk, optic nerves, or ventricles. They may show a dural attachment or are centered in the leptomeninges, thus the historical assignment of such tumors into the realm of vascular meningiomas. Multiple spinal hemangioblastomas may be indicative of VHL disease, and are most common in the cervical and thoracic regions. Some hemangioblastomas may occur in the retina and when found in conjunction with other similar tumors in the nervous system, it is presumed to be a manifestation of VHL disease. The radiographic image of hemangioblastomas, particularly in the cerebellum, is highly suggestive, usually showing a hyperdense mural tumor nodule and a large adjacent cyst.

VHL disease is an autosomal-dominant familial tumor predisposition syndrome due to germline mutations in the VIIL gene, in which the aforementioned nervous system hemangioblastomas may be associated with systemic extraneural tumors and cysts including renal cell carcinoma and cysts; pancreatic neuroendocrine tumors, microcystic adenoma and cysts, pheochromocytoma, and paragangliomas; endolymphatic sac tumor of the middle ear (Chapter 3, page 324); and epididymal or mesosalpingeal papillary cystadenoma.

Pathology

The intraoperative gross appearance of these lesions usually involves the recognition of a well-circumscribed highly vascularized red nodule at the edge of the cyst. The tumor nodule may show yellow areas due to focal lipid accumulation.

The microscopic appearance in typical forms consists of two main components: stromal cells that are large and vacuolated and sometimes markedly pleomorphic, and abundant benign-appearing vascular cells (Figure 3.216). Cellularity and stromal fibrosis may vary considerably. Evidence of previous hemorrhage may exist as well as regions of extensive sclerosis.

Adjacent compressed brain often contains Rosenthal fibers as evidence of chronic fibrillary gliosis. The vacuoles in the stromal cells are due to lipid accumulation, which is dissolved in paraffin embedding. The resulting clear cell morphology may be highly reminiscent of renal clear cell carcinoma, and indeed

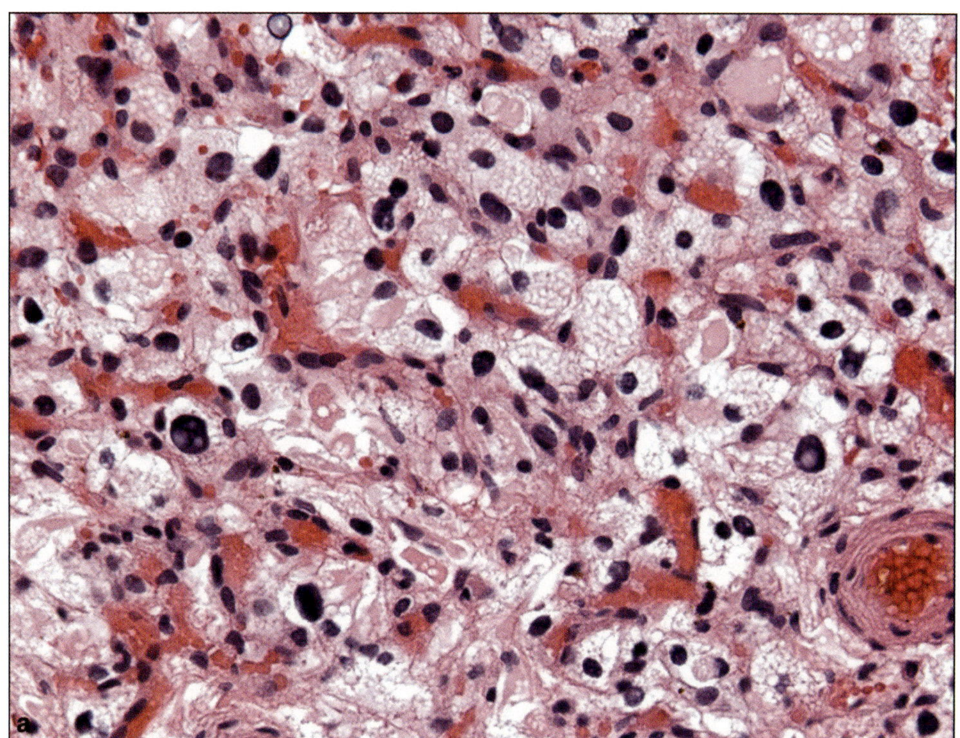

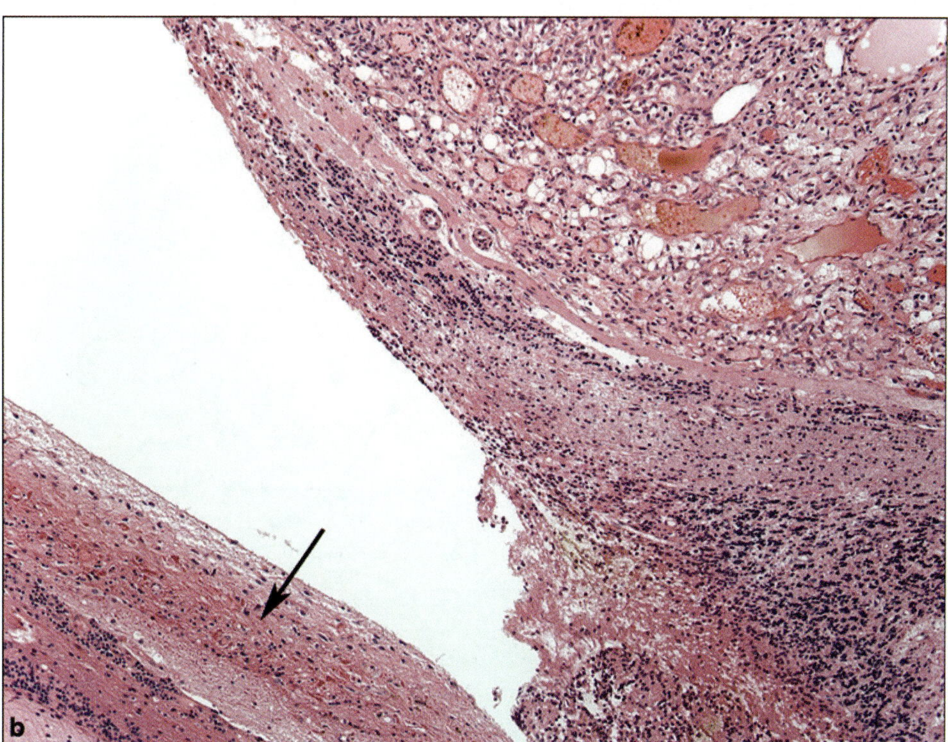

Figure 3.216. (a) Typical appearance of capillary hemangioblastoma, composed of extensively vacuolated stronal cells and a rich capillary network.
(b) Capillary hemangioblastomas typically compress surrounding neural tissue, either directly or through formation of a cyst, causing gliosis with Rosenthal formation (arrow).

a low threshold of suspicion should be maintained for this occurrence; renal imaging is often indicated to allow for either circumstance and for the possibility that extraneural manifestations of VHL disease (including renal cell carcinoma) be revealed. The phenomenon of renal cell carcinoma metastatic

Figure 3.216. *continued* (c) Tumor cells can be markedly pleomorphic. (d) CD34 immunohistochemistry highlights the vascular component. Tumor cells may be (e) inhibin or (f) neuron-specific enolase immunopositive.

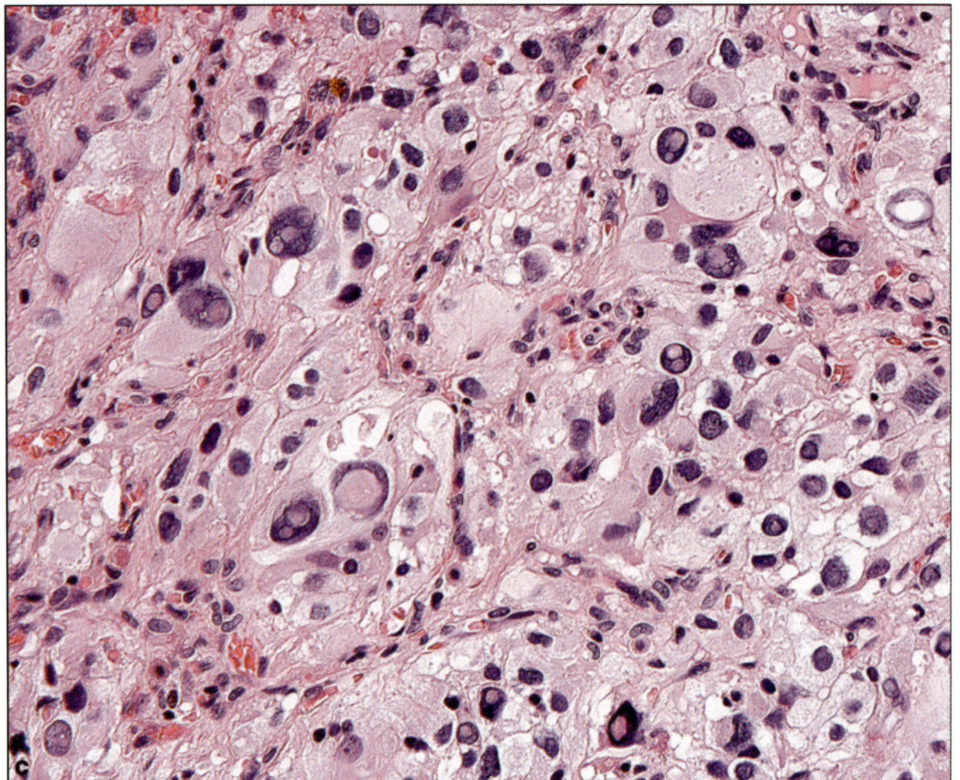

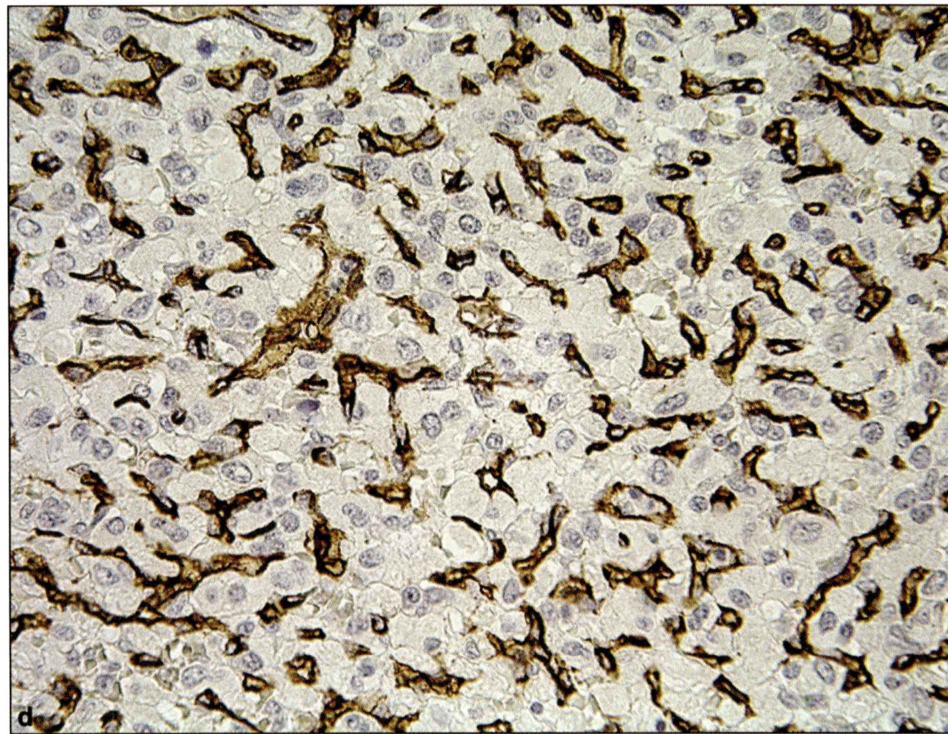

to cerebellar capillary hemangioblastoma has been described (Polydorides et al., 2007).

Immunohistochemical studies have revealed a number of stromal cell markers of varying expressivity and disappointing specificity, including S-100,

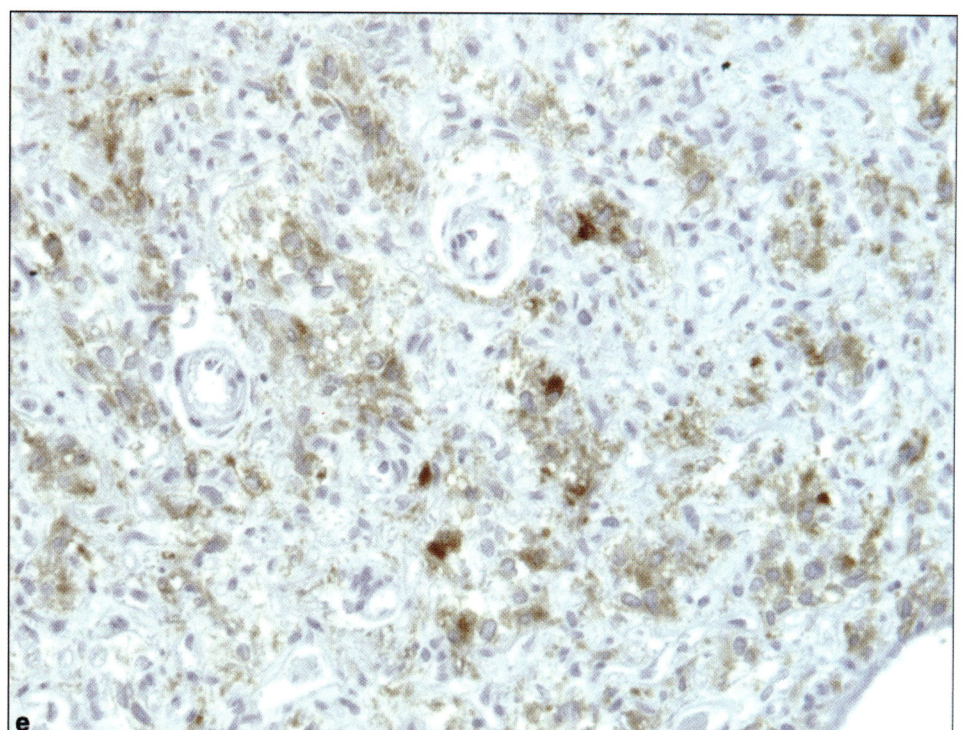

Figure 3.216. *continued.*

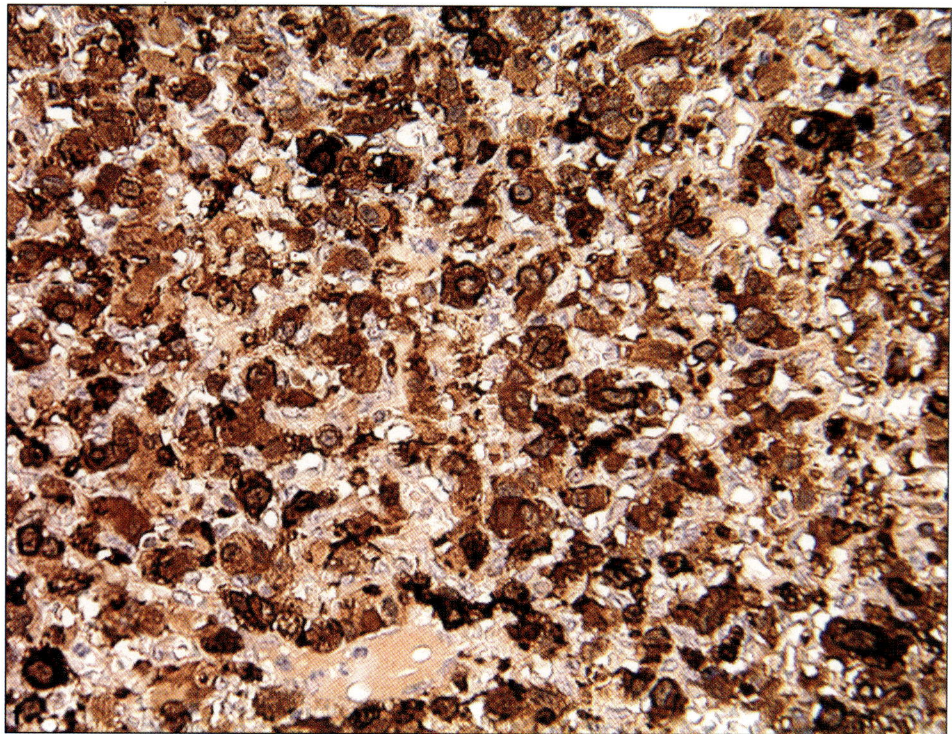

neuron-specific enolase, CD56, and vimentin. Anti-inhibin has been discovered to be a relatively consistent if not focal marker of stromal cells (Hoang and Amirkhan, 2003; Takei et al., 2007). When differentiating possible metastatic renal cell carcinoma from hemangioblastoma, the former may be identified with antibodies to CAM 5.2, RCC antigen, CD10, and EMA while these are negative in hemangioblastomas.

Kaposi Sarcoma

Clinical Features

Brain involvement by Kaposi sarcoma has only been reported in patients with AIDS and as a metastatic lesion (Bahat et al., 2002; Levy et al., 1984). The development of this cancer presumes infection with Kaposi's sarcoma herpesvirus/human herpesvirus-8 (KSHV/HHV8) (Douglas et al., 2007).

Pathology

Kaposi sarcoma may show a number of pathological patterns; however, the unifying feature is vascular proliferation forming somewhat irregular vascular spaces with intermixed collagen. There may be a sparse lymphocytic or plasma cellular infiltrate. There are frequently extravasated erythrocytes and deposits of hemosiderin around vascular structures. Hyaline bodies may be seen in within the tumor cells. CD34 immunohistochemistry identifies the tumor cells.

OTHER NEOPLASMS

Ewing Sarcoma – Peripheral Primitive Neuroectodermal Tumor

Clinical Features

This highly malignant neoplasm is most commonly considered as a bone tumor and is the second most common sarcoma in bone and soft tissue in children. There is a predilection for males and nearly 80% of patients are younger than 20 years of age. The vast majority occur as bone tumors (Desai et al., 2000). However, extraskeletal Ewing's sarcoma involving the CNS occurs as either a primary dural neoplasm (Kazmi et al., 2007) or by direct extension from contiguous bone or soft tissue such as from the skull, vertebral bodies, or paraspinal soft tissues. Parameningeal examples may mimic meningioma radiologically.

These tumors are defined by a genetic alteration involving a recurrent t(11;22)(q24;q12) chromosomal translocation, detectable in approximately 90% of cases by cytogenetic and molecular analysis (Riggi and Stamenkovic, 2007). Intracranial examples have not been as extensively tested to be conventional Ewing sarcoma/peripheral primitive neuroectodermal tumor (pPNET) for the characteristic translocation.

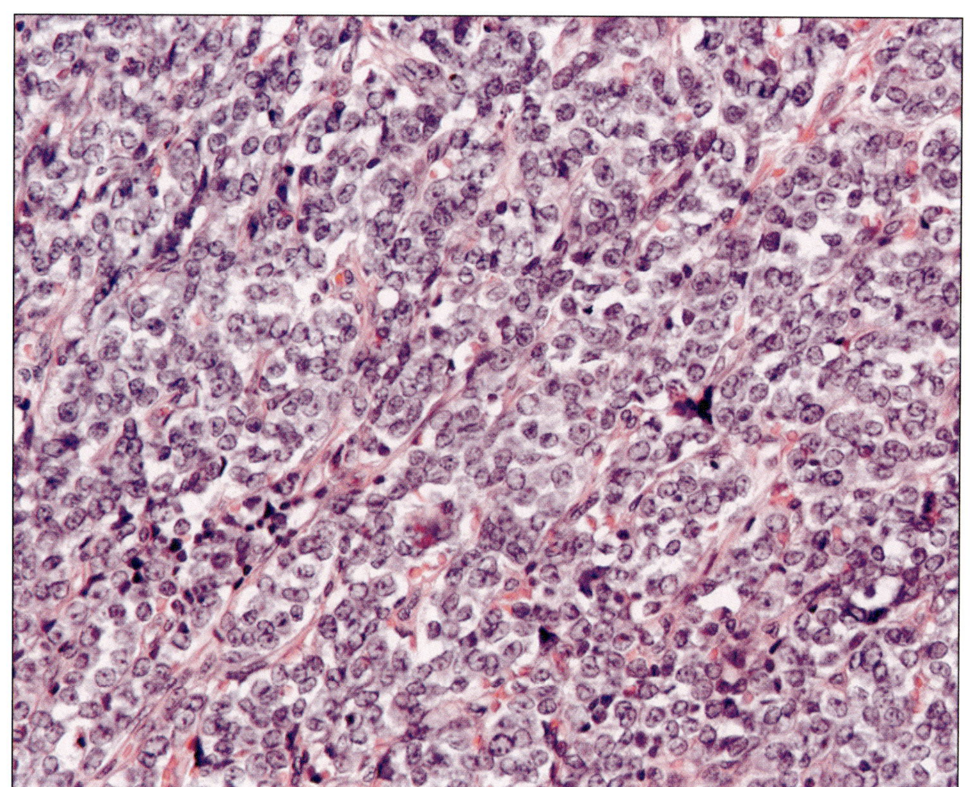

Figure 3.217. Ewing sarcoma.

Pathology

The histopathology of intracranial Ewing sarcoma/pPNET is essentially identical to that of bone or soft tissue examples. They show sheets of undifferentiated small round primitive cells (Figure 3.217) within rims of PAS-positive, diastase-sensitive, glycogen-rich cytoplasm. Homer Wright rosettes may be seen. The majority stain for neuronal markers such as synaptophysin and are immunonegative for cytokeratin. There is strong CD99 cell membrane staining yielding a honeycomb-like pattern.

Synovial Sarcoma

Intracranial examples are extraordinarily rare, having been reported in the sellar region (Kleinschmidt-DeMasters et al., 1998) and in a separate single report within a series of primary sarcomas of the brain in an unspecified location (Oliveira et al., 2002). A lumbar spinal example (Greene et al., 2006) and a particularly hemorrhagic metastasis (Przkora et al., 2003) have been reported.

Pathology

The monophasic synovial sarcoma consists of ovoid or spindle cells in fascicles, and the biphasic variant has discernible glandular or solid epithelial structures. Most synovial sarcomas are immunoreactive for cytokeratin, EMA, and bcl-2 protein, and are negative for CD34. Some may express S-100 protein and CD99. Nearly all synovial sarcomas have a specific t(X;18) (p11.2;q11.2) chromosomal abnormality, resulting in fusion of either of two variants of the SSX gene with the SYT gene (Sandberg and Bridge, 2002).

MELANOCYTIC TUMORS

Diffuse Melanocytosis and Melanomatosis

Clinical Features

This unusual entity is linked with neurocutaneous melanosis (Makkar and Frieden, 2004), a rare neurocutaneous syndrome of childhood that usually presents before the age of 2 years. Symptoms may arise due to hydrocephalus or focal compressive effects on brain parenchyma inducing intracranial hypertension. This entity would not normally provoke surgical biopsy; however, it is important to recognize the normal presence of meningeal melanocytes or "melanophores" within the leptomeninges that may give rise to the melanocytic tumors (Chang et al., 1997; Wang et al., 2007).

Pathology

Diffuse melanocytosis and melanomatosis involve the superior and infratentorial leptomeninges and underlying superficial brain parenchyma, was variable focal intensity, highest in the cerebellum, pons, medulla, and temporal lobes. Microscopy reveals a proliferation of meningeal melanocytes with otherwise bland features (Slaughter et al., 1969). They may extend into parenchymal Virchow–Robin spaces.

Melanocytoma

Clinical Features

Melanocytomas occur at all ages, but most frequently in the fifth decade with a slight female predominance (Fagundes-Pereyra et al., 2005). They mostly arise in the extramedullary intradural compartment of the cervical and thoracic spinal cord and may be dural-based or associated with nerve roots or spinal foramina (Ahluwalia et al., 2003). Melanocytomas are benign tumors that can be cured by complete surgical resection alone.

Pathology

These are noninvasive low-grade solitary tumors. Melanocytomas show nests of pigmented low-grade spindle cells of varying cellularity and intervening stroma (Figure 3.218). Melanin-containing macrophages may be numerous. Some cells may show eosinophilic cytoplasm with small amounts of fine

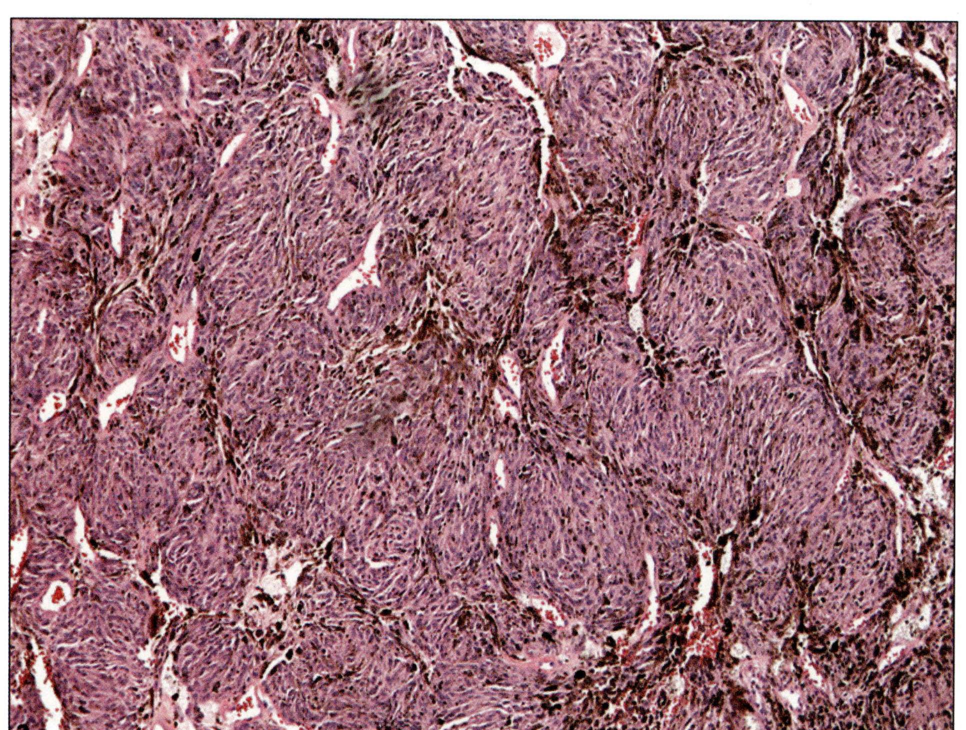

Figure 3.218. Melanocytoma: nested spindle cells with abundant pigmentation.

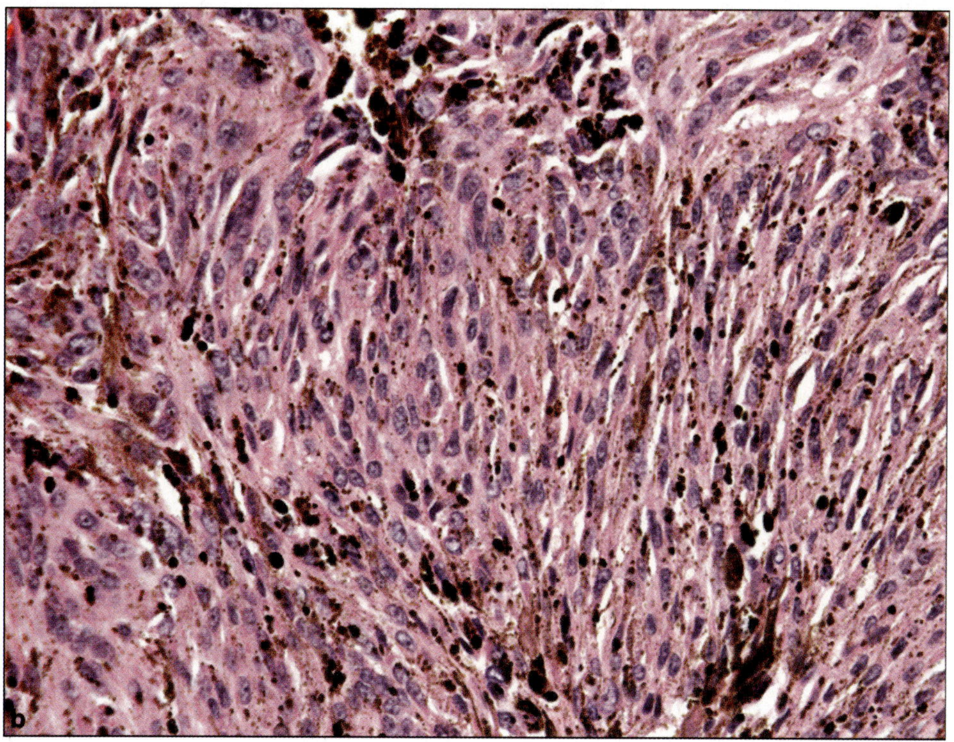

pigment. Nuclei are cytologically bland and mitoses are generally absent. The differential diagnosis with malignant melanoma might be problematic in cases with cytological atypia and increased proliferative activity. Cases of malignant transformation of melanocytomas have been reported (Wang et al., 2007).

Malignant Melanoma

Clinical Features

Primary melanomas occur at ages ranging from the teens to older adulthood. They may occur throughout the CNS with a slight predilection for the spinal cord and posterior fossa (Singhal et al., 1991). They present with signs of local mass effect.

Pathology

The microscopic features of primary malignant melanomas of the CNS leptomeninges are essentially identical to those of melanomas in other sites. They are composed of anaplastic spindle-shaped or epithelioid cells, arranged in nests, fascicles, or sheets, with variable amounts of cytoplasmic melanin, including amelanotic forms (Figure 3.219). Bizarre and pleomorphic nuclei with prominent nucleoli, cellular cannibalism, and frequent typical and especially atypical mitotic figures are other characteristic microscopic features. Also analogous to extraneural melanomas, the tumors usually react with anti-HMB45 or melan-A, and usually express S-100 protein. It is important to realize that several other primary brain tumors may show significant pigmentation, including schwannomas, medulloblastomas, paragangliomas, and some gliomas. Metastatic melanoma must; of course; also be excluded.

Figure 3.219. Examples of primary leptomeningeal melanomas with diagnostic immunohistochemistry. (a) Sheets of large neoplastic cells with prominent nucleoli, immunopositive for (b) Melan A.

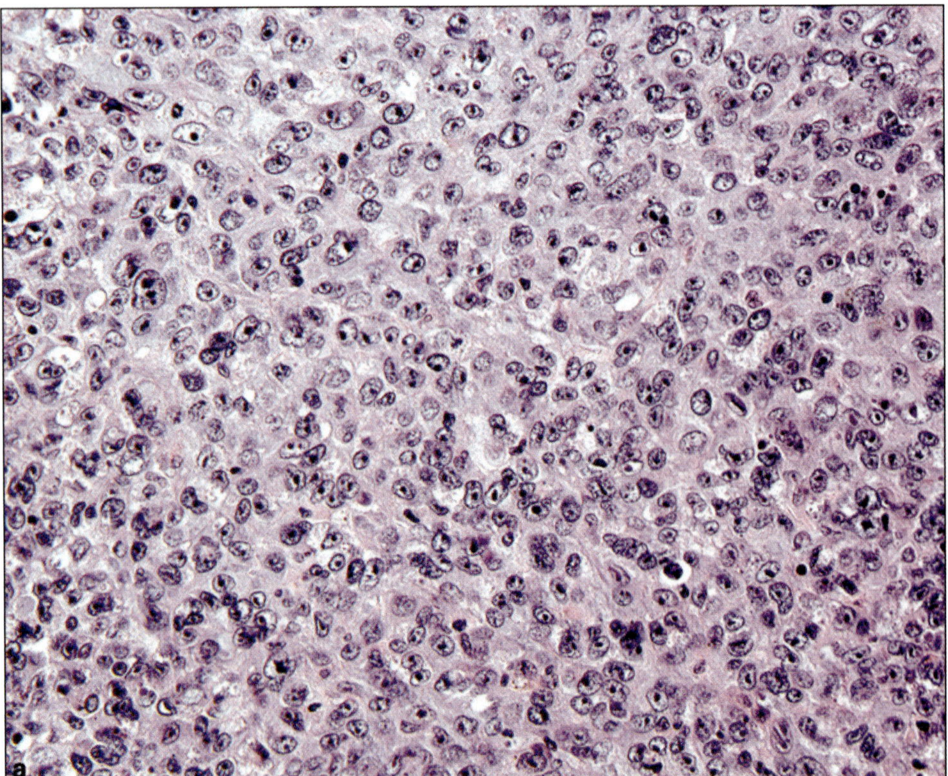

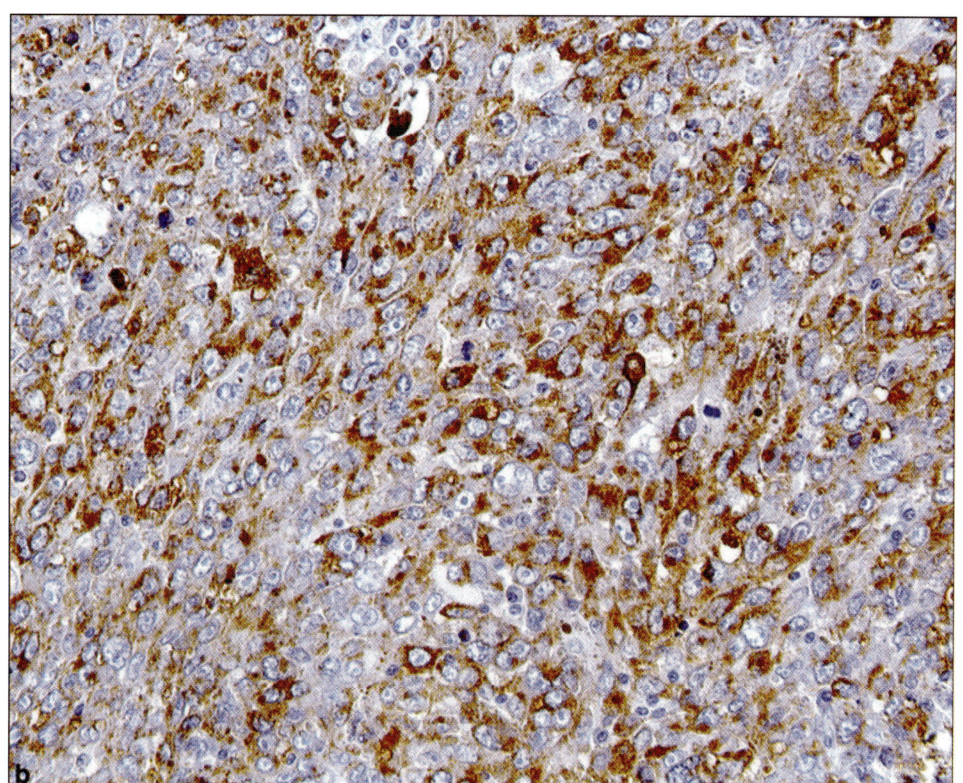

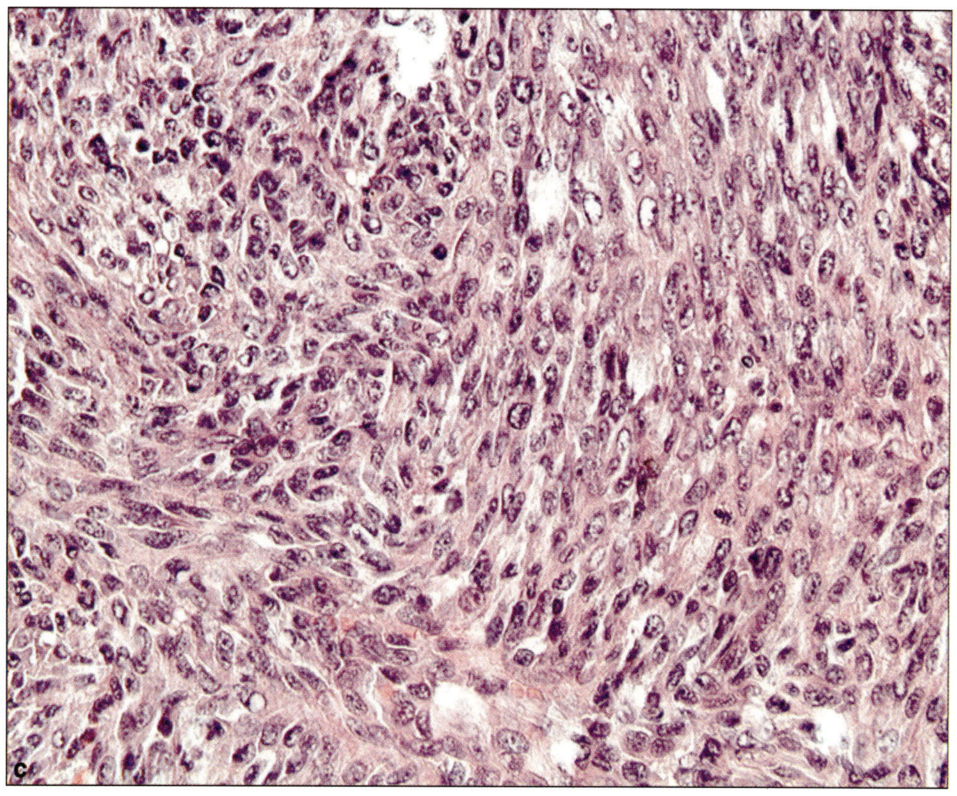

Figure 3.219. *continued* (c) Spindle-cell melanoma, sometimes difficult to distinguish from other primary or metastatic neoplasms, labeled for (d) S-100 and (e) HMB45.

Figure 3.219. *continued.*

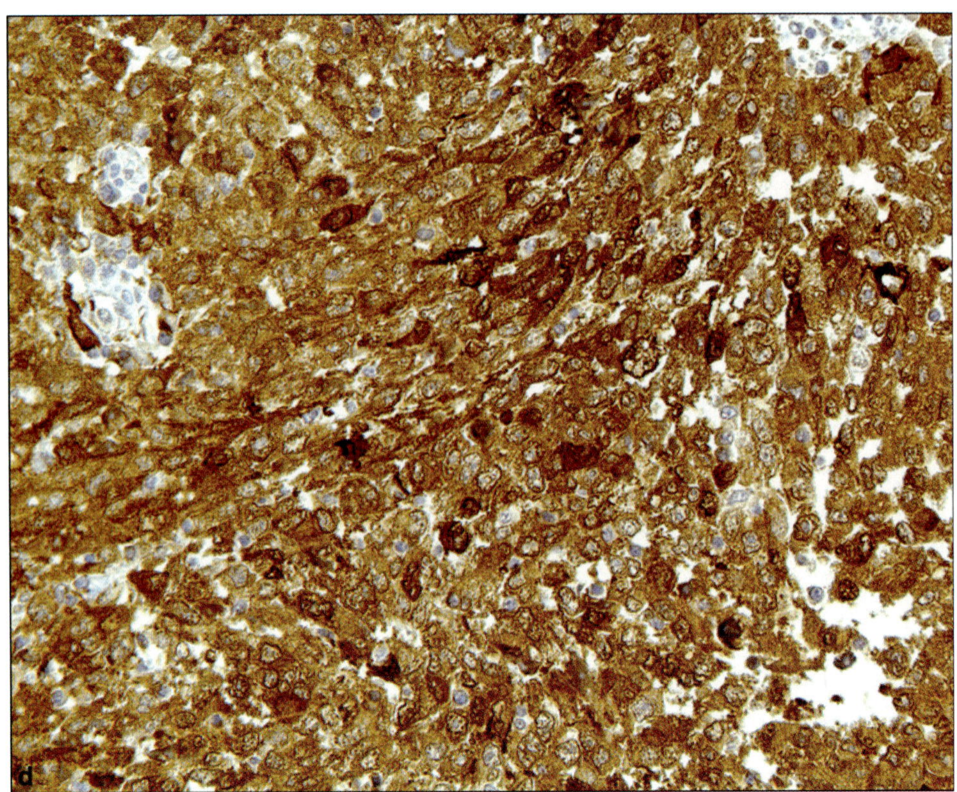

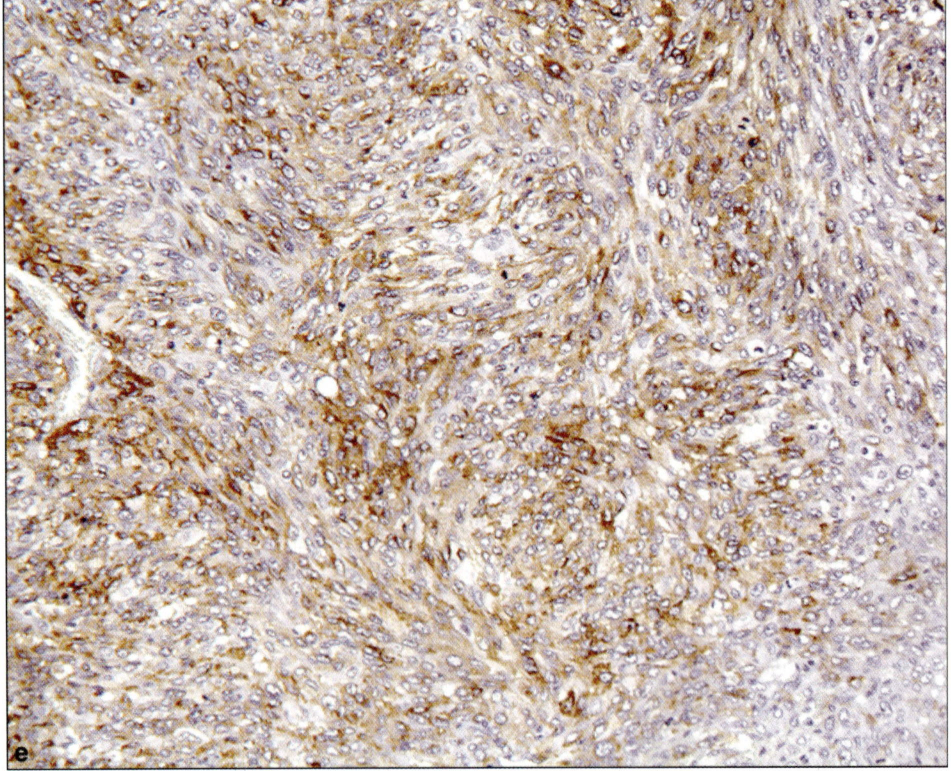

REFERENCES

Ahluwalia S, Ashkan K, Casey AT. Meningeal melanocytoma: clinical features and review of the literature. *Br J Neurosurg* 2003; 17: 347–51.

Akhaddar A, Ennouali H, Gazzaz M, Naama O, Elmostarchid B, Boucetta M. Idiopathic spinal epidural lipomatosis without obesity: a case with relapsing and remitting course. *Spinal Cord.* 2008; 46: 243–4.

Alessi G, Lemmerling M, Vereecken L, De Waele L. Benign metastasizing leiomyoma to skull base and spine: a report of two cases. *Clin Neurol Neurosurg* 2003; 105: 170–4.

Ali AE, Fazl M, Bilbao JM. Primary intracranial leiomyoma: a case report and literature review. *Virchows Arch* 2006; 449: 382–4.

Baehring JM, Dickey PS, Bannykh SI. Epithelioid hemangioendothelioma of the suprasellar area: a case report and review of the literature. *Arch Pathol Lab Med* 2004; 128: 1289–93.

Bahat E, Akman S, Karpuzoglu G, Aktan S, Ucar T, Arslan AG, et al. Visceral Kaposi's sarcoma with intracranial metastasis: a rare complication of renal transplantation. *Pediatr Transplant* 2002; 6: 505–8.

Bargiela A, Rey JL, Diaz JL, Martinez A. Meningeal leiomyoma in an adult with AIDS: CT and MRI with pathological correlation. *Neuroradiology* 1999; 41: 696–8.

Bauman GS, Wara WM, Ciricillo SF, Davis RL, Zoger S, Edwards MS. Primary intracerebral osteosarcoma: a case report. *J Neurooncol* 1997; 32: 209–13.

Bilkay U, Erdem O, Ozek C, Helvaci E, Kilic K, Ertan Y, et al. Benign osteoma with Gardner syndrome: review of the literature and report of a case. *J Craniofac Surg* 2004; 15: 506–9.

Bingaman KD, Alleyne CH, Jr., Olson JJ. Intracranial extraskeletal mesenchymal chondrosarcoma: case report. *Neurosurgery* 2000; 46: 207–11; discussion 211–12.

Broniscer A, Ke W, Fuller CE, Wu J, Gajjar A, Kun LE. Second neoplasms in pediatric patients with primary central nervous system tumors: the St. Jude Children's Research Hospital experience. *Cancer* 2004; 100: 2246–52.

Budka H. Intracranial lipomatous hamartomas (intracranial "lipomas"). A study of 13 cases including combinations with medulloblastoma, colloid and epidermoid cysts, angiomatosis and other malformations. *Acta Neuropathol* 1974; 28: 205–22.

Cagli S, Oktar N, Dalbasti T, Islekel S, Demirtas E, Ozdamar N. Intravascular papillary endothelial hyperplasia of the central nervous system – four case reports. *Neurol Med Chir (Tokyo)* 2004; 44: 302–10.

Cai N, Kahn LB. A report of primary brain fibrosarcoma with literature review. *J Neurooncol* 2004; 68: 161–7.

Celli P, Cervoni L, Maraglino C. Primary rhabdomyosarcoma of the brain: observations on a case with clinical and radiological evidence of cure. *J Neurooncol* 1998; 36: 259–67.

Cessna MH, Zhou H, Perkins SL, Tripp SR, Layfield L, Daines C, et al. Are myogenin and myoD1 expression specific for rhabdomyosarcoma? A study of 150 cases, with emphasis on spindle cell mimics. *Am J Surg Pathol* 2001; 25: 1150–7.

Chang CS, Hsieh PF, Chia LG, Chen CC, Pan ST, Wang YC. Leptomeningeal malignant melanoma arising in neurocutaneous melanocytosis: a case report. *Zhonghua Yi Xue Za Zhi (Taipei)* 1997; 60: 316–20.

Chitoku S, Kawai S, Watabe Y, Nishitani M, Fujimoto K, Otsuka H, et al. Intradural spinal hibernoma: case report. *Surg Neurol* 1998; 49: 509–12; discussion 512–13.

Coffin CM, Watterson J, Priest JR, Dehner LP. Extrapulmonary inflammatory myofibroblastic tumor (inflammatory pseudotumor). A clinicopathologic and immunohistochemical study of 84 cases. *Am J Surg Pathol* 1995; 19: 859–72.

Coffin CM, Dehner LP, Meis-Kindblom JM. Inflammatory myofibroblastic tumor, inflammatory fibrosarcoma, and related lesions: an historical review with differential diagnostic considerations. *Semin Diagn Pathol* 1998; 15: 102–10.

Coffin CM, Hornick JL, Fletcher CD. Inflammatory myofibroblastic tumor: comparison of clinicopathologic, histologic, and immunohistochemical features including ALK expression in atypical and aggressive cases. *Am J Surg Pathol* 2007; 31: 509–20.

de Ruiter GC, Scheithauer BW, Amrami KK, Spinner RJ. Benign metastasizing leiomyomatosis with massive brachial plexus involvement mimicking neurofibromatosis type 1. *Clin Neuropathol* 2006; 25: 282–7.

Desai KI, Nadkarni TD, Goel A, Muzumdar DP, Naresh KN, Nair CN. Primary Ewing's sarcoma of the cranium. *Neurosurgery* 2000; 46: 62–8; discussion 68–9.

Deyrup AT, Lee VK, Hill CE, Cheuk W, Toh HC, Kesavan S, et al. Epstein–Barr virus-associated smooth muscle tumors are distinctive mesenchymal tumors reflecting multiple infection events: a clinicopathologic and molecular analysis of 29 tumors from 19 patients. *Am J Surg Pathol* 2006; 30: 75–82.

Diaz R, Segura A, Calderero V, Cervera I, Aparicio J, Jorda MV, et al. Central nervous system metastases of a pulmonary epitheloid haemangioendothelioma. *Eur Respir J* 2004; 23: 483–6.

Dickerman RD, Bennett MT. Acute spinal cord compression caused by vertebral hemangioma. *Spine J* 2005; 5: 582–4; author reply 584.

Donati F, Vassella F, Kaiser G, Blumberg A. Intracranial lipomas. *Neuropediatrics* 1992; 23: 32–8.

Douglas JL, Gustin JK, Dezube B, Pantanowitz JL, Moses AV. Kaposi's sarcoma: a model of both malignancy and chronic inflammation. *Panminerva Med* 2007; 49: 119–38.

Eghwrudjakpor PO, Kurisaka M, Fukuoka M, Mori K. Intracranial lipomas. *Acta Neurochir (Wien)* 1991; 110: 124–8.

Ellegala DB, Kligori C, Vandenberg S, Dumont A, Shaffrey ME. Intracranial metastasis of a primary scalp angiosarcoma. Case illustration. *J Neurosurg* 2002; 97: 725.

Endo T, Su CC, Numagami Y, Shirane R. Malignant intracranial epithelioid hemangioendothelioma presumably originating from the lung: case report. *J Neurooncol* 2004; 67: 337–43.

Fagundes-Pereyra WJ, de Sousa L, Carvalho GT, Pittella JE, de Sousa AA. Meningeal melanocytoma of the posterior fossa: case report and literature review. *Surg Neurol* 2005; 63: 269–73; discussion 273–4.

Fan CY, Wang ST, Liu CL, Chang MC, Chen TH. Idiopathic spinal epidural lipomatosis. *J Chin Med Assoc* 2004; 67: 258–61.

Fernandes AL, Ratilal B, Mafra M, Magalhaes C. Aggressive intracranial and extracranial epithelioid hemangioendothelioma: a case report and review of the literature. *Neuropathology* 2006; 26: 201–5.

Fletcher CDM, Unni KK, Mertens F, World Health Organization, International Agency for Research on Cancer. *Pathology and Genetics of Tumours of Soft Tissue and Bone.* Lyon: IARC Press, 2002.

Fogel GR, Cunningham PY, 3rd, Esses SI. Spinal epidural lipomatosis: case reports, literature review and meta-analysis. *Spine J* 2005; 5: 202–11.

Friede RL, Pollak A. Neurosurgical desmoid tumors: presentation of four cases with a review of the differential diagnoses. *J Neurosurg* 1979; 50: 725–32.

Fuse T, Takagi T, Hirose M. Primary intracranial epithelioid angiosarcoma – case report. *Neurol Med* Chir (Tokyo) 1995; 35: 364–8.

Gaspar LE, Mackenzie IR, Gilbert JJ, Kaufmann JC, Fisher BF, Macdonald DR, et al. Primary cerebral fibrosarcomas. Clinicopathologic study and review of the literature. *Cancer* 1993; 72: 3277–81.

Gengler C, Guillou L. Solitary fibrous tumour and haemangiopericytoma: evolution of a concept. *Histopathology* 2006; 48: 63–74.

Gold JS, Antonescu CR, Hajdu C, Ferrone CR, Hussain M, Lewis JJ, et al. Clinicopathologic correlates of solitary fibrous tumors. *Cancer* 2002; 94: 1057–68.

Granter SR, Renshaw AA, Fletcher CD, Bhan AK, Rosenberg AE. CD99 reactivity in mesenchymal chondrosarcoma. *Hum Pathol* 1996; 27: 1273–6.

Gray MH, Rosenberg AE, Dickersin GR, Bhan AK. Cytokeratin expression in epithelioid vascular neoplasms. *Hum Pathol* 1990; 21: 212–17.

Greene S, Hawkins DS, Rutledge JC, Tsuchiya KD, Douglas J, Ellenbogen RG, et al. Pediatric intradural extramedullary synovial sarcoma: case report. *Neurosurgery* 2006; 59: E1339; discussion E1339.

Hamlat A, Casallo-Quilliano C, Saikali S, Lesimple T, Brassier G. Epithelioid hemangioendothelioma of the infundibular–hypothalamic region: case report and literature review. *J Neurooncol* 2004; 67: 361–6.

Harrison MJ, Mitnick RJ, Rosenblum BR, Rothman AS. Leptomyelolipoma: analysis of 20 cases. *J Neurosurg* 1990; 73: 360–7.

Higashida T, Sakata K, Kanno H, Tanabe Y, Kawasaki T, Yamamoto I. [Intracranial chondroma arising from the skull base: two case reports featuring the image findings for differential diagnosis]. *No Shinkei Geka* 2007; 35: 495–501.

Hoang MP, Amirkhan RH. Inhibin alpha distinguishes hemangioblastoma from clear cell renal cell carcinoma. *Am J Surg Pathol* 2003; 27: 1152–6.

Hussein MR. Cranial fasciitis of childhood: a case report and review of literature. *J Cutan Pathol* 2008; 35: 212–14.

Ito T, Tsutsumi T, Ohno K, Takizawa T, Kitamura K. Intracranial angiosarcoma arising from a schwannoma. *J Laryngol Otol* 2007; 121: 68–71.

Jattiot F, Goupille P, Azais I, Roulot B, Alcalay M, Jeannou J, et al. Fourteen cases of sarcomatous degeneration in Paget's disease. *J Rheumatol* 1999; 26: 150–5.

Jeon YK, Chang KH, Suh YL, Jung HW, Park SH. Inflammatory myofibroblastic tumor of the central nervous system: clinicopathologic analysis of 10 cases. *J Neuropathol Exp Neurol* 2005; 64: 254–9.

Kan P, Schmidt MH. Osteoid osteoma and osteoblastoma of the spine. *Neurosurg Clin N Am* 2008; 19: 65–70.

Karsdorp N, Elderson A, Wittebol-Post D, Hene RJ, Vos J, Feldberg MA, et al. Von Hippel–Lindau disease: new strategies in early detection and treatment. *Am J Med* 1994; 97: 158–68.

Kazmi SA, Perry A, Pressey JG, Wellons JC, Hammers Y, Palmer CA. Primary Ewing sarcoma of the brain: a case report and literature review. *Diagn Mol Pathol* 2007; 16: 108–11.

Kim KJ, Lee JY, Lee SH. Spinal intradural capillary hemangioma. *Surg Neurol* 2006; 66: 212–14.

Kleinschmidt-DeMasters BK, Mierau GW, Sze CI, Breeze RE, Greffe B, Lillehei KO, et al. Unusual dural and skull-based mesenchymal neoplasms: a report of four cases. *Hum Pathol* 1998; 29: 240–5.

Kothandaram P. Dural liposarcoma associated with subdural hematoma. Case report. *J Neurosurg* 1970; 33: 85–7.

Kriss TC, Warf BC. Cervical paraspinous desmoid tumor in a child: case report. *Neurosurgery* 1994; 35: 956–9; discussion 959.

Kristof RA, Van Roost D, Wolf HK, Schramm J. Intravascular papillary endothelial hyperplasia of the sellar region. Report of three cases and review of the literature. *J Neurosurg* 1997; 86: 558–63.

Kroe DJ, Hudgins WR, Simmons JC, Blackwell CF. Primary intrasellar leiomyoma. Case report. *J Neurosurg* 1968; 29: 189–91.

Kulkarni V, Rajshekhar V, Chandi SM. Orbital apex leiomyoma with intracranial extension. *Surg Neurol* 2000; 54: 327–30.

Lach B, Duncan E, Rippstein P, Benoit BG. Primary intracranial pleomorphic angioleiomyoma – a new morphologic variant. An immunohistochemical and electron microscopic study. *Cancer* 1994; 74: 1915–20.

Lach B, Lesiuk H. Intracranial suprasellar angiolipoma: ultrastructural and immunohistochemical features. *Neurosurgery* 1994; 34: 163–7.

Lam RM, Malik GM, Chason JL. Osteosarcoma of meninges: clinical, light, and ultrastructural observations of a case. *Am J Surg Pathol* 1981; 5: 203–8.

Larrea-Oyarbide N, Valmaseda-Castellon E, Berini-Aytes L, Gay-Escoda C. Osteomas of the craniofacial region. Review of 106 cases. *J Oral Pathol Med* 2008; 37: 38–42.

Lee JW, Cho EY, Hong SH, Chung HW, Kim JH, Chang KH, et al. Spinal epidural hemangiomas: various types of MR imaging features with histopathologic correlation. *AJNR Am J Neuroradiol* 2007; 28: 1242–8.

Lee YY, Van Tassel P, Raymond AK. Intracranial dural chondrosarcoma. *AJNR Am J Neuroradiol* 1988; 9: 1189–93.

Levy RM, Pons VG, Rosenblum ML. Central nervous system mass lesions in the acquired immunodeficiency syndrome (AIDS). *J Neurosurg* 1984; 61: 9–16.

Loddenkemper T, Morris HH, 3rd, Diehl B, Lachhwani DK. Intracranial lipomas and epilepsy. *J Neurol* 2006; 253: 590–3.

Makkar HS, Frieden IJ. Neurocutaneous melanosis. *Semin Cutan Med Surg* 2004; 23: 138–44.

Martinez-Salazar A, Supler M, Rojiani AM. Primary intracerebral malignant fibrous histiocytoma: immunohistochemical findings and etiopathogenetic considerations. *Mod Pathol* 1997; 10: 149–54.

Mentzel T, Katenkamp D. Intraneural angiosarcoma and angiosarcoma arising in benign and malignant peripheral nerve sheath tumours: clinicopathological and immunohistochemical analysis of four cases. *Histopathology* 1999; 35: 114–20.

Mitchell A, Scheithauer BW, Ebersold MJ, Forbes GS. Intracranial fibromatosis. *Neurosurgery* 1991; 29: 123–6.

Miyamori T, Mizukoshi H, Yamano K, Takayanagi N, Sugino M, Hayase H, et al. Intracranial chondrosarcoma – case report. *Neurol Med Chir (Tokyo)* 1990; 30: 263–7.

Nakashima Y, Unni KK, Shives TC, Swee RG, Dahlin DC. Mesenchymal chondrosarcoma of bone and soft tissue. A review of 111 cases. *Cancer* 1986; 57: 2444–53.

Neumann HP, Eggert HR, Weigel K, Friedburg H, Wiestler OD, Schollmeyer P. Hemangioblastomas of the central nervous system. A 10-year study with special reference to von Hippel–Lindau syndrome. *J Neurosurg* 1989; 70: 24–30.

Nora FE, Scheithauer BW. Primary epithelioid hemangioendothelioma of the brain. *Am J Surg Pathol* 1996; 20: 707–14.

Oliveira AM, Scheithauer BW, Salomao DR, Parisi JE, Burger PC, Nascimento AG. Primary sarcomas of the brain and spinal cord: a study of 18 cases. *Am J Surg Pathol* 2002; 26: 1056–63.

Oruckaptan HH, Berker M, Soylemezoglu F, Ozcan OE. Parafalcine chondrosarcoma: an unusual localization for a classical variant. Case report and review of the literature. *Surg Neurol* 2001; 55: 174–9.

Paradowski B, Zub W, Sasiadek M, Markowska-Wojciechowska A, Paradowski M. Intraosseous hemangioma in parietal bone. *Neurology* 2007; 68: 44.

Pirotte B, Krischek B, Levivier M, Bolyn S, Brucher JM, Brotchi J. Diagnostic and microsurgical presentation of intracranial angiolipomas. Case report and review of the literature. *J Neurosurg* 1998; 88: 129–32.

Polydorides AD, Rosenblum MK, Edgar MA. Metastatic renal cell carcinoma to hemangioblastoma in von Hippel–Lindau disease. *Arch Pathol Lab Med* 2007; 131: 641–5.

Porter DG, Martin AJ, Mallucci CL, Makunura CN, Sabin HI. Spinal cord compression due to Masson's vegetant intravascular hemangioendothelioma. Case report. *J Neurosurg* 1995; 82: 125–7.

Przkora R, Vogel P, Ullrich OW, Knuchel R, Jauch KW, Bolder U. Synovial sarcoma – unusual presentation with cerebral hemorrhage. *Arch Orthop Trauma Surg* 2003; 123: 376–8.

Quint DJ, Boulos RS, Sanders WP, Mehta BA, Patel SC, Tiel RL. Epidural lipomatosis. *Radiology* 1988; 169: 485–90.

Raghavendra S, Krishnamoorthy T, Ashalatha R, Kesavadas C. Spinal angiolipoma with acute subarachnoid hemorrhage. *J Clin Neurosci* 2007; 14: 992–4.

Rathore PK, Mandal S, Meher R, Subhalakshmi R, Chauhan V, Singh S. Giant ossifying chondroma of skull. *Int J Pediatr Otorhinolaryngol* 2005; 69: 1709–11.

Riggi N, Stamenkovic I. The Biology of Ewing sarcoma. *Cancer Lett* 2007; 254: 1–10.

Rushing EJ, Armonda RA, Ansari Q, Mena H. Mesenchymal chondrosarcoma: a clinicopathologic and flow cytometric study of 13 cases presenting in the central nervous system. *Cancer* 1996; 77: 1884–91.

Rutigliano MJ, Pollack IF, Ahdab-Barmada M, Pang D, Albright AL. Intracranial infantile myofibromatosis. *J Neurosurg* 1994; 81: 539–43.

Sandberg AA, Bridge JA. Updates on the cytogenetics and molecular genetics of bone and soft tissue tumors. gastrointestinal stromal tumors. *Cancer Genet Cytogenet* 2002; 135: 1–22.

Sarangarajan R, Dehner LP. Cranial and extracranial fasciitis of childhood: a clinicopathologic and immunohistochemical study. *Hum Pathol* 1999; 30: 87–92.

Shah JA, Flynn P, Choudhari KA. Idiopathic spinal epidural lipomatosis. *Br J Neurosurg* 2005; 19: 265–7.

Sima A, Kindblom LG, Pellettieri L. Liposarcoma of the meninges. A case report. *Acta Pathol Microbiol Scand [A]* 1976; 84: 306–10.

Singhal S, Singh K, Fernandes P, Sharma S, Chander S, Rath GK, et al. Primary melanoma of the central nervous system: report of a case and review of the literature. *Indian J Cancer* 1991; 28: 92–8.

Sipos EP, Tamargo RJ, Epstein JI, North RB. Primary intracerebral small-cell osteosarcoma in an adolescent girl: report of a case. *J Neurooncol* 1997; 32: 169–74.

Slaughter JC, Hardman JM, Kempe LG, Earle KM. Neurocutaneous melanosis and leptomeningeal melanomatosis in children. *Arch Pathol* 1969; 88: 298–304.

Summers LE, Florez L, Berberian ZJ, Bhattacharjee M, Walsh JW. Postoperative cranial fasciitis. Report of two cases and review of the literature. *J Neurosurg* 2007; 106: 1080–5.

Takei H, Bhattacharjee MB, Rivera A, Dancer Y, Powell SZ. New immunohistochemical markers in the evaluation of central nervous system tumors: a review of 7 selected adult and pediatric brain tumors. *Arch Pathol Lab Med* 2007; 131: 234–41.

Tammam AG, Lewis PD, Crockard HA. Cerebello-pontine angle epithelioid haemangioendothelioma in a 4-year-old boy. *Childs Nerv Syst* 1997; 13: 648–50.

Taratuto AL, Molina HA, Diez B, Zuccaro G, Monges J. Primary rhabdomyosarcoma of brain and cerebellum. Report of four cases in infants: an immunohistochemical study. *Acta Neuropathol* 1985; 66: 98–104.

Taricco MA, Vieira JO, Jr., Machado AG, Ito FY. Intravascular papillary endothelial hyperplasia causing cauda equina compression: case report. *Neurosurgery* 1999; 45: 1478–80.

Templin CR, Stambough JB, Stambough JL. Acute spinal cord compression caused by vertebral hemangioma. *Spine J* 2004; 4: 595–600.

Truwit CL, Barkovich AJ. Pathogenesis of intracranial lipoma: an MR study in 42 patients. *AJR Am J Roentgenol* 1990; 155: 855–64; discussion 865.

Vandewalle G, Brucher JM, Michotte A. Intracranial facial nerve rhabdomyoma. Case report. *J Neurosurg* 1995; 83: 919–22.

Vilela P, Saraiva P, Goulao A. Intracranial angiolipoma as cause of subarachnoid haemorrhage. Case report and review of the literature. *Neuroradiology* 2005; 47: 91–6.

Wang F, Li X, Chen L, Pu X. Malignant transformation of spinal meningeal melanocytoma. Case report and review of the literature. *J Neurosurg Spine* 2007; 6: 451–4.

Zimmerman HM. *Progress in Neuropathology*. New York: Raven Press, 1979.

VASCULAR MALFORMATIONS

Arteriovenous Malformation

Clinical and Radiological Features

Arteriovenous malformations (AVMs) occur at almost any age but are most common in the third and fourth decades and are slightly more common in men. They result in symptoms either due to hemorrhage into brain parenchyma or the subarachnoid space, or by producing focal ischemia. Unlike some cavernous malformations, they are rarely familial. AVMs are typically well characterized by angiographic studies, having defined feeding arteries and draining veins. They are the most common type of central nervous system (CNS) malformation seen as surgical specimens (Hang et al., 1996).

Pathology

Low-power microscopy will show a torturous and disorganized aggregate of vascular channels of varying diameter and wall thicknesses, some containing laminated thrombi (Figure 4.1). "Cushions" formed through intimal hyperplasia associated with nonlaminar blood flow may be a valuable histologic finding in distinguishing the blood vessels of an AVM from a merely ectatic native blood vessel, particularly problematic when sectioning normal blood vessels of the subarachnoid space. Intervening brain tissue may show significant gliosis, macrophage accumulation, and evidence of recent and remote hemorrhage with hemosiderin deposition. Calcification may be seen in both parenchymal and vascular components of an AVM.

Figure 4.1. Arteriovenous malformation AVM. a) Abnormally large vessels with intervening gliotic brain tissue represent the typical microscopic appearance, b) with the EVG stain highlighting irregularities of the internal elastic lamina, focally duplicated or disappearing entirely.

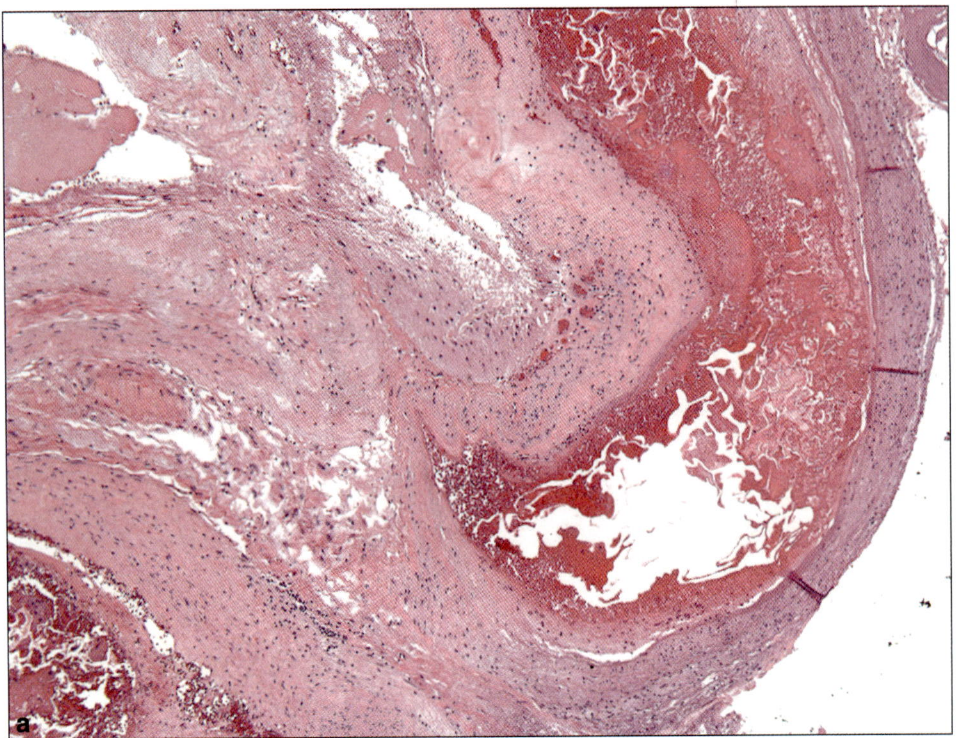

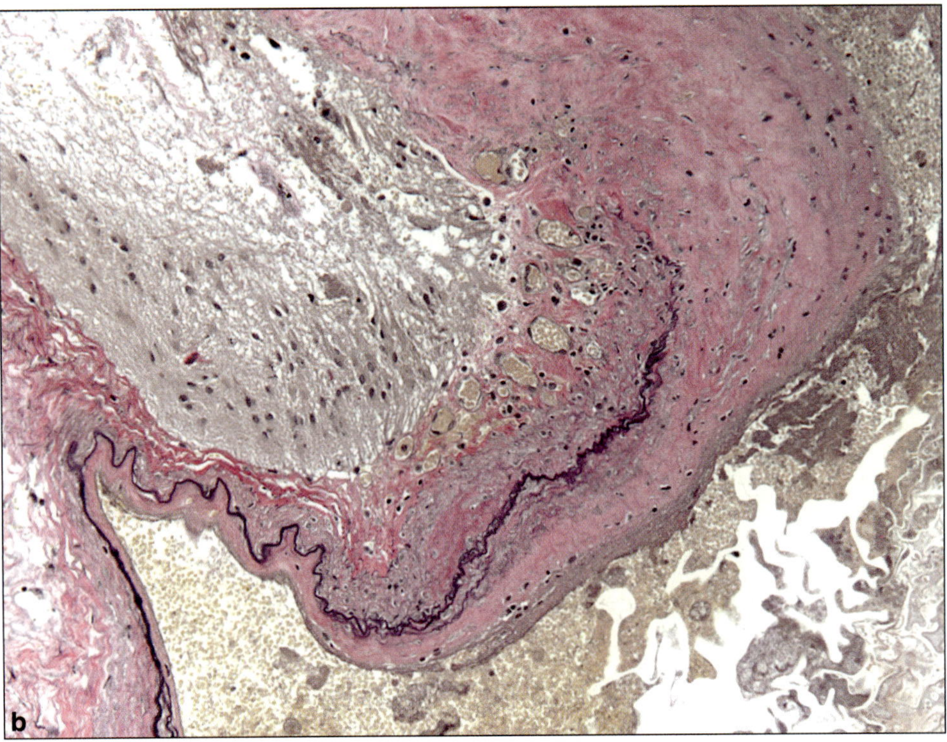

An important adjunct to the diagnosis is the elastin van Giesen stain (EVG), which will highlight the internal elastic lamina of arterial blood vessels. AVMs characteristically show vessels with discontinuous, duplicated, or otherwise incomplete presence of elastica in blood vessels that may be considered "arterialized" veins.

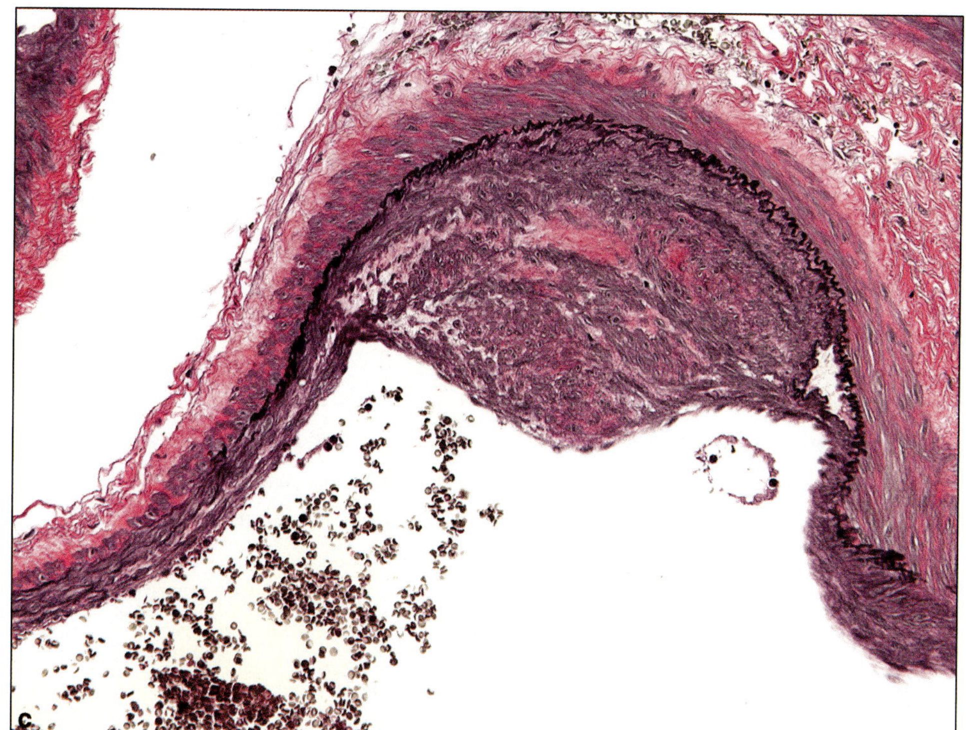

Figure 4.1. *continued*
c) Intimal "cushions" are indicative of nonlaminar blood flow through AVMs and can be a useful finding in adding evidence for a vascular malformation since they are not found in vessels which may be deceptively large in some planes of section.
d) Brain tissue adjacent to AVMs is usually gliotic and often contains hemosiderin-laden macrophages as evidence of prior hemorrhage.

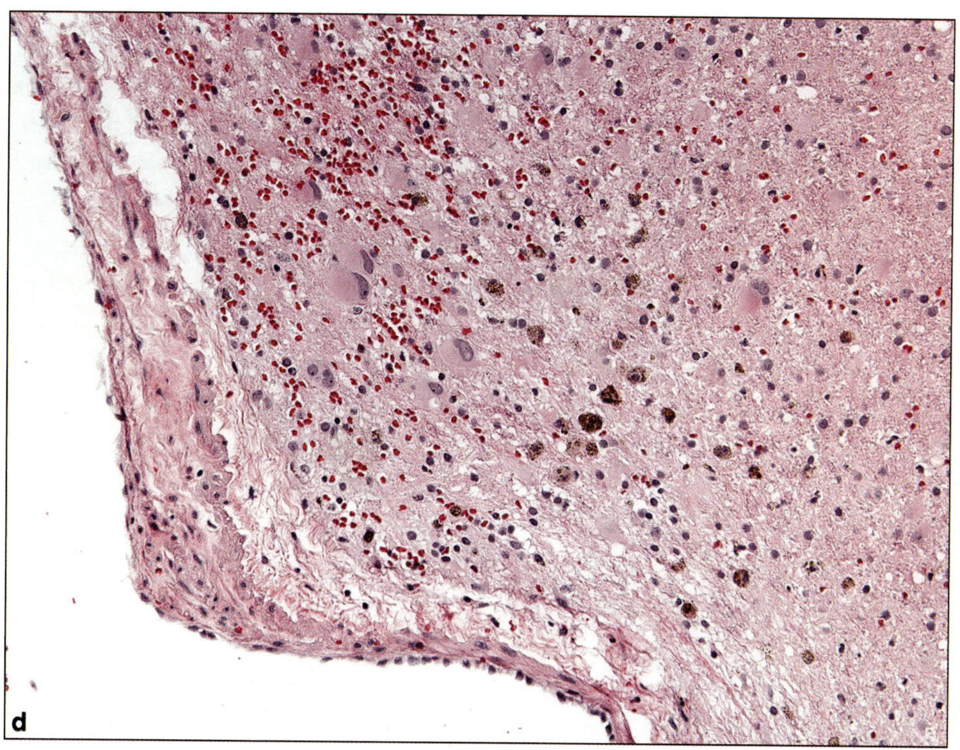

Cavernous Malformation

Clinical and Radiological Features

These are also known as cavernous hemangiomas or cavernomas. Most cases are sporadic, but some occur as a familial disorder in which they may be multiple. A number of genetic loci have been linked with familial cavernous malformations (Mindea et al., 2006) including linkage of a Mexican kindred to a locus at proximal 7q (Gunel et al., 1996; Marchuk et al., 1995).

These lesions are far less likely to be detected by angiography than AVMs and are traditionally revealed by characteristic appearance on computed tomography (CT) or magnetic resonance imaging (MRI) scans (Figure 4.2a). Neuroimaging may show multiple signal intensities, reflecting hemorrhage in various stages of evolution.

Pathology

Cavernous malformations are classically described as a tightly packed array of ectatic vessels with variable hyalinization of the walls (Figure 4.2b–d). They may often be surrounded by abundant old hemorrhage and reactive gliosis. The lack of intervening brain tissue between abnormal blood vessels has been considered a distinguishing feature from AVMs; however, exceptions exist.

CEREBRAL AMYLOID ANGIOPATHY

Clinical and Radiological Features

This condition may represent the second most common cause of primary nontraumatic intracranial hemorrhage, accounting for as many as 10–15% of cases. Its presence may exceed 50% in autopsy series of the elderly (Yamada et al., 1987). Cerebral amyloid angiopathy is most commonly associated with Alzheimer's disease (Yamada, 2002) but may exist in its absence (Vinters and Gilbert, 1983) or various causes of systemic amyloidosis. The hemorrhages are almost always supratentorial, originating in superficial cortical or subcortical locations with frequent rupture into the subarachnoid space (Gilbert and Vinters, 1983) as opposed to deeper hypertensive intracerebral hemorrhages, which tend to rupture into cerebral ventricles. The frontal and occipital lobes are particularly prone to involvement (Attems et al., 2007; Xu et al., 2003; Yamada et al., 1987). Neuroimaging may show ischemic lesions of varying ages (Figure 4.3a).

Pathology

The pathological evaluation of any intracerebral hematoma evacuation specimen in a patient over 60 years of age, or even younger (Campbell et al., 2008), should prompt careful scrutiny for the presence of small fragments of brain tissue or even isolated vascular fragments showing the characteristic homogeneous eosinophilic hyaline material, which is congophilic and immunopositive for beta-amyloid (Figure 4.3b,c).

SUBDURAL HEMORRHAGE

Clinical Features

Subdural hemorrhages are most accurately described as intradural in origin since there is no subdural "space" associated with the normal dura mater (Fuller

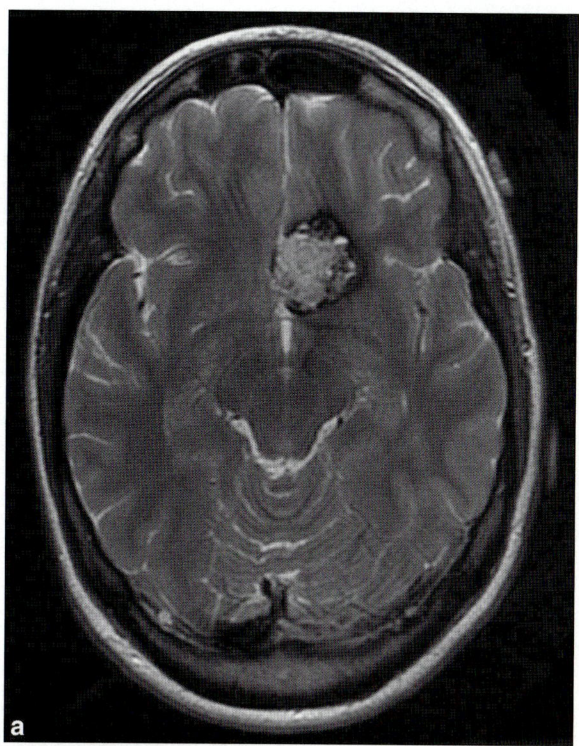

Figure 4.2. Cavernous malformation. (a) An axial T2-weighted image shows a popcorn-like mass in the inferior left frontal lobe. The mass has a ring of surrounding low intensity from hemosiderin deposition. The ring of hemosiderin and the popcorn-like appearance of cavernous malformations are fairly specific for a cavernous malformation; occasionally, other hemorrhagic neoplasms can have a similar MR appearance. Approximately half of cavernous malformations are calcified on CT. (b) Typical appearance of a cavernous malformation with crowded vessels and no intervening brain tissue.

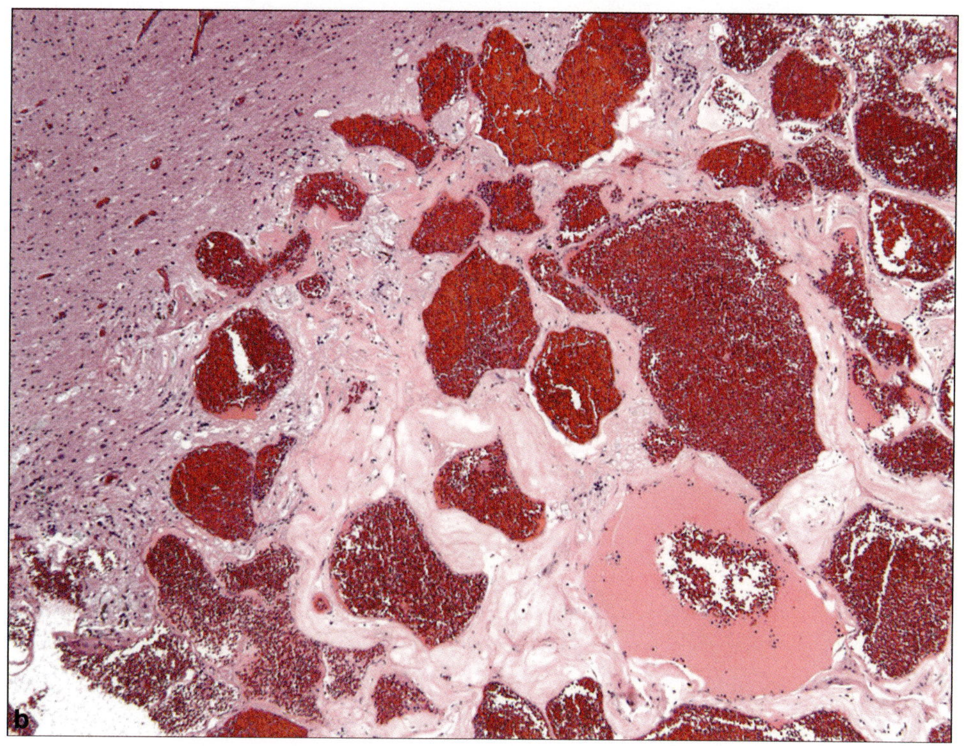

and Burger, 2007). They are usually the result of trauma although when they occur in the elderly, the minor degree of trauma may have gone unnoticed or seemed nonthreatening. It occurs with the rupture of veins, traversing the inner surface of the dura and the brain and significant cerebral atrophy may potentiate this occurrence.

Figure 4.2. *continued*
(c) with the EVG stain
showing no "arterial"
component as is seen in an
AVM. (d) A significant
proportion of cavernous
malformations diagnosed
radiographically and
pathologically may have brain
tissue intervening between the
abnormal vessels.

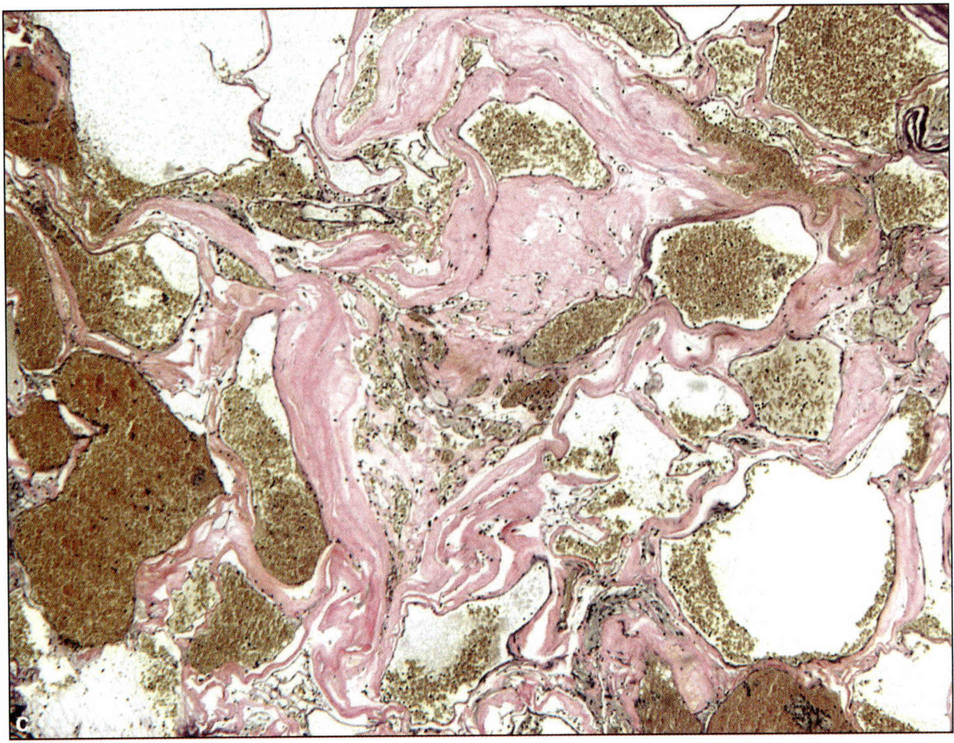

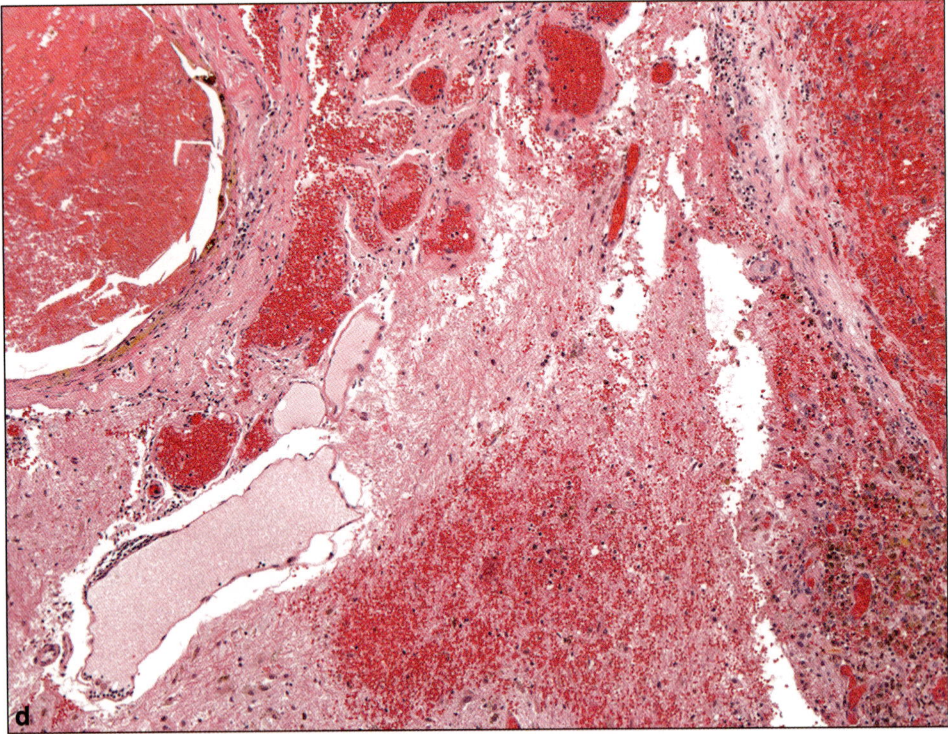

By the time they present as a lesion requiring surgical recourse, they may
have undergone some degree of organization and possible rehemorrhage. They
may also occur in association with dural neoplasms such as meningiomas or
metastases.

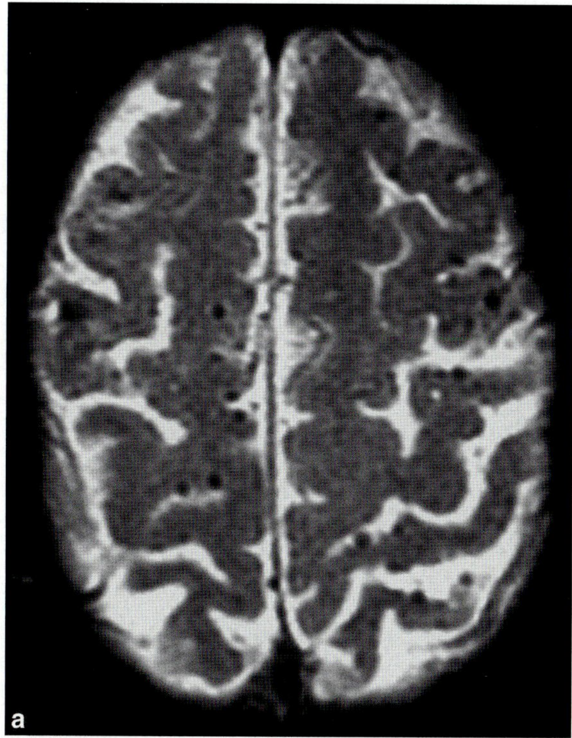

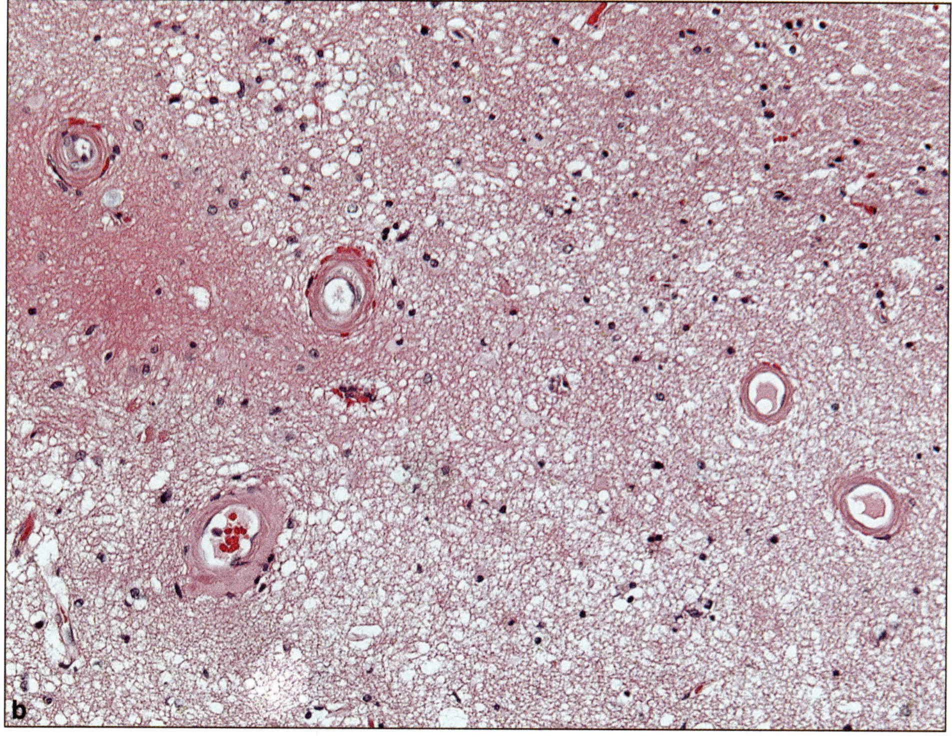

Figure 4.3. Amyloid angiopathy. (a) A T2 (gradient) image shows numerous subcortical punctate areas of hypointensity, typical of amyloid angiopathy. These areas of hypointensity represent areas of hemosiderin deposition from numerous remote microhemorrhages. T2 or GRE imaging is very sensitive in detecting the field distortions caused by hemosiderin deposition. Cavernous malformations, diffuse hemorrhagic metastases, hypertensive microhemorrhages, and diffuse axonal injury can also cause numerous foci of low signal on T2 GRE imaging. Clinical history and the distribution of the hypointensities can help to distinguish these entities from one another. (b) Fragment of brain from a hematoma evacuation in an older adult in which the eosinophilic hyaline vascular transformation is noted, and (c) confirmed with the highly sensitive anti-β amyloid immunohistochemistry.

Pathology

In their acute form, subdural hematomas possess no distinguishing features from other blood collections. With the passage of 24–48 hours, red blood cells undergo lysis and there is early fibroblast activation and infiltration. Macrophages also appear within 24–48 hours and persist well beyond 10 days

Figure 4.3. *continued.*

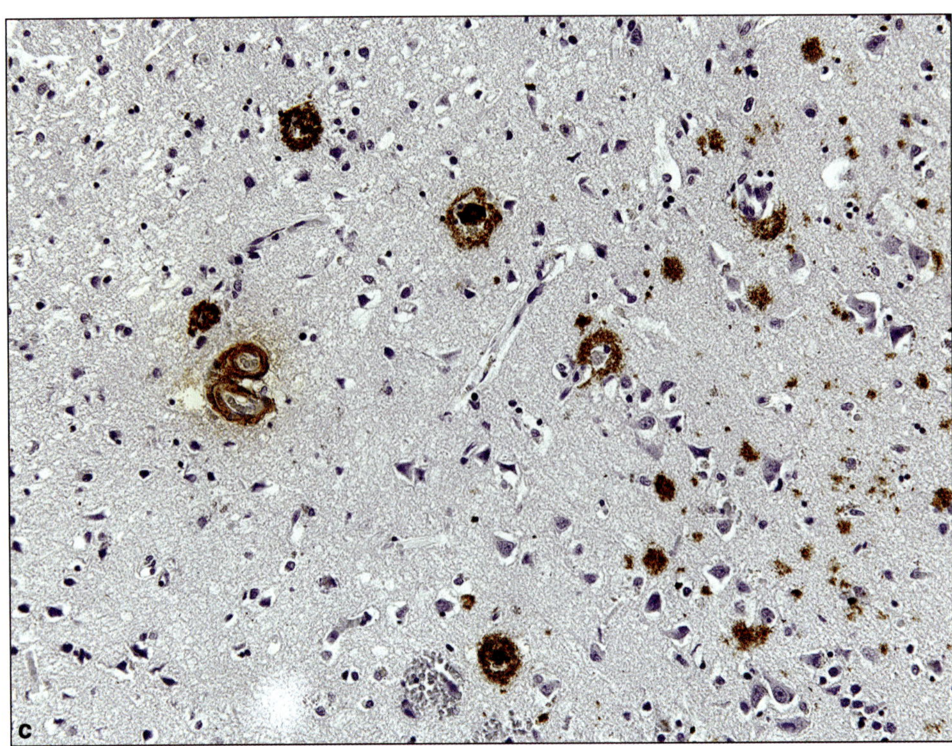

(Al-Sarraj et al., 2004). Hemosiderin-laden macrophages may occur as early as 5 days (Oehmichen et al., 2006). There ensues a brisk process of organization, featuring an influx of inflammatory cells including eosinophils with extramedullary hematopoiesis, new blood vessels, and pseudomembrane formation (Figure 4.4a). Because subdural hematomas may be associated with primary or metastatic neoplasms, the pathologist should carefully exclude this possibility (Figure 4.4b).

CEREBRAL INFARCTIONS

Cerebral infarctions are only rarely encountered by surgical biopsy, usually through misdiagnosis of a neoplasm or abscess, especially in younger individuals. They are composed of a variable mixture of macrophages, prominent capillaries, and reactive astrocytes (Figure 4.5a). It is not unusual to identify evidence of chronic hypertensive arteriopathy, with vascular fibrotic thickening. Some recent infarctions result in a form of inflammation affecting blood vessels that may mimic cerebral vasculitis (Figure 4.5b), which is in turn sometimes a diagnostic consideration among possible causes of cerebral infarctions.

CADASIL

Clinical Features

CADASIL (cerebral autosomal dominant arteriopathy with subcortical infarcts and leukoencephalopathy) is the result of missense mutations of the notch 3

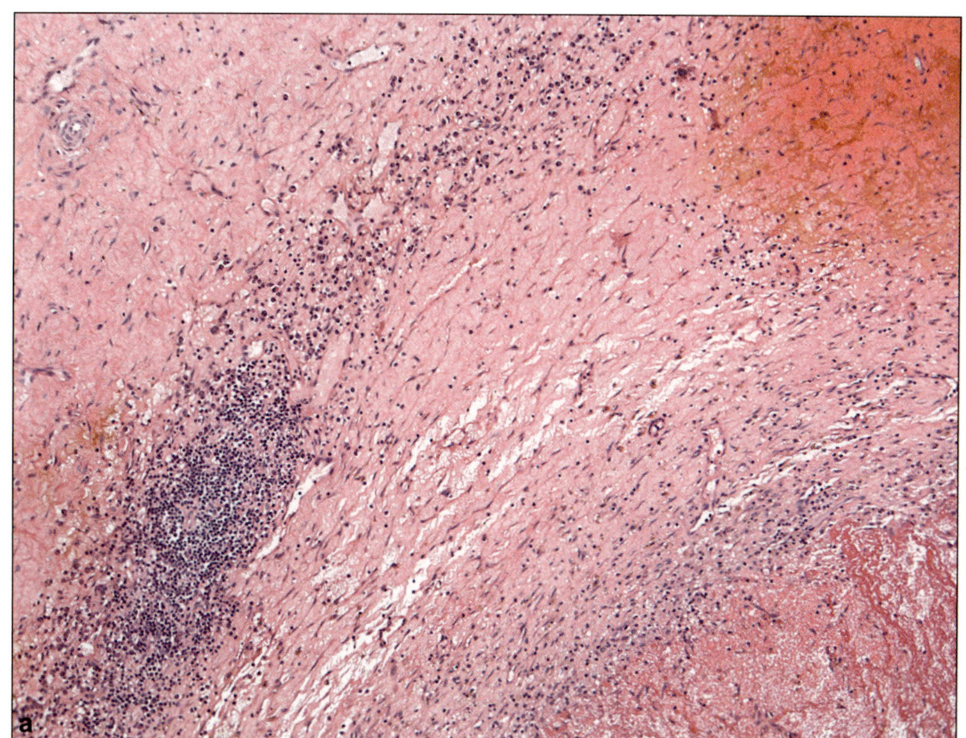

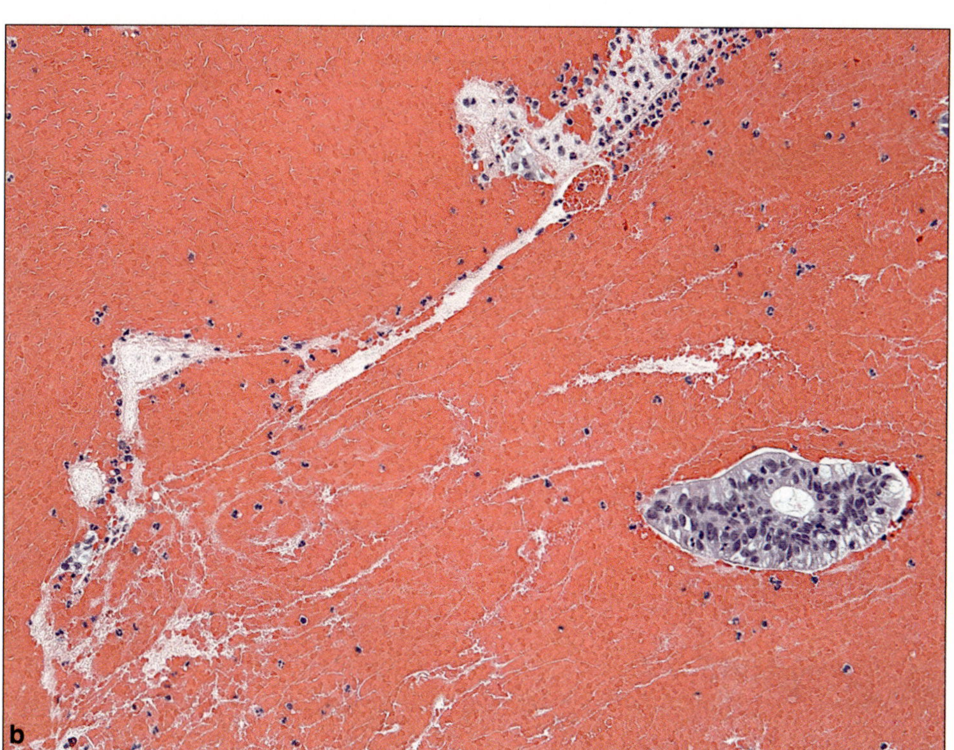

Figure 4.4. Subdural hemorrhage. (a) An organizing subdural hematoma may show conspicuous reactive inflammation including extramedullary hematopoiesis, and often shows evidence of more recurrent hemorrhages of varying ages. (b) Subdural hemorrhage specimens should be carefully examined for associated metastatic disease, as in this case of metastatic colon carcinoma to the dura leading to subdural hemorrhage.

gene on chromosome 19 (Thomas et al., 2000). It usually presents in the fifth or sixth decade with over 90% of patients suffering migraine headaches, and repeated subcortical ischemic infarctions with dementia. Brain biopsy is not indicated because of the relative ease of skin biopsy in making the diagnosis.

Figure 4.5. (a) Characteristic reactive pattern in an organizing infarction, including macrophages, gliosis, and reactive vascular hyperplasia. (b) Infarcted brain tissue may cause acute inflammation and necrosis of blood vessels that mimics the true fibrinoid change of a necrotizing vasculitis.

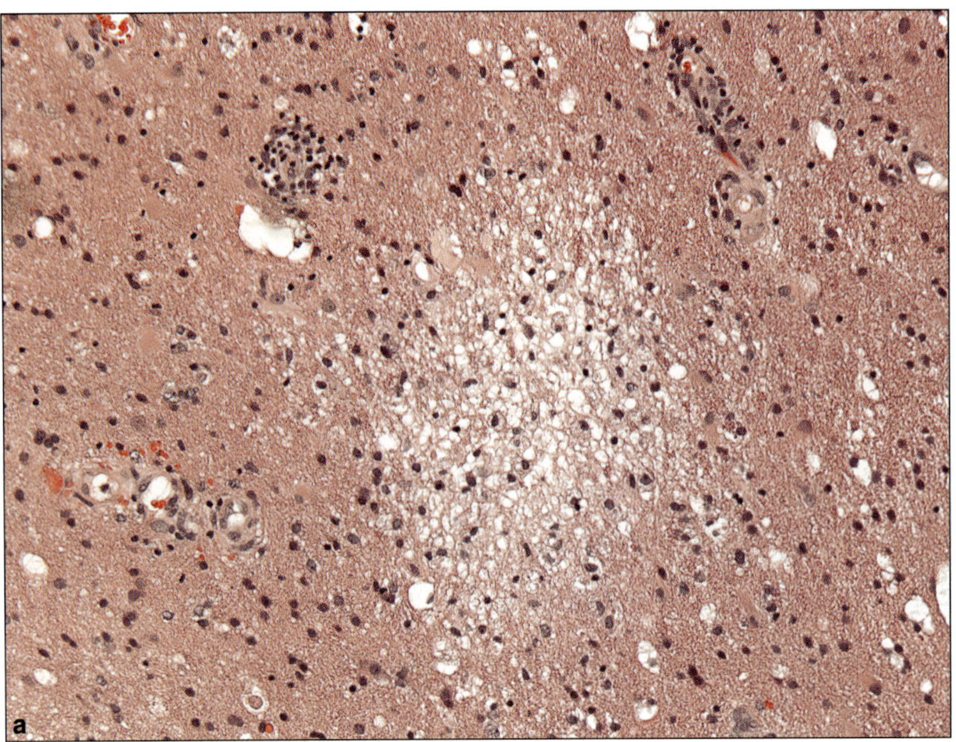

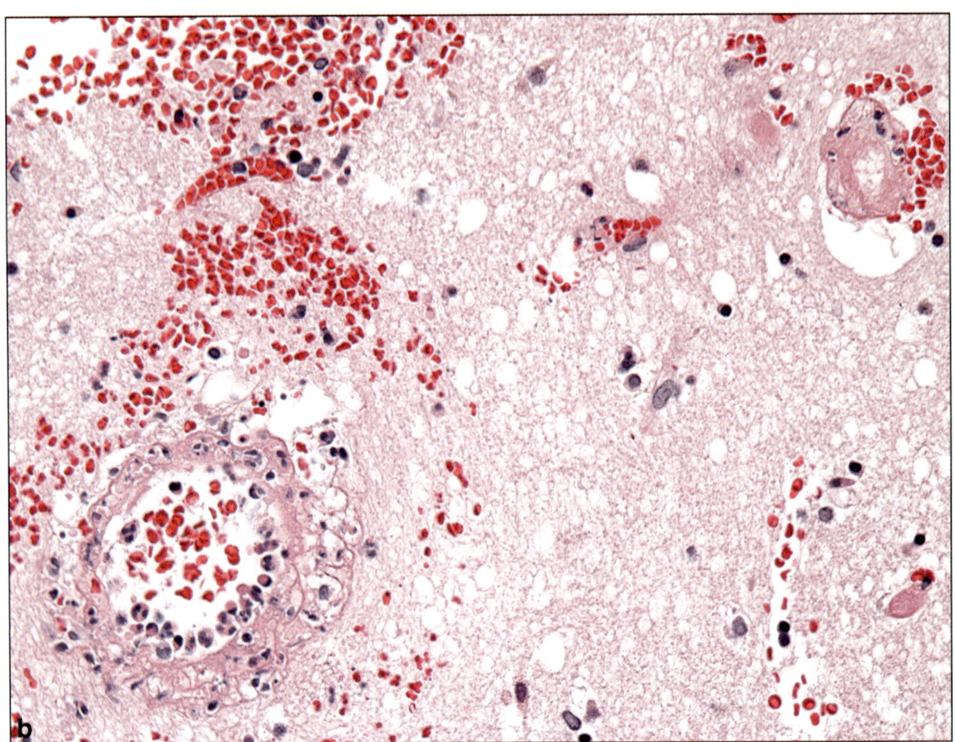

Pathology

Dermal arterioles may be examined for the same sort of perivascular smooth muscle degeneration and granular osmiophilic deposits as is seen in brain pathology (Figure 4.6). Abnormalities are considered 100% specific for the

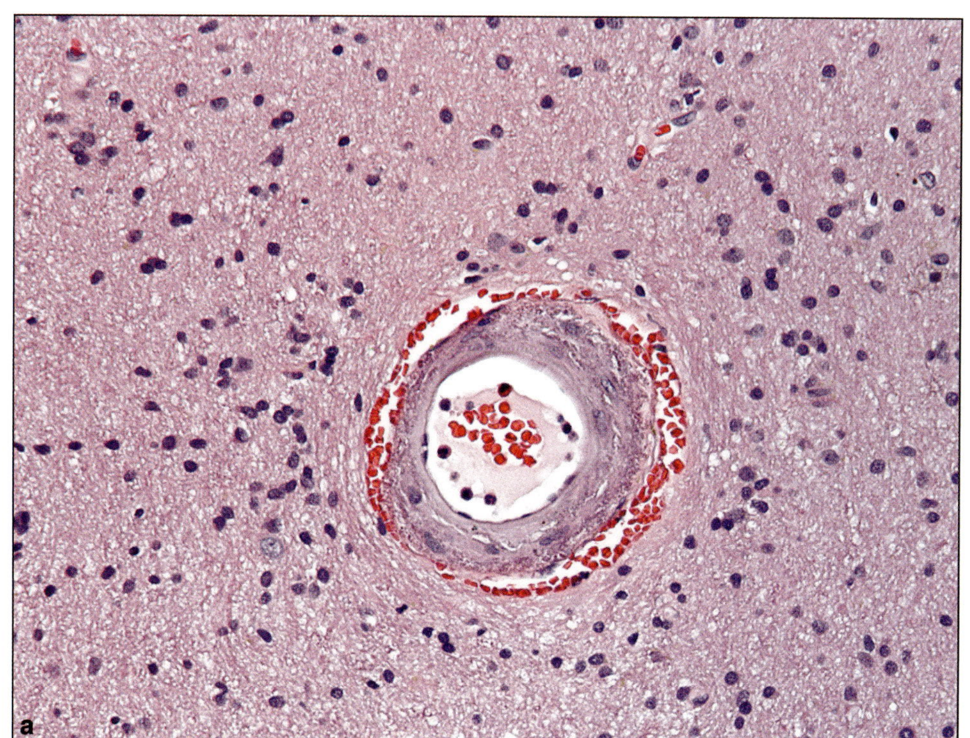

Figure 4.6. CADASIL. (a) H&E appearance of affected cerebral white matter arterial blood vessel in an earlier phase of development, with concentric sclerosis of the wall, (b) finely granular Periodic acid–Schiff positive material surrounding the arterial wall (arrow).

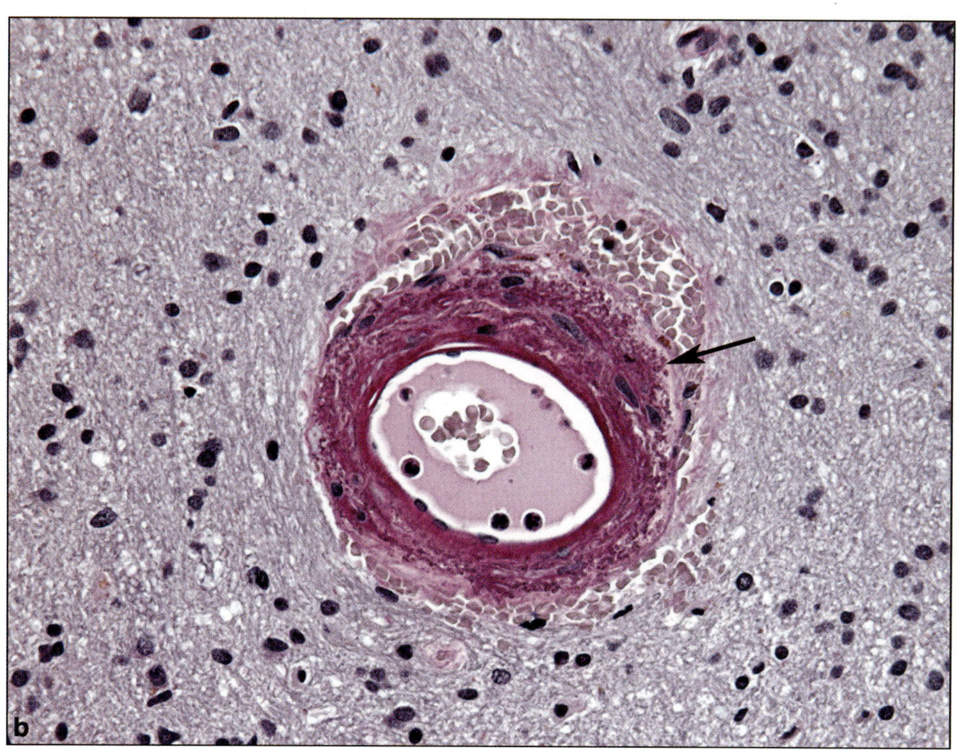

disease but sensitivity may be considerably less owing to the subtle changes and their focal nature. In order to increase sensitivity, some reports included the examination of six different arterioles within the same skin biopsy.

Figure 4.6. *continued* (c) Smooth muscle actin immunohistochemistry shows abnormal discontinuities in the vascular wall reflecting smooth muscle degeneration. (d) Electron microscopy shows osmiophilic globular bodies.

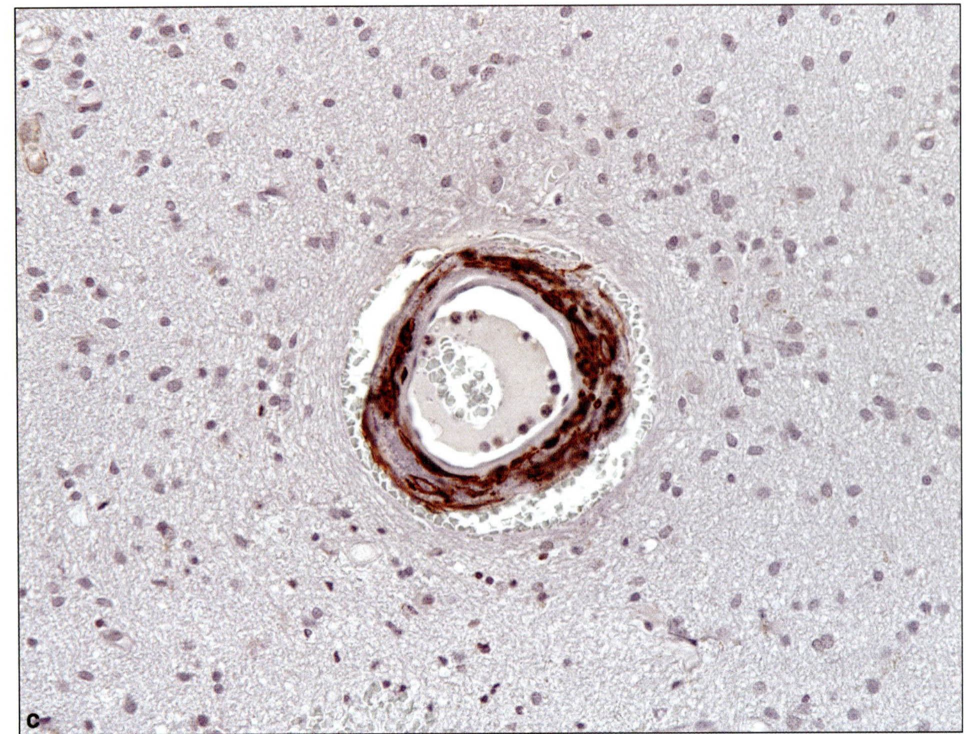

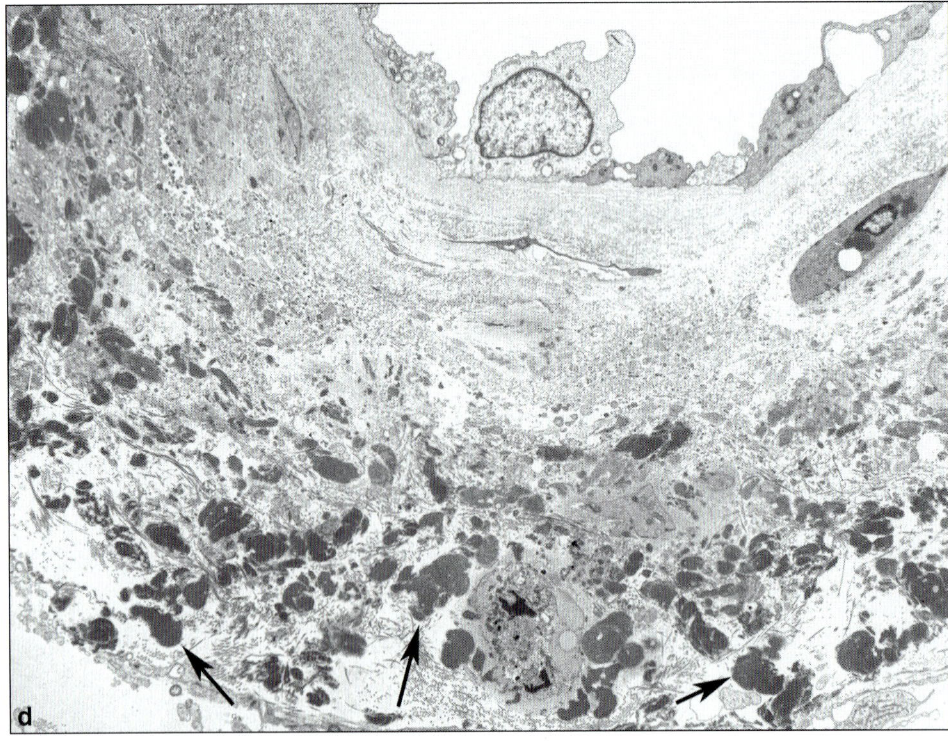

VASCULITIS

Cerebral vasculitis is considered far more frequently on clinical and radiological grounds than is actually confirmed by biopsy. It occurs either as a part of systemic and multiorgan disease or limited to the CNS. As in all inflammatory conditions, an infectious etiology must be considered. Surgical biopsies are only done in extraordinary situations in which the clinical, laboratory, and radiological evaluation points to no leading diagnosis, a circumstance in which vasculitis is almost invariably under consideration.

Polyarteritis nodosa involves the CNS in 20–40% of patients and the peripheral nervous system in over 50% of patients. It is associated with hepatitis B antigenemia in 10–50% of patients, and seropositivity for hepatitis C virus in 20% of patients. CNS involvement is considered more common in later stages of the disease and is the second most common cause of death among patients with polyarteritis nodosa (Travers et al., 1979).

It causes necrotizing lesions in medium-sized and small arteries with distal spread into arterioles. The lesions are typically patchy and discontinuous with a predilection for involvement of vascular branch. Active lesions show fibrinoid necrosis of the blood vessel wall with neutrophil infiltration, followed by fibrous scarring or lymphocytic infiltration in the healing phase.

Wegener's granulomatosis may involve cerebral blood vessels accompanied by necrotizing lesions of the respiratory tract, usually in middle-aged adults but rarely in children (Bajema et al., 1997; Ulinski et al., 2005). The diagnosis is usually confirmed by the serological detection of antineutrophil cytoplasmic autoantibodies (C-ANCA).

Other immune mediated systemic conditions that may result in CNS vasculitis are the *allergic angiitis and granulomatosis (Churg–Strauss) syndrome* (Chang et al., 1993; Liou et al., 1997; Louthrenoo et al., 1999; Tyvaert et al., 2004), *Sjogren's syndrome* (Alexander et al., 1986; Berman et al., 1990; Niemela and Hakala, 1999), and *Behcet's syndrome* (Diri and Espinoza, 2006; Siva et al., 2004).

Vasculitis limited to the CNS includes *primary* or *granulomatous angiitis of the CNS*, a condition with male predominance that tends to occur in the middle aged and elderly, presenting with a wide range of neurologic symptoms including headaches, other diffuse neurologic abnormalities, and ischemic or hemorrhagic infarctions. This is characterized by segmental granulomatous inflammation of leptomeningeal and parenchymal blood vessels (Figure 4.7). The granulomas usually contain giant cells, and fibrinoid necrosis is common. Neurosarcoidosis and infectious granulomatous diseases must be excluded. The lesion may also be especially difficult to distinguish from primary CNS lymphoma with a minor granulomatous component, or *lymphomatoid granulomatosis* (Figure 4.8). Both entities may have in common the distinctive perivascular arrangement of atypical cells causing concentric perivascular reticulin deposition and often accompanied by necrosis seen in CNS lymphomas. Lymphomatoid granulomatosis is also characterized by the presence of Epstein–Barr virus (EBV).

Figure 4.7. Granulomatous angiitis, seen involving a blood vessel in the superficial cortex extending into leptomeninges, a typical location for this disease process.

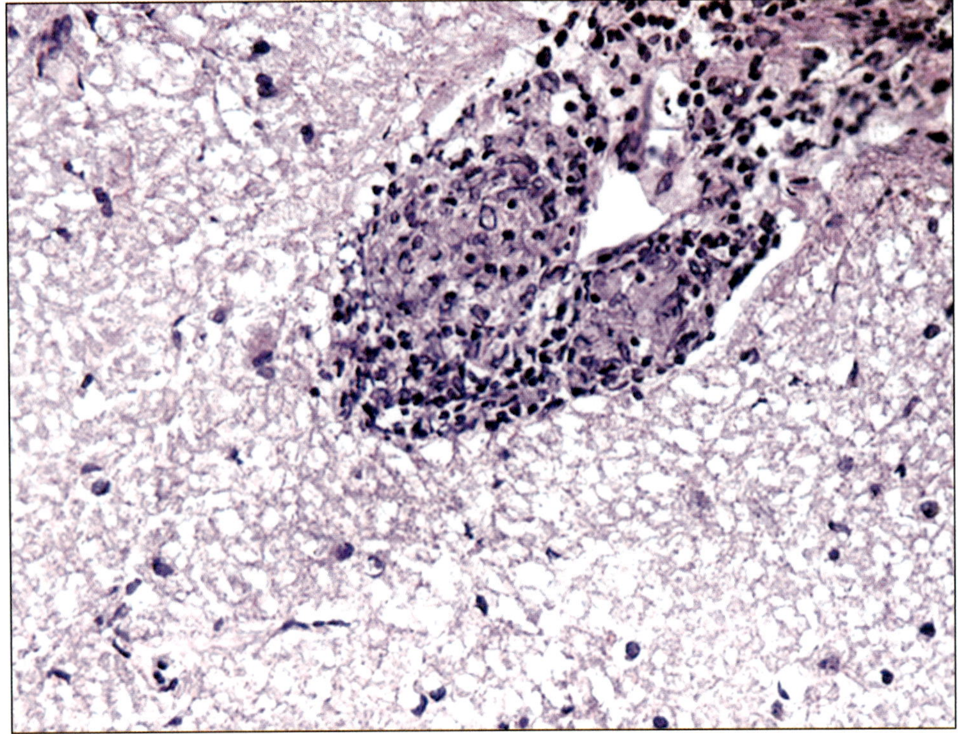

Figure 4.8. Lymphomatoid granulomatosis, with nodular vasocentric mixed granulomatous infiltrate and surrounding gliotic brain tissue which may contain foci of necrosis.

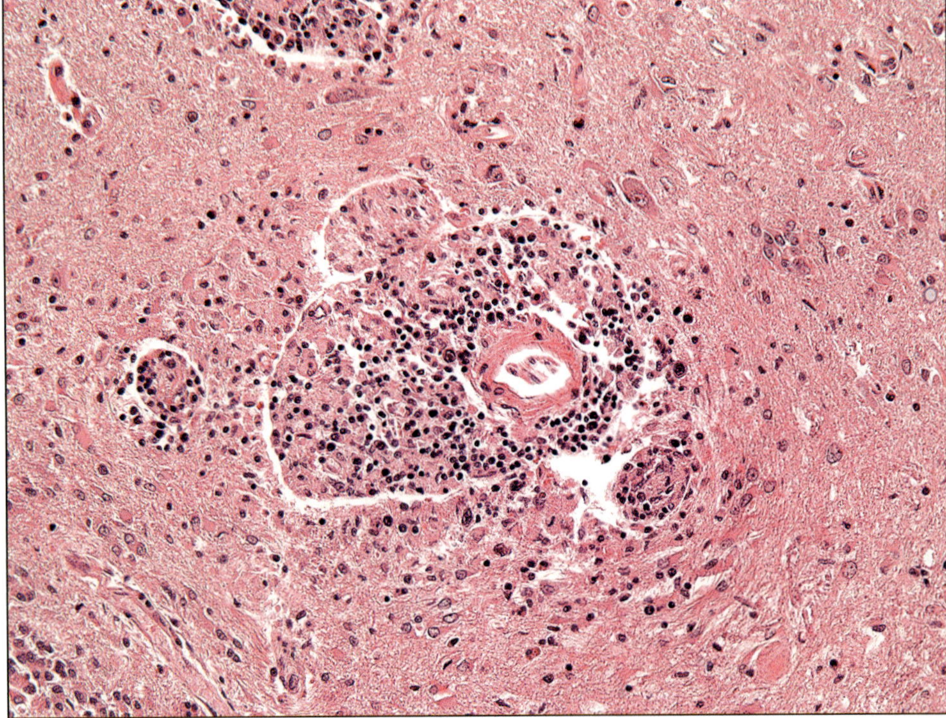

REFERENCES

Al-Sarraj S, Mohamed S, Kibble M, Rezaie P. Subdural hematoma (SDH): assessment of macrophage reactivity within the dura mater and underlying hematoma. *Clin Neuropathol* 2004; 23: 62–75.

Alexander EL, Malinow K, Lejewski JE, Jerdan MS, Provost TT, Alexander GE. Primary Sjogren's syndrome with central nervous system disease mimicking multiple sclerosis. *Ann Intern Med* 1986; 104: 323–30.

Attems J, Quass M, Jellinger KA, Lintner F. Topographical distribution of cerebral amyloid angiopathy and its effect on cognitive decline are influenced by Alzheimer disease pathology. *J Neurol Sci* 2007; 257: 49–55.

Bajema IM, Hagen EC, Weverling-Rijnsburger AW, van der Pijl H, van Dorp WT, van Ravenswaay Claasen HH, et al. Cerebral involvement in two patients with Wegener's granulomatosis. *Clin Nephrol* 1997; 47: 401–6.

Berman JL, Kashii S, Trachtman MS, Burde RM. Optic neuropathy and central nervous system disease secondary to Sjogren's syndrome in a child. *Ophthalmology* 1990; 97: 1606–9.

Campbell DM, Bruins S, Vogel H, Shuer LM, Wijman CA. Intracerebral hemorrhage caused by cerebral amyloid angiopathy in a 53-year-old man. *J Neurol* 2008; 597–8.

Chang Y, Kargas SA, Goates JJ, Horoupian DS. Intraventricular and subarachnoid hemorrhage resulting from necrotizing vasculitis of the choroid plexus in a patient with Churg-Strauss syndrome. *Clin Neuropathol* 1993; 12: 84–7.

Diri E, Espinoza LR. Neuro-Behcet's syndrome: differential diagnosis and management. *Curr Rheumatol Rep* 2006; 8: 317–22.

Fuller GN, Burger PC. Central nervous system. In: Mills SE, editor. *Histology for Pathologists*. Philadelphia: Lippincott Williams & Wilkins, 2007.

Gilbert JJ, Vinters HV. Cerebral amyloid angiopathy: incidence and complications in the aging brain. I. Cerebral hemorrhage. *Stroke* 1983; 14: 915–23.

Gunel M, Awad IA, Finberg K, Anson JA, Steinberg GK, Batjer HH, et al. A founder mutation as a cause of cerebral cavernous malformation in Hispanic Americans. *N Engl J Med* 1996; 334: 946–51.

Hang Z, Shi Y, Wei Y. [A pathological analysis of 180 cases of vascular malformation of brain]. *Zhonghua Bing Li Xue Za Zhi* 1996; 25: 135–8.

Liou HH, Liu HM, Chiang IP, Yeh TS, Chen RC. Churg-Strauss syndrome presented as multiple intracerebral hemorrhage. *Lupus* 1997; 6: 279–82.

Louthrenoo W, Norasetthada A, Khunamornpong S, Sreshthaputra A, Sukitawut W. Childhood Churg–Strauss syndrome. *J Rheumatol* 1999; 26: 1387–93.

Marchuk DA, Gallione CJ, Morrison LA, Clericuzio CL, Hart BL, Kosofsky BE, et al. A locus for cerebral cavernous malformations maps to chromosome 7q in two families. *Genomics* 1995; 28: 311–4.

Mindea SA, Yang BP, Shenkar R, Bendok B, Batjer HH, Awad IA. Cerebral cavernous malformations: clinical insights from genetic studies. *Neurosurg* Focus 2006; 21: e1.

Niemela RK, Hakala M. Primary Sjogren's syndrome with severe central nervous system disease. *Semin Arthritis Rheum* 1999; 29: 4–13.

Oehmichen M, Auer R, König HG. *Forensic Neuropathology and Associated Neurology*. Berlin, New York: Springer, 2006.

Siva A, Altintas A, Saip S. Behcet's syndrome and the nervous system. *Curr Opin Neurol* 2004; 17: 347–57.

Thomas NJ, Morris CM, Scaravilli F, Johansson J, Rossor M, De Lange R, et al. Hereditary vascular dementia linked to notch 3 mutations. CADASIL in British families. *Ann N Y Acad Sci* 2000; 903: 293–8.

Travers RL, Allison DJ, Brettle RP, Hughes GR. Polyarteritis nodosa: a clinical and angiographic analysis of 17 cases. *Semin Arthritis Rheum* 1979; 8: 184–99.

Tyvaert L, Devos P, Deloizy M, Belhadia A, Stekelorom T. [Peripheral and central neurological manifestations in a case of Churg Strauss syndrome]. *Rev Neurol (Paris)* 2004; 160: 89–92.

Ulinski T, Martin H, Mac Gregor B, Dardelin R, Cochat P. Fatal neurologic involvement in pediatric Wegener's granulomatosis. *Pediatr Neurol* 2005; 32: 278–81.

Vinters HV, Gilbert JJ. Cerebral amyloid angiopathy: incidence and complications in the aging brain. II. The distribution of amyloid vascular changes. *Stroke* 1983; 14: 924–8.

Xu D, Yang C, Wang L. Cerebral amyloid angiopathy in aged Chinese: a clinico-neuropathological study. *Acta Neuropathol* 2003; 106: 89–91.

Yamada M. Risk factors for cerebral amyloid angiopathy in the elderly. *Ann N Y Acad Sci* 2002; 977: 37–44.

Yamada M, Tsukagoshi H, Otomo E, Hayakawa M. Cerebral amyloid angiopathy in the aged. *J Neurol* 1987; 234: 371–6.

5 INFECTIONS OF THE CNS

Almost any infectious process may involve the brain, its vasculature, cerebrospinal fluid (CSF), or coverings and bony surroundings. This section will describe infectious diseases that are more commonly under consideration through surgical biopsy. The differential diagnosis in many surgical specimens with inflammation involves closely intertwined infectious and noninfectious inflammatory disorders as described in **Inflammatory Diseases.**

BACTERIAL INFECTIONS

Abscess

Clinical and Radiological Features

Brain abscesses represent the second most common infection of the nervous system after meningitis (Brown and Gray, 2008). Because of advances in radiographic imaging in the proper clinical context, many cases are successfully treated with antibiotics and do not involve biopsy (Bernardini, 2004). In fact, some neuropathologists will encounter brain abscesses more frequently as an unexpected diagnosis when a ring-enhancing tumor constitutes the prebiopsy diagnosis (Figure 5.1).

The usual antecedent predisposing clinical condition involves hematogenous spread of septic emboli, chiefly from bacterial endocarditis, suppurative lung diseases, or in congenital heart diseases with right-to-left shunts, pericranial infections of soft tissue and bone such as sinusitis, otitis media, mastoiditis, and infected dentition. More recently, there has been a decline in the incidence of brain abscesses related to otitis media and congenital heart disease and an increase in examples related to trauma or neurosurgery (Carpenter et al., 2007).

Epidural and subdural abscesses may follow infection of nearby soft tissue or bone. Vertebral epidural abscesses are more common than their intracranial counterparts, and their incidence has increased in the past decade. Spinal epidural abscess is a potentially life-threatening condition that can cause paralysis by the accumulation of purulent material in the epidural space. These lesions are sometimes the consequence of a trivial skin infection. They have numerous associations, including long-term corticosteroid use, degenerative joint disease, diabetes mellitus, intravenous drug abuse, end-stage renal disease, and others. Spinal epidural abscesses may be localized or diffuse depending on the extent of fibrous adhesions. If surgical intervention does not occur emergently, regional thrombosis of spinal blood vessels may occur along with spinal cord compression (Darouiche, 2006).

The most common causative organisms are *Staphylococcus aureus*, accounting for approximately 70% of cases followed by *Streptococcus* species; gram-negative bacilli are frequently isolated from intravenous drug abusers. *Mycobacterium tuberculosis*, Brucella species, fungal species, and parasitic organisms are rare causes of spinal epidural abscess. Up to 40% of cultures in some series are sterile.

Pathology

Most brain abscesses due to hematogenous spread occur in the distribution of the middle cerebral artery followed by the anterior cerebral artery and then within the posterior circulation. By the time of diagnosis, most abscesses will have progressed through a series of stages, often beginning as a microabscess in the gray–white junction. These lesions progress to form a necrotic and purulent lesion surrounded by the abscess capsule made up of granulation tissue and a mixed inflammatory infiltrate. The wall of a purulent abscess contains reactive astrocytes and proliferating blood vessels to the extent that it may be confused with a high-grade glial neoplasm (Figure 5.2).

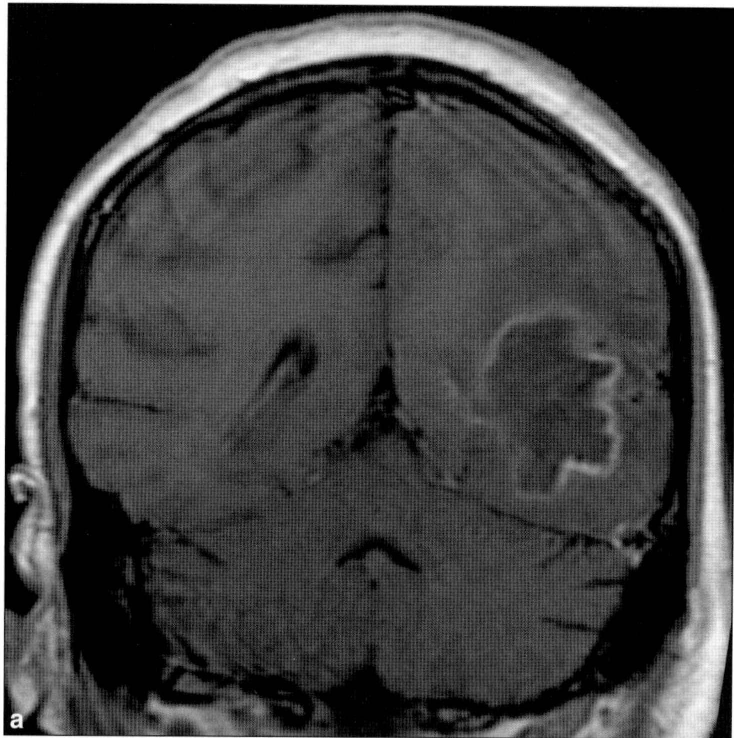

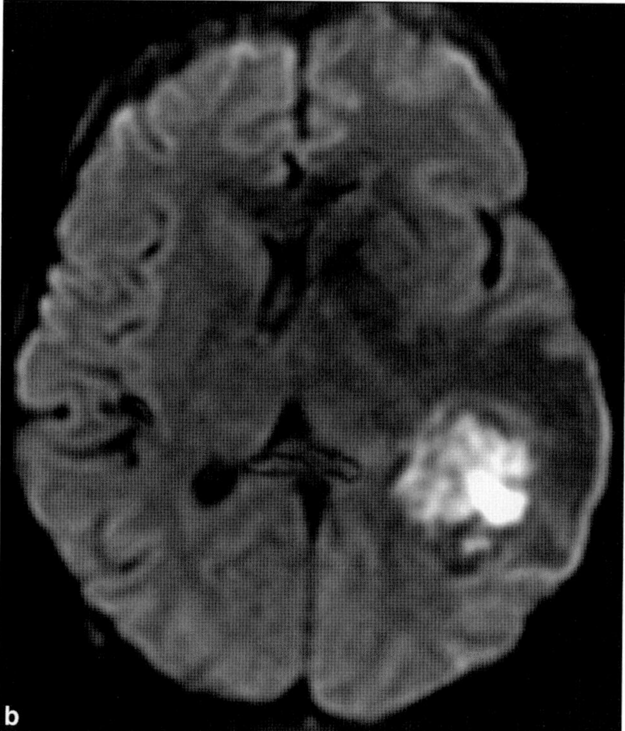

Figure 5.1. Brain abscess. (a) A coronal contrast enhanced MR shows a peripherally enhancing mass centered in the left temporal lobe. There is extensive surrounding vasogenic edema. The ring of enhancement is thicker on the side of the mass closest to the cortex. A thicker rim of enhancement on the cortical compared to the ventricular side of abscesses is common and can help to differentiate abscesses from other ring-enhancing masses. The thickness of the enhancing abscess wall may be related to differences in perfusion to the cortical and ventricular sides of the abscess. (b) An axial diffusion-weighted image MR of the same patient shows that the mass has restricted diffusion centrally. The viscous and highly cellular pus-filled core of abscesses restricts the diffusion of water unlike the necrotic core of most ring-enhancing neoplasms.

The histology of the epidural abscess is similar to that of brain abscesses. Very chronic epidural infections may spread to the extent that the original source is not obvious and produce a prominent pachymeningitis (Riggs and Schlezinger, 1953).

Figure 5.2. (a) Low-power image of wall of brain abscess mimics the appearance of a high-grade glial neoplasm, with vascular proliferation and glial proliferation. (b) Higher-power view reveals neutrophils, granular mitosis (arrow), and lipid-laden macrophages (arrowhead), each of which should raise suspicion of a nonneoplastic, reactive process.

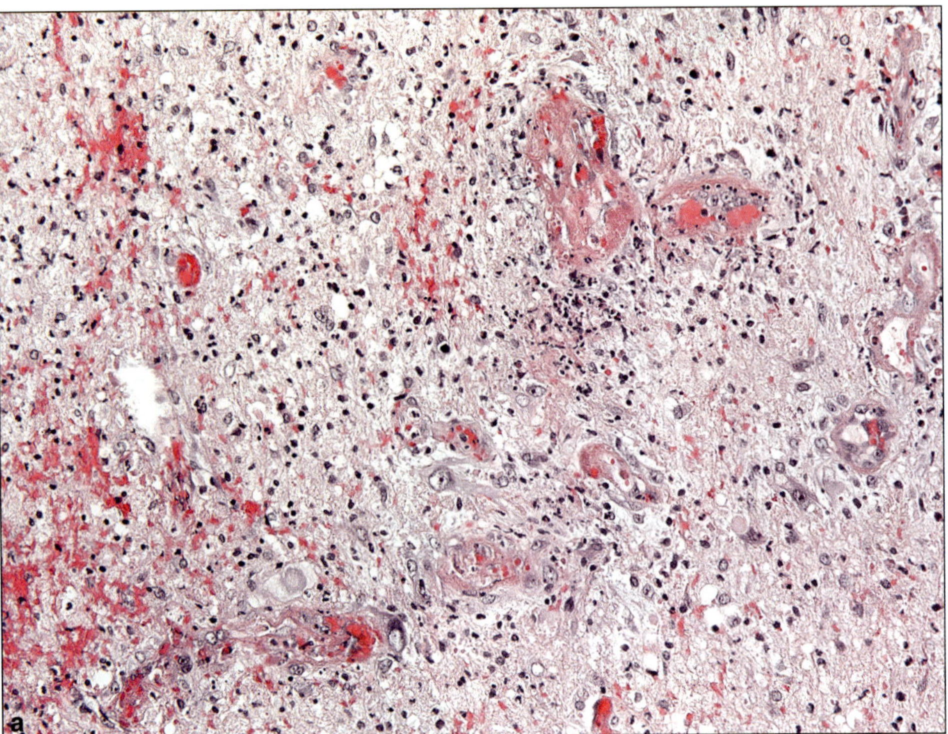

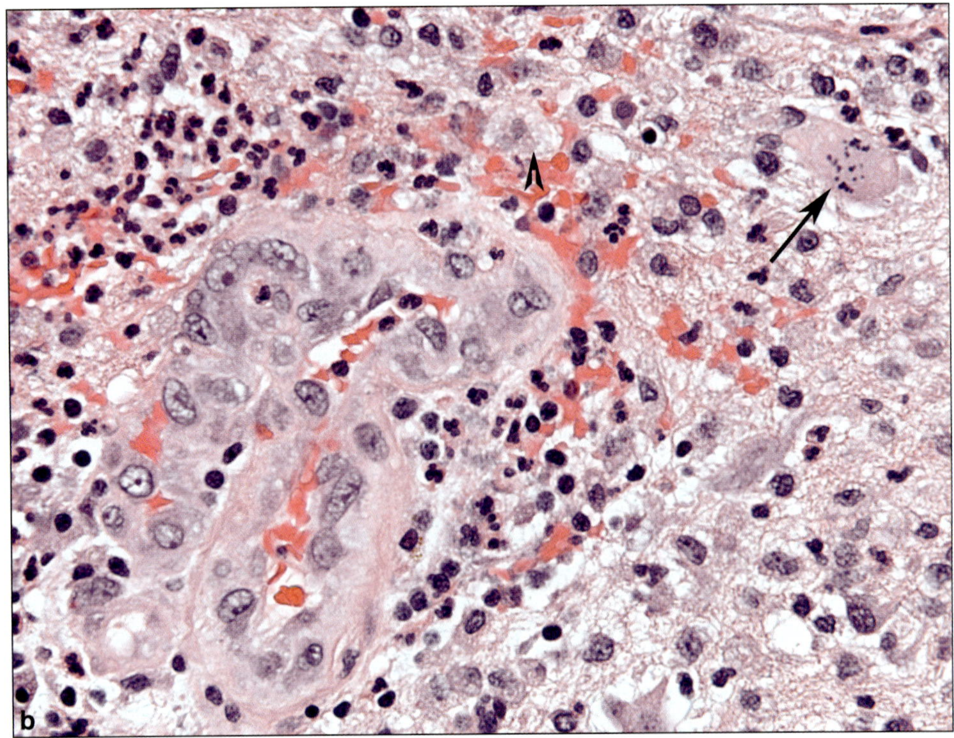

Tuberculosis

From the standpoint of the surgical neuropathologist, tuberculosis is most often encountered as an unusual form of meningitis, epidural, subdural, or cerebral tuberculous abscess, or tuberculoma of the brain and spinal cord.

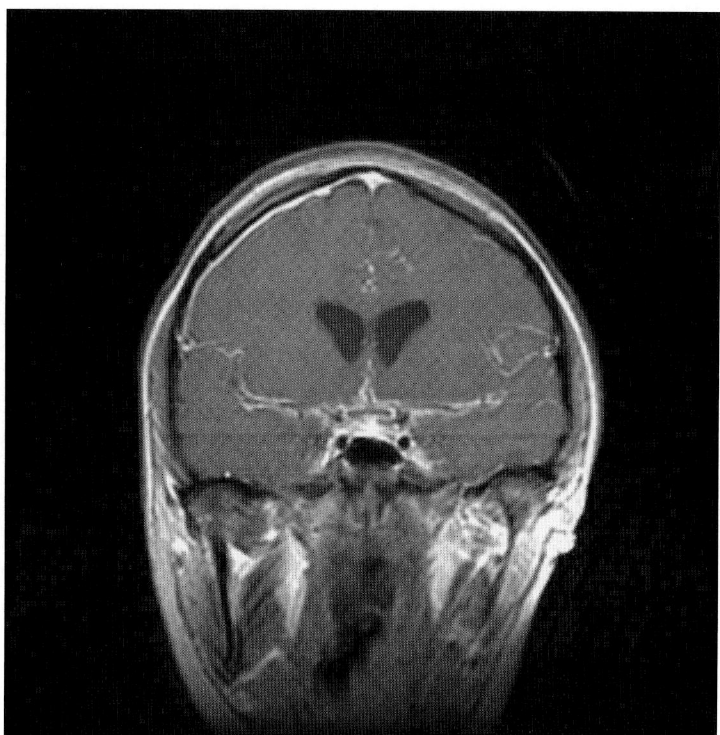

Figure 5.3. Tuberculous meningitis, with thickening of basilar meninges and spread into Sylvian fissures bilaterally, evidenced by leptomeningeal contrast enhancement.

Tuberculous meningitis is the most common manifestation of tuberculosis affecting the central nervous system (Brown and Gray, 2008). It may arise in association with small tuberculous lesions of the meninges, brain, or spinal cord, and may also be seen in miliary tuberculosis. Symptoms include the subacute or slow onset of symptoms of chronic meningitis, including fever, headache, neck stiffness, or alterations in mental status.

The pathologist should be diligent and pursuing a possible history of exposure to tuberculosis in the patient or other supportive data such as evidence of pulmonary tuberculosis, a positive skin test, or the characteristic CSF findings in which there is a mixed mononuclear inflammatory infiltrate, increased total protein, and a conspicuously low glucose concentration. Experience dictates that this supportive data is sometimes nonexistent because the diagnosis was not considered preoperatively. Mycobacterial organisms are identified by the Ziehl–Nielsen or Fite stains.

Tuberculous meningitis preferentially involves the base of the brain but may extend laterally into the Sylvian fissures (Figure 5.3) or into the posterior fossa. The inflammatory process follows penetrating vasculature, particularly striate arteries supplying subcortical gray matter and branches of the basilar artery penetrating the pons. An occlusive process due to vasculitis results in small vascular infarctions in these regions. Microscopic examination of affected medium- and large-sized arterial blood vessels demonstrates the process of endarteritis obliterans whereby there is impressive intimal proliferation in association with perivascular inflammation to the extent that the vascular lumen is occluded (Figure 5.4).

Figure 5.4. Tuberculous meningitis (a) with prominent thickening of the leptomeninges by the exudative inflammatory process accompanied by endarteritis obliterans and (b) Langhans cell with adjoining caseous necrosis.

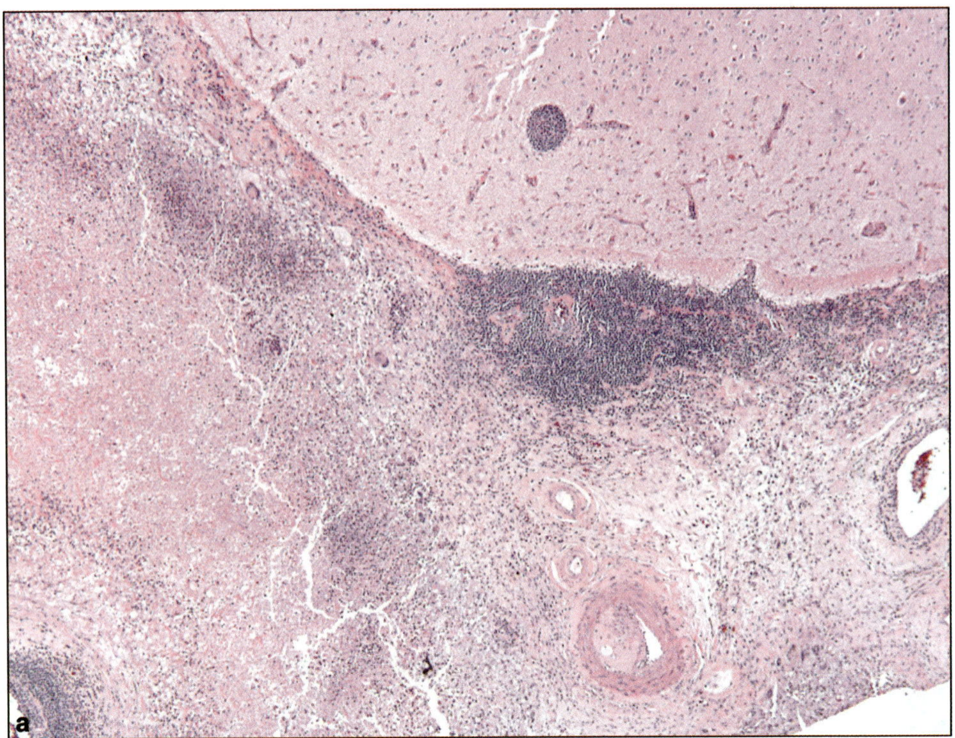

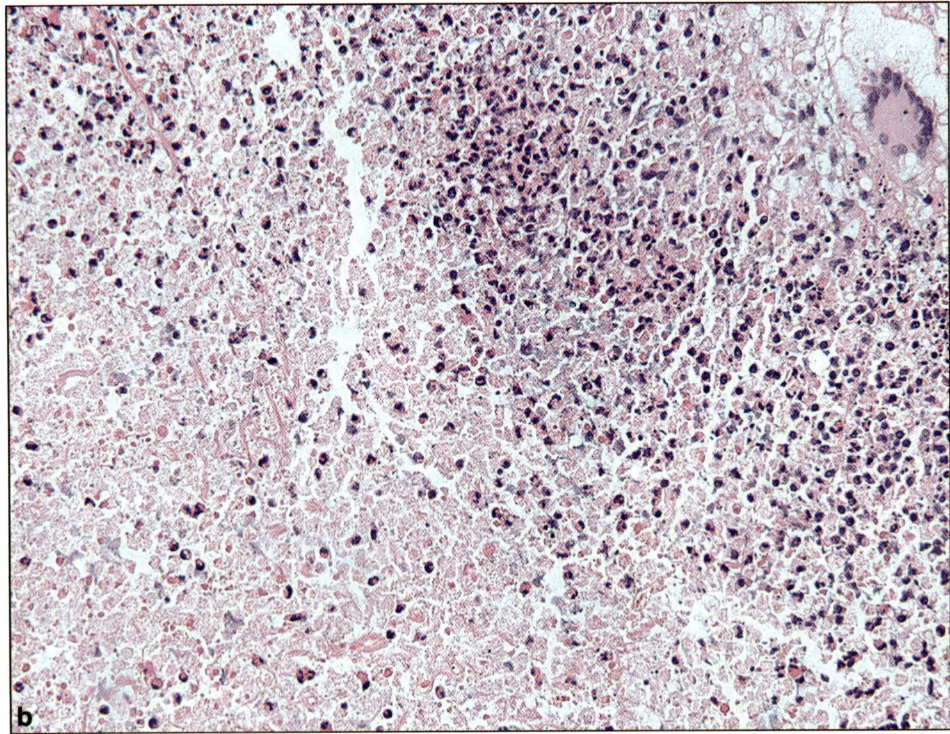

Abscesses due to tuberculosis occur most commonly as spinal epidural or subdural abscesses. Epidural examples are usually a complication of tuberculosis of the spine (Pott's disease) involving vertebral bodies or the intervertebral disks, and complications include spinal cord compression. Tuberculous abscesses of the brain, unlike tuberculomas, contain a necrotic center with purulent material and abundant *M. tuberculosis* organisms without the characteristic inflammatory reaction, including Langhans giant cells formed through the fusion of epithelioid macrophages. They are considered more frequent in the immunocompromised states such as with acquired immunodeficiency syndrome (AIDS) (Berenguer et al., 1992).

Tuberculomas are relatively rare in areas in which tuberculosis is well-controlled; however, they represent causes of brain masses where tuberculosis is more common. They may be single but are more often multiple. They occur most frequently in the cerebellum, the tegmentum of the pons, and the pericentral lobule (Isenmann et al., 1996). Unlike tuberculous abscesses, these have a more firm consistency with a gray gelatinous rim and minimal associated edema. Microscopic examination shows the typical caseous necrosis with a granulomatous reaction that includes Langhans giant cells, lymphocytes, and fibrosis. With time, the lesions become fibrotic and calcified and *M. tuberculosis* organisms may be impossible to demonstrate.

Neurosyphilis

Neurosyphilis is caused by the spirochete *Treponema pallidum*, the incidence of which fell dramatically with effective recognition and treatment of systemic disease and is thus not likely to be a viable consideration for the surgical neuropathologist. However, in the context of the AIDS epidemic, there has been a rise in the number of cases which may manifest as an especially aggressive form (Gordon et al., 1994). CSF infection actually occurs early in the disease and may be a frequent but asymptomatic feature of tertiary stage neurosyphilis.

Symptomatic neurosyphilis occurs in two predominant forms, *meningovascular* and *parenchymatous*. *Meningovascular syphilis* is composed of a chronic inflammatory infiltrate including lymphocytes and plasma cells, which may be diffuse or localized to the base of the brain. Inflammation may spread around small blood vessels accompanied by fibrillary astrocytosis extending into the pia arachnoid. Endarteritis obliterans also occurs in association with penetrating vessels in the base of the brain, reminiscent of tuberculosis or other types of basilar meningitis. Foci of reticulin-rich necrosis forming a mass may arise in the leptomenges or dura and are known as cerebral *gummas*. Spirochete microorganisms may be exceedingly difficult to demonstrate in any lesion of neurosyphilis. Specific silver impregnation techniques may be used but are difficult to interpret because of the nonspecific staining of structures, which may mimic spirochetes. Immunofluorescence (Handsfield et al., 1983) and the polymerase chain reaction (Horowitz et al., 1994) represent more sensitive methods.

Parenchymatous syphilis manifests as either dementia due to parenchymatous changes related to chronic meningeal inflammation or as *tabes dorsalis*. In the latter, there is selective degeneration of posterior spinal nerve roots with involvement of the dorsal root ganglia and secondary Wallerian degeneration of the posterior columns of the spinal cord.

Lyme Disease

Lyme disease due to the spirochete *Borrelia burgdorferi* is a multisystemic disorder usually diagnosed after recognition of skin lesions following a tick bite, representing the first stage of the disease. In the second stage, 15% of cases may develop neurological symptoms including meningitis, cranial neuritis, and radiculoneuritis. The details of neuropathological examinations are rare but include perivascular or vasculitic inflammation (Bertrand et al., 1999; Miklossy et al., 1990; Oksi et al., 1996). The organism is demonstrable with Dieterle's silver impregnation.

Cat Scratch Disease

This infection is caused by the gram-negative bacillus *Bartonella henselae* following transmission by cats, usually kittens, and resulting in a self-limited case of regional lymphadenopathy. Neurological complications are rare, occurring approximately 2–5 weeks after adenopathy with an acute encephalopathy, sometimes with seizures, which are very rarely fatal. Autopsy pathology has revealed perivascular lymphocytic infiltrates and microglial nodules (Fouch and Coventry, 2007). Vertebral osteomyelitis with epidural abscess has also been reported (Abdel-Haq et al., 2005).

Whipple's Disease

Clinical Features

This condition almost invariably involves symptomatic involvement of the gastrointestinal tract resulting in malabsorption and weight loss, usually occurring in the fourth to seventh decades. Arthralgias, lymphadenopathy, and hyperpigmentation may also occur, and almost any organ system may be involved. A minority of patients develop neurologic signs including dementia, ophthalmoplegia, hypothalamic and pituitary dysfunction, and myoclonus. Neurologic findings, said to be pathognomonic in Whipple's disease, are convergent nystagmus associated with abnormal palatal, tongue, and mandibular movements, called oculomasticatory myorhythmia. The causative organism is *Tropheryma whippelii*. A fatal outcome will generally occur within 6–12 months in untreated cases.

Pathological Features

Because of usual concomitant involvement of the intestine, a jejunal biopsy will usually demonstrate macrophages containing periodic acid–Schiff (PAS)-positive rod-shaped structures, and the diagnosis may be aided by polymerase chain reaction (PCR)-based assays even in the absence of overt pathological abnormalities. In cases with predominantly neurological manifestations, diagnostic approaches include the detection of abnormal macrophages in CSF or by PCR analysis of CSF. Brain biopsy will demonstrate perivascular and

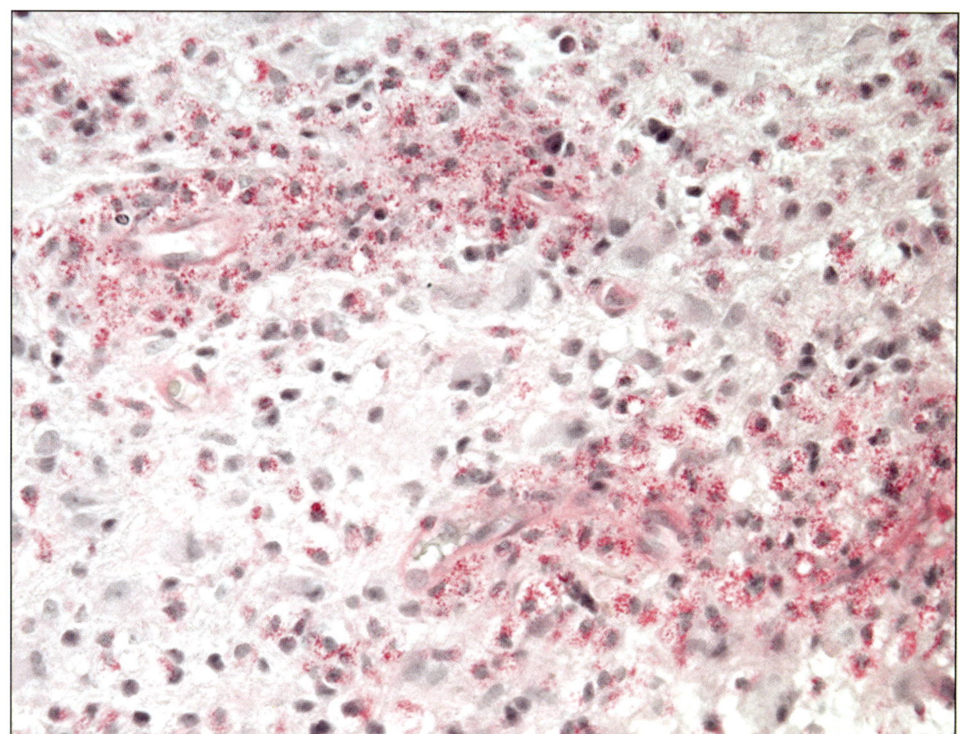

Figure 5.5. Whipple's disease. The brain parenchyma is gliotic and there is a striking accumulation of macrophages with granular PAS positivity around blood vessels.

parenchymal macrophages containing gram-positive and PAS-positive cytoplasmic inclusions in a background of reactive gliosis and a lymphoplasmacytic inflammatory infiltrate (Figure 5.5).

VIRAL INFECTIONS

Brain biopsies may be done on rare occasions for suspected viral infection. It is most frequently a diagnostic consideration when the neuropathologist is confronted with the otherwise nonspecific histologic features of viral meningoencephalitis followed by the often fruitless attempt at identifying the pathogenic cause. Examples of biopsied viral meningoencephalitis for which a causative organism was identified include those listed below as well as *La Crosse encephalitis* (McJunkin et al., 1997), *parvovirus B-19* (Druschky et al., 2000), and *coxsackie B virus*.

Whatever viral infection is under consideration, it is important to reserve material for diagnostic molecular genetic testing at public health laboratories suitably equipped for this purpose. Otherwise, diagnostic consideration should be given to endemic conditions that may favor certain diagnoses, for example, arboviral or enteroviral encephalitis.

Herpes Simplex Encephalitis

Clinical and Radiological Features

Herpes simplex encephalitis is the most common cause of acute necrotizing encephalitis in immunocompetent persons. The disease may occur at all ages

Figure 5.6. Adult herpes encephalitis. (a) An axial fluid-attuned inversion recovery FLAIR MR shows high signal in the right medial temporal lobe with minimal mass effect. (b) An axial diffusion-weighted image shows restricted diffusion in the same location as the abnormal signal on the FLAIR image. High signal on diffusion-weighted images is often the most striking imaging finding in early herpes encephalitis and can be used to help distinguish herpes encephalitis from an infiltrative temporal lobe tumor. In addition to the medial temporal lobe, the insula and cingulate gyri are often involved in herpes encephalitis. Purely unilateral disease is unusual.

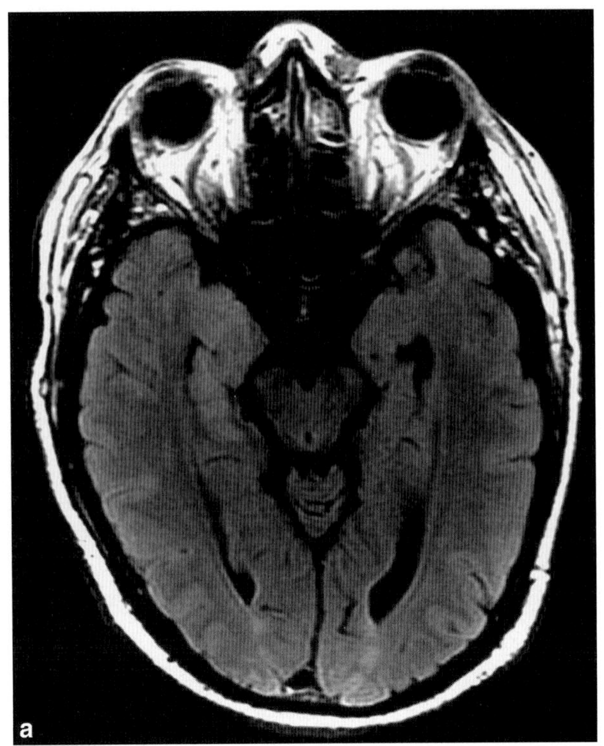

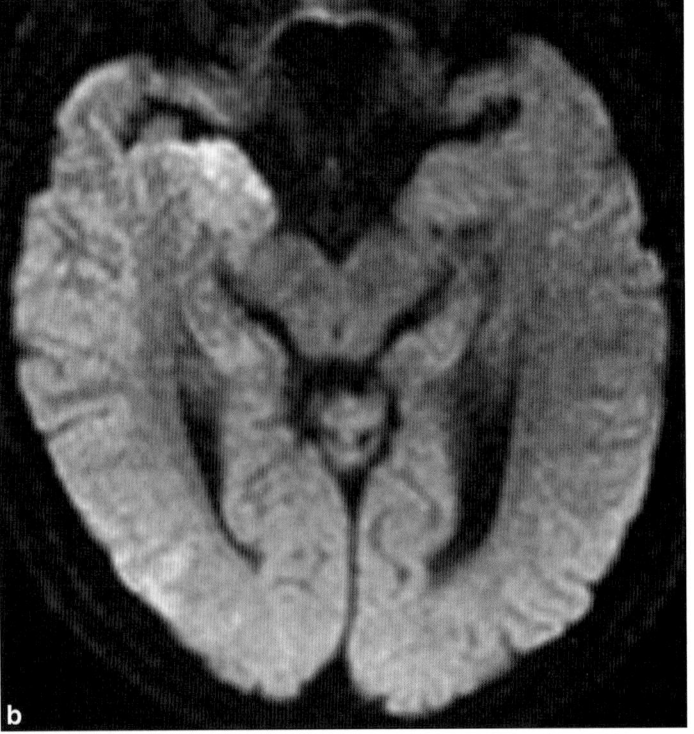

and is acquired through contact with respiratory secretions or saliva. The route of infection is believed to be either by spread along olfactory nerve tracts, reactivation of latent virus in the trigeminal ganglia, or within the brain. Symptoms may develop acutely or over several days and typically reflect involvement of the temporal and frontal lobes. There is fever, headache, confusion, sometimes after a prodrome of personality changes and behavioral abnormalities lasting several days. Focal neurological deficits include seizures. CSF contains a moderate number of leukocytes, red blood cells, with elevation of protein although it may be normal in early stages. Neuroimaging (Figure 5.6) and electroencephalograms (EEG) typically reveal focal abnormalities in either unilateral or bilateral temporal lobes.

Untreated cases are usually fatal or marked by significant neurologic injury and disability. Morbidity and mortality has a significantly improved with antiviral therapy.

Pathology

Brain biopsy is currently done with much less frequency now that PCR-based methods for detecting virus in cerebrospinal fluid are used. Herpes encephalitis should be considered when there is a significant inflammatory infiltrate extending from the pia through gray matter and into white matter, beginning with perivascular neutrophils and lymphocytes, which grow in numbers with progression of the infection. Infected neurons may gradually develop the recognizable eosinophilic nuclear inclusions, superficially resembling hypoxic/ischemic eosinophilic neurons. Hemorrhage may be conspicuous, reflecting the gross observation of hemorrhagic necrosis. Otherwise, the pathologic features include nonspecific changes seen in many forms of viral meningoencephalitis including perivascular lymphocytic cuffing, with microglial activation and microglial nodules. Immunohistochemistry for herpes simplex virus will clearly label infected cells although the number of such cells declines after about 2 weeks of infection.

Progressive Multifocal Leukoencephalopathy

Clinical and Radiological Features

This opportunistic infection was first reported in association with chronic lymphocytic leukemia and Hodgkin disease (Astrom et al., 1958). It remained a rarity until the AIDS epidemic as well as the rise in the iatrogenically immuno-compromised patient population. It is caused by the polyoma JC virus and presumes latent infection, which becomes clinically significant in the context of immunodeficiency. This includes the recent occurrence of progressive multi-focal leukoencephalopathy (PML) in patients treated with natalizumab as an immunosuppressive agent directed at T-cell migration for multiple sclerosis and Crohn's disease (Bartt, 2006). The prognosis in PML is usually fatal unless immune reconstitution is possible.

Patients usually present with focal neurologic deficits including weakness, cognitive and visual deficits. Results of radiographic studies are of particular importance in the setting of evaluating neurological deficits in the immuno-compromised patient since the differential diagnosis includes other infections such as toxoplasmosis, central nervous system (CNS) lymphoma, or other forms of primary demyelinating disease. Neuroimaging typically reveals

Figure 5.7. Progressive multifocal leukoencephalopathy (PML). (a) An axial T1 MR with contrast enhancement shows an area of low intensity within the right frontal lobe white matter. There is minimal enhancement at the margin of the lesion. (b) By T2-weighted MR, the lesion displays high signal and no mass effect. The area of abnormal signal extends all the way to the gray–white matter junction giving the cortex a scalloped appearance, which is often seen in PML.

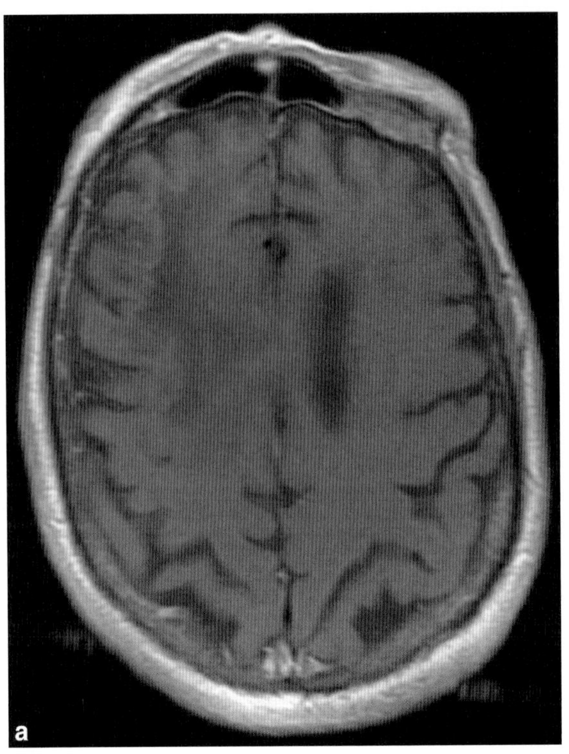

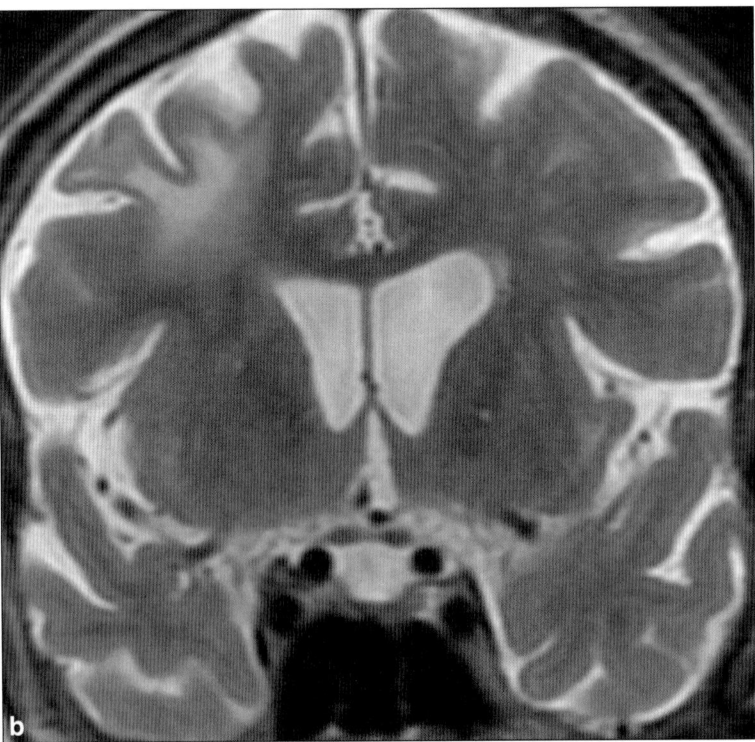

multifocal lesions with hyperintense signal abnormalities of the white matter on T2-weighted magnetic resonance imaging (MRI) with variable contrast enhancement, often faint and peripheral when present (Figure 5.7). JC virus DNA may be detected in the CSF by PCR.

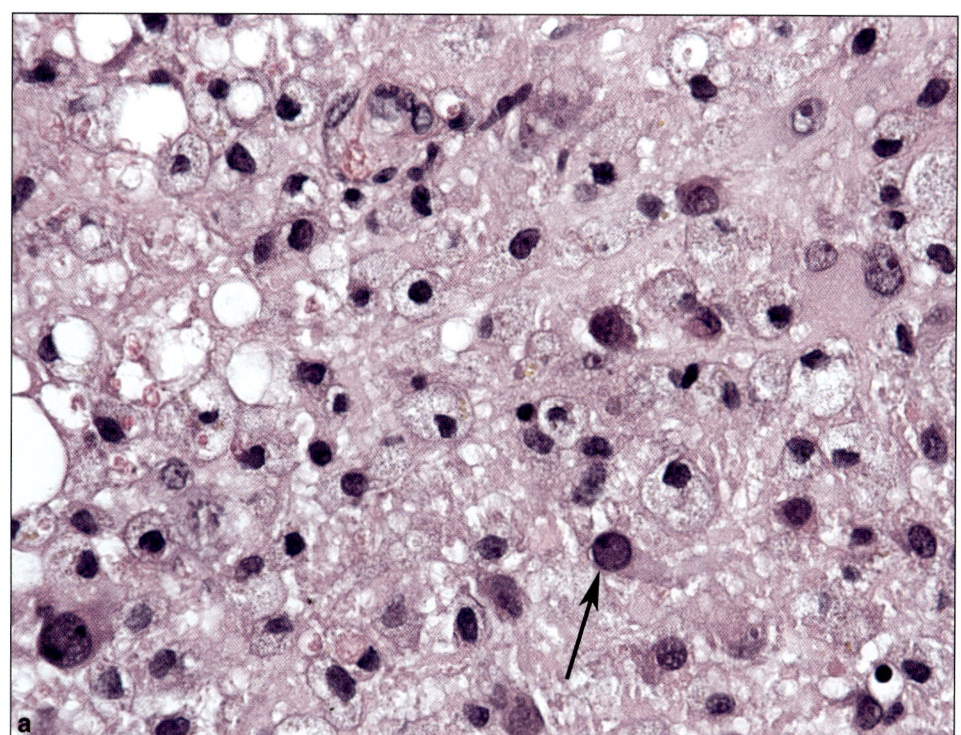

Figure 5.8. PML with (a) scattered macrophages, reactive astrocytes, and enlarged oligodendroglial nuclei with "ground" glass appearance and margination of chromatin (arrow). (b) Infected cells show nuclear positivity for JC virus, or as demonstrated here, reactivity for anti-SV40 virus antibody as a surrogate antibody for diagnosing PML.

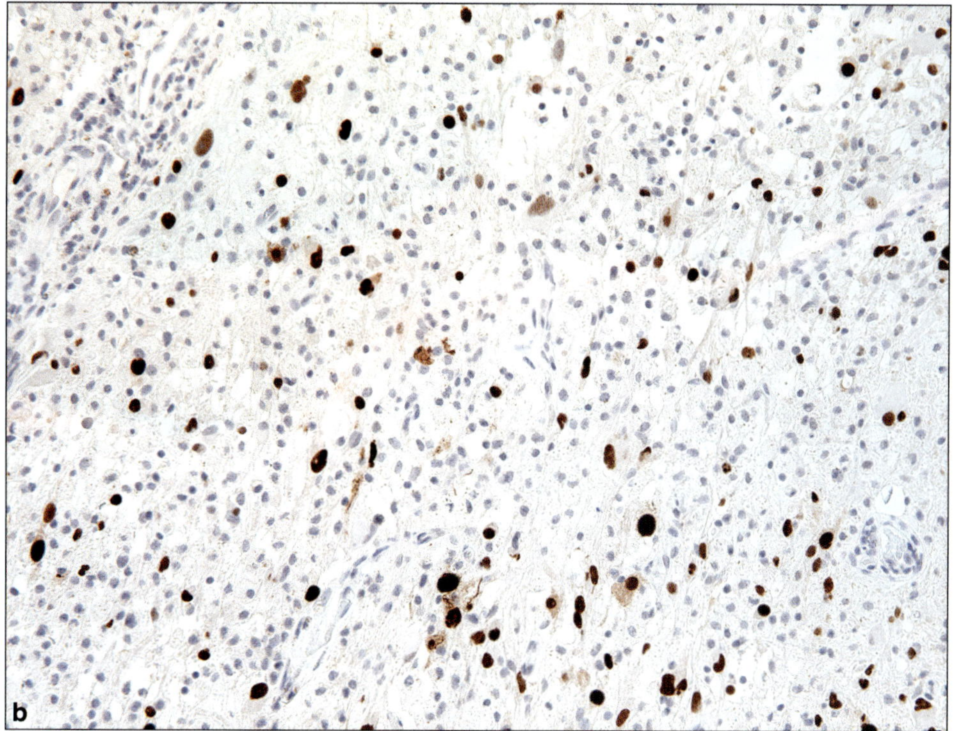

Pathology

Lesions may occur in diverse subcortical white matter regions with a predilection for the parietal occipital regions. Examples of brainstem and cerebellar involvement are also reported.

Microscopic examination reveals a loss of myelin accompanied by reactive astrocytosis and the presence of lipid-laden macrophages (Figure 5.8). Astrocytes are occasionally quite atypical, with lobulated and hyperchromatic nuclei. In some patients who retain an adequate degree of immune function, a conspicuous mononuclear inflammatory infiltrate may be seen, representing the so-called inflammatory form of PML. Enlarged oligodendroglial nuclei showing viral proliferation display a ground glass appearance with unapparent or marginated chromatin. Such nuclei will be highlighted by immunohistochemical staining or in situ hybridization for JC or SV40 virus.

Subacute Sclerosing Panencephalitis

Clinical and Radiological Features

Subacute sclerosing panencephalitis (SSPE) is a notably rare condition occurring in immunocompetent individuals, manifesting years after initial infection by measles virus. Thus, neurologists and neuropathologists should be attuned to the possible occurrence of SSPE with a latency averaging 7 years following an outbreak of measles. The risk is especially high in patients who contract measles during the first year of life and is reduced significantly by measles vaccination (Modlin et al., 1979). The disease occurs as a result of mutations in the viral genome that result in proliferation of virus without cytotoxic effect.

The clinical progression in SSPE is insidious and marked by the additional development of intellectual impairment and behavioral abnormalities, followed by visual disturbances in at least 50% of patients. Intellectual decline then accelerates with the onset of motor disturbances including myoclonic jerks and characteristic EEG changes. The final stages may last for months to years in which the patient becomes uncommunicative with severe movement disorders including ataxia, spasticity, choreoathetosis, and dystonia.

Pathology

Microscopic features of SSPE include nonspecific leptomeningeal, perivascular, and parenchymal infiltration by lymphocytes and macrophages. Affected gray matter shows conspicuous microglial activation, gliosis, with loss of neurons and occasional neuronophagia. Nuclear inclusions may be easily found in some cases that conform to the characteristics of a Cowdry Type A nuclear inclusion, consisting of an eosinophilic globule with surrounding halo and margination of chromatin to the nuclear membrane (Figure 5.9). These inclusions may react to antibodies to measles virus antigen. Interestingly, intraneuronal neurofibrillary tangles may be seen in long-standing cases.

HIV and AIDS

Clinical and Radiological Features

The incidence of neurological disease in AIDS due to human immunodeficiency virus (HIV)-1 infection approaches 100%. This includes *primary HIV encephalitis* and *aseptic meningitis*, which may occur as subclinical infections. In

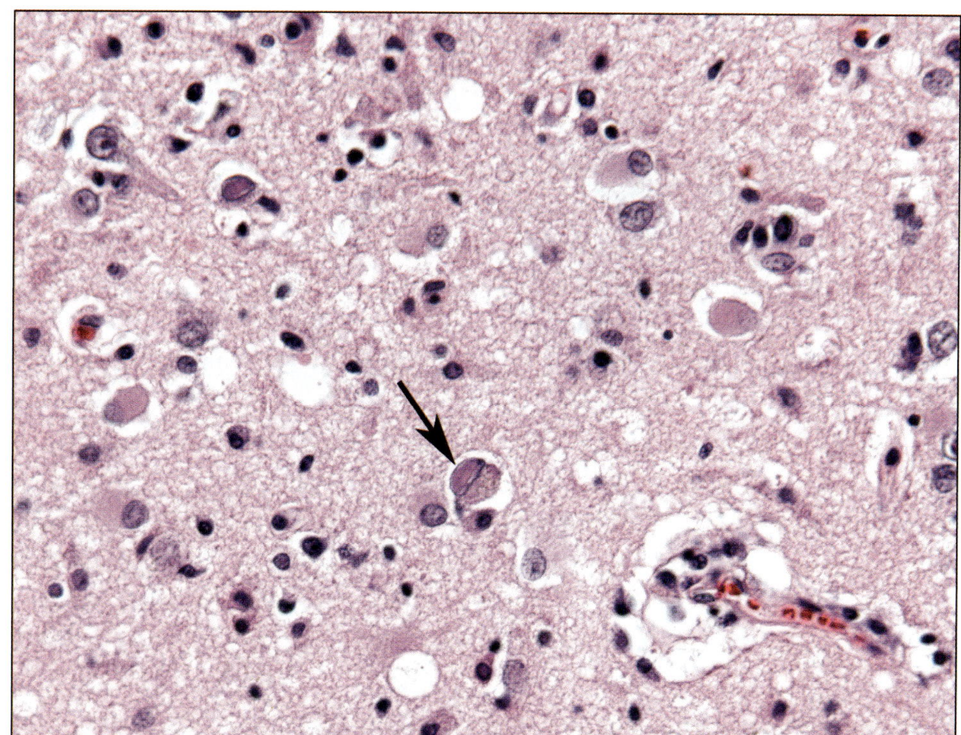

Figure 5.9. SSPE is characterized by a mixed chronic inflammatory infiltrate, reactive gliosis and occasionally prominent intraneuronal nuclear Cowdry Type A inclusions.

the late stages of the disease, between 20% and 30% of patients develop motor and cognitive deficits that are not attributable to opportunistic infection. This comprises the AIDS dementia complex/HIV-associated dementia complex, marked by memory loss, apathy, ataxia, leg weakness, and tremor. A *vacuolar myelopathy* may occur manifesting as leg weakness, spastic paraparesis, sensory ataxia, and incontinence. Peripheral neuropathies and myopathies have also been described. However, these examples of HIV-1 infection essentially never provide the motivation for surgical biopsy.

In contrast, a large number of opportunistic infections and neoplasms are well associated with AIDS and form the basis for this necessity of radiological and pathological expertise in evaluating these sometimes coexisting processes.

The most common secondary infections occurring in AIDS include the fungi *Cryptococcus neoformans* affecting up to 5–10% of patients, and less frequently *Aspergillus fumigatus* and *Coccidioides* species in regions where this fungal infection is endemic such as the southwestern United States and the Central Valley of California. Cytomegalovirus (CMV) is the most common viral opportunistic infection of the CNS in AIDS and manifestations may range from low-grade to a severe necrotizing encephalitis or ventricular ependymitis. CMV meningoradiculitis and myelitis were among the first opportunistic infections recognized in AIDS. *Varicella zoster* may also cause a severe leukoencephalitis, ventriculitis, or vasculitis affecting large vessels at the base of the brain, which may result in infarction or aneurysm formation.

The most common parasitic infection in AIDS is toxoplasmosis, usually resulting in large necrotic brain abscesses, which may be multiple and which often result in a difficult differential diagnosis between toxoplasmosis and CNS lymphoma. Specific treatment may result in a marked diminution in identifiable organisms in biopsies.

The most common bacterial infections of the CNS in AIDS are due to acid fast bacilli including *Mycobacterium avium intracellulare* and *M. tuberculosis*. Neurosyphilis also has an increased incidence in AIDS and is associated with an especially aggressive course.

Neoplasms of the CNS in AIDS include the meningeal spread of systemic lymphoma and Epstein–Barr virus related primary CNS lymphoma in addition to the fact that non-Hodgkin lymphomas are many times more common in patients with AIDS than in the general population. The diagnostic algorithm when dealing with neurological disease in an AIDS patient and focal lesions by neuroimaging usually includes steps to avoid biopsy such as examination of CSF or serologic markers for Epstein–Barr virus, JC virus, and *Toxoplasma gondii* in the appropriate clinical setting. When the differential diagnosis exists between toxoplasmosis and primary CNS lymphoma, a trial of therapy for toxoplasmosis may be undertaken and biopsy performed when no therapeutic response is noted. Studies have shown a high rate of diagnostic yield when undertaken; however, this patient population is more prone to complications of biopsy (Antinori et al., 2000) and in general should be restricted to patients who can tolerate therapy for the suspected diagnostic entity (Hornef et al., 1999).

FUNGAL INFECTIONS

Fungal infections are increasing in frequency because of the widespread use of immunosuppressive drugs, the spread of AIDS, and the aging of populations in which relative immunodeficiency and incidence of cancer becomes more prevalent. The surgical diagnosis of CNS fungal infection may be unexpected in the setting of a mass lesion otherwise suspected to be a neoplasm. Necrotic capillary blood vessels may mimic the appearance of branched fungi. Fungal infection may also affect the CNS as basilar meningitis and thus be amenable to diagnosis by CSF examination.

Aspergillosis

This is a common infection of the CNS and is closely associated with immunosuppression. It follows hematogenous dissemination, often from the lungs, typically leading to multiple lesions in the anterior and middle cerebral artery distributions although any other portion of the brain, cerebellum, and brainstem may be involved. They are characterized by direct infiltration of blood vessels by fungal hyphae with vascular thrombosis, hemorrhage, and infarction.

The organisms grow as branched septated hyphae that appear in sections as homogeneous and uniform, measuring 3–6 μm in width and a progressive arboreal pattern of branching (Figure 5.10). The organisms are visible in

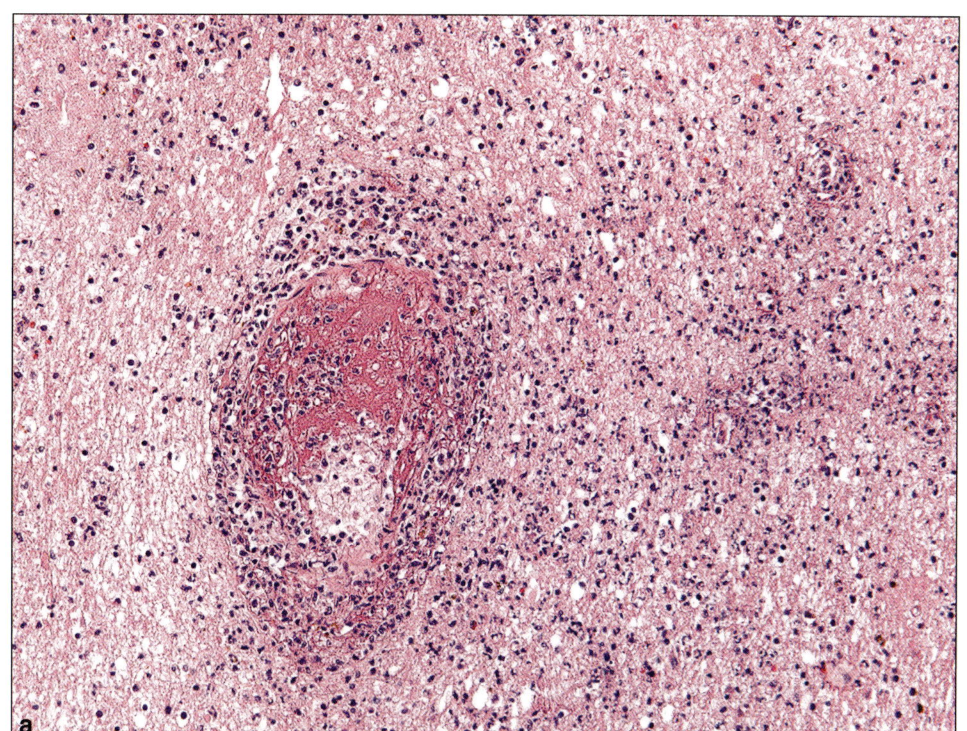

Figure 5.10. (a) Aspergillosis causes a necrotizing and hemorrhagic cerebritis with a distinct propensity for vascular thrombosis, which is related to the organism's tendency to invade vessel walls, as highlighted by the GMS stain (b).

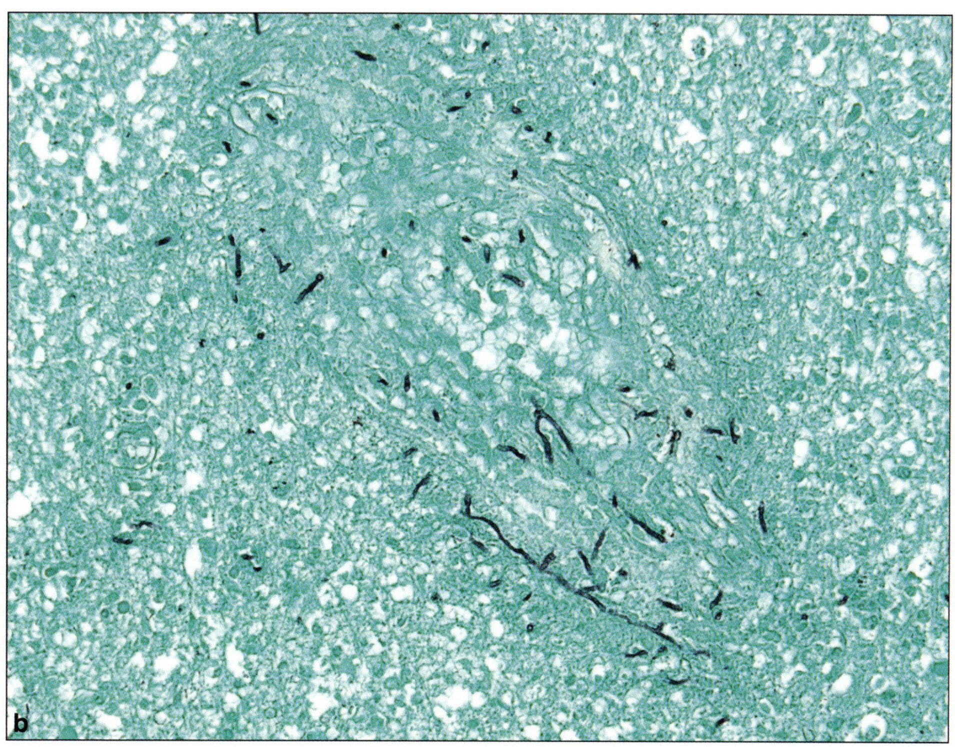

hematoxylin and eosin-stained sections but are highlighted by special stains for fungi such as Gomori methenamine silver (GMS). The accompanying inflammatory infiltrate is variable, marked by neutrophils early in the disease and macrophages in later stages. Granulomatous lesions may occur including multinucleated giant cells.

Blastomycosis

North American blastomycosis is caused by *Blastomyces dermatitis*, which predominantly affects men, is not associated with immunosuppression, and is endemic in the southeastern United States. The CNS is only rarely involved, usually due to hematogenous spread from the lungs. CNS infection is usually paralleled by symptoms of meningitis but occasionally patients develop focal abscesses or granulomas, which are caused focal neurologic signs and increased intracranial pressure.

Blastomycosis usually involves a mixed granulomatous and purulent reaction surrounding necrotic tissue with a variable number of yeast forms. These lesions may resemble the central caseous necrosis of tuberculous granulomas. The organism is a dimorphic fungus, which appears in H&E-stained sections as yeastlike cells with a distinctive spherical hyaline structure 8–15 μm in diameter, which are multinucleated and have vacuolated cytoplasm and thick double-contoured walls. The organisms are highlighted with GMS and other special stains for fungi and are sometimes lightly colored with mucin stains such as mucicarmine, Alcian blue, and colloidal iron.

Coccidiomycosis

Coccidiomycosis is caused by *Coccidioides immitis* and has a distinctive geographic distribution related to arid and dusty regions of Argentina, Paraguay, and Mexico in Latin America and the southwestern United States, particularly the Central Valley of California. African American adults are particularly prone to severe illness. The disease begins as a mild febrile illness due to the lung infection or more rarely as a primary skin infection. The nervous system may be involved in up to one-third of cases, often as a terminal event resulting from hematogenous spread. The majority of these cases involve basilar meningitis followed by acute communicating hydrocephalus. Occasionally vasculitis of penetrating blood vessels of the base of the brain and brainstem may occur. Less commonly, large granulomatous lesions may occur within the parenchyma of the brain, cerebellum, or spinal cord, sometimes to such an extent as to produce spinal cord compression. An especially fulminant form of the disease is associated with AIDS.

Histologic sections show a granulomatous and necrotic response to the organisms, which are recognizable as large round spherules or spore-producing structures, which are 20–35 μm in diameter and have a thick refractile capsule. Within the spherules are endospores, which are 2–5 μm in diameter and released into tissue when the spherules rupture (Figure 5.11).

Candidiasis

This is the most common yeast infection of the CNS, while normally causing infections of the skin, oral cavity, vagina, or visceral organs. In the individuals

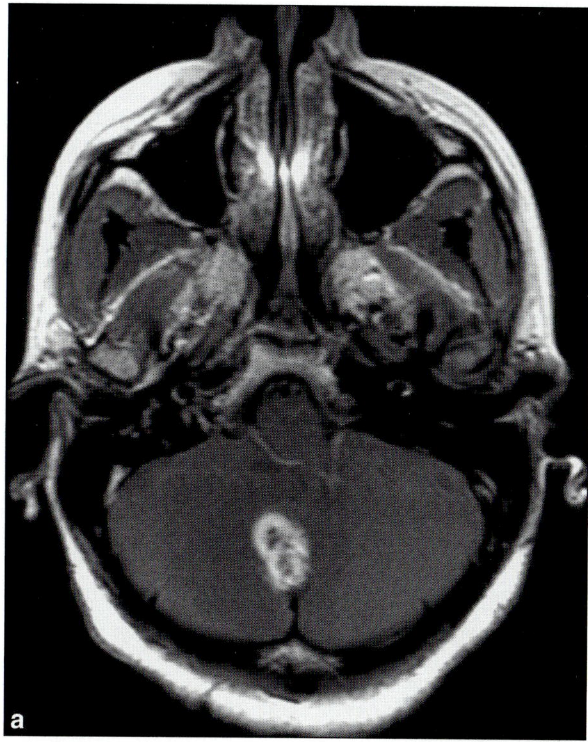

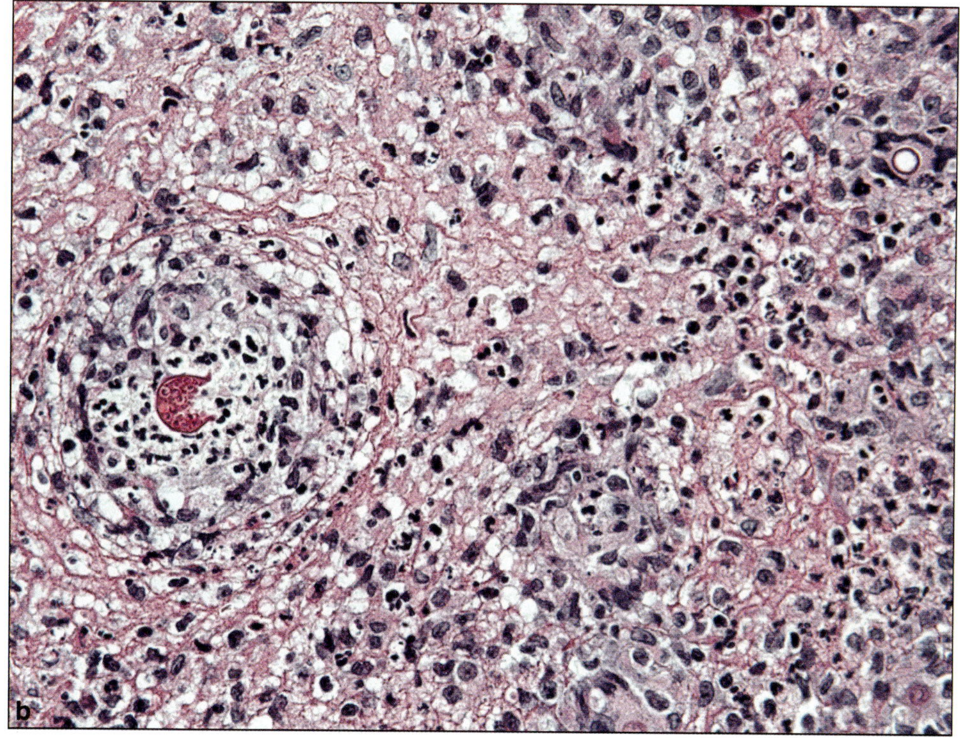

Figure 5.11. Intraparenchymal coccidiomycosis. (a) Axial T1 contrast-enhanced MR shows a ring-enhancing mass centered in the cerebellar vermis with surrounding vasogenic edema. Although this patient presented with an intraparenchymal mass, leptomeningeal coccidiomycosis is more prevalent. (b) Coccidiomycosis of the CNS parenchyma results in a chronic inflammatory process with abscess formation. The organisms are highlighted by the PAS stain, one of which is in the process of rupture in this photomicrograph.

with intestinal overgrowth of Candida associated with antibiotics, immunosuppression, or other debilitating conditions, the fungus may travel to other organs by a hematogenous route and this is usually associated with cardiac and renal lesions. CNS candidiasis is usually represented by low-grade meningitis or multifocal abscesses.

The organisms are seen as 2- to 3-μm budding yeasts and pseudohyphae, which are faintly basophilic by H&E staining but intensely PAS positive as well as GMS positive. The accompanying inflammatory reaction varies from an absent or scanty response to the formation of small granulomas composed of lymphocytes, macrophages, plasma cells, and occasional multinucleated giant cells.

Mucormycosis

Mucormycosis is a general term for infections caused by pathogens belonging to the order Mucorales with the most frequent agent of mucormycosis in humans being *Rhizopus arrhizus*. These infections are contained within a greater unifying entity known as Zygomycosis. These infections occur predominantly in patients with ketoacidosis, the immunocompromised, and those with leukemia or lymphoma. The infection is acquired by exposure to sporangiospores, which may be inhaled, ingested, or deposited onto sites of mucocutaneous injury, especially burns. The infection is actually rare in AIDS except with a history of intravenous drug use.

Several clinical manifestations of mucormycosis are recognized but the form, which typically involves the brain, is known as rhinoorbitalcerebral mucormycosis. This fulminant infection involves the nasal cavity, paranasal sinuses, and orbit from where it may extend to the meninges and brain. Uncontrolled diabetes mellitus with acidosis and severe immunocompromise are especially associated with this condition.

The typical hyphae of these agents have a characteristic appearance in tissue sections. They hyphae are broad, 5–20 μm or more in width, irregular in contour, and pleomorphic (Figure 5.12). They are classically described as nonseptate, however, they may be rarely observed in tissue sections to be simulated by folds in the hyphal walls. Hyphal branching is irregular and nonprogressive, arising at right angles from the parent hyphae. The thin walls appear as basophilic or amphophilic in H&E-stained sections and stain weakly with Gomori methenamine silver impregnation. The accompanying inflammatory infiltrate is variable to absent depending on the degree of immunocompromise in a patient.

The organisms are aggressively angioinvasive, resulting in thrombosis and infarction of affected tissues. In this respect, mucormycosis and aspergillosis may resemble each other; however, the two infections should be easily distinguished by hyphal morphology. Occasionally however, Aspergillus hyphae are swollen or degenerated and resemble those of mucormycosis and conversely in some instances of zygomycosis the hyphae were relatively uniform and parallel with occasional septa. Some authorities urge caution in assigning a definitive microbiological name to a fungal infection in the absence of confirmatory culture.

Cryptococcosis

This infection is most commonly caused by *C. neoformans*, a fungus that is usually found in soil and bird manure. Cryptococcosis is found worldwide,

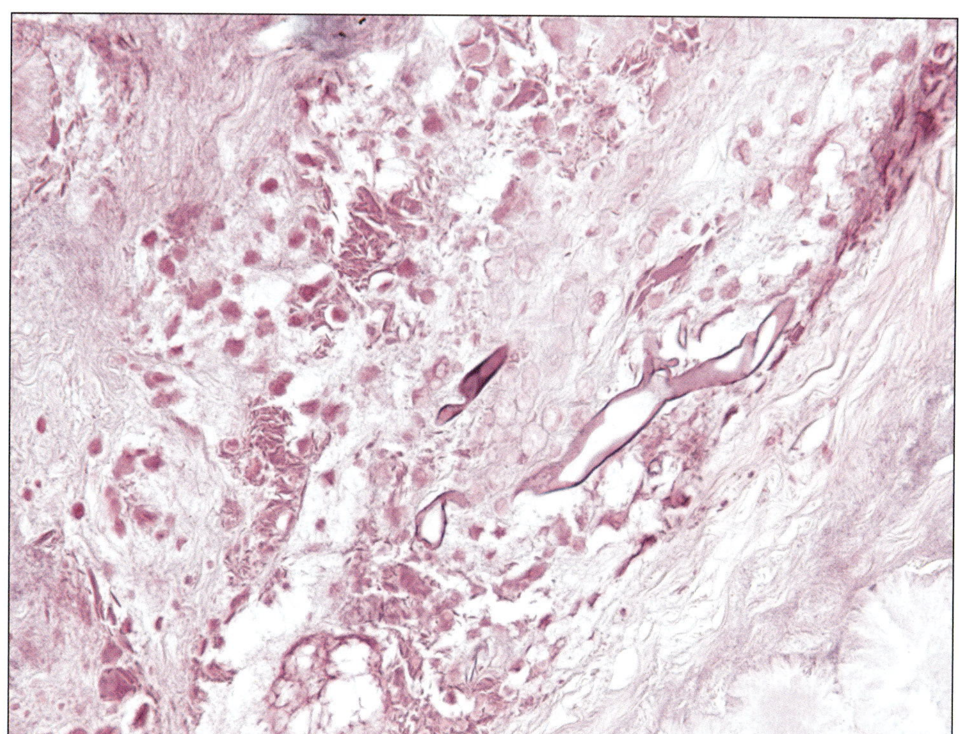

Figure 5.12. Mucormycosis, with broad nonseptate hyphae.

however, is most frequent in the southern United States and in Australia. The disease affects predominantly males and 85% of the cases are associated with debilitating conditions including cancer, alcoholism, malnutrition, and AIDS. The *C. neoformans* variant *gattii* is far less prevalent however has recently been identified as a cause of disease including pulmonary and brain abscesses in immunocompetent individuals (Colom et al., 2005).

Cryptococcosis occurs in two basic forms: pulmonary cryptococcosis and by hematogenous or lymphatic dissemination, cerebral meningeal cryptococcosis. Other examples of soft tissue infection from hematogenous spread include skin and bone. Cerebral meningeal cryptococcosis is the most common form of cryptococcosis in patients with AIDS as a manifestation of a neurotrophic tendency in *C. neoformans*. The clinical course is typically fulminant and fatal if untreated.

The diagnosis is usually made in a straightforward manner by the demonstration of the organism in tissue sections or by India ink preparations of CSF in which the abundant capsule is seen as optically clear. This classic test has been somewhat supplanted by the more sensitive latex agglutination detection of cryptococcal polysaccharide antigen in the CSF.

In histological sections, the organisms appear as round bodies 4–7 μm in diameter surrounded by a capsule 3–5 μm in thickness. Small buds may be seen attached to the main body by a thin neck. Because of the optically empty capsule, aggregates of organisms in the leptomeninges or perivascular spaces invoke the term "soap bubble" in describing the low-power appearance. The organisms are readily highlighted with GMS or Mayer's mucicarmine stain.

PROTOZOAL INFECTIONS

Amebiasis

Cerebral amebiasis occurs in three forms associated with separate species of ameba. Cerebral amebic abscesses are caused by *E. histolytica;* primary amebic meningoencephalitis is caused by *Naegleria fowleri;* and granulomatous amebic encephalitis may be caused by either *Acanthamoeba* species or *Balamuthia mandrillaris,* the latter originally classified as a Leptomyxid amoeba (Visvesvara et al., 1990). Amebic disease of the nervous system of any cause is a serious and likely fatal infection and is thus not often the diagnostic objective of a timely surgical biopsy.

Cerebral amebic abscess due to *Entamoeba histolytica* is usually a rare and late complication of intestinal, pulmonary, or hepatic amebiasis and is also usually fatal. These lesions may occur as single or multiple abscesses involving the cortex, the gray–white matter junction, or basal ganglia, with hemorrhagic purulent cavities. As in all amebic infections, trophozoites may be difficult to distinguish from macrophages. The organisms are spherical or oval, 5–25 μm in diameter, and have vacuolated cytoplasm with a single nucleus (Figure 5.13). The PAS stain may show the organism but to no great advantage over H&E.

Primary amebic encephalitis due to *N. fowleri* is most often contracted by swimming in brackish fresh water containing the organisms. The amebae enter the nasal cavity and spread into the central nervous system through the cribriform plate. The infection manifests as a precipitous and fulminant disease in immunocompetent children or young adults due to a rapidly progressive meningitis causing coma and death within 48–72 hours.

Microscopy shows a scanty mononuclear inflammatory infiltrate with extensive necrosis. The amoeba are typically present in the subarachnoid space and around blood vessels, are 8–15 μm in diameter and like *E. histolytica* can be distinguished from macrophages by their vesicular nucleus and large central nucleolus.

Granulomatous amebic encephalitis was originally associated with *Acanthamoeba* species but essentially identical clinical and pathologic features may be seen with infection by *B. mandrillaris* (Deol et al., 2000; Rowen et al., 1995). Infection usually occurs through hematogenous spread from the respiratory tract or skin and usually occurs in immunocompromised or debilitated patients. Symptoms are gradual in onset and usually referable to meningeal or brain infection with headache, fever, stiff neck, and possibly focal neurologic abnormalities including seizures. The infected brain is swollen, softened, hemorrhagic, and necrotic.

Microscopically, the lesions show chronic inflammation around blood vessels including lymphocytes, macrophages, plasma cells, and multinucleated giant cells. In spite of the name, well-formed granulomas are not part of the typical microscopic findings. The *Acanthamoeba* or *Balamuthia* trophozoites may be found in and around the walls and blood vessels and in areas remote from inflammation. The two species are indistinguishable morphologically

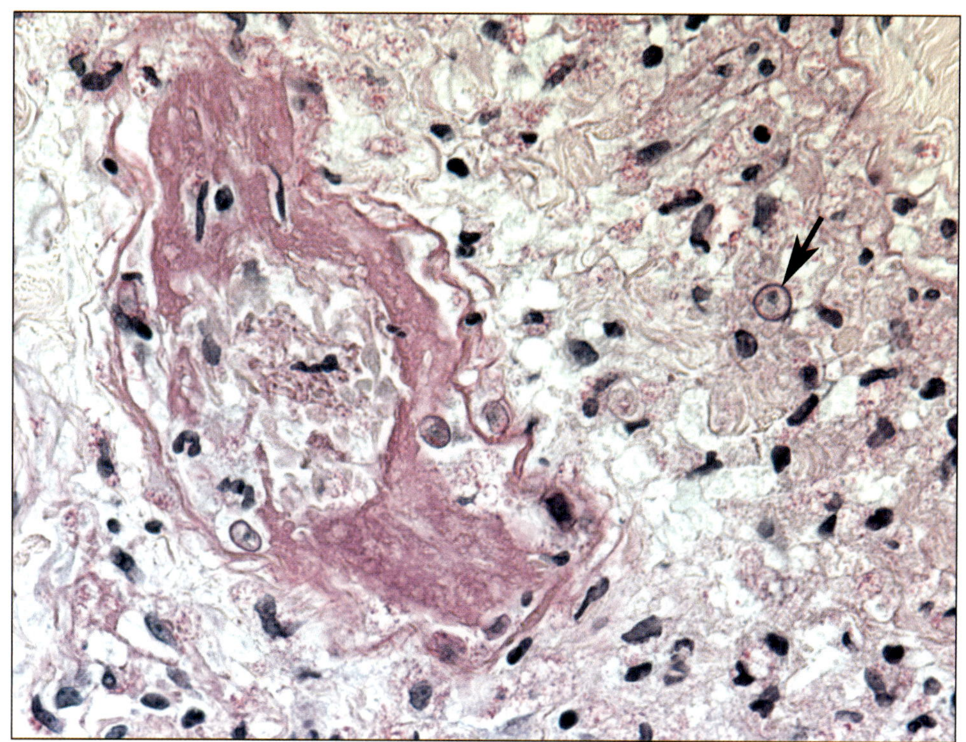

Figure 5.13. Ameba are easily missed in histological sections since in a mixed inflammatory infiltrate with necrosis, they may be assumed to be macrophages. When the plane of section includes a prominent single nucleolus, the organism is more easily identifiable (arrow) and may be slightly more obvious with this PAS with diastase digestion stain than H&E.

however may be separately identified by immunohistochemical means. They are 15–40 μm in diameter with a prominent vesicular nucleus and dense central nucleolus. Cysts are surrounded by a double membrane.

Toxoplasmosis

Clinical and Radiological Features

Cerebral toxoplasmosis is caused by *T. gondii*, and is most frequently acquired by the ingestion of undercooked beef or exposure to cat feces containing parasitic cysts. The infection is usually asymptomatic in immunocompetent individuals, or may result in a benign febrile illness with lymphadenopathy. Symptomatic and progressive neurologic disease is much more commonly associated with immunosuppression and particularly in AIDS in which there is reactivation of dormant infection (Bertoli et al., 1995).

Cerebral toxoplasmosis commonly presents as solitary or multifocal necrotic abscesses in any part of the brain (Carrazana et al., 1989), but may also produce diffuse encephalitis without focal lesions, or a predominantly meningeal-based infection. Therefore, the clinical manifestations are widely varied, ranging from nonlocalizing symptoms such as headaches, drowsiness, and disorientation to focal neurologic deficits. Neuroimaging usually reveals contrast-enhancing lesions by computed tomography (CT) or MRI (Figure 5.14a).

Pathology

Cerebral toxoplasmosis results in hemorrhagic process of infected tissue, accompanied by a lymphocytic and macrophage infiltrate with microglial activation.

Figure 5.14. (a) Toxoplasmosis. A sagittal T1 contrast-enhanced MR shows ring-enhancing masses in the frontal lobe and cerebellar hemisphere with surrounding vasogenic edema. Toxoplasmosis typically produces several ring–enhancing lesions with a predilection for the basal ganglia and thalamus. In the immunocompromised patient, lymphoma and tuberculomas can appear similar to toxoplasmosis on T1 contrast-enhanced MR imaging. Cerebral toxoplasmosis appears microscopically as (b) nonspecific necrosis, a mixed chronic inflammatory infiltrate. A distinctive microscopic feature is a prominent sclerosing reaction in vascular walls.

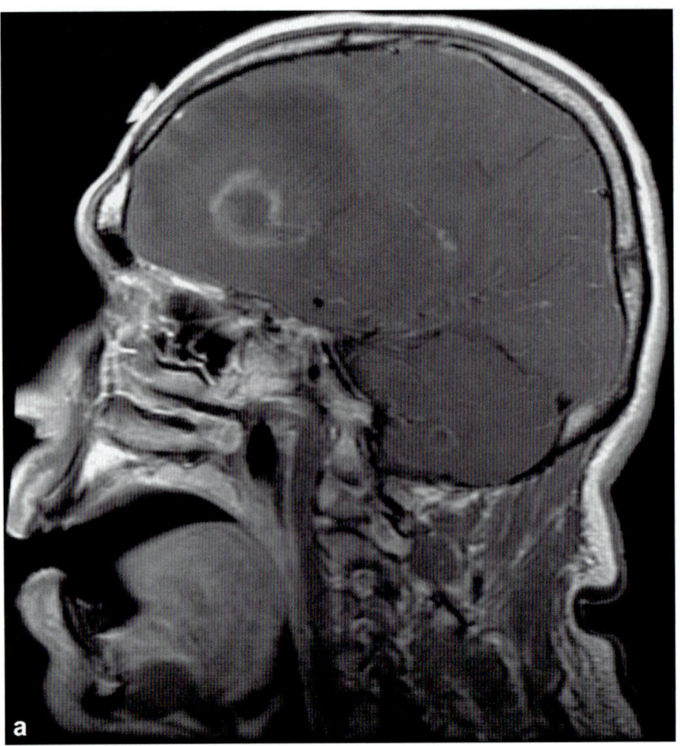

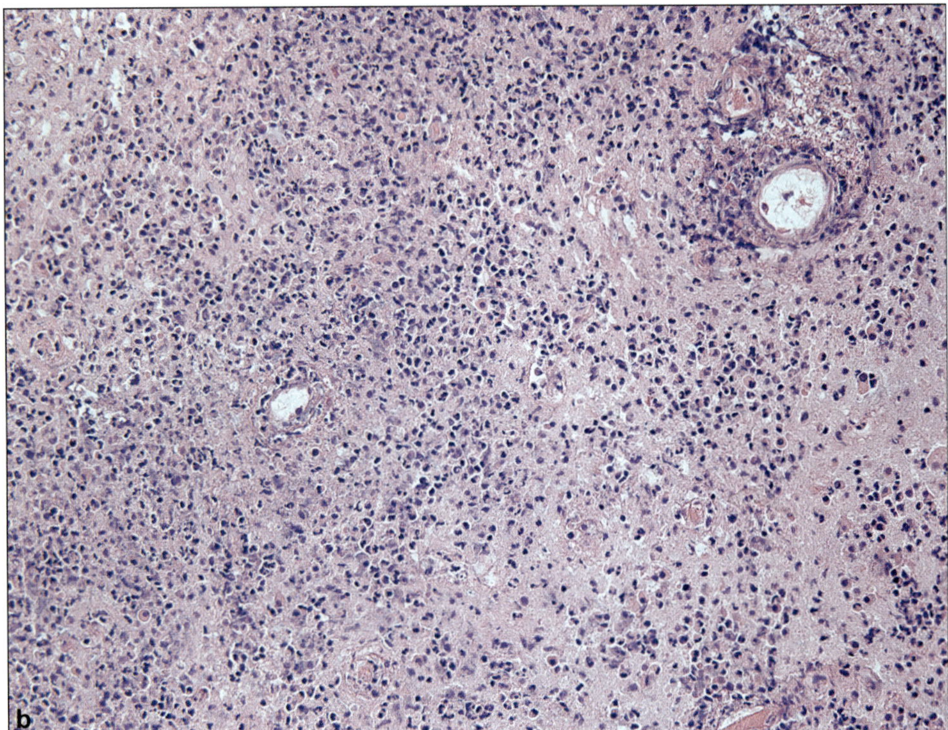

A distinctive form of fibrinoid vascular necrosis may be present (Figure 5.14b). The organisms may be seen in two forms and are usually abundant. Encysted intracellular bradyzoites or individual extracellular Toxoplasma tachyzoites are oval or crescent shaped structures measuring 2–4 μm by 4–8 μm. They are easily

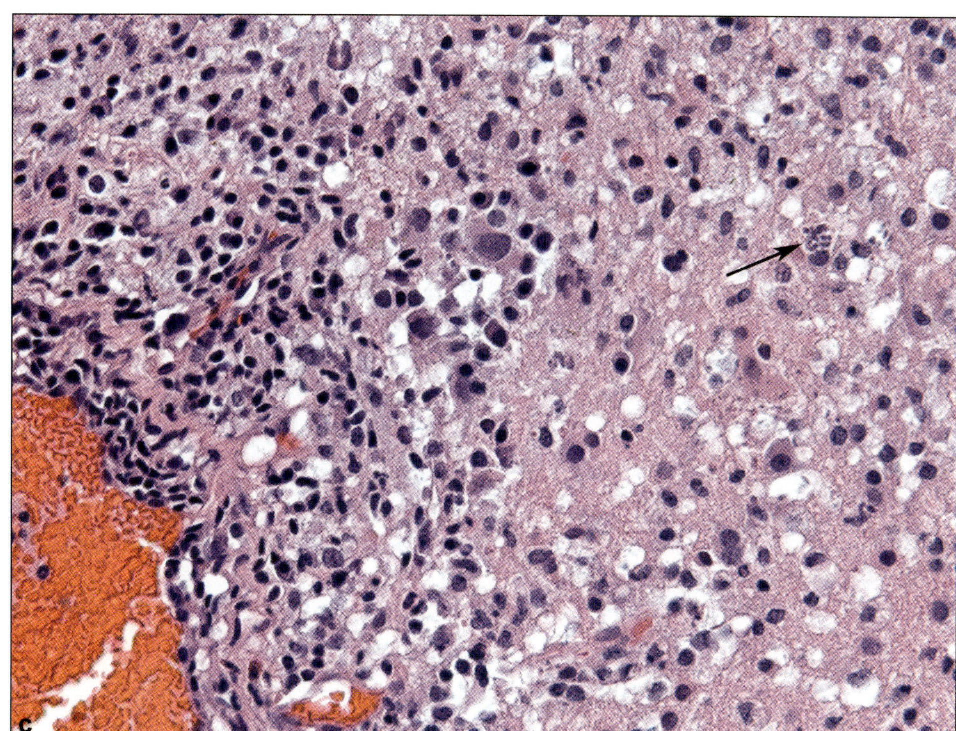

Figure 5.14. *continued* (c) Encysted bradyzoites (arrow) and single tachyzoites in untreated cases or those in early phases of therapy. (d) Immunohistochemistry is mandatory in excluding toxoplasmosis in the appropriate clinical setting and this microscopic setting.

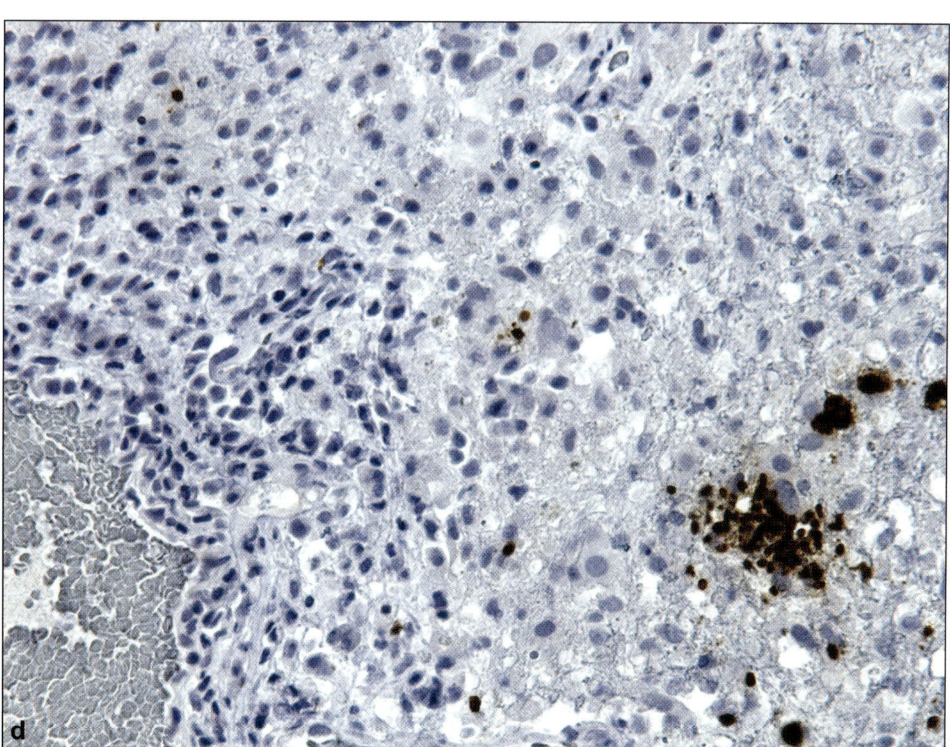

seen with H&E-staining (Figure 5.14c) but are readily identifiable by immuno-histochemistry (Figure 5.14d). Chronic lesions may show a lesser number of organisms, and effective treatment may also decrease the number of identifiable organisms.

Figure 5.15. Cerebral malaria, essentially never the diagnostic goal of a brain biopsy, is characterized by intravascular parasites within erythrocytes, which may lead to microthromboses and perivascular hemorrhages.

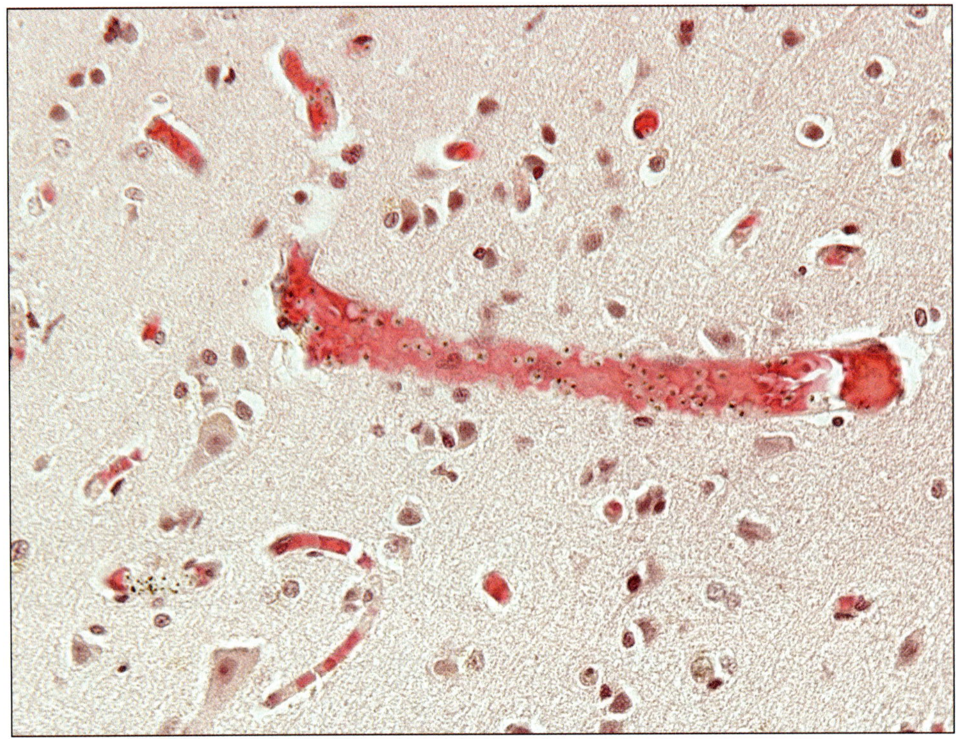

Cerebral Malaria

Cerebral malaria occurs in 1–10% of patients infected with *Plasmodium falciparum* and most commonly affects young children and travelers to an endemic region, both groups lacking immunity. The condition is marked by severe and progressive generalized neurologic deficit (Lou et al., 2001; Newton and Warrell, 1998). It is almost exclusively a postmortem diagnosis and as such rarely if ever the object of a surgical biopsy.

When viewed microscopically, the parasites are sequestered in vessels (Figure 5.15), later resulting in characteristic perivascular ring hemorrhages (Turner, 1997). In patients who survive for at least 10 days of cerebral malaria, areas of softening, demyelination, and glial proliferation may be noted around small vessels, known as Dürck's granulomas.

HELMINTHIC INFECTIONS

Cysticercosis

Human cysticercosis is invasion of tissues by the larval stage of the pork tapeworm *Taenia solium*, and represents the most common helminth with nervous system involvement. It represents a significant public health issue in certain parts of the world, particularly Latin America, India, and sporadically in Europe and Australia (Turner and Scaravilli, 2002; Lucas et al., 2008). When cysticercosis is seen in industrialized countries, it is usually in immigrants. The adult *T. solium* lives in the human intestine. Gravid segments (proglottids) of the tapeworm are shed in stool from which eggs are expelled and contaminate the ground. Eggs may then be ingested by pigs, which in turn hatch into larvae (oncospheres). These burrow through the wall of the gut, enter the circulation, encyst in soft tissues, and mature into cysticerci. When humans eat poorly cooked pork containing viable cysticerci, they encyst in the small intestine and attach to the wall of the jejunum. They grow into adult tapeworms in about 3 months at which time they begin to shed proglottids, thus completing the life cycle.

Humans develop cysticercosis by consuming the eggs, whether in situations involving poor personal hygiene or sewage disposal and thus ingesting eggs in their own feces, or from eggs shed from domestic food handlers (Schantz et al., 1992), and rarely through the process of regurgitation of proglottids from the small intestine into the stomach. Once larvae gain hematogenous access to soft tissues, the brain, skeletal muscle, the eyes, and subcutaneous tissues are the most commonly affected. A wide latency exists between infection and symptoms, between 2 months and 30 years.

MR imaging is a sensitive way to detect to lesions (Figure 5.16a). A typical pattern of evolution has been described in which the initial appearance of edema and contrast enhancement is followed by cyst and early capsule formation. With degeneration of the organism, there is loss of cystic features and eventual calcification (Dumas et al., 1997).

Virtually any portion of the nervous system may be involved but there is a predilection for the brain with only rare involvement of the spinal cord. In the majority of individuals, the CNS cysticercosis is asymptomatic. The most common symptoms in decreasing order are seizures, leptomeningitis, often basilar with ensuing hydrocephalus, and intraventricular, especially the fourth ventricle (McCormick et al., 1982; Sotelo et al., 1985). Cerebrovascular localization, disseminated forms, and encephalitis related to the immune reaction are rarer manifestations. Regardless, the symptoms usually herald the reaction to death of the organism, since while alive they deploy mechanisms that block the host's inflammatory response.

Cysticercosis presents to the surgical neuropathologist usually in one of two forms: as intact single or multiple cysts sometimes withdrawn from a ventricular space, most commonly the fourth ventricle in order to relieve obstruction or as a resection specimen intended to remove an epileptogenic focus. The wall of the parasite displays three distinct layers: an outer or cuticular layer about 3 μm thick, a middle cellular layer, and an inner reticular or fibrillary layer (Figure 5.16b).

After the death of the larva, the organism may retain some architectural features and upon degeneration, there is a reaction including neutrophils, mononuclear and foreign body giant cells, and eosinophils with later granulation tissue formation (Figure 5.16e).

Echinococcal Cyst

Echinococcal infection producing hydatid disease occurs where people live in close proximity to dogs (Taratuto and Venturiello, 1997). The disease is endemic

Figure 5.16.
Neurocysticercosis. (a) An
axial T1 contrast-enhanced
MR image shows
a peripherally enhancing,
left parietal lobe cyst at the
gray–white matter junction.
There is surrounding
vasogenic edema. The
enhancing dot within the
center of the mass is the dead
scolex. Typically, cysticercosis
cysts only enhance and elicit
surrounding vasogenic edema
after the scolex dies and
degenerates (colloidal stage).
Neurocysticercosis cysts can
also occur in the ventricles
and in the subarachnoid
space. (b) In the live parasite,
sometimes extracted from a
ventricular space to relieve
acute obstructive
hydrocephalus, the
characteristic three layers of
the wall are the outer or
cuticular layer, a middle
cellular layer, and an inner
reticular or fibrillary layer.
In parenchymal resections,
careful comparison with
adjacent host tissue will
reveal the comparatively
much smaller nuclear size of
the parasite's nuclei.

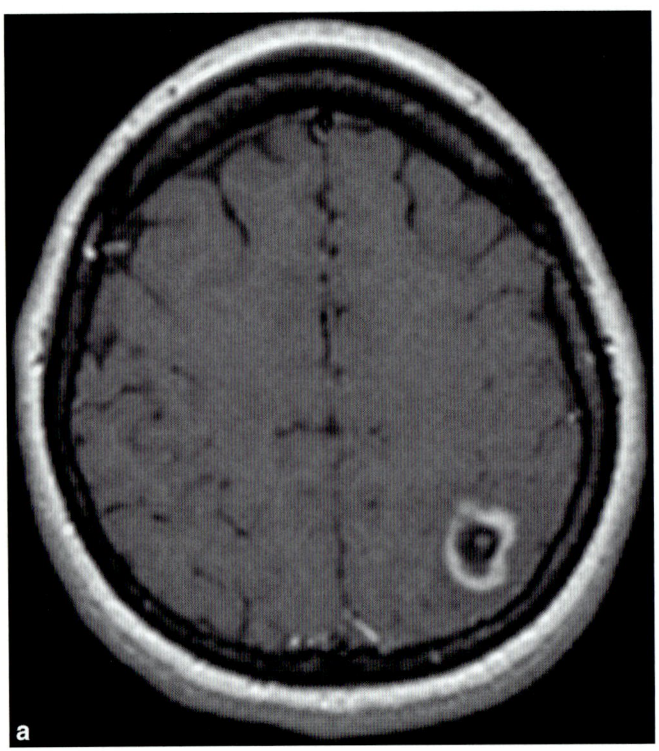

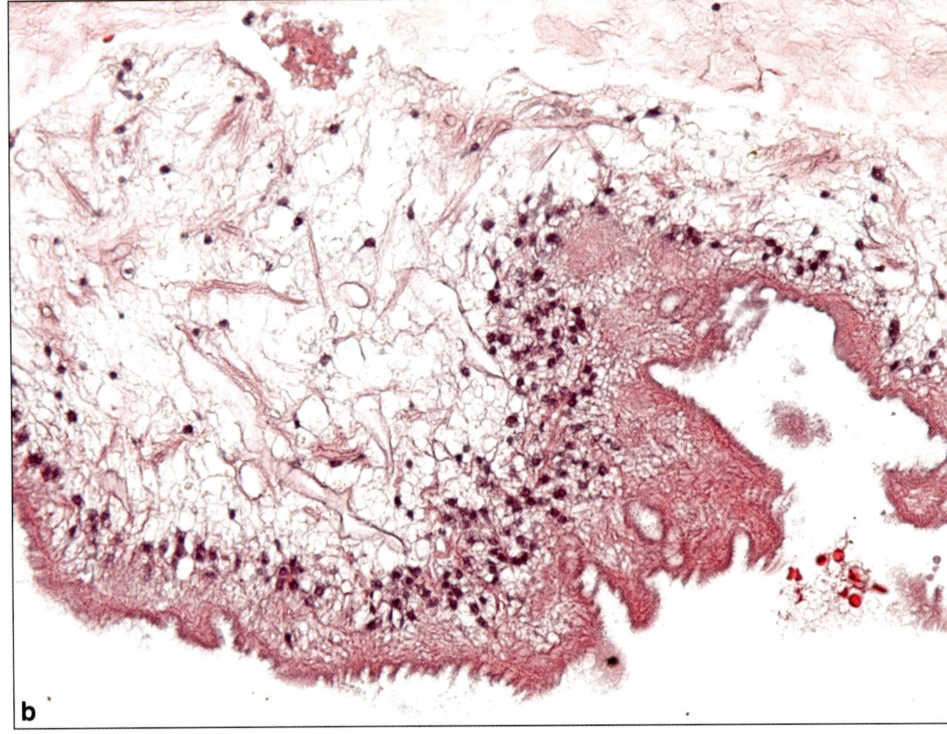

in Mediterranean regions and the Middle East, parts of South America and the British Isles. Dogs become definitive hosts when they become infected after eating a hydatid cyst in uncooked sheep or goat meat. Human infection occurs with ingestion of food contaminated with dog feces and presupposes the frequent and intimate contact with dogs. The infection is rare in infants and most common in children up to the age of 15 years.

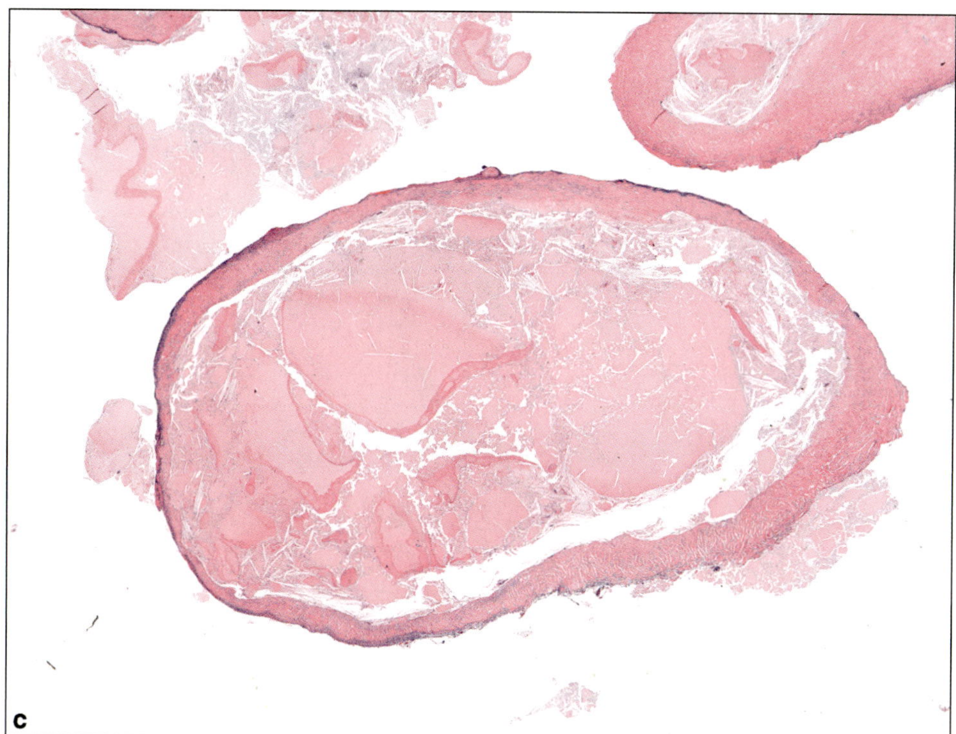

Figure 5.16. *continued* (c) Example of an intraventricular sclerotic cyst with the remnants of the dead parasite in the center, (d) seen at higher magnification.

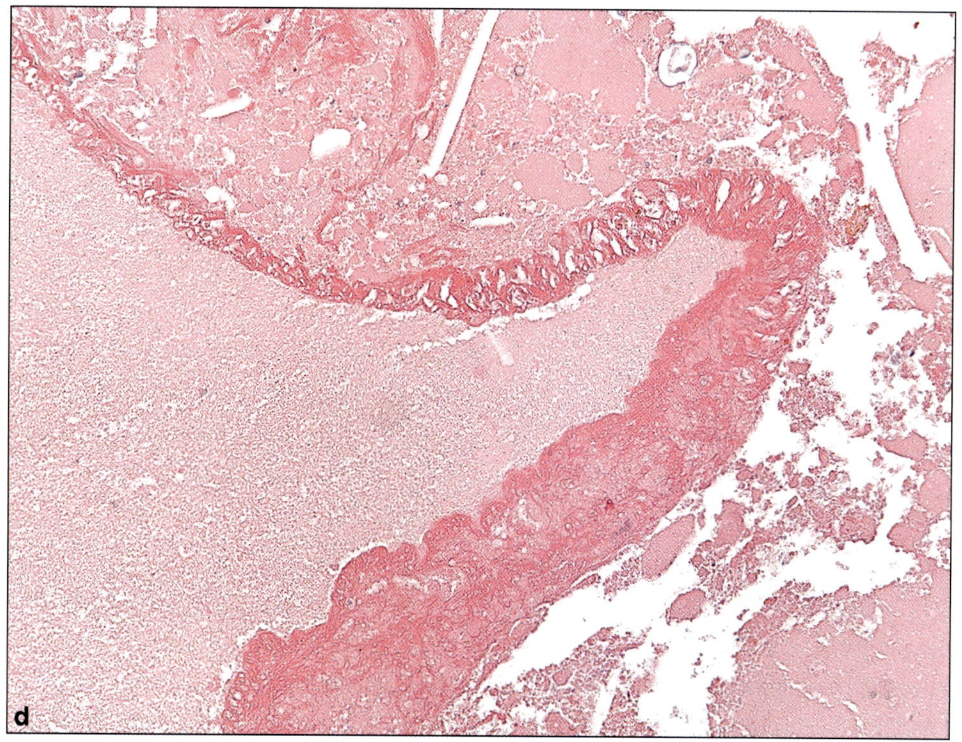

As in cysticercosis, eggs hatch in the small intestine, releasing larvae to penetrate the mucosa whereupon they are transported by hematogenous and lymphatic routes to the liver, lungs, and other organs. The brain is involved in less than 1% of cases (Canbolat et al., 1994). In most cases, the cyst is solitary. Spinal cord compression may occur as a consequence of vertebral involvement.

Figure 5.16. *continued*
(e) Months or years after
death of the parasite,
a surgical resection specimen
of an unknown brain mass
may show a sclerotic lesion
with a variable chronic
inflammatory infiltrate and
even granulomatous
components.

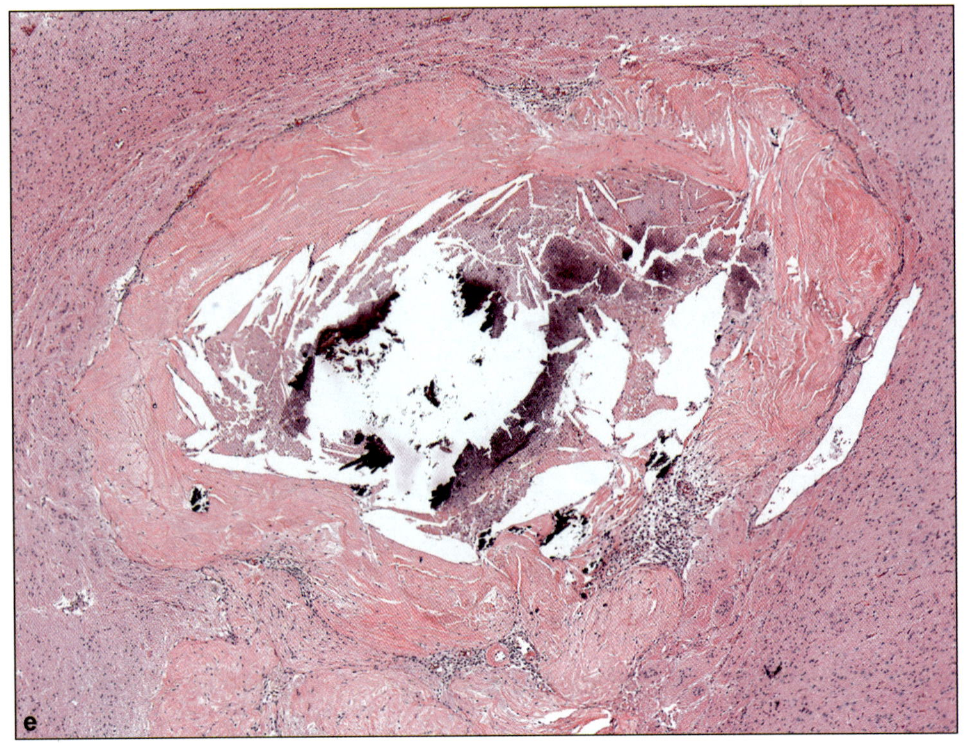

CT imaging in the appropriate clinical context will suggest the diagnosis. Aspiration of cyst fluid may reveal hooklets or vesicles.

The cysts are typically large, up to 10 cm in diameter, producing cortical compression or the risk of intraventricular rupture. The cyst contains clear colorless fluid. Microscopy of the cyst wall shows an outer laminated chitinous or cuticular layer and an inner layer to which oval vesicles are usually attached. Sections may show the scolex with four spherical suckers and a double ring of hooklets. The adjacent brain may show a mild inflammatory reaction, limited by similar anti-inflammatory strategies as seen in cysticercosis.

PRION DISEASES

Clinical and Radiological Features

Creutzfeldt–Jacob disease (CJD) is the prototypic prionopathy, mostly sporadic yet a transmissable disease, causing in most cases a course of rapid dementia over weeks or months, accompanied by myoclonus, characteristic electroencephalographic changes and radiographic changes (Figure 5.17). Many cases are diagnosed through clinical and laboratory examination, including CSF positivity for elevated 14-3-3 protein. However, atypical cases occur that lead to brain biopsy.

Pathology

Surgical brain biopsies for suspected CJD may be compromised by sampling issues. Radiographically, abnormal cortex should be biopsied if possible. Early stages of the disease may produce only very subtle changes. The complete

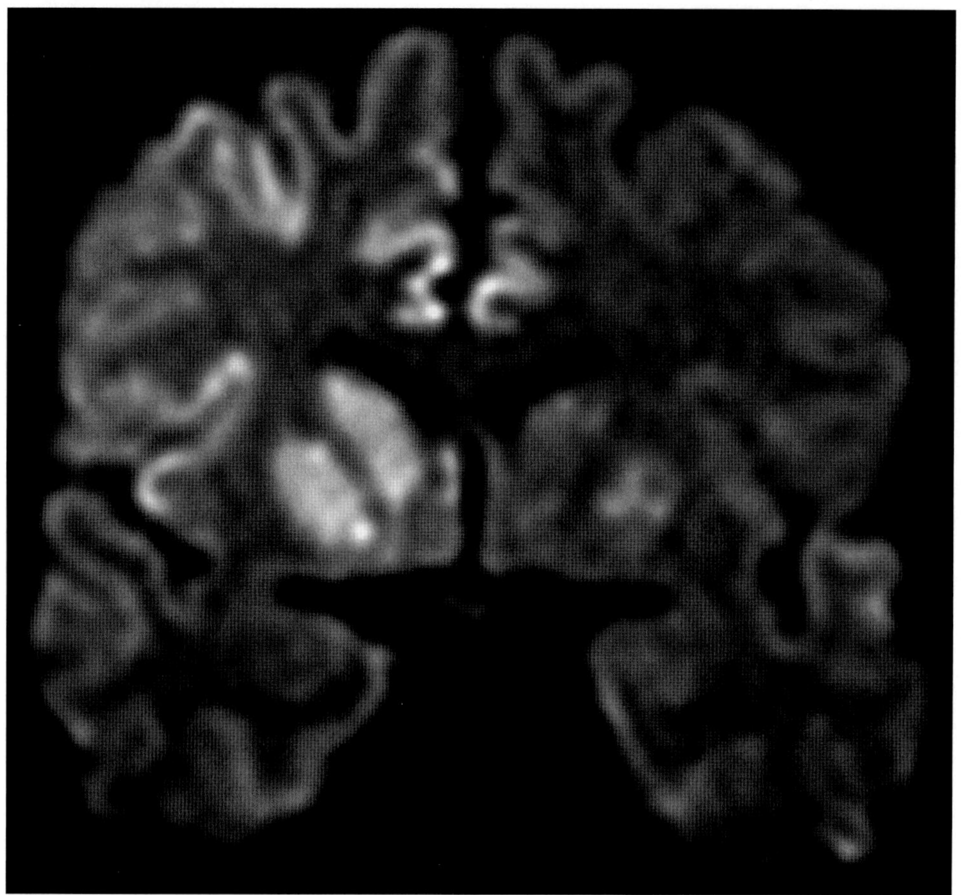

Figure 5.17. Creutzfeldt–Jakob disease (CJD). A coronal diffusion-weighted image shows high signal within the basal ganglia and within multifocal areas of cortex. Progressive diffusion restriction and abnormal signal on T2-weighted MR within the basal ganglia, thalamus, and cortex are nearly diagnostic of Creutzfeldt–Jakob disease in the setting of an adult with rapidly progressive dementia.

pathological entity is comprised of spongiform change, neuronal loss, and gliosis (Figure 5.18). Spongiform change may be the earliest subtle finding, and while fully developed cases show involvement of the entire cortical thickness, early disease may preferentially involve deeper cortical layers only. Spongiform changes are notoriously mimicked by other conditions, including autolysis (not usually an issue with surgical specimens), and even status epilepticus as may manifest in some patients with prion diseases.

Recommendations Regarding the Diagnosis of Prion Diseases

The pathologist should be vigilant in considering almost any case involving brain biopsy for an unexplained neurodegenerative disease as potentially CJD. The following background and guidelines are advisable in handling tissue in suspected cases in order to minimize the possible risk of transmission of infection and ensure the accurate diagnosis of prion-related disease.

1. Prions are nonviral, nonbacterial infectious proteins that are extremely resistant to normal decontamination and sterilization methods.
2. Prions have long incubation periods, ranging from 1 year to over 35 years.
3. Disease caused by prions includes CJD and other diseases classified as spongiform encephalopathies.

Figure 5.18. (a) Spongiform
encephalopathy of confirmed
CJD in which status
spongiosis exists for the entire
thickness of the cortex.
(b) Status spongiosis is not
entirely specific for prion
diseases; however,
perineuronal vacuoles may be
suggestive (arrow).

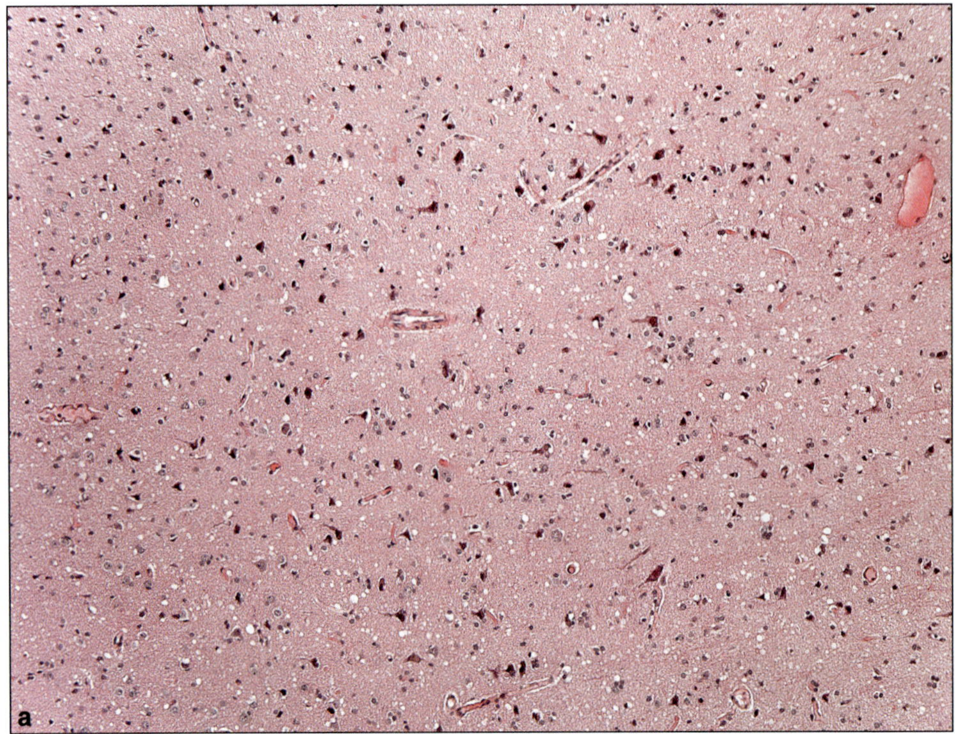

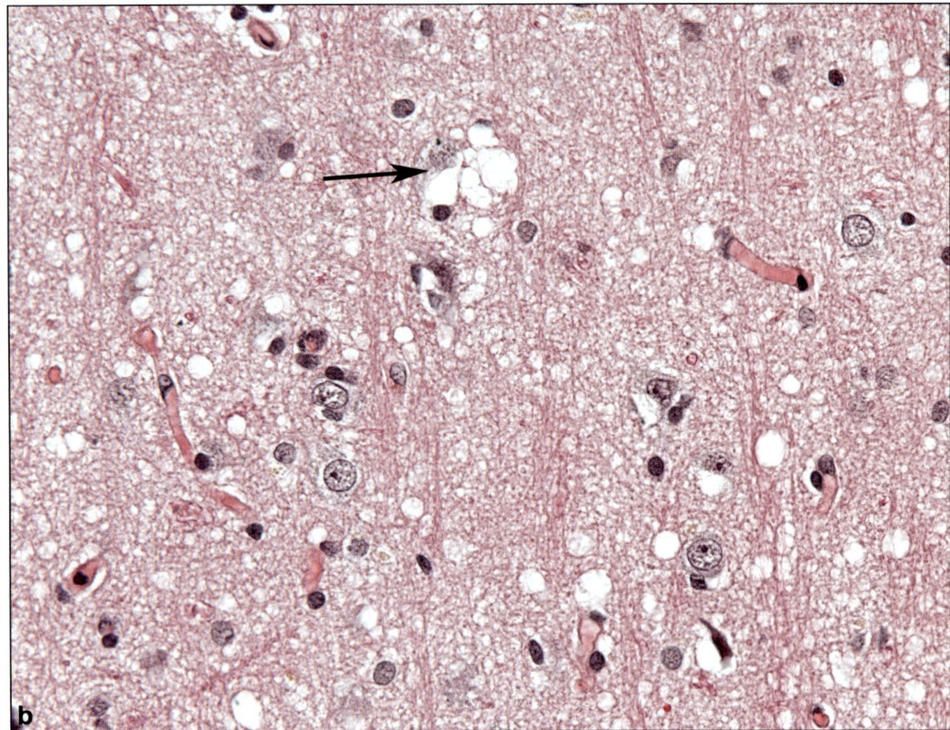

4. Known sources of transmission include: Tissue for transplantation
   (cornea, dura mater and pericardial homografts), pituitary hormones removed during autopsy, neurosurgical instruments, neurological electrodes. Note: to date, no cases of prion disease have
   been documented to be attributable to the handling of surgical or
   postmortem tissues.

5. Tissues and body fluids were classified into 4 classes of infectivity according to specific measures taken by the EU to prevent spread of animal-derived disease:
    - high infectivity: CNS tissues (brain, spinal cord) and adjacent tissues (eyes);
    - medium infectivity: lymphoid tissues (spleen, lymph nodes, tonsils), internal organs with lymphatic component (e.g. ileum, proximal colon), placenta, pituitary gland, dura mater and CSF;
    - low infectivity: peripheral nerves, bone marrow, liver, lung, pancreas, thymus;
    - no detectable infectivity: muscle, kidney, fat, bone, blood, milk, bile.
6. Prions are NOT decontaminated by
    standard steam sterilization settings,
    ethylene oxide sterilization,
    formalin/formaldehyde,
    glutaraldehyde,
    phenolics,
    iodophors,
    alcohol,
    hydrogen peroxide, and
    peracetic acid
7. There is no reason to refuse a biopsy (or an autopsy) on a patient with suspected transmissible spongiform encephalopathy. Moreover, obtaining a definite diagnosis is of utmost importance not only for research into these enigmatic diseases, but also for epidemiological and public health reasons.
8. The National Prion Disease Pathology Surveillance Center (NPDPSC) was established in 1997 with the endorsement and support of the American Association of Neuropathologists, Centers for Diseases Control and Prevention (CDC), and later on of the U.S. Congress. The purpose of the NPDPSC is to diagnose prion diseases following tissue examination to monitor not only their incidence but also to timely detect forms of high public health concern. Prion surveillance is especially important because of the insidious infectivity of prion diseases that make them transmissible from human to human and from animals to humans. More recently, it became clear that a variant of Creutzfeldt–Jakob disease (vCJD) can be acquired by eating contaminated beef products. A special concern in the United States is the possible occurrence of the human prion disease acquired from elk or deer affected by chronic wasting disease, a prion disorder. The Surveillance Center performs histopathology, immunocyto-chemistry, Western blot, and prion gene analysis in autopsy and

biopsy tissues to establish the diagnosis and to determine the type of prion disease. CSF is also examined for the presence of the CJD protein marker 14-3-3. Test results are reported in a timely manner and free of charge to the sender of the sample, and to CDC. Remaining tissues are stored and made available for research. Information about the NPDPSC and specimen collection and shipping instructions can be obtained by calling 216-368-0587 or visiting its Web site at www.cjdsurveillance.com. All correspondence and shipments should be addressed to: Pierluigi Gambetti, M.D. Division of Neuropathology, Room 419 Case Western Reserve University 2085 Adelbert Road Cleveland, Ohio 44106 Telephone: 216-368-0587 For shipping: Federal Express Acct. # 1153-2834-4

It is strongly recommended that a portion of the tissue obtained either at biopsy or autopsy be frozen as the diagnostic study of prion disease is fully reliable and complete only after immunodiagnostic and genetic analysis of the prion protein. It is important that available clinical history be shared with the Surveillance Center in every referred case.

Protocol and Procedure: Surgical Specimens

1. All neuropathology faculty and fellowship trainees, as well as the general surgical pathology faculty, will be made aware of the following protocol involving diagnostic central nervous system biopsies in all clinically suspected cases of prion disease. The protocol will be followed even if prion disease is not the leading clinical diagnosis but is stated in a differential diagnosis of the patient's illness, or if circumstances listed below are applicable.
2. Neuropathology faculty on service will hold primary responsibility for the proper immediate handling of such tissue, whereby no frozen section is to be performed or intraoperative diagnostic maneuver such as would risk contamination of shared equipment, solutions, etc.
3. A portion of the biopsy should be snap frozen in an appropriately marked sealed container and triple bagged and placed at −80°, and the remainder placed in 10% buffered formalin for 24 hours, followed by 1 hour immersed in 100% formic acid. The tissue and suspected agent is then considered nontransmissable and may be processed in a routine manner for paraffin embedding and slide preparation.
4. All disposable containers, instruments, blades, gloves, etc. should be bagged as medical waste for incineration and brought to the morgue for appropriate handling. Instruments that were contaminated by formaldehyde-fixed, nonformic acid–treated tissue are not

decontaminated by autoclaving but should instead be immersed in 2 N NaOH for 1 hour.

5. Frozen and fixed tissue samples will be shipped to the National Prion Disease Pathology Surveillance Center, which will provide containers and instructions for shipment. If paraffin sections are submitted, please cut 1 section 5-μm thick (for H.E.) and three sections 8-μm thick (for PrP immunohistochemistry).

Postexposure Management

a. Mucous membrane or other splash exposure should be managed by rinsing area with copious amounts of water.

b. For a percutaneous exposure, rinse-injured area with 5% solution of sodium hypochlorite (undiluted bleach), followed by washing with soap and water.

c. Notify the infection control practitioner (Employee Health), as soon as possible after any exposures.

REFERENCES

Abdel-Haq N, Abuhammour W, Al-Tatari H, Asmar B. Disseminated cat scratch disease with vertebral osteomyelitis and epidural abscess. *South Med J* 2005; 98: 1142–5.

Antinori A, Ammassari A, Luzzati R, Castagna A, Maserati R, Rizzardini G, et al. Role of brain biopsy in the management of focal brain lesions in HIV-infected patients. Gruppo Italiano Cooperativo AIDS & Tumori. *Neurology* 2000; 54: 993–7.

Astrom KE, Mancall EL, Richardson EP, Jr. Progressive multifocal leuko-encephalopathy; a hitherto unrecognized complication of chronic lymphatic leukaemia and Hodgkin's disease. *Brain* 1958; 81: 93–111.

Bartt RE. Multiple sclerosis, natalizumab therapy, and progressive multifocal leukoencephalopathy. *Curr Opin Neurol* 2006; 19: 341–9.

Berenguer J, Moreno S, Laguna F, Vicente T, Adrados M, Ortega A, et al. Tuberculous meningitis in patients infected with the human immunodeficiency virus. *N Engl J Med* 1992; 326: 668–72.

Bernardini GL. Diagnosis and management of brain abscess and subdural empyema. *Curr Neurol Neurosci Rep* 2004; 4: 448–56.

Bertoli F, Espino M, Arosemena JRt, Fishback JL, Frenkel JK. A spectrum in the pathology of toxoplasmosis in patients with acquired immunodeficiency syndrome. *Arch Pathol Lab Med* 1995; 119: 214–24.

Bertrand E, Szpak GM, Pilkowska E, Habib N, Lipczynska-Lojkowska W, Rudnicka A, et al. Central nervous system infection caused by Borrelia burgdorferi. Clinico-pathological correlation of three post-mortem cases. *Folia Neuropathol* 1999; 37: 43–51.

Brown E, Gray F. Bacterial infections. In: Greenfield JG, Love S, Louis DN, Ellison D, editors. *Greenfield's Neuropathology*. London: Hodder Arnold, 2008.

Canbolat A, Onal C, Kaya U, Coban TE. Intracranial extradural hydatid cysts: report of three cases. *Surg Neurol* 1994; 41: 230–4.

Carpenter J, Stapleton S, Holliman R. Retrospective analysis of 49 cases of brain abscess and review of the literature. *Eur J Clin Microbiol Infect Dis* 2007; 26: 1–11.

Carrazana EJ, Rossitch E, Jr., Samuels MA. Cerebral toxoplasmosis in the acquired immune deficiency syndrome. *Clin Neurol Neurosurg* 1989; 91: 291–301.

Colom MF, Frases S, Ferrer C, Jover A, Andreu M, Reus S, et al. First case of human cryptococcosis due to Cryptococcus neoformans var. gattii in Spain. *J Clin Microbiol* 2005; 43: 3548–50.

Darouiche RO. Spinal epidural abscess. *N Engl J Med* 2006; 355: 2012–20.

Deol I, Robledo L, Meza A, Visvesvara GS, Andrews RJ. Encephalitis due to a free-living amoeba (Balamuthia mandrillaris): case report with literature review. *Surg Neurol* 2000; 53: 611–16.

Druschky K, Walloch J, Heckmann J, Schmidt B, Stefan H, Neundorfer B. Chronic parvovirus B-19 meningoencephalitis with additional detection of Epstein–Barr virus DNA in the cerebrospinal fluid of an immunocompetent patient. *J Neurovirol* 2000; 6: 418–22.

Dumas JL, Visy JM, Belin C, Gaston A, Goldlust D, Dumas M. Parenchymal neurocysticercosis: follow-up and staging by MRI. *Neuroradiology* 1997; 39: 12–18.

Fouch B, Coventry S. A case of fatal disseminated Bartonella henselae infection (cat-scratch disease) with encephalitis. *Arch Pathol Lab Med* 2007; 131: 1591–4.

Gordon SM, Eaton ME, George R, Larsen S, Lukehart SA, Kuypers J, et al. The response of symptomatic neurosyphilis to high-dose intravenous penicillin G in patients with human immunodeficiency virus infection. *N Engl J Med* 1994; 331: 1469–73.

Handsfield HH, Lukehart SA, Sell S, Norris SJ, Holmes KK. Demonstration of Treponema pallidum in a cutaneous gumma by indirect immunofluorescence. *Arch Dermatol* 1983; 119: 677–80.

Hornef MW, Iten A, Maeder P, Villemure JG, Regli L. Brain biopsy in patients with acquired immunodeficiency syndrome: diagnostic value, clinical performance, and survival time. *Arch Intern Med* 1999; 159: 2590–6.

Horowitz HW, Valsamis MP, Wicher V, Abbruscato F, Larsen SA, Wormser GP, et al. Brief report: cerebral syphilitic gumma confirmed by the polymerase chain reaction in a man with human immunodeficiency virus infection. *N Engl J Med* 1994; 331: 1488–91.

Isenmann S, Zimmermann DR, Wichmann W, Moll C. Tuberculoma mimicking meningioma of the falx cerebri. PCR diagnosis of mycobacterial DNA from formalin-fixed tissue. *Clin Neuropathol* 1996; 15: 155–8.

Lou J, Lucas R, Grau GE. Pathogenesis of cerebral malaria: recent experimental data and possible applications for humans. *Clin Microbiol Rev* 2001; 14: 810–20, table of contents.

Lucas S, Bell J, Chimelli L. Parasitic and fungal infections. In: Greenfield JG, Love S, Louis DN, Ellison D, editors. *Greenfield's Neuropathology*. London: Hodder Arnold, 2008.

McCormick GF, Zee CS, Heiden J. Cysticercosis cerebri. Review of 127 cases. *Arch Neurol* 1982; 39: 534–9.

McJunkin JE, Khan R, de los Reyes EC, Parsons DL, Minnich LL, Ashley RG, et al. Treatment of severe La Crosse encephalitis with intravenous ribavirin following diagnosis by brain biopsy. *Pediatrics* 1997; 99: 261–7.

Miklossy J, Kuntzer T, Bogousslavsky J, Regli F, Janzer RC. Meningovascular form of neuroborreliosis: similarities between neuropathological findings in a case of

Lyme disease and those occurring in tertiary neurosyphilis. *Acta Neuropathol* 1990; 80: 568–72.

Modlin JF, Halsey NA, Eddins DL, Conrad JL, Jabbour JT, Chien L, et al. Epidemiology of subacute sclerosing panencephalitis. *J Pediatr* 1979; 94: 231–6.

Newton CR, Warrell DA. Neurological manifestations of falciparum malaria. *Ann Neurol* 1998; 43: 695–702.

Oksi J, Kalimo H, Marttila RJ, Marjamaki M, Sonninen P, Nikoskelainen J, et al. Inflammatory brain changes in Lyme borreliosis. A report on three patients and review of literature. *Brain* 1996; 119(Pt 6): 2143–54.

Riggs H, Schlezinger NS. Clinical pathologic conference on myelomalacia due to hypertrophic pachymeningitis secondary to epidural abscess; etiologic possibilities. *Neurology* 1953; 3: 148–53.

Rowen JL, Doerr CA, Vogel H, Baker CJ. Balamuthia mandrillaris: a newly recognized agent for amebic meningoencephalitis. *Pediatr Infect Dis J* 1995; 14: 705–10.

Schantz PM, Moore AC, Munoz JL, Hartman BJ, Schaefer JA, Aron AM, et al. Neurocysticercosis in an Orthodox Jewish community in New York City. *N Engl J Med* 1992; 327: 692–5.

Sotelo J, Guerrero V, Rubio F. Neurocysticercosis: a new classification based on active and inactive forms. A study of 753 cases. *Arch Intern Med* 1985; 145: 442–5.

Taratuto AL, Venturiello SM. Echinococcosis. *Brain Pathol* 1997; 7: 673–9.

Turner G. Cerebral malaria. *Brain Pathol* 1997; 7: 569–82.

Turner G, Scaravilli F. Parasitic and fungal diseases. In: Greenfield JG, Graham DI, Lantos PL, editors. *Greenfield's Neuropathology*. London, New York: Arnold, 2002.

Visvesvara GS, Martinez AJ, Schuster FL, Leitch GJ, Wallace SV, Sawyer TK, et al. Leptomyxid ameba, a new agent of amebic meningoencephalitis in humans and animals. *J Clin Microbiol* 1990; 28: 2750–6.

6 INFLAMMATORY DISEASES

An inflammatory cell reaction may be present in the histopathological profile of virtually all diseases of the central nervous system (CNS), including neoplasms, and hypoxic/ischemic, neurodegenerative, and metabolic diseases. Preneoplastic or neoplastic inflammatory cell diseases may be difficult to distinguish from purely reactive infiltrates. Some of the most common pitfalls in dealing with inflammatory lesions lie in the failure to recognize primary demyelinating disease from atypical or neoplastic lymphoproliferative disease.

The nature of the inflammatory infiltrate may provide a clue as to the type of inflammatory disease. *Neutrophils* predominate in abscesses, most forms of meningitis except viral and fungal infections, and in toxoplasmosis and acute hemorrhagic leukoencephalitis. *Lymphocytes* predominate in viral meningitis, encephalitis, some chronic bacterial infections including rickettsial and Lyme disease and a number of immune-mediated disorders including Rasmussen's encephalitis, paraneoplastic encephalitis, lymphocytic hypophysitis, and others. *Plasma cells* are frequent in neurosyphilis, subacute sclerosing panencephalitis (SSPE), inflammatory pseudotumor and Castleman's disease. *Epithelioid cells, giant cells,* and *granulomas* should provoke the consideration of infections such as tuberculosis, mycotic infections, amebiasis due to Acanthameba, human immunodeficiency virus (HIV), and other immunologic disorders including sarcoidosis, granulomatous angiitis, rheumatoid nodules, particularly in para-spinal lesions, and Wegener's granulomatosis. Macrophages are frequent in demyelinating processes, progressive multifocal leukoencephalopathy, Whipple's disease, histoplasmosis, Rosai–Dorfman disease, and various xanthomatous lesions. *Eosinophils* are sometimes but all not always indicative of parasitic diseases, Langerhans cell histiocytosis, and are found in subdural hematomas. *Microglial activation* is common in viral encephalitis, Rasmussen's encephalitis but may also be conspicuous histologic component of infiltrating gliomas.

DEMYELINATING DISEASES

This term implies the selective destruction of myelin with relative preservation of axons and is to be distinguished from axonal degeneration with secondary demyelination or dysmyelination in which myelin is not normally formed. Axonal and gray matter injury is an increasingly appreciated aspect of primary demyelinating diseases, however, the histopathological diagnosis of these conditions usually requires the conventional demonstration of demyelination with preservation of axons in white matter lesions.

Multiple Sclerosis

Clinical and Radiological Features

Multiple sclerosis is the most common demyelinating disease of the CNS (Sobel and Moore, 2008). It is typically multifocal with lesions of different ages. Its prevalence varies geographically, being most common in northern portions of the northern hemisphere and least common in Asia, Africa, and northern South America. Migration from a high to a low prevalence area before the age of 15 years reduces the likelihood of developing multiple sclerosis (MS) and migration after 15 years of age from a low to high prevalence area increases the risk of developing MS. MS is more common in men than women, and the peak age of onset is between 20 and 40 years. The risk of developing MS is increased 15- to 20-fold in first-degree relatives of patients with this disease and shows a high concordance rate in monozygotic twins as compared with dizygotic twins. Various epigenetic associations may affect the incidence and severity of the disease. The prevailing opinion regarding the etiology of MS is that it is an autoimmune condition, perhaps precipitated by a viral infection.

MS commonly presents with focal motor or sensory deficits involving one or more limbs, optic neuritis, diplopia, lack of coordination, or vertigo. Cognitive impairment and seizures are indicative of gray matter involvement in spite of the previously conventional view of MS as a disease of white matter. The disease may progress in a highly variable matter ranging from mild relapses with long intervening asymptomatic periods to fulminant progression; however, it is usually marked by a steadily relapsing and remitting course.

Figure 6.1.
(a) Ring-enhancing or tumefactive multiple sclerosis. A coronal T1 contrast-enhanced MR image shows circular lesions with abnormally low signal in the center and with surrounding incomplete rings of enhancement. Areas of enhancement are thought to correlate with areas of active demyelination. When multiple sclerosis presents in its tumefactive ring-enhancing form, it can mimic neoplastic disease and lead to a biopsy. More frequently, multiple sclerosis presents as multiple solid ovoid lesions orientated along the axis of the medullary veins, and a tentative diagnosis of demyelinating disease can be made based on imaging. Sarcoidosis can appear nearly identical to MS on MR imaging. (b) Low magnification appearance of MS, showing perivascular lymphocytic infiltrates, gliosis, macrophages, particularly in the region of relative pallor.

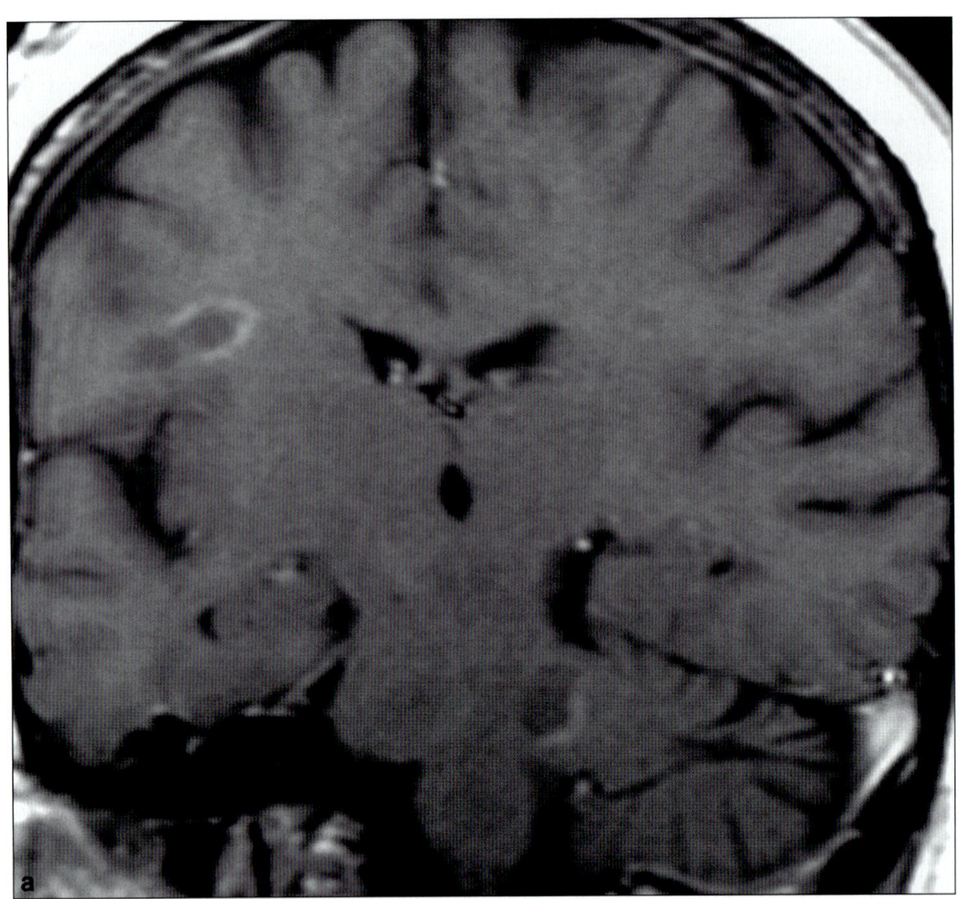

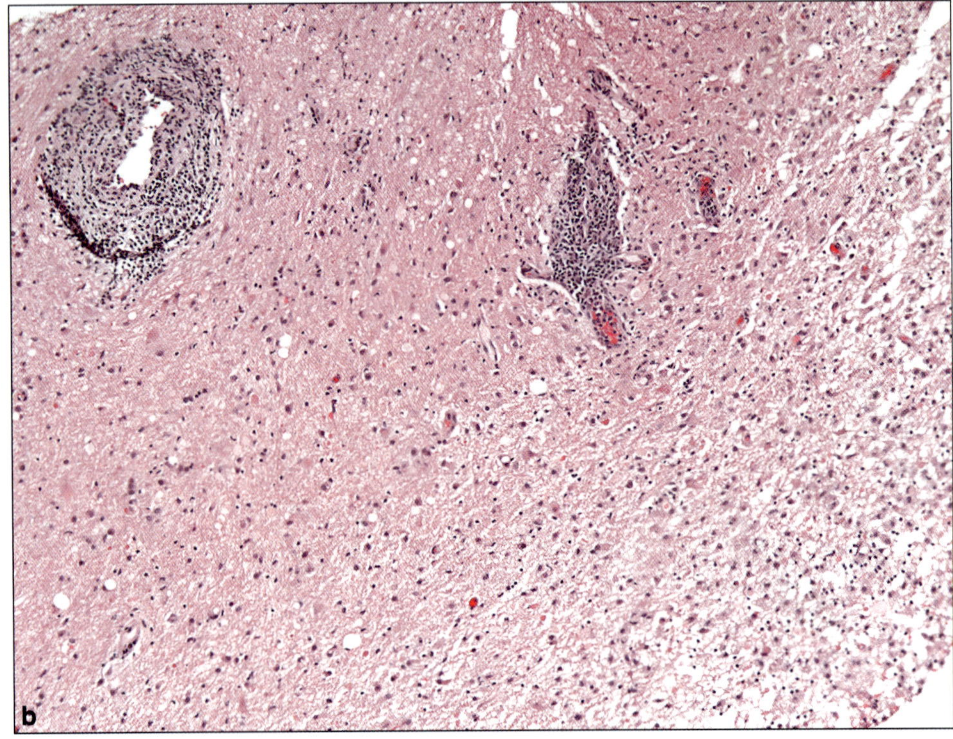

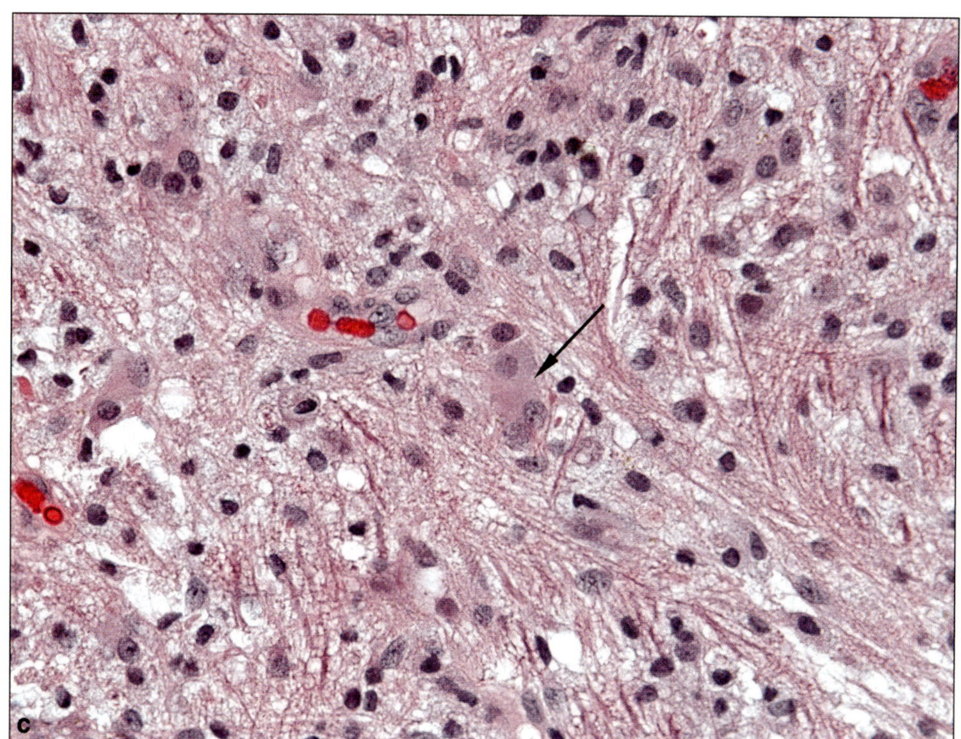

Figure 6.1. *continued* (c) A distinctive feature of active demyelination is the Creutzfeldt astrocyte, a multinucleated reactive cell (arrow). (d) The Luxol fast blue stain for myelin indicates loss of myelin, while an adjacent section shows relative although not complete preservation of axons within the same demyelinated area.

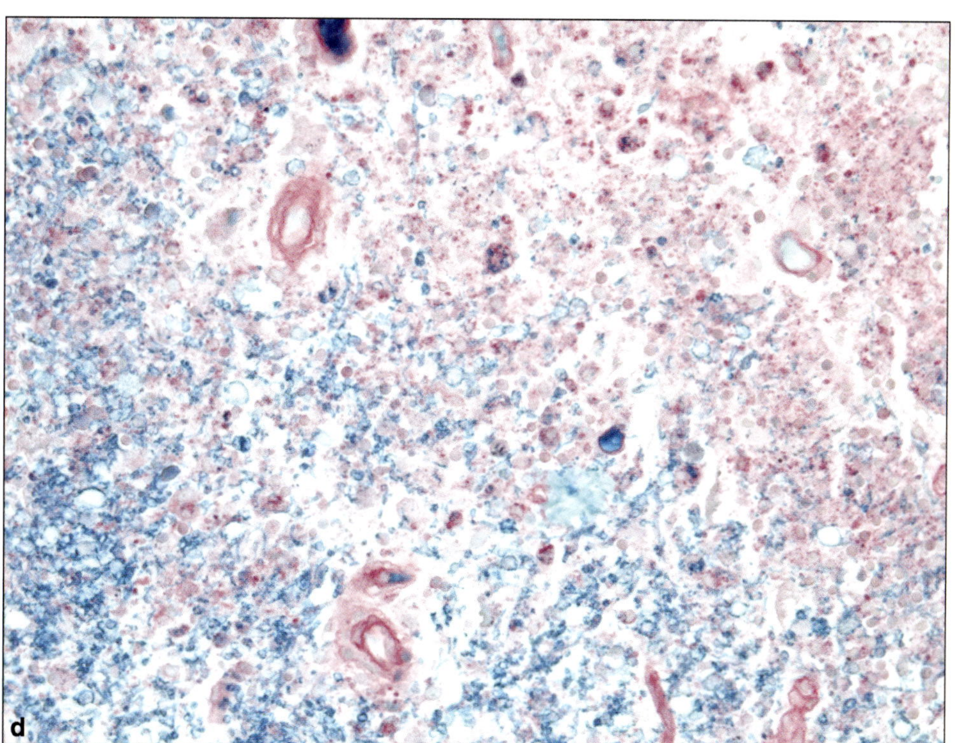

Demyelinating foci are usually readily demonstrable by magnetic resonance imaging (MRI); however, it is of paramount importance to recognize the existence of tumefactive MS, which may mimic a primary glial neoplasm, especially when present as a single lesion. This is one of the most treacherous pitfalls in diagnostic surgical neuropathology. T1-weighted images with intravascular

Figure 6.1. *continued*
(e) Immunophenotyping is not called for in the routine diagnosis of a demyelinating process, however immunohistochemistry for (f) CD68 can reveal a surprising number of macrophages and activated microglial cells, which should always prompt the strong consideration of a nonneoplastic disease.

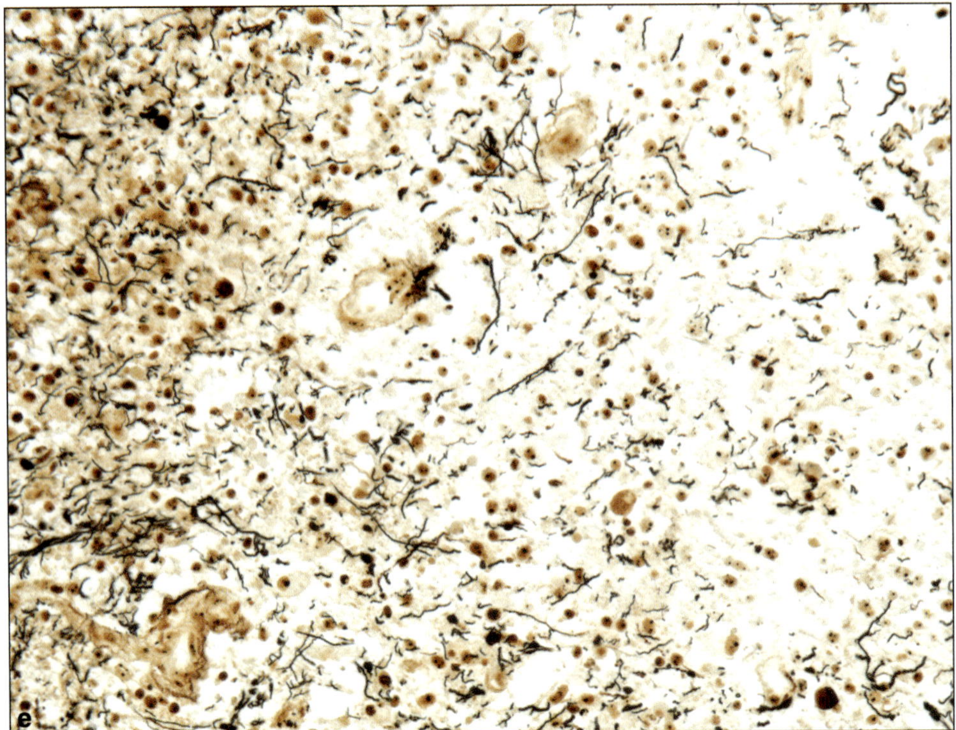

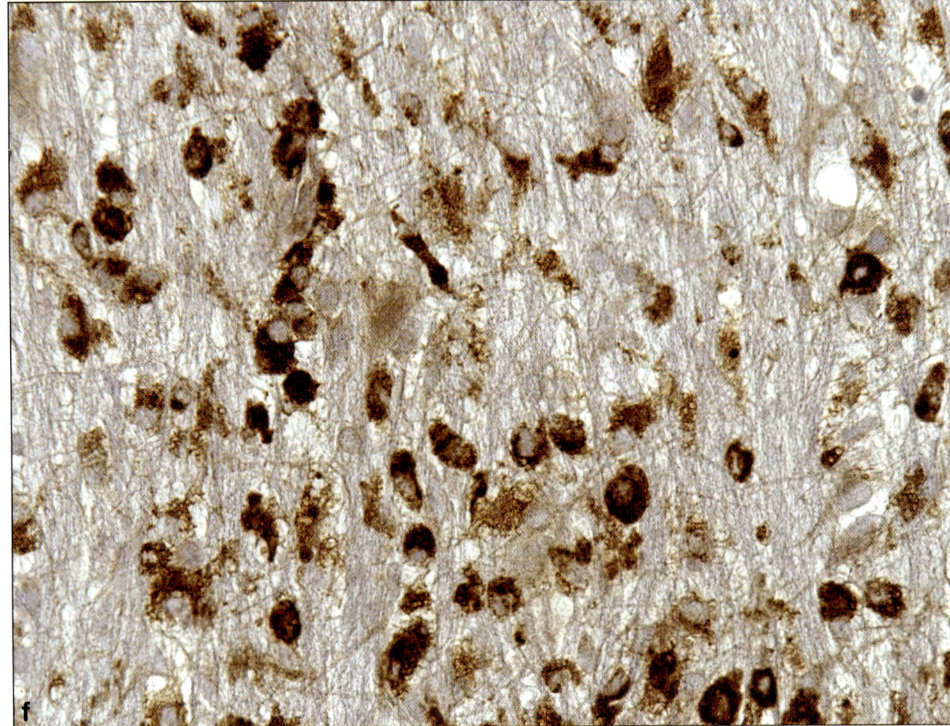

contrast show an interesting tendency to incomplete horseshoe or C-shaped ring enhancement (Figure 6.1a). A series of patients with this condition included a majority with single lesions but almost one-fourth had multiple lesions, mimicking metastatic disease. Because some patients never developed subsequent lesions and some were temporally associated with recent vaccination or possible infections, it was speculated that this form of tumefactive MS may in some instances be a postinfectious phenomenon (Kepes, 1993).

When the visual system is involved, delayed visual evoked responses may be noted. The cerebrospinal fluid (CSF) may show oligoclonal bands of immunoglobulins on electrophoresis; however, this may be present in a number of other conditions including 100% of patients with SSPE, 50% of patients with bacterial, viral, fungal, and spirochetal CNS infections, and a variety of CNS inflammatory disorders including sarcoidosis, CNS vasculitis, CNS lupus erythematosus, Behçet disease, and Guillain–Barré syndrome.

There are four clinical types of MS: classic, acute, neuromyelitis optica, and concentric sclerosis.

Classic (Charcot type) MS is characterized by patches of demyelination, which appear gray in fixed sections and while they may occur anywhere within white matter, they are more commonly found at the lateral angles of the lateral ventricles and olfactory tracts and optic nerves and cerebellar white matter. Such typical lesions with a suggestive clinical and laboratory profile will not lead to biopsy. However, a solitary lesion with mass effect leading to biopsy should include consideration of a demyelinating lesion.

Pathology

Microscopic features of the type of plaque that would more likely be the object of surgical biopsy would be those of an active lesion: hypercellular lesions containing a relatively dense perivascular and parenchymal infiltrate of macrophages and mostly perivascular lymphocytes (Figure 6.1b). Scattered reactive astrocytes may be quite pleomorphic, multinucleated, or contain multiple irregular nuclear fragments along with glassy eosinophilic cytoplasm, known as a granular mitosis or Creutzfeldt astrocyte (Figure 6.1c). These cells are particularly associated with reactive or demyelinating conditions, thus when faced with numerous macrophages, Creutzfeldt cells, other reactive astrocytes, and variable perivascular lymphocytic infiltrates, extreme caution should be exercised in rendering the intraoperative diagnosis.

Macrophages are sometimes not easily recognizable in cryostat sections but are usually identifiable because of their small centrally placed nucleus in a vacuolated cytoplasm. Infarcts, corticosteroid-treated lymphoma, some infections such as herpes simplex encephalitis may mimic this appearance, and even in exceptional examples of some especially high-grade gliomas in which significant necrosis with macrophage infiltration has occurred.

The conventional and generally reliable histological method of demonstrating a demyelinating process is by performing a myelin stain, most commonly the Luxol fast blue (LFB)–periodic acid–Schiff and an axonal stain such as by the Bielschowsky silver impregnation (Figure 6.1d,e). In a selective demyelinating process, there is loss of myelin with relative preservation of axons. The border of demyelination is often abrupt and the region of demyelination may contain macrophages and reactive astrocytes in abundance. Careful scrutiny of

Figure 6.2. Acute disseminated encephalomyelitis. (a) Low magnification suggests a process selectively involving white matter. (b) LFB myelin stains indicates perivenous demyelination.

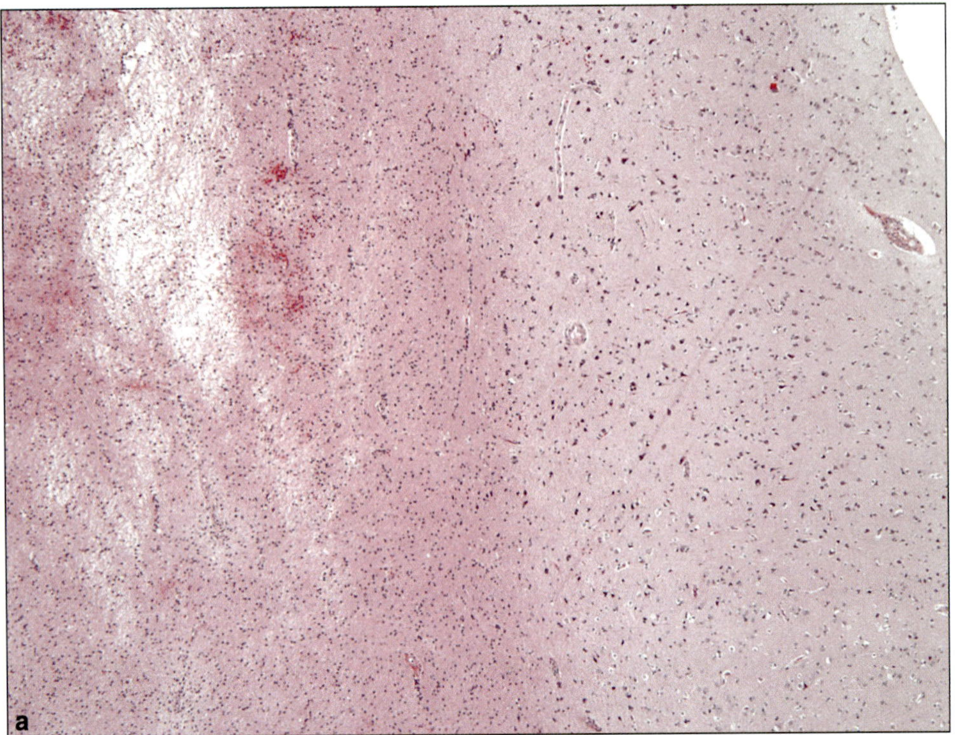

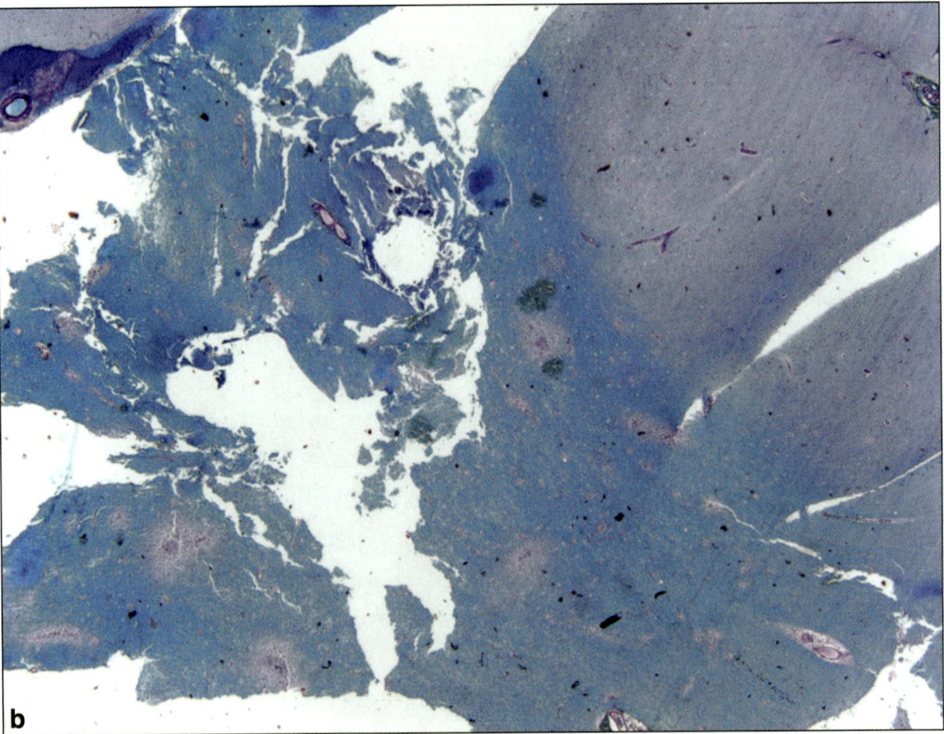

the axonal stain may reveal irregularities in axonal profiles with small varicosities or discontinuities; however a hypoxic/ischemic, neoplasm, or other destructive lesion will show axonal loss commensurate with demyelination.

Immunohistochemistry is not usually necessary to strengthen the diagnosis. Macrophage markers such as CD68 or CD163 (Figure 6.1f) will show abundant

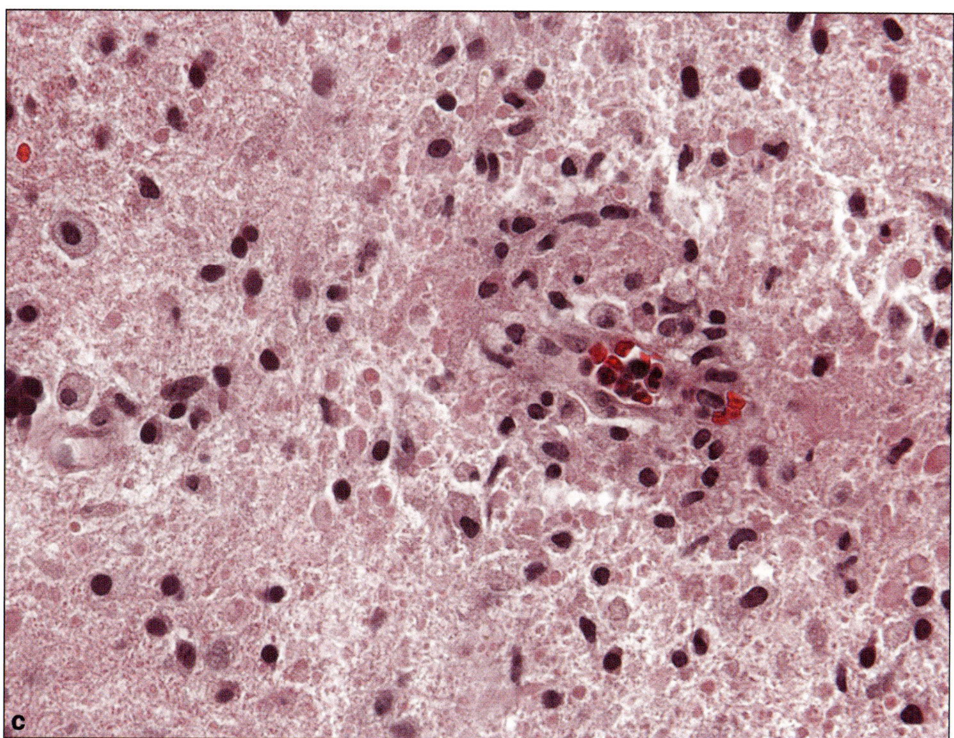

Figure 6.2. *continued*
(c) Higher magnification shows numerous lipid-laden macrophages and microglial cell activation. (d) LFB myelin stain, and
(e) Bielschowsky silver impregnation show loss of perivenous myelin with axonal preservation.

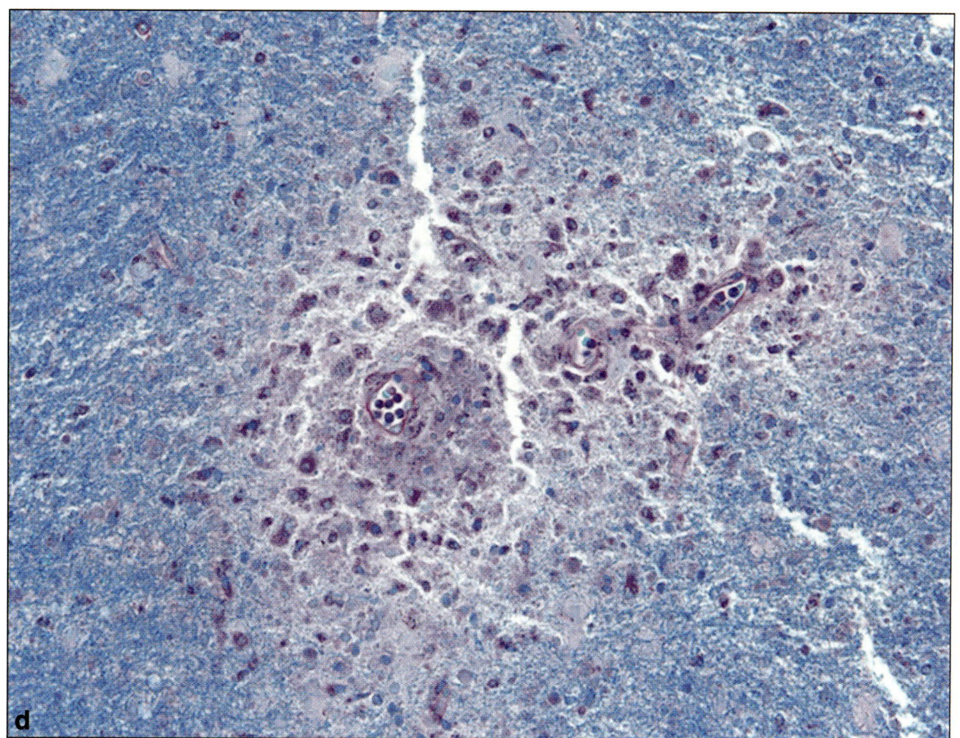

macrophages and glial fibrillary acid protein (GFAP) will identify reactive astrocytes with their characteristically slender and delicate processes. Leukocyte markers will reveal a predominance of T lymphocytes in both the perivascular and interstitial infiltrates.

Figure 6.2. *continued.*

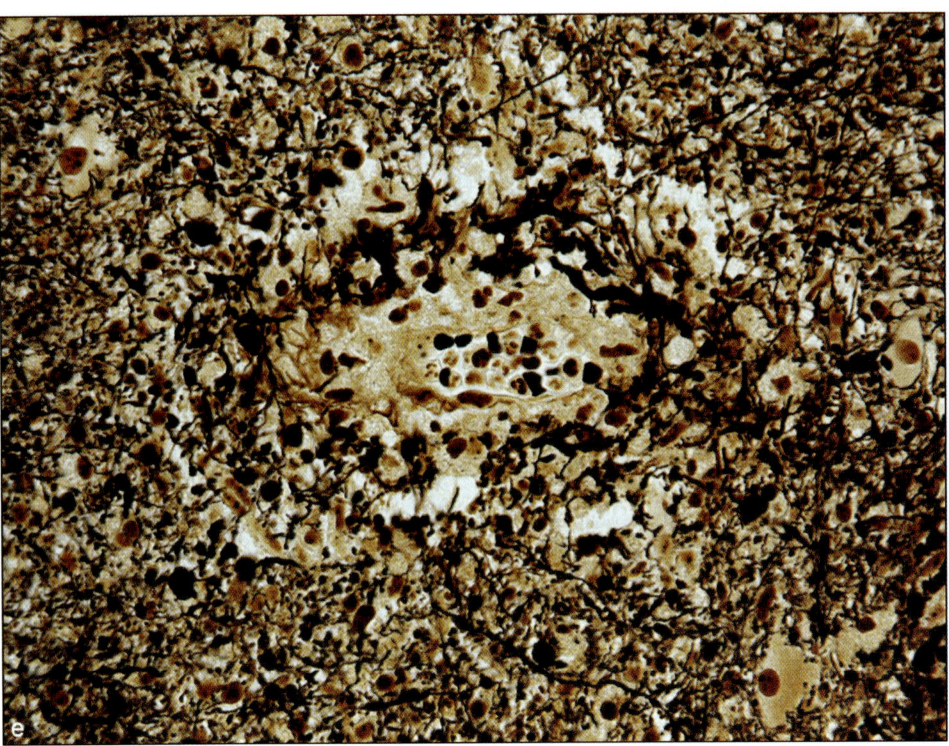

An entity, which is somewhat similar to MS, is the monophasic acute disseminated encephalomyelitis (ADEM). This is a para- or postinfectious auto-immune demyelinating disease with the highest incidence occurring in childhood (Menge et al., 2007). Viral infections commonly associated with ADEM include influenza, measles, mumps, rubella, Varicella zoster, Epstein–Barr virus, cytomegalovirus (CMV), herpes simplex, hepatitis A, enterovirus, and coxsackievirus. Bacterial associations include *Mycoplasma pneumoniae*, *Borrelia burgdorferi* (Lyme disease), leptospirosis, and beta-hemolytic *Streptococcus* (Krupp et al., 2007).

This disease rarely results in biopsy since it is usually diagnosed on combined clinical and radiologic evidence. However, pathologic reports indicate features similar to those of MS, sometimes with a distinct perivenous pattern of demyelination (Figure 6.2).

NEUROSARCOIDOSIS

Clinical and Radiological Features

Sarcoidosis is usually diagnosed between the ages of 20 and 40 years and has a predilection for some racial groups including West Africans. Typically, it a systemic disease, which may rarely occur in an isolated form involving the CNS. The most common neurological manifestations are cranial neuropathies, particularly affecting cranial nerve VII being unilateral in 65% and bilateral in 35% of the patients, but also including seizures, chronic meningitis, and the focal effects of a mass lesion (Joseph and Scolding, 2007). A highly suggestive

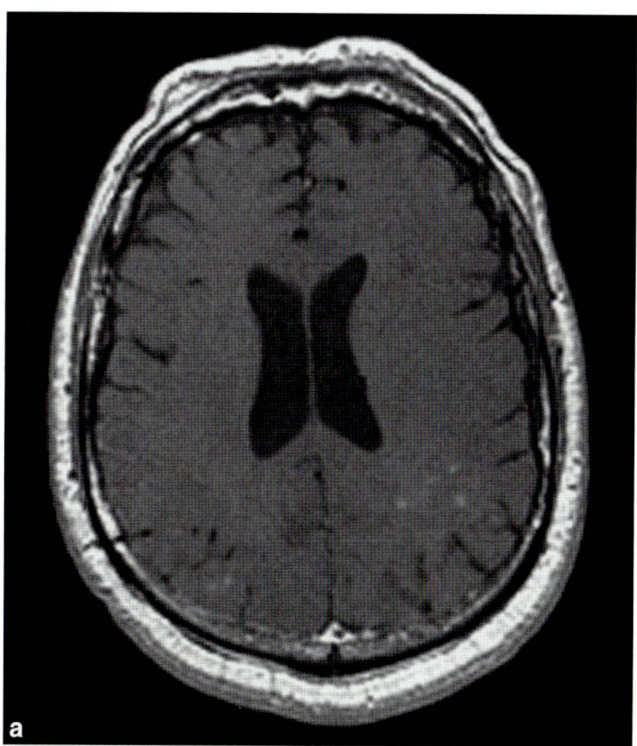

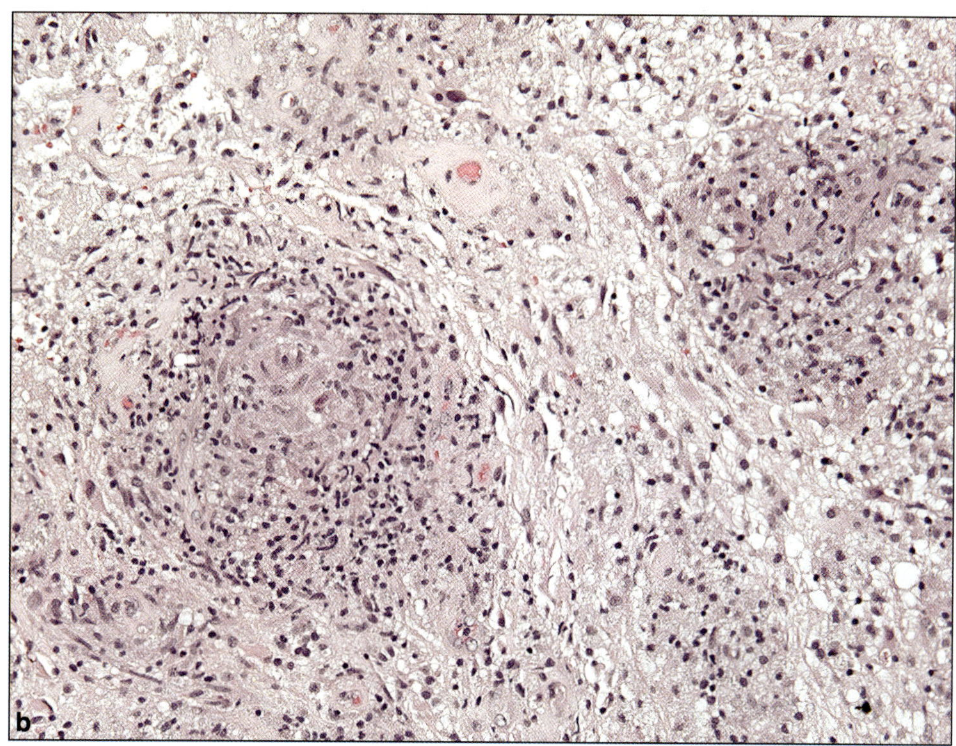

Figure 6.3. Neurosarcoidosis. There is a wide spectrum of neuroimaging abnormalities in neurosarcoidosis. Forty percent of patients with neurosarcoidosis have either leptomeningeal enhancement or (a) multiple white matter lesions in a periventricular distribution that may be difficult to distinguish from those seen in multiple sclerosis. (b) Typical noncaseating granulomas of sarcoidosis, lacking any features specific to the diagnosis, consisting of epithelioid cells and macrophages in the center surrounded by lymphocytes, plasma cells, and mast cells.

symptom complex is uveitis, parotid gland enlargement, fever, and cranial neuropathy (Heerfordt's syndrome).

When neurosarcoidosis occurs, it is often early in the course of the disease and thus may lead to diagnostic confusion. Seizures are more ominous feature of neurosarcoidosis, may be the initial presenting manifestation, and are usually of the tonic clonic type. They are poorly responsive to therapy and usually indicative of parenchymal involvement, vasculopathy, or hydrocephalus. Either acute or chronic meningitis may occur, associated with elevated CSF protein and lowered glucose in some cases. Mass lesions may occur in any part of the CNS, however, there is a predilection for involvement of the base of the brain, hypothalamus, and pituitary gland resulting in endocrinopathies. Involvement of spinal cord, peripheral muscle, or nerves may be seen and other manifestations include psychiatric and movement disorders.

MRI with enhancement is a highly sensitive but often nonspecific indicator of CNS involvement by sarcoidosis. Forty percent of patients may have leptomeningeal enhancement, mimicking chronic meningitis or meningeal neoplasms, or periventricular white matter lesions resembling those seen in MS (Figure 6.3a).

Pathology

While the clinical, radiological, and laboratory findings may be highly suggestive of sarcoidosis, biopsy is conceivably the only way of proving the diagnosis. The usual rationale for biopsy is in the face of isolated CNS disease and the prospect of using significant immunosuppressant therapy. The lesions are composed of granulomas formed by macrophages and epithelioid cells forming a nonnecrotic center surrounded by lymphocytes, plasma cells, and mast cells (Figure 6.3b). Other causes of granulomatous infection must be carefully excluded with special stains for microorganisms in the morphologic exclusion of neoplasms.

LANGERHANS CELL HISTIOCYTOSIS

Clinical and Radiological Features

This term, formerly nearly synonymous with histiocytosis X, encompasses a group of sometimes overlapping syndromes forming a spectrum from uni- or multifocal eosinophilic granuloma of bone to Hand–Schüller–Christian disease, defined as multifocal unisystem disease usually represented in bone, to a multifocal multisystem and potentially fatal disease with bone, skin, liver, spleen, and lymph node involvement (Letterer–Siwe disease).

The CNS is involved in approximately 25% of patients with systemic disease. The most common manifestations are diabetes insipidus, being caused by compression of the pituitary stalk and neurohypophysis by bone disease, extension of the inflammatory infiltrate into the pituitary gland, or direct involvement of the hypothalamic–pituitary axis. When involving the parenchyma of the brain, the hypothalamic–pituitary axis and base of the brain are most commonly involved, disease may also occur in the cerebral hemispheres, choroid plexus, and even the brainstem (Grois et al., 1993, 2005).

Patients with unifocal disease are usually children or young adults with a lytic lesion of bone and occasional extranodal sites such as skin. When the skull is involved, there may be exophthalmos, diabetes insipidus, and tooth loss. Patients with multisystem disease usually present with fever, hepatosplenomegaly, lymphadenopathy, bone and skin lesions, and pancytopenia.

Radiographic imaging of bone will show discrete punched out lesions. MRI may be used to reveal contrast enhancing parenchymal lesions within the brain or as lytic bone lesions (Figure 6.4a,b).

Pathology

Given ample clinical and radiologic suspicion, the microscopic diagnosis is not usually overchallenging, by virtue of identifying the key diagnostic feature, the Langerhans cell. They are approximately 10–15 μm in diameter and marked by grooved, folded, indented, or lobulated nuclei with fine chromatin, inconspicuous nucleoli, and thin nuclear membranes (Figure 6.4c–e). Frank nuclear atypia is usually absent. Mitotic activity is variable. The characteristic but variable background cytological milieu consists of eosinophils, histiocytes, sometimes multinucleated, with neutrophils and small lymphocytes. Langerhans cells are easily identifiable by anti-CD1a immunohistochemistry as well as S-100 protein immunopositivity although the former is usually sufficient to confirm the diagnosis. The classical ultrastructural feature of Langerhans cells is the cytoplasmic Birbeck granule, a parallel structure with a bulbous end resembling a tennis racquet, measuring about 200 to 400 nm in length.

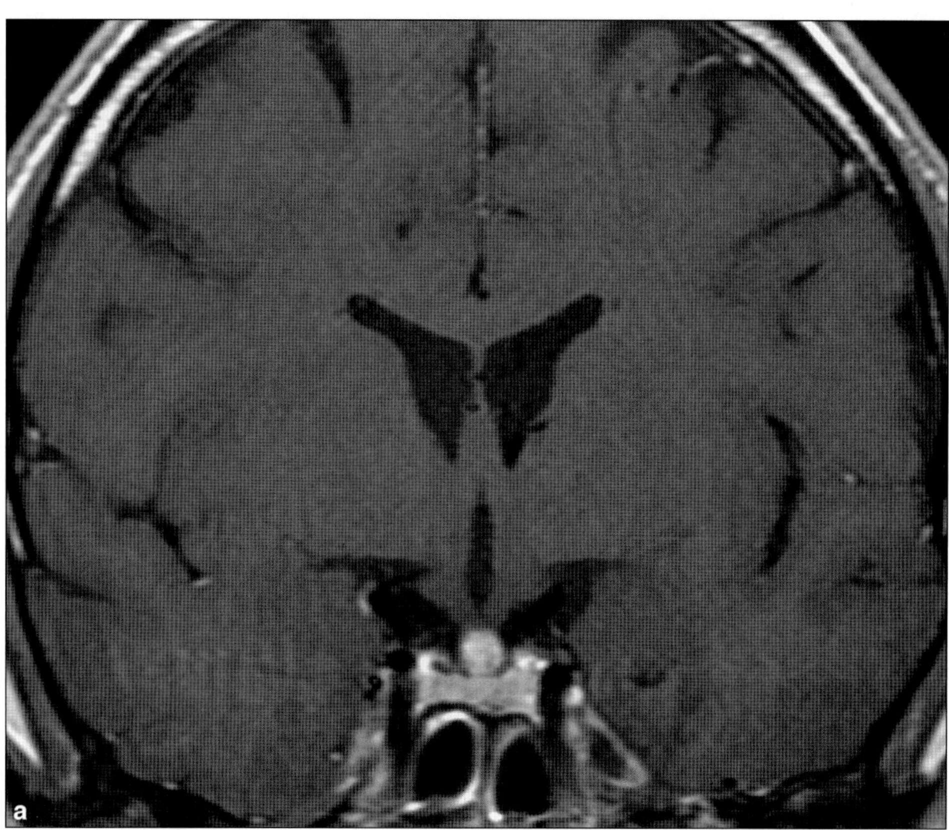

Figure 6.4. Langerhans cell histiocytosis. (a) A coronal T1 MR with contrast image shows an enhancing nodule involving the pituitary infundibulum in this case of biopsy proven Langerhans cell histiocytosis. Patients with Langerhans cell histiocytosis often present with diabetes insipidus, because the disease process interferes with the normal passage of antidiuretic hormone-containing vesicles from the hypothalamus to the posterior pituitary gland. Germ cell neoplasms, lymphoma, sarcoidosis, gliomas, lymphocytic hypophysitis and metastases could have similar imaging appearances to suprasellar Langerhans cell histiocytosis.

Figure 6.4. *continued*
(b) Langerhans cell histiocytosis also commonly involves the skull base and calvarium where it produces lytic masses. Rhabdomyosarcoma, metastases (commonly neuroblastoma), fibrous dysplasia, and severe mastoiditis could have a similar imaging appearance to temporal bone Langerhans cell histiocytosis. (c) Squash preparation showing the typical cellular elements, including nuclear grooves in the histiocytes seen to great advantage, along with eosinophils.

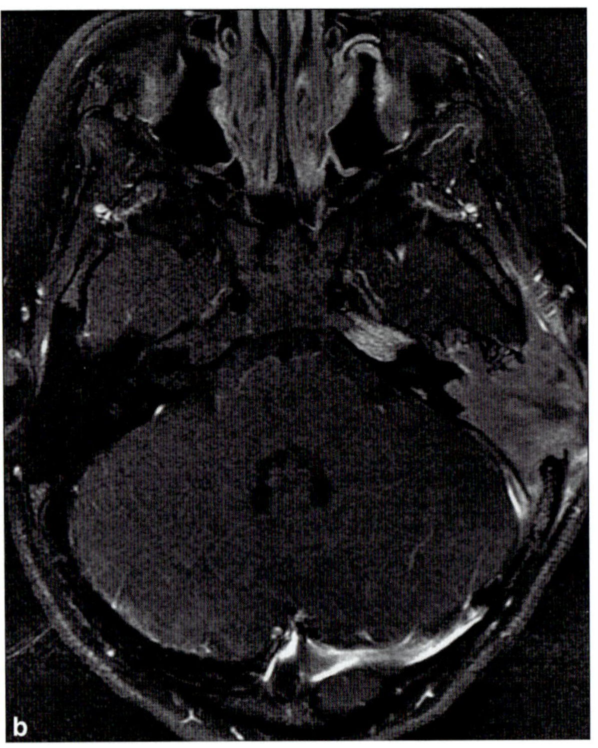

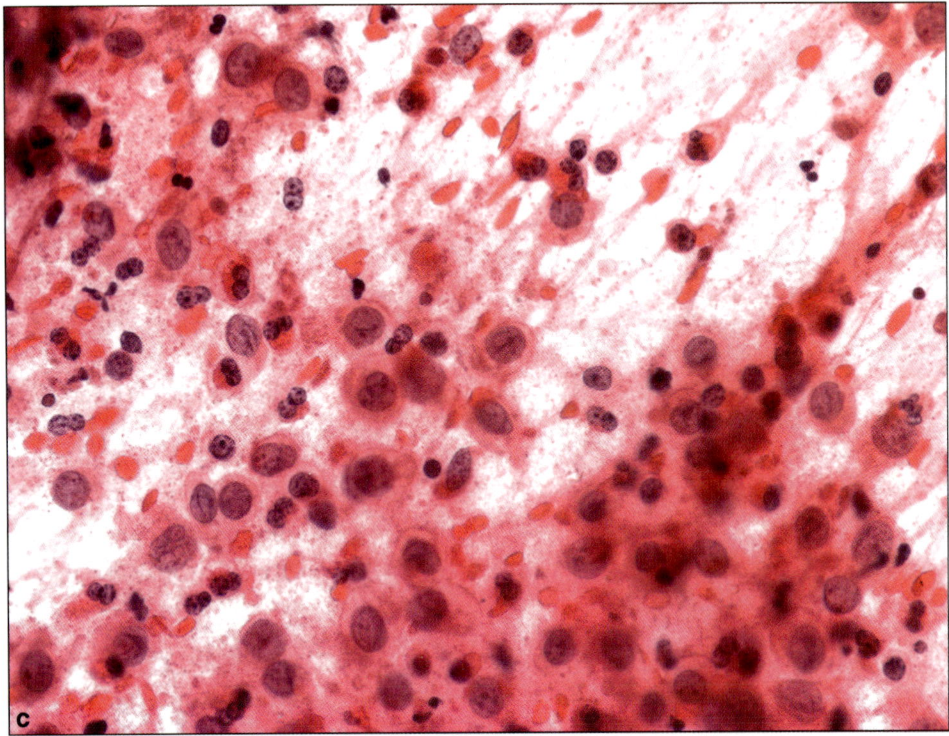

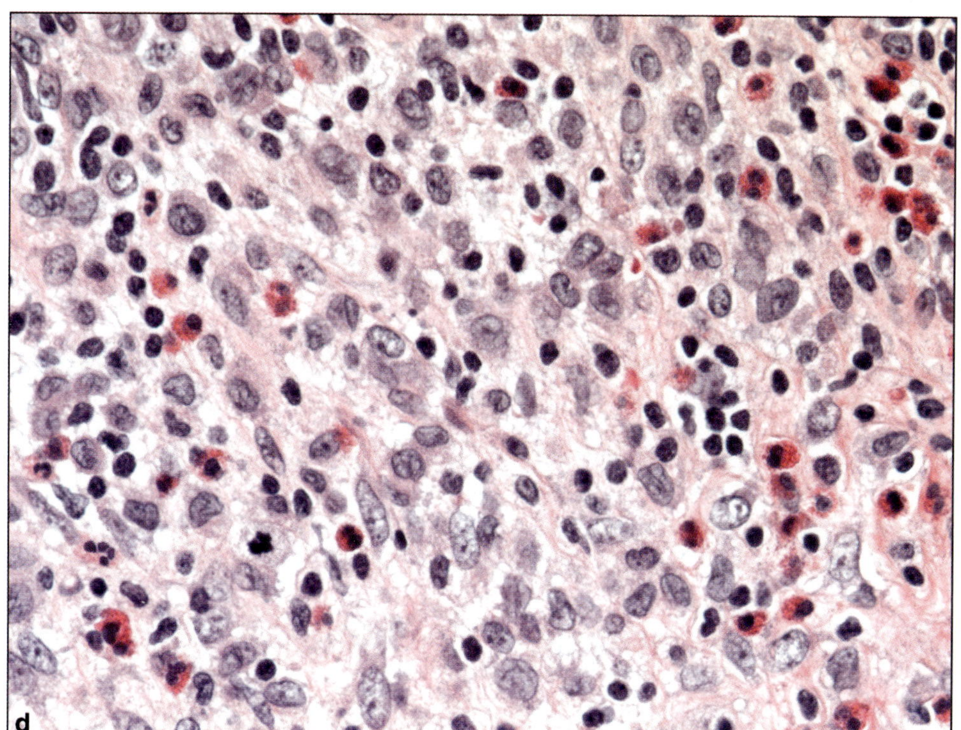

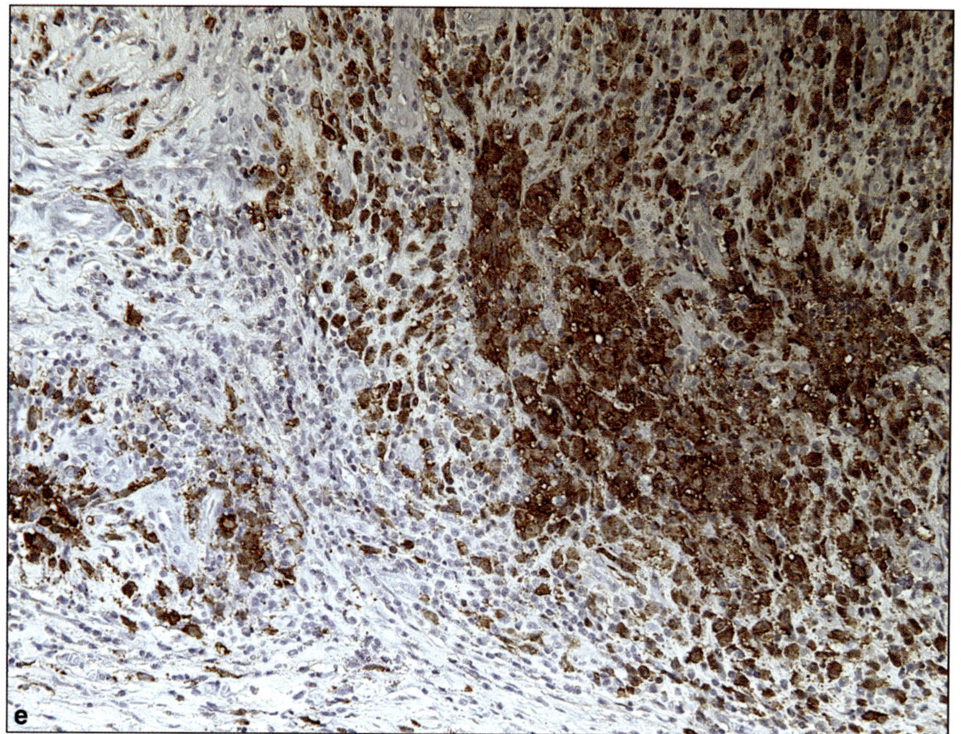

Figure 6.4. *continued*
(d) Histological section from the same case, (e) with the histiocytes immunolabeled with anti-CD1a.

RASMUSSEN'S ENCEPHALITIS

Clinical and Radiological Features

This is a rare condition of childhood producing a gradual loss of motor function, cognitive ability, and an extremely refractory seizure disorder known as epilepsy partialis continua. There is a particular tendency for unilateral hemispheric involvement. Because of the inexorable course of the disease, partial but nonetheless impressive corticectomies have been required in some cases. The etiology remains unknown although some experimental evidence to suggest autoimmune mechanisms directed at neurons (Granata, 2003) or astrocytes (Bauer et al., 2007). Radiologically, the process results in diffuse unilateral hemispheric atrophy with compensatory ventricular dilatation.

Pathology

The histological features of Rasmussen's encephalitis include an inflammatory infiltrate that mimics features of viral encephalitis, namely perivascular lymphocytic cuffing, microglial activation, and nodular aggregates, with reactive gliosis and neuronal loss. Lymphocytes are mostly of T-cell specificity. Leptomeningeal inflammation may also occur. Immunohistochemistry is no additional diagnostic value other than highlighting microglia, lymphocytes, and reactive astrocytes.

ERDHEIM–CHESTER DISEASE

This is an exceedingly rare condition representing a non-Langerhans cell histiocytosis with primary involvement of bones, visceral organs, and fatty tissues. Cerebellar and pyramidal symptoms are said to be the most common signs of CNS involvement (Lachenal et al., 2006). Most pathological descriptions have originated in autopsy studies thus the disease has not been a consideration for surgical biopsy. The neuropathology consists of multiple xanthogranulomas including multinucleated (Touton-like) cells and infrequent eosinophils, involving a cerebral hemispheres, hypothalamus, cerebellum, and brainstem (Adle-Biassette et al., 1997).

ROSAI–DORFMAN DISEASE (SINUS HISTIOCYTOSIS WITH MASSIVE LYMPHADENOPATHY)

This disease often presents with massive painless bilateral lymph node involvement in the neck and mediastinum accompanied by fever. Extranodal disease without concomitant lymph node involvement is uncommon. Intracranial disease may mimic meningioma and multiple lesions have been described they also mimic meningiomas by contrast enhancement with MR imaging and a broad dural base.

Rosai–Dorfman disease is characterized by a lymphoplasmacytic proliferation with focal aggregates or sheets of pale, often multinucleated histiocytes. There may be variable fibrosis. An interesting feature, which is from a diagnostic standpoint unfortunately less frequent than in nodal disease, is engulfment by histiocytes of viable lymphocytes and plasma cells known as emperipolesis. The histiocytes are strongly S-100 protein positive but CD1a negative, which along with the lack of eosinophils help to distinguish this process from Langerhans cell histiocytosis.

PLASMA CELL GRANULOMA

These are benign nonneoplastic lesions referring to masses that are usually dural based, composed of lymphocytes and plasma cells, often containing Russell bodies (Breidahl et al., 1996; Gochman et al., 1990; Hirohata et al., 1996; Murakami et al., 2003). Concurrent lung involvement has been reported (Greiner et al., 2003; Malhotra et al., 1991). Surgical excision is curative. Actual granulomas are not a histological feature of this lesion. Germinal centers may be present. There is some diagnostic overlap with an entity known as inflammatory myofibroblastic pseudotumor, which is marked by large numbers of myofibroblasts. Meningeal cells may be seen in some lesions; however, they should be distinguished from actual lymphoplasmacytoid meningiomas.

RADIATION INJURY

Clinical and Radiological Features

Radiation injury to the brain is a common and somewhat unpredictable consequence of irradiation for brain tumors or in other examples of head, neck, and spinal region radiotherapy. It exists in acute, early delayed and, late delayed forms (Ellison et al. 2008). The younger the patient, the more is the susceptibily to radiation-induced neurotoxicity, including cognitive deficits.

Radiation necrosis gains particular importance when a mass arises in a region exposed to large amounts of therapeutic radiation, generally cumulative doses greater than 50–60 Gy to the brain or 45 Gy to the spinal cord, and biopsy or resection is necessary to both exclude the possibility of recurrent neoplasm and to relief the mass effect than even pure radiation necrosis may produce. Various neuroimaging strategies may allow for a presumptive preoperative diagnosis (Figure 6.5a).

Pathology

In a large resection, the degree of selective vulnerability of white matter to radiation toxicity is striking, in which white matter shows large infarct-like regions of necrosis and hypocellularity, sometimes with dystrophic calcification (Figure 6.5b–d). Blood vessels show distinctive telangiectatic, hyaline, or necrotic changes, which may lead to an occlusive vasculopathy. Endothelial cells often show atypicality without proliferation. Such specimens should be carefully inspected for the concurrent presence of residual glioma. Radiation necrosis tends to be a hypocellular process without the proliferative, infiltrative, and atypical cytomorphological aspects of recurrent glioma.

Figure 6.5. Radiation necrosis. (a) An axial T1 contrast-enhanced MR shows a shaggy-edged ring enhancing mass with extensive surrounding edema centered within the left temporal lobe. Centrally, the mass has a bubbly appearance. This is fairly typical appearance for radiation necrosis. Radiation necrosis can be extremely difficult to distinguish from metastases and recurrent primary brain neoplasms by anatomic imaging techniques. FDG-PET, cerebral perfusion imaging, and MR spectroscopy have had variable success. This patient underwent whole brain radiation followed by stereotactic radiosurgery for a small left temporal lobe choriocarcinoma metastasis. The area of radiation necrosis was resected shortly after this MR. (b) Low-magnification view of a cerebral resection specimen of radiated brain shows the dramatic vulnerability of white matter to injury while overlying cortex may appear almost normal.

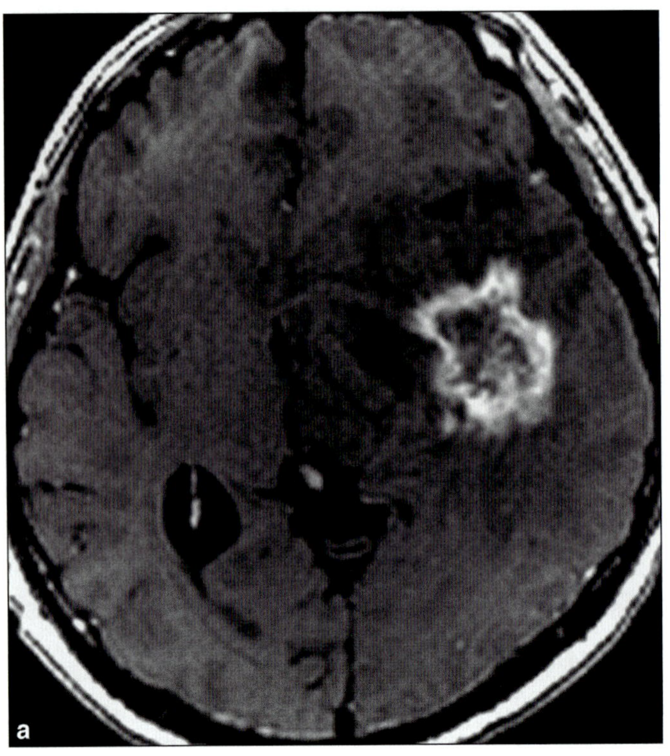

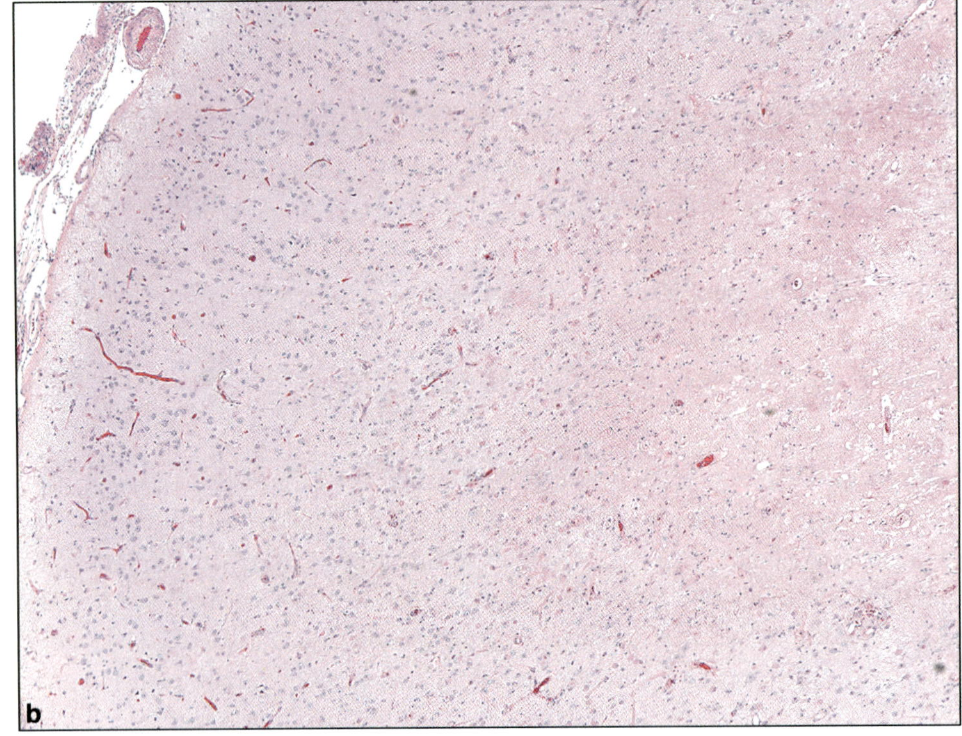

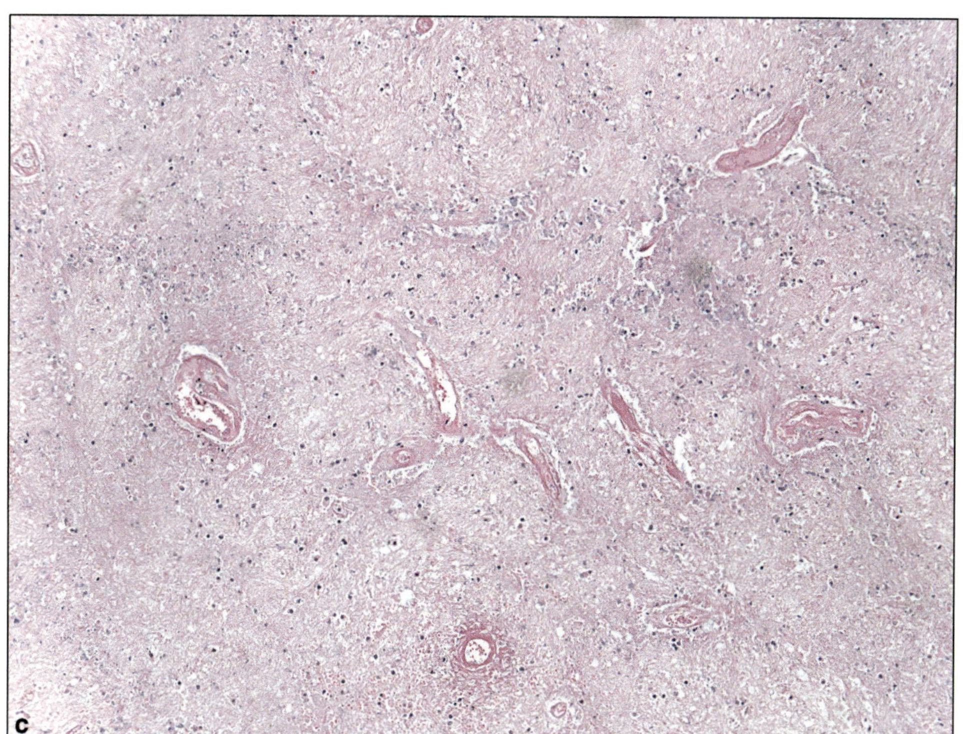

Figure 6.5. *continued* (c) Higher magnification of severely affected white matter shows coagulative necrosis and interspersed fibrosed blood vessels. (d) Atypicality without proliferation is the hallmark of radiation-induced vascular endothelial pathology.

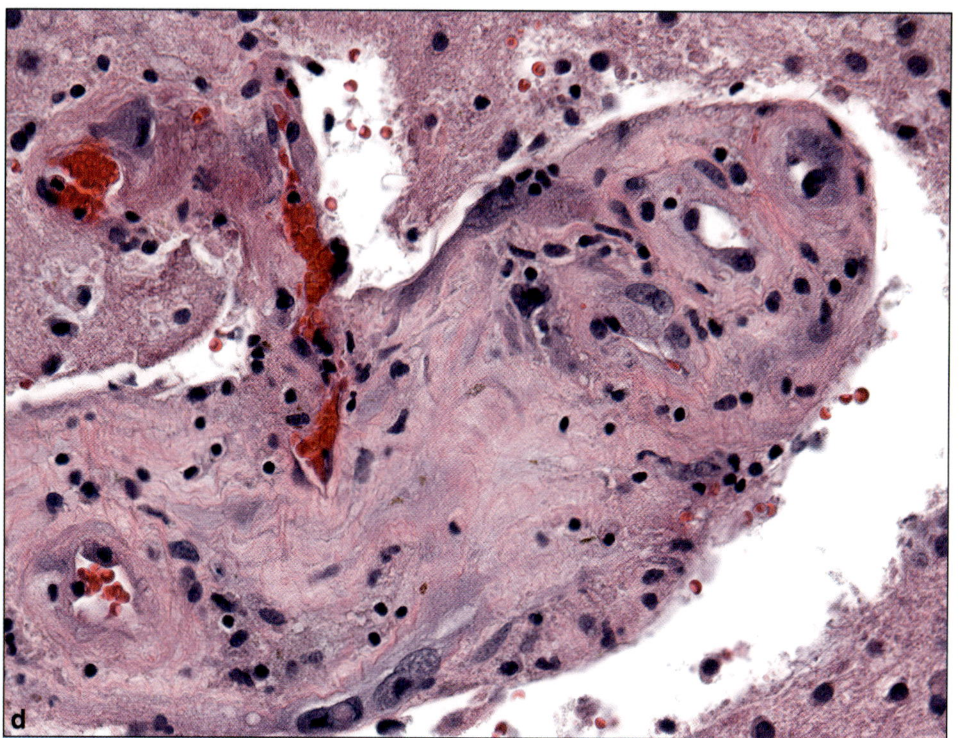

REFERENCES

Adle-Biassette H, Chetritt J, Bergemer-Fouquet AM, Wechsler J, Mussini JM, Gray F. Pathology of the central nervous system in Chester–Erdheim disease: report of three cases. *J Neuropathol Exp Neurol* 1997; 56: 1207–16.

Bauer J, Elger CE, Hans VH, Schramm J, Urbach H, Lassmann H, et al. Astrocytes are a specific immunological target in Rasmussen's encephalitis. *Ann Neurol* 2007; 62: 67–80.

Breidahl WH, Robbins PD, Ives FJ, Wong G. Intracranial plasma cell granuloma. *Neuroradiology* 1996; 38 Suppl. 1: S86–9.

Ellison DW, Perry A, Rosenblum M, Asa S, Reid R, Louis DN. Tumours: non-neuroepithelial tumours and secondary effects. In: Greenfield JG, Love S, Louis DN, Ellison D, editors. *Greenfield's Neuropathology*. London: Hodder Arnold, 2008.

Gochman GA, Duffy K, Crandall PH, Vinters HV. Plasma cell granuloma of the brain. *Surg Neurol* 1990; 33: 347–52.

Granata T. Rasmussen's syndrome. *Neurol Sci* 2003; 24 Suppl. 4: S239–43.

Greiner C, Rickert CH, Mollmann FT, Rieger B, Semik M, Heindel W, et al. Plasma cell granuloma involving the brain and the lung. *Acta Neurochir (Wien)* 2003; 145: 1127–31.

Grois N, Barkovich AJ, Rosenau W, Ablin AR. Central nervous system disease associated with Langerhans' cell histiocytosis. *Am J Pediatr Hematol Oncol* 1993; 15: 245–54.

Grois N, Prayer D, Prosch H, Lassmann H. Neuropathology of CNS disease in Langerhans cell histiocytosis. *Brain* 2005; 128: 829–38.

Hirohata M, Sasaguri Y, Sugita Y, Tokutomi T, Kobayashi S, Morimatsu M, et al. Intracranial plasma-cell granuloma: a case report. *Noshuyo Byori* 1996; 13: 133–8.

Joseph FG, Scolding NJ. Sarcoidosis of the nervous system. *Pract Neurol* 2007; 7: 234–44.

Kepes JJ. Large focal tumor-like demyelinating lesions of the brain: intermediate entity between multiple sclerosis and acute disseminated encephalomyelitis? A study of 31 patients. *Ann Neurol* 1993; 33: 18–27.

Krupp LB, Banwell B, Tenembaum S. Consensus definitions proposed for pediatric multiple sclerosis and related disorders. *Neurology* 2007; 68: S7–12.

Lachenal F, Cotton F, Desmurs-Clavel H, Haroche J, Taillia H, Magy N, et al. Neurological manifestations and neuroradiological presentation of Erdheim–Chester disease: report of 6 cases and systematic review of the literature. *J Neurol* 2006; 253: 1267–77.

Malhotra V, Tatke M, Malik R, Gondal R, Beohar PC, Kumar S, et al. An unusual case of plasma cell granuloma involving lung and brain. *Indian J Cancer* 1991; 28: 223–7.

Menge T, Kieseier BC, Nessler S, Hemmer B, Hartung HP, Stuve O. Acute disseminated encephalomyelitis: an acute hit against the brain. *Curr Opin Neurol* 2007; 20: 247–54.

Murakami M, Hashimoto N, Kimura S, Hosokawa Y, Kakita K. Intracranial plasma cell granuloma with genetic analysis. *Acta Neurochir (Wien)* 2003; 145: 221–5; discussion 225.

Sobel RA, Moore GRW. Demyelinating diseases. In: Greenfield JG, Love S, Louis DN, Ellison D, editors. *Greenfield's Neuropathology*. London: Hodder Arnold, 2008.

7 SURGICAL NEUROPATHOLOGY OF EPILEPSY

Josef Zámečník and Hannes Vogel

Neurosurgical resection has been increasingly applied to patients who have intractable epilepsy in recent years. It has resulted in a notable increase in knowledge of pathological changes in epileptogenic tissues, as well as of the corresponding neuroimaging findings. Furthermore, these surgical specimens involve refined approaches toward a greater understanding of pathophysiological alterations in the diseased tissue, thus providing new insights into the pathogenesis of intractable epilepsy (Beck et al., 2000; Becker et al., 2002).

The findings in surgical neuropathology of epilepsy may be divided into several groups:

A. Temporal lobe epilepsy (TLE), mainly associated with hippocampal sclerosis (HS).
B. Malformative lesions:
   1. Neuronal migration disorders (NMD) – mainly focal cortical dysplasia, but also including tuberous sclerosis complex (TSC), hemimegalencephaly (HMC), etc.
   2. Vascular malformations including Sturge–Weber syndrome (see page 461).
C. Epilepsy-associated brain tumors – the most frequent entities are ganglion cell tumors (Chapter 3, page 97), dysembryoplastic neuroepithelial tumor (DNET) (Chapter 3, page 93), pilocytic astrocytoma (Chapter 3, page 40), and pleomorphic xanthoastrocytoma (Chapter 3, page 58). Recently, several new entities of epilepsy-associated central nervous system (CNS) neoplasms have been recognized, such as angiocentric neuroepithelial tumor or angiocentric glioma (Chapter 3, page 116).

D. Rassmussen's syndrome.

E. Posttraumatic and postinflammatory changes.

TEMPORAL LOBE EPILEPSY

Patients with intractable TLE are the most common candidates for surgical treatment. TLE is characterized mainly by recurrent complex partial seizures (with loss of consciousness) preceded in a variable percentage of cases by epileptic auras that represent simple partial seizures (Serrano-Castro et al., 1998).

TLE is divided into two main groups: Approximately 65% of temporal lobes resected from refractory TLE patients harbor the lesion pattern of HS also called mesial temporal sclerosis or Ammon's horn sclerosis. A second group, representing approximately 30% of TLE patients, exhibits focal lesions within the temporal lobe, which usually do not involve the hippocampus proper. The condition of TLE having both hippocampal sclerosis and lateral temporal lesions is called "dual pathology."

TLE with HS: Mesial Temporal Lobe Epilepsy

Clinical Features

Complex partial seizures originate principally in the temporal medial structures such as the hippocampus, entorhinal cortex, amygdala, and parahippocampal gyrus.

Neuroimaging

Magnetic resonance imaging (MRI) can detect HS, a condition typically revealed as an atrophic hippocampal formation with high signal intensity change on T2-weighted or fluid-attenuated inversion recovery (FLAIR)images. In cases in which differences in hippocampal size are difficult to judge visually, quantitative volumetric techniques may be employed. There are also additional changes on the affected side such as atrophy of the fornix and loss of the gray–white matter differentiation in the anterior temporal lobe (Camacho and Castillo, 2007).

Neuropathology

Histopathologically, HS is characterized by segmental pyramidal cell loss in CA1 (Sommer's sector) and CA4 (hilus, endfolium) (Figures 7.1–7.3). CA3 is often also affected, whereas CA2 pyramidal cells (the so-called resistant zone) are relatively spared (Blümcke et al., 2002). Dense fibrillary astrogliosis and sclerosis of the tissue are present in all the segments that display prominent neuronal cell loss. This may be highlighted by the use of the Luxol fast blue– periodic acid– Schiff stain whereby gliosis is accompanied by a prominent and abnormal increase in corpora amylacea (Chung and Horoupian, 1996).

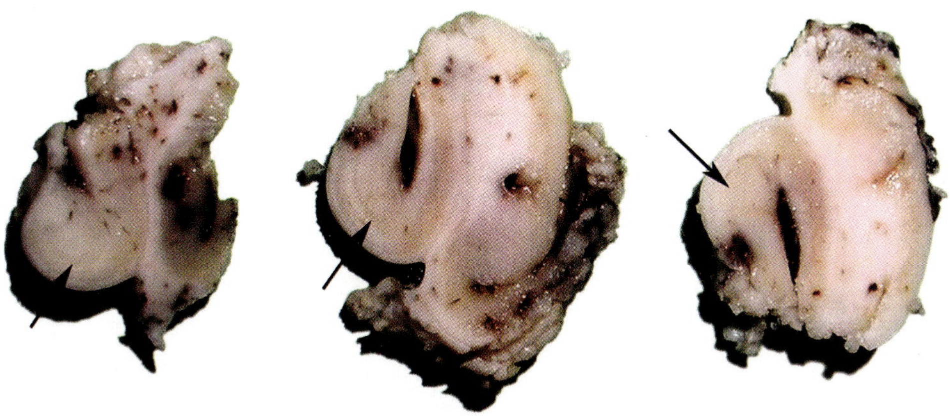

Figure 7.1. Resection specimen of hippocampus in serial sections in which the characteristic morphology of Ammon's horn is ideally recognized, thus allowing cross-sections of a properly oriented section of hippocampus in which the dentate gyrus and sectors 1–4 of the pyramidal cell layers may be recognized (arrows).

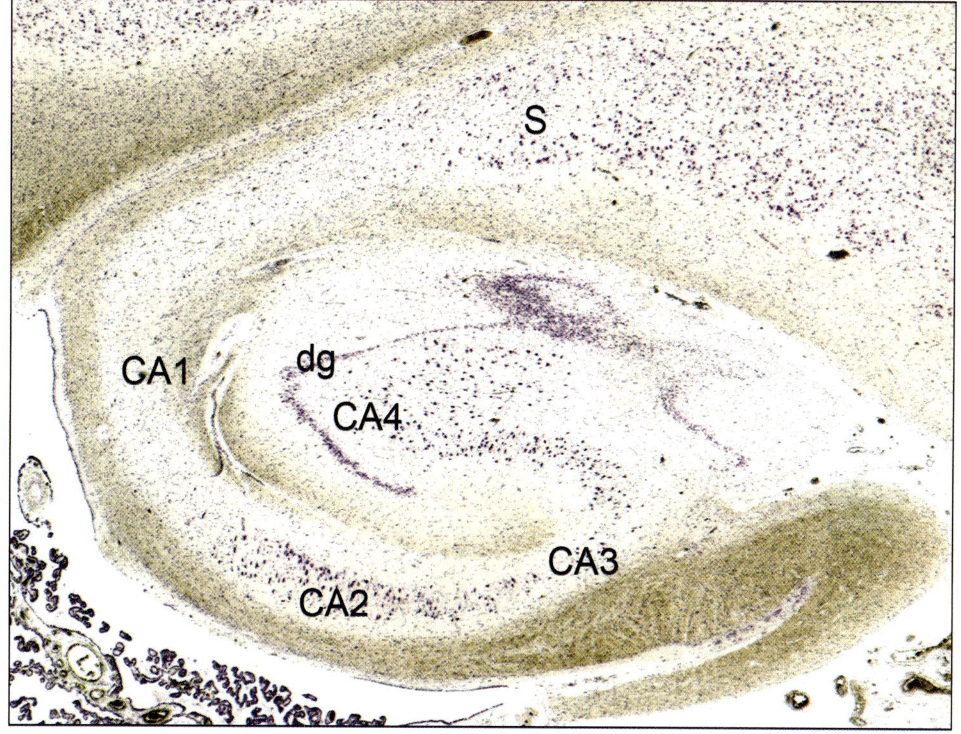

Figure 7.2. Microscopy of hippocampus in hippocampal sclerosis: localization of hippocampal subfields of Ammon's horn (CA 1–4), subiculum (S), and dentate gyrus (dg). This example shows loss of pyramidal neurons in CA1 and CA3, and the characteristic preservation of CA2 neurons. CA4 neurons are usually also diminished in number although are relatively preserved in this example (see Figure 7.3). Nissl stain.

Semiquantitative grading schemes for HS based on the variation in the extent of principle neuronal loss in hippocampal subfields have been proposed (Proper et al., 2001; Watson et al., 1996); however, they are not in common use. The prosubiculum, subiculum, and presubiculum are strangely free from histological abnormalities; in fact, the preservation of the subiculum is characteristic of hippocampal sclerosis and is never observed in other hippocampal changes such as from anoxic injury. In contrast, the entorhinal cortex and amygdala nuclei appear to be severely affected in many, although not in all, HS patients (Yilmazer-Hanke et al., 2000).

In the dentate gyrus, distinct cytoarchitectural abnormalities have been described in HS, which include seizure-associated postnatal neurogenesis and "dispersion of the granular cell layer" (Figure 7.4). The significance and mechanism of the latter pathological phenomenon are still unclear (Camacho and Castillo, 2007; Lurton et al., 1997).

Figure 7.3. Loss of pyramidal neurons within CA4 in hippocampal sclerosis (right) in comparison with normal density of pyramidal neurons (left). Note the thinning and dispersion of granular cell layer in the dentate gyrus (dg).

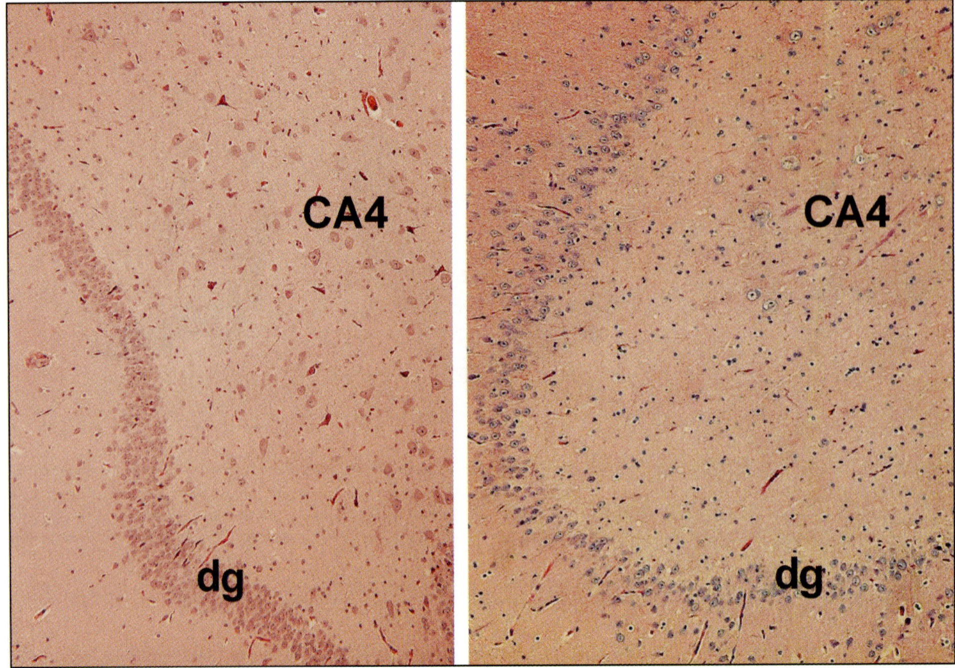

Figure 7.4. Hippocampal sclerosis. Dispersion of the granular cell layer in the dentate gyrus.

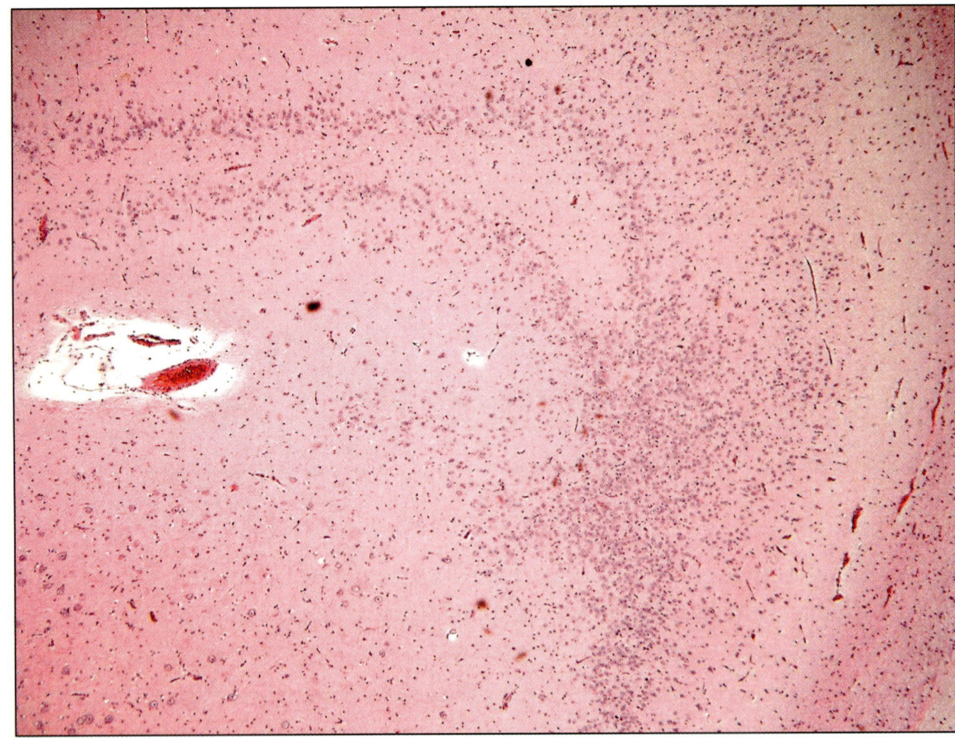

HS in "dual pathology" TLE: There is some evidence that less severe hippocampal neuronal loss occurs when a second pathology is present (Mathern et al., 1997).

TLE without HS: Lateral Temporal Lobe Epilepsy

The second type of TLE is the "lateral" or "neocortical" TLE, in which the temporal neocortex is affected, which includes the superior, medial, and inferior temporal gyri, the temporal–occipital and temporal–parietal junctions, and the associated sensory areas for hearing, visual, and language functions.

Generally, hippocampi in lesion-associated TLE do not show pronounced segmental neuronal cell loss and substantial structural reorganization, whereas variable astrogliosis is frequently observed (Blümcke et al., 2002). Focal lesions include low-grade glial and glioneuronal neoplasms as well as glioneuronal malformations (NMD) that include focal cortical dysplasias.

MALFORMATIVE LESIONS

NMD can be defined as cerebral malformations characterized by malpositioning and faulty differentiation of cortical gray matter. Clinically and pathologically, the spectrum of NMD is complex. NMD can uniformly affect broad regions of the cerebral cortex as in classical lissencephaly and HMC, or may be restricted to focal areas such as tubers in the TSC or focal cortical dysplasia (FCD).

NMD may also exhibit large collections of heterotopic neurons, as in syndromes of subcortical band heterotopia and periventricular nodular heterotopia. Over the years, there were several attempts by different expert panels to come up with a uniform nomenclature of malformations of cortical development, which variously addressed specific aspects of these disorders, for example, their embryology, imaging features, histopathology, and genetic background. One of the more comprehensive classification attempts was introduced by Barkovich et al. (2001, 2005).

Virtually all seizure subtypes, for example, generalized tonic–clonic, complex partial, atonic, myoclonic, atypical absence seizures, and infantile spasms, have been described when the totality of NMD is considered.

Surgical treatment is inappropriate for brain anomalies such as lissencephalies, though functional hemispherectomy might be applicable to unilateral hemispheric lesions such as HMC or Sturge–Weber syndrome. Most commonly, the neuropathologist deals with focal malformative lesions, mainly with focal cortical dysplasias and TSC.

Focal Cortical Dysplasia

Terminology: General Comment

The terminology and classification of these lesions is confusing. "Cortical dysplasia" was previously used as a generic term to describe a variety of focal malformations of cortical development, including heterotopias and polymicrogyria, whereas the term "focal cortical dysplasia" was generally reserved for the cortical malformation described by Taylor et al. (1971), one feature of which is the presence of balloon cells (the so-called "FCD-Taylor type"). Milder microscopic dysplasias with subtler cytopathology were variously termed microdysgenesis, mild focal dysplasia, "non-Taylor" dysplasia, architectural dysplasia, cytoarchitectural dysplasia, or glioneuronal hamartias.

Epidemiology and Genetics

The incidence of cortical dysplasias in epilepsy surgical series varies from 12% to 40% (Prayson et al., 2002). The so-called "dual pathology" (a second epileptogenic pathology) may be present. The combination of FCD, in particular between a mild NMD and FCD type I and hippocampal sclerosis is well recognized (Blümcke et al., 2002; Tassi et al., 2002). Furthermore, cortical dysplasia is often noted in proximity to low-grade glioneuronal tumors like DNET and gangliogliomas, suggesting a common etiology (Daumas-Duport et al., 1999).

There has been an explosive growth of information on the genetics of malformations of cortical development over the past 10 years with many of the genes responsible for a number of malformations (e.g., TSC1, TSC2, LIS-1, DCX, and FLN1) having been cloned successfully (Crino, 2005). However, FCD is mostly a sporadic disorder in contrast to some of the other malformations of cortical development associated with epilepsy, such as lissencephalies and heterotopias (Hua and Crino, 2003).

Neuroimaging

Cases with focal cortical dysplasia manifest blurring of the gray matter–white matter junction on T2-weighted or FLAIR images, abnormal signal intensity in the white matter, and thickness of the cortical gyri; however, in many cases, the pathological changes are not detectable by MRI. These pathologies include FCD type I and mild NMD. Functional neuroimaging by positron emission tomography (PET) and single-photon emission computed tomography (SPECT) is useful for detecting epileptic foci, even in cases with a normal MRI (Maehara, 2007).

Neuropathology

Surgical specimens in FCD may appear normal macroscopically, but in some cases, widening of the cortex with poor demarcation from the underlying white matter is noted. The dysplastic region may be firmer to the touch (Urbach et al., 2002).

A spectrum of changes is recognized microscopically. Palmini et al. (2004) proposed the grading system of FCD (Figure 7.5). The issue of "milder forms of FCD" is a matter of ongoing debate (Arai et al., 2007; Kasper, 2005; Rickert, 2006).

FCD type I
    Type IA: Cortical dislamination only
    Type IB: Cortical dislamination + additional giant or immature neurons
FCD type II (Taylor-type)
    Type IIA: Cortical dislamination + additional dysmorphic neurons
    Type IIB: Cortical dislamination + dysmorphic neurons and additional balloon cells.

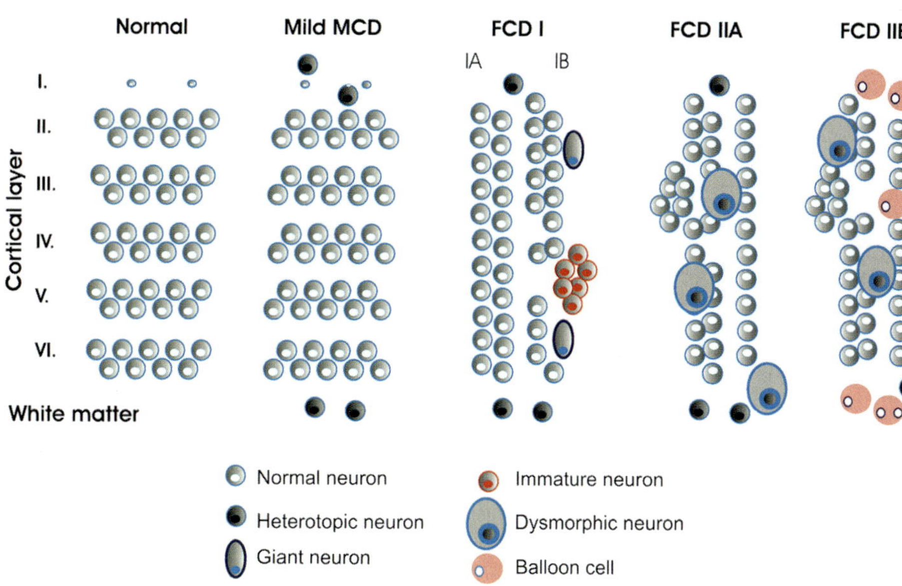

Figure 7.5. Classification scheme of focal cortical dysplasias (FCD). Malformations of cortical development (MCD).

"Mild malformation of cortical development"
    Type I - heterotopic or excess neurons in layer I
    Type II - heterotopic or excess neurons outside layer I

In FCD type I, the main pathological feature is disorganization of the cortical architecture ("dislamination") with less striking neuronal and glial cytopathology. They are mostly reported in the lateral temporal lobe in association with mesial temporal sclerosis, but may be widespread and involve other regions like the frontal and occipital cortex (Tassi et al., 2002). Microscopic evaluation shows an excess of neurons in layer I, clusters of neurons, marginal glioneuronal heterotopias, and a persistent subpial granule cell layer. In many cases however, layer I remains hypocellular. The borders between cortical layers may be ill defined, and abnormal cortical cytoarchitecture with persistent columnar alignment of neurons was described (Kasper et al., 1999; Thom et al., 2000) (Figure 7.6). An excess of white matter neurons (Figure 7.7) and perineuronal satellitosis was reported, particularly in patients with TLE.

In FCD type IB, additional aberrant cytology of individual neurons is observed, which may also be displaced in the underlying white matter. Giant neurons are of increased size compared with layer V pyramidal neurons (50–80 μm) and contain central nuclei while preserving an overall pyramidal morphology with normal orientation. They are can be identified in other cortical layers, particularly in the upper half of the cortex (Figure 7.8). Immature neurons are round or oval homogeneous cells with a large, immature nucleus, and thin rim of cytoplasm (Figure 7.9). They are the most common cell type in macroscopically visible heterotopic nodules.

The hallmarks of FCD type II are major changes in the cytology of individual neurons in addition to the aberrant laminar architecture of the cortex. Dysmorphic neurons (typical for FCD type IIA) are misshapen cells with

Figure 7.6. Disruption of cortical laminar organization in a case of type I focal cortical dysplasia with cluster of aberrantly oriented with a somewhat columnar arrangement of neurons.

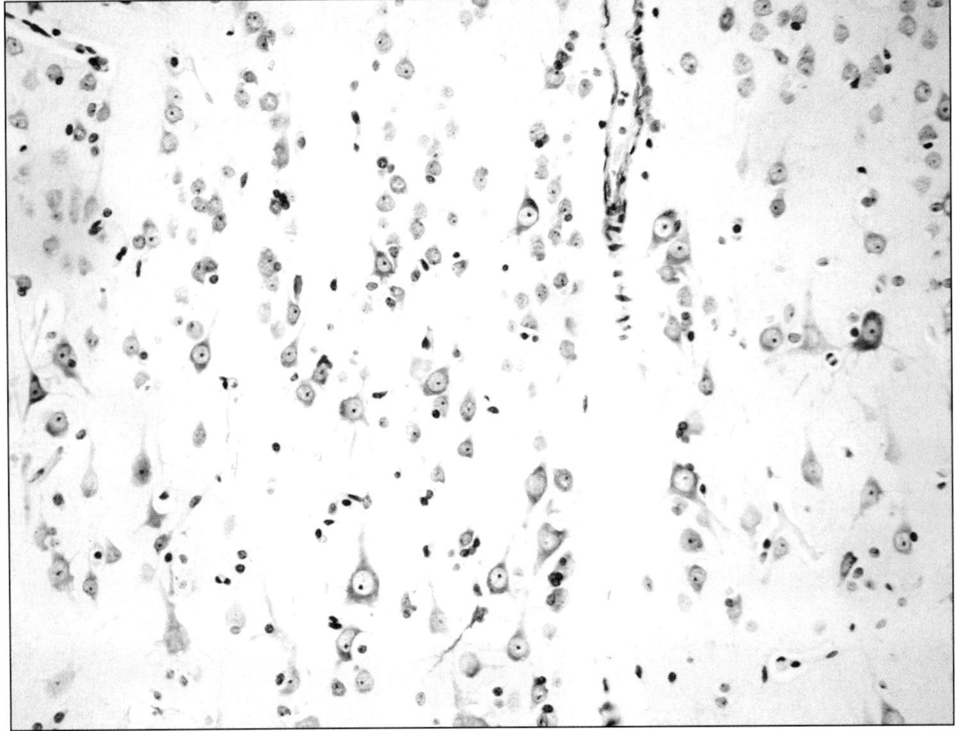

Figure 7.7. TLE may be associated with heterotopic dysmorphic neurons in subjacent white matter; however, this determination may be difficult since the normal temporal lobe contains more mature neurons within white matter than in other lobes of the brain. Nissl stain.

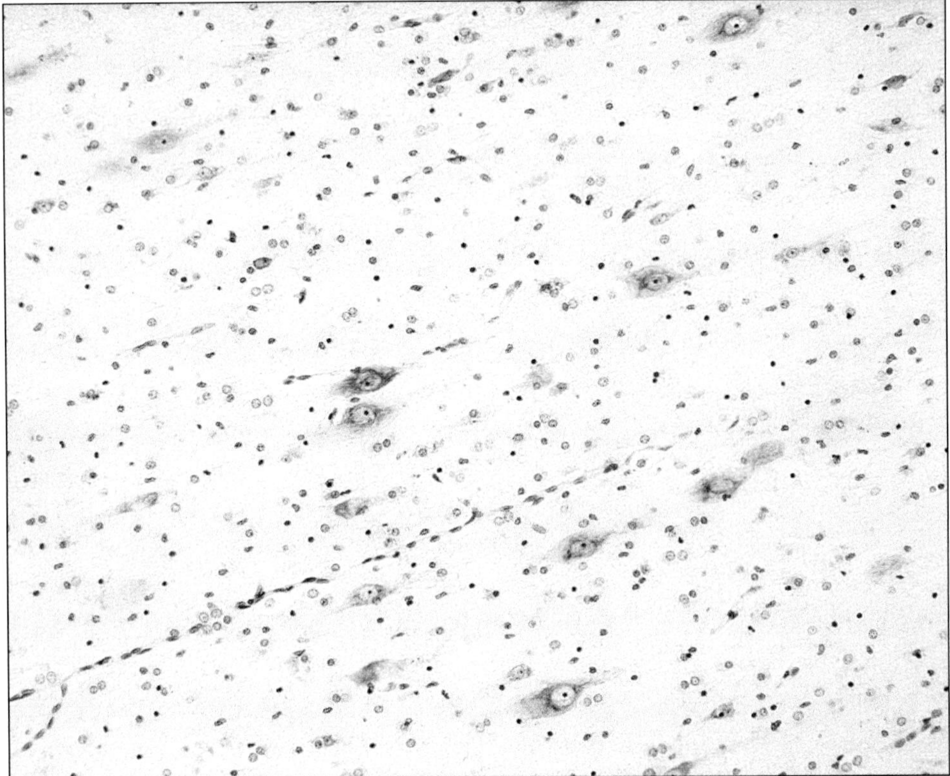

abnormal size, cytoskeletal structure, somal and dendritic morphology, and random orientation in the cortex (Figure 7.10). Their Nissl staining is coarse and a thickening of the nuclear membrane may be appreciated. The dysplastic region may be relatively sharply demarcated from adjacent cortex; however,

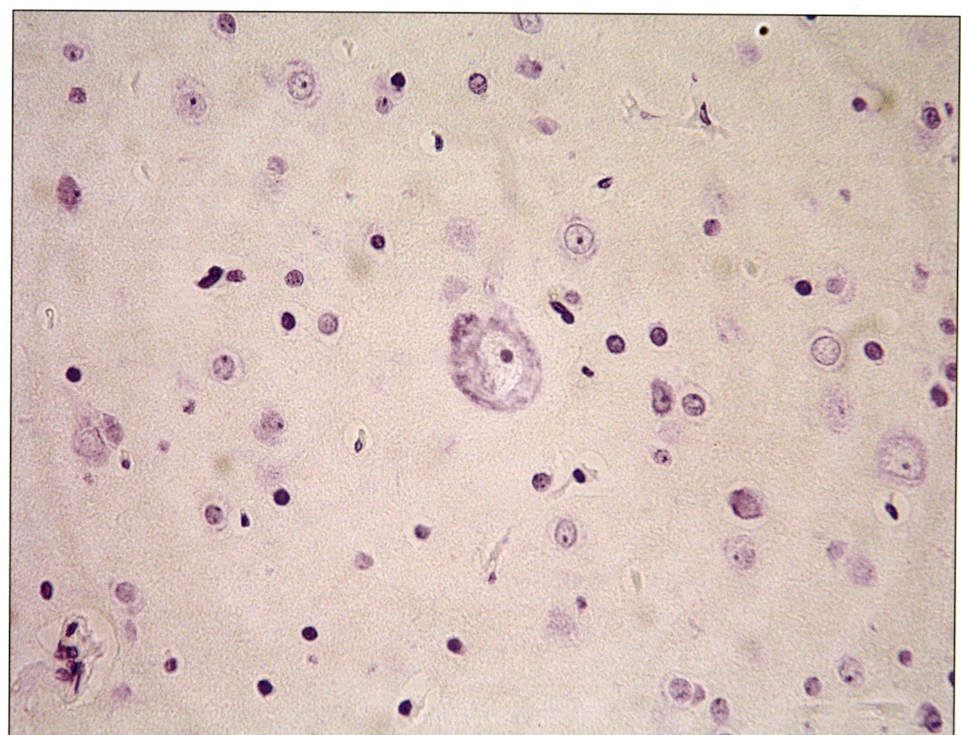

Figure 7.8. FCD type IB: giant neuron, characteristically found in the upper half of the cortex.

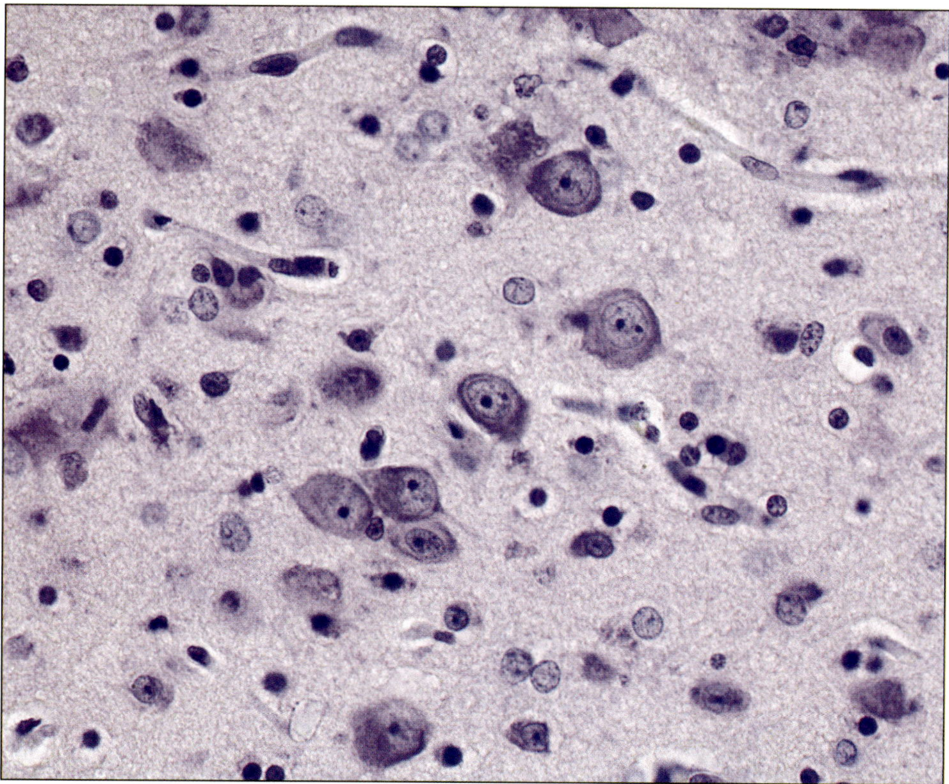

Figure 7.9. Immature neurons of FCD type IB are sometimes loosely clustered.

discontinuous or "skip" lesions of dysplasia with intervening normal cortex may also be seen.

The pathognomonic cell type associated with FCD type IIB is the balloon cell, an abnormally large cell (80–100 μm) with a thin membrane, pale glassy

Figure 7.10. FCD type IIA: dysmorphic neuron in the center.

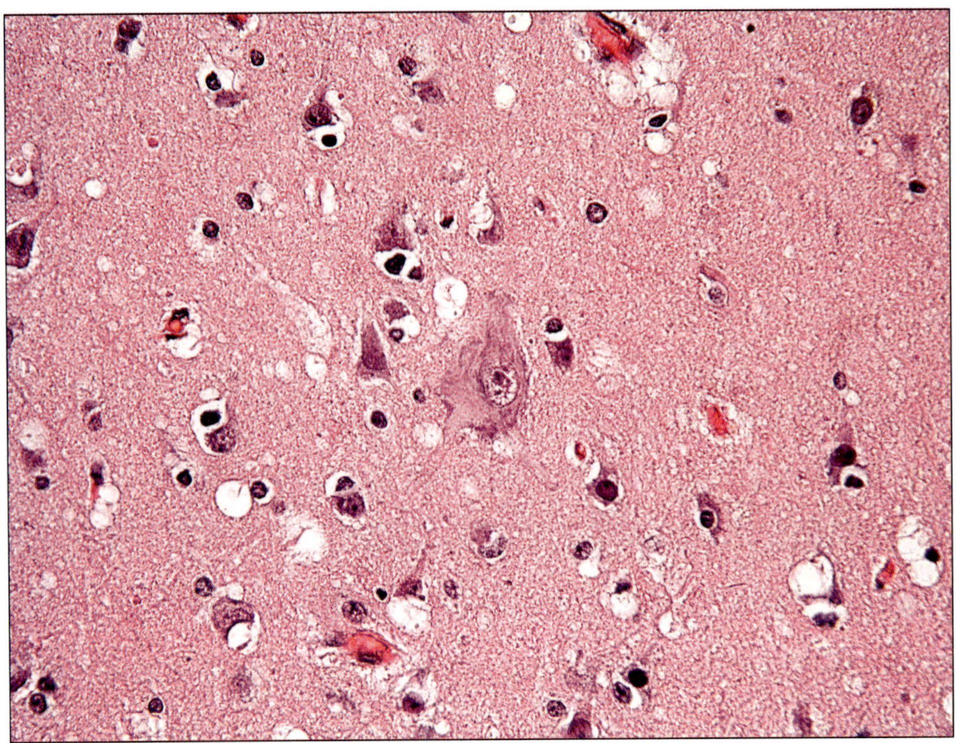

Figure 7.11. FCD type IIB: the balloon cells.

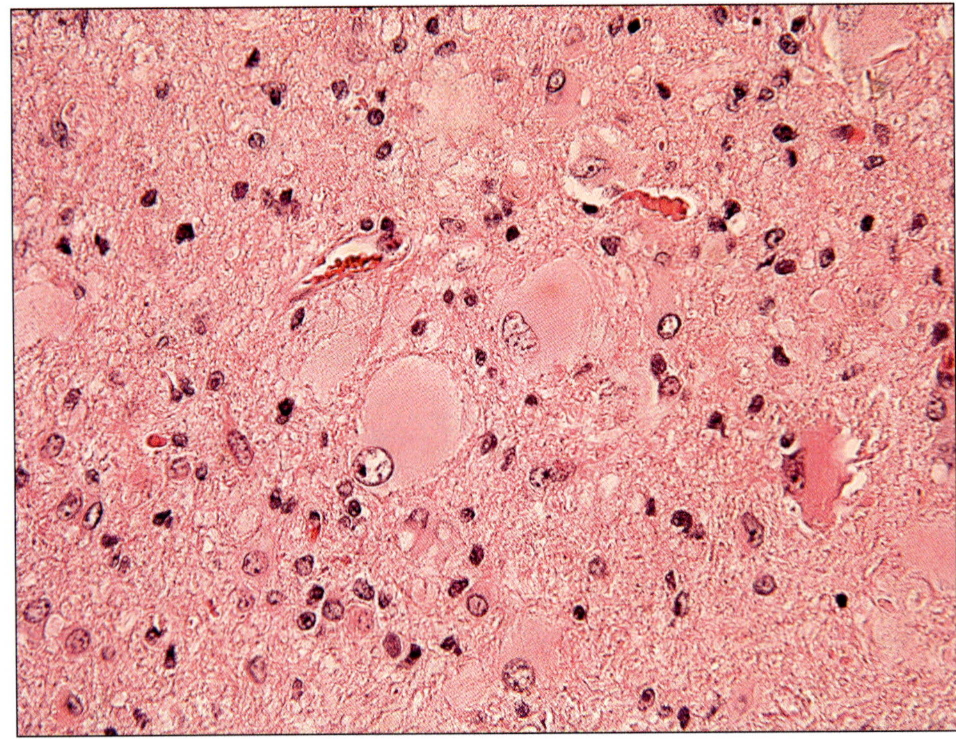

eosinophilic cytoplasm lacking cellular processes, and eccentric nucleus (or nuclei), found in the molecular layer, deeper cortex, and underlying white matter (Figure 7.11).

Abnormal cortical cytoarchitecture, calcification, small infarcts, and chronic inflammation were also reported in FCD (Crino et al., 2002). Surprisingly, a

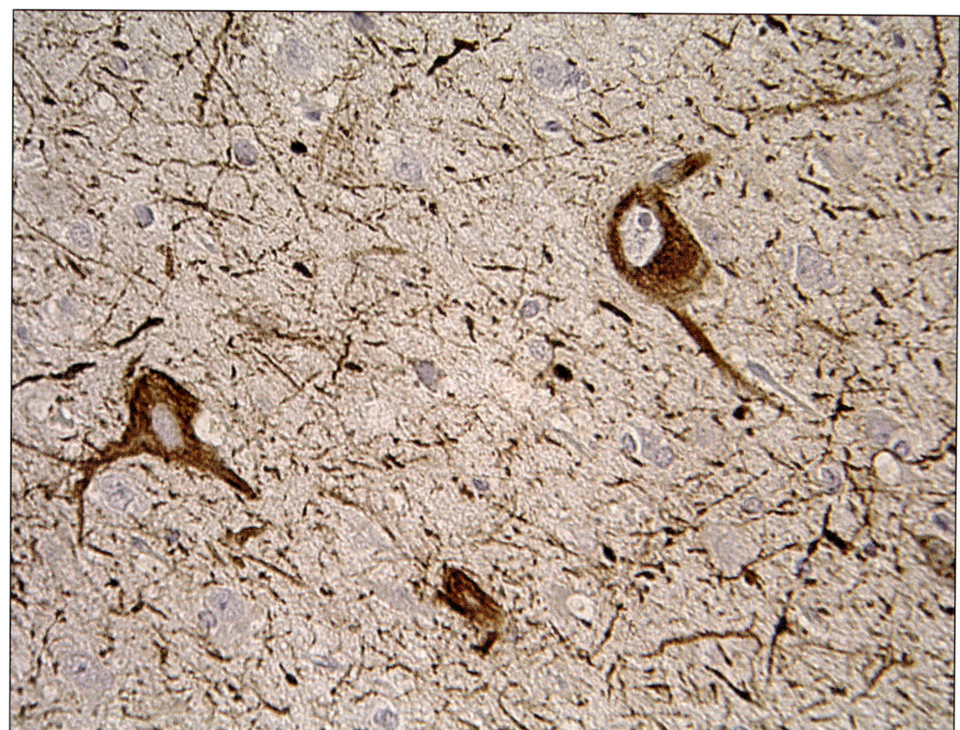

Figure 7.12. FCD type II: dysmorphic neurons; immunohistochemistry against nonphosphorylated neurofilaments.

significant reduction in neuronal density in the region of dysplasia compared to the adjacent unaffected cortex has been identified (Thom et al., 2005).

Immunohistochemistry is not essential in making the diagnosis of FCD but allows further characterization of cell types. A portion of dysmorphic neurons show intense labeling for phosphorylated and nonphosphorylated neurofilament of both high and low molecular weights (Figure 7.12). Immunohistochemistry for tau is negative. The majority of balloon cells show variable expression of the glial fibrillary acidic protein (GFAP) (Figure 7.13); coexpression of neuronal proteins like neurofilament and synaptophysin may be present. Expression of developmentally related proteins indicating impaired maturation in FCD was demonstrated with many balloon cells being positive for nestin, CD34, and embryonal neural cell adhesion molecule (NCAM, CD56). Increased expression of microtubule associated proteins MAP-2, MAP-1B, and MAP-2c was also shown in dysplastic neurons. Selective reduction of inhibitory neurons can be demonstrated by immunohistochemistry for parvalbumin (Figure 7.14), calbindin, and calretinin.

Tuberous Sclerosis

Tuberous sclerosis (TSC) is a multisystem disorder caused by a mutation in either of two tumor suppressor genes, *TSC1* (on chromosome 9q34) or *TSC2* (on 16p13.3) with variable phenotypic expression (Jozwiak et al., 2008). Two-thirds of the patients have TSC as a result of spontaneous genetic mutations while in one-third of the patients the disorder is inherited in an autosomal dominant manner. A prevalence of 1:30, 000–50, 000 has been reported. The brain is the

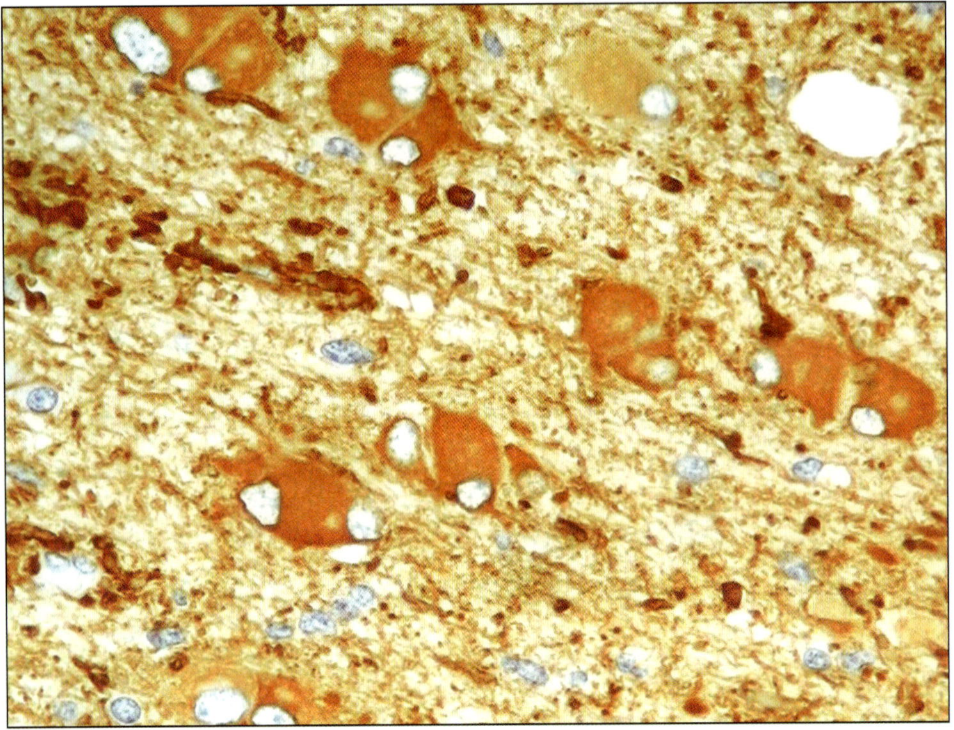

Figure 7.13. FCD type II: dysmorphic neurons; immunohistochemistry for GFAP.

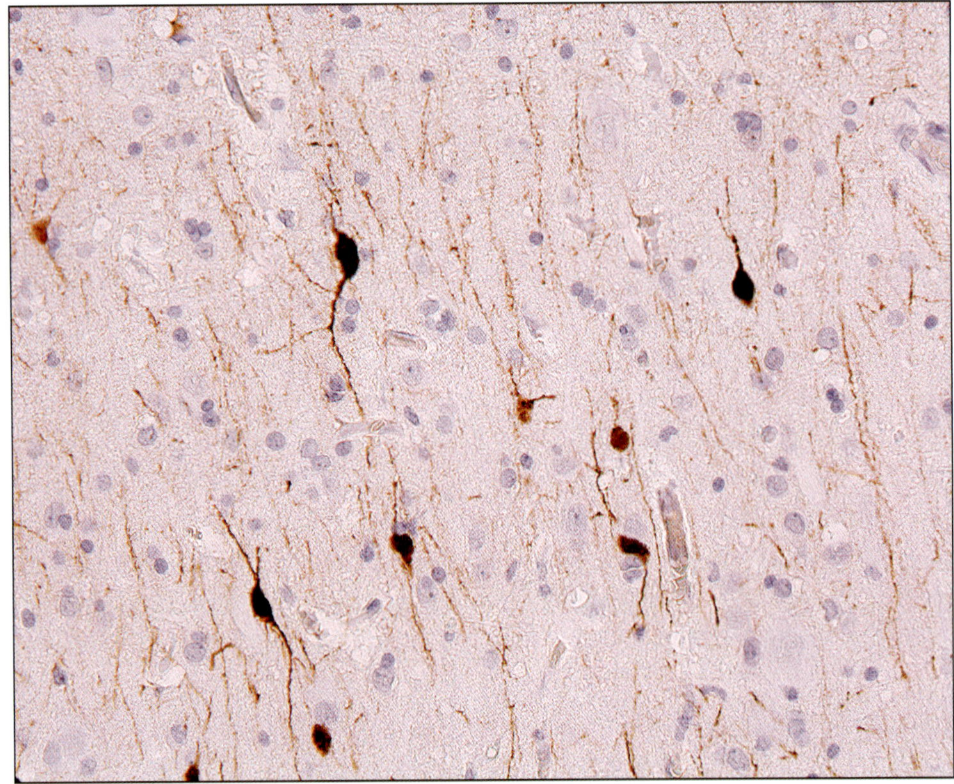

Figure 7.14. Inhibitory GABAergic interneurons, which may be reduced in epileptogenic foci; immunohistochemistry for parvalbumin.

most frequently affected organ in TSC; however, hamartomas may also arise in other organs such as the kidney (renal angiomyolipomas) and heart (cardiac rhabdomyomas). Neurological signs include epilepsy, mental retardation, autism, and attention deficit/hyperactivity disorder.

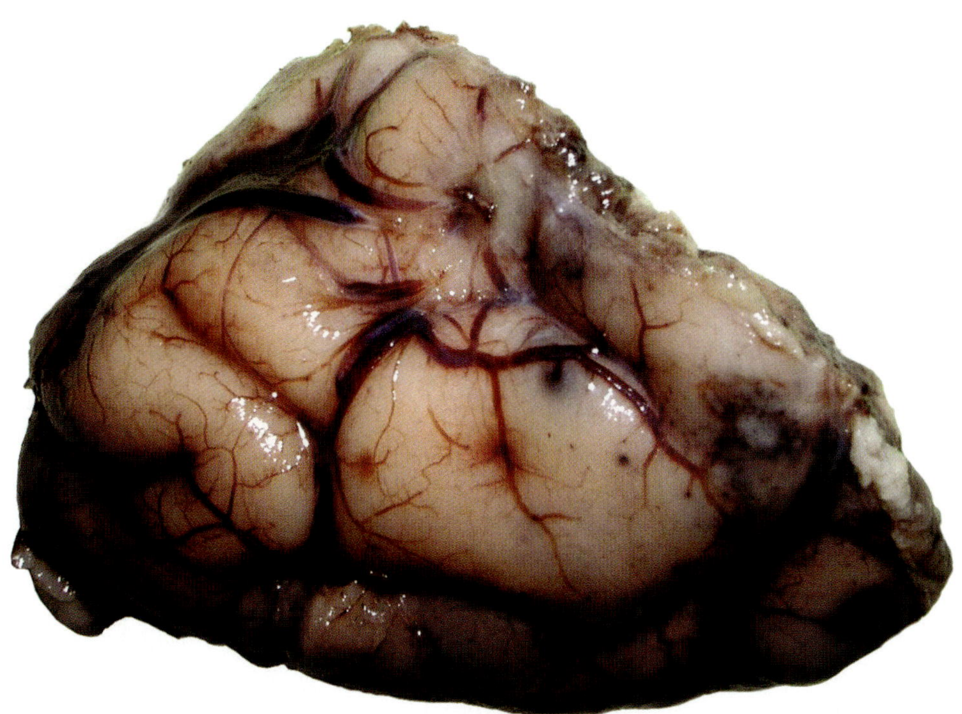

Figure 7.15. Tuberous sclerosis: resection specimen. Note the enlargement of a gyrus affected by a tuber in the center.

Neuropathology

TSC has three different pathological profiles in the brain: two types of lesions, cortical tubers and subcortical heterotopic nodules, are static. The latter, subependymal nodules, are often progressive, hence the term subependymal giant cell astrocytoma (SEGA) (see Chapter 3, page 46). All are detectable by CT or MRI with ease (Luat et al., 2007).

Cortical tubers are focal enlargements of gyri (Figure 7.15), firm to palpation. They vary in number from single to multiple, range from microscopic to several centimeters in size, and may span part of a gyrus, the entire gyrus, or extend across the adjacent gyri. Neuropathological diagnosis of cortical tuber is not difficult (Mizuguchi and Takashima, 2001; Richardson, 1991): normal neuronal lamination is lost and cytologically abnormal giant neurons are present (Figure 7.16). The giant neurons are abnormally oriented, have prominent nucleoli, multiple nuclei, aberrant dendritic arborization, abnormal shape, and accumulation of perikaryal fibrils (Figure 7.17). Giant bizarre cells with abundant eosinophilic cytoplasm and eccentric nuclei are also present in the tuber and in the underlying white matter (Figure 7.18). The cortex adjacent to the tuber usually demonstrates a normal cytoarchitecture. Marked subpial gliosis (Figure 7.19) might be of diagnostic help since the latter is never observed in either FCD or HMC. Heterotopic clusters of dysplastic neurons and giant cells in the subcortical areas give rise to subcortical heterotopic nodules (Figure 7.20).

Numerous immunohistochemical studies have been undertaken to characterize the bizarre giant cells in tuberous sclerosis. In contrast to a paucity of staining of the cells for GFAP in the subependymal giant cells of SEGAs, several studies have shown higher proportion of GFAP-positive cells in the subcortical

Figure 7.16. Tuberous sclerosis: normal neuronal lamination is lost and abnormal giant neurons are present.

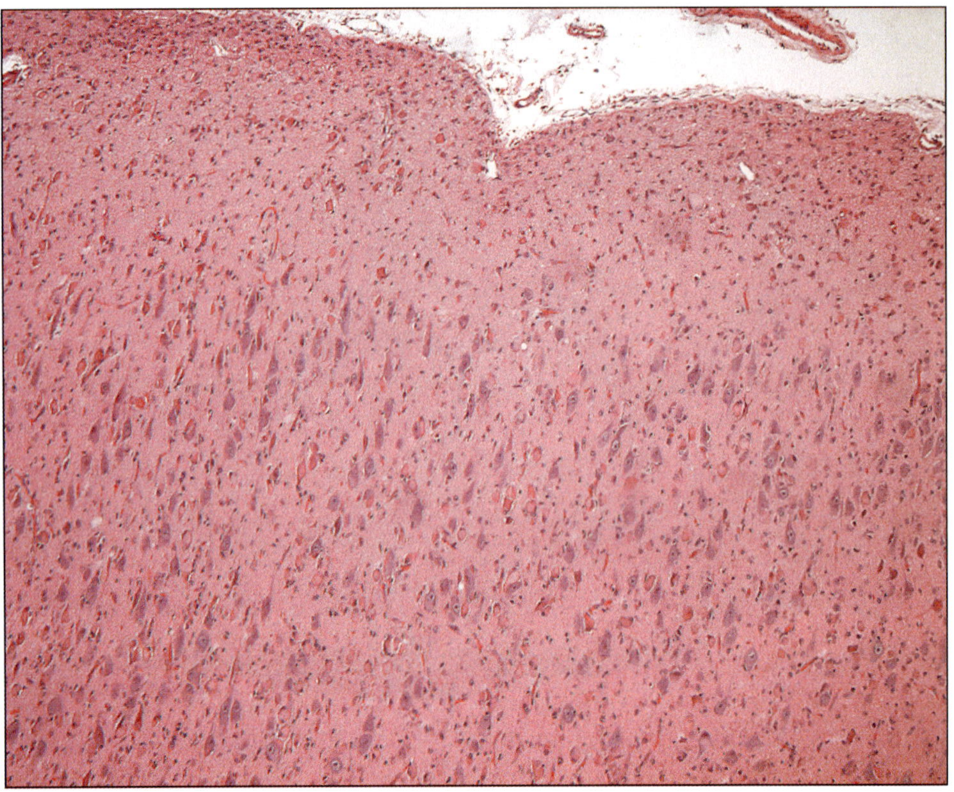

Figure 7.17. Tuberous sclerosis: the giant neurons in a tuber.

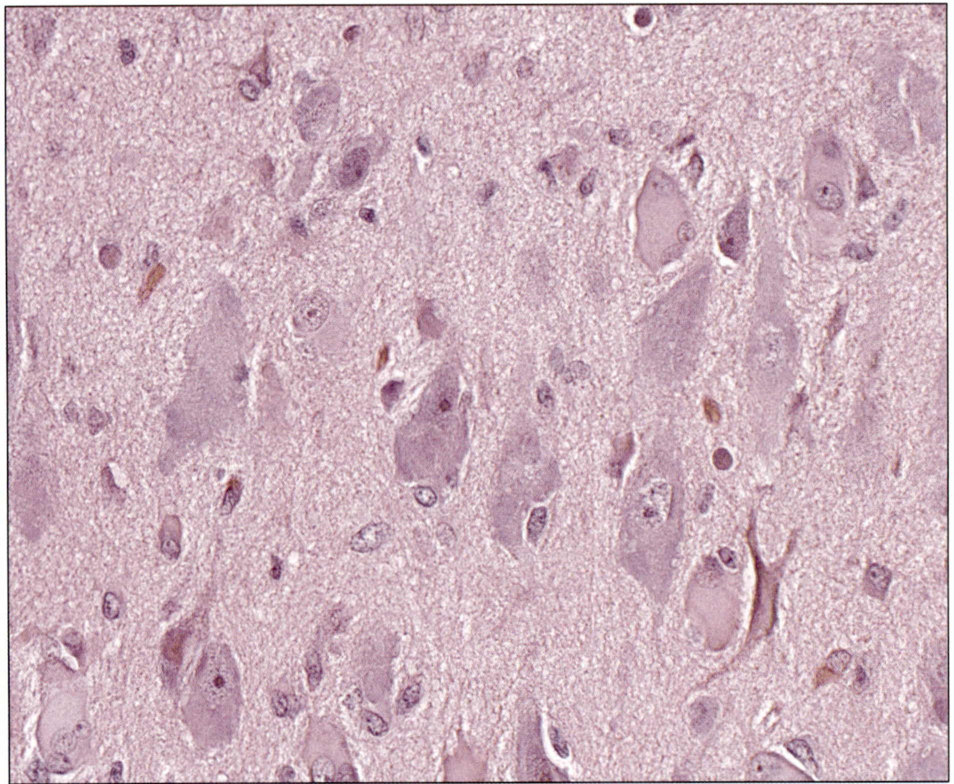

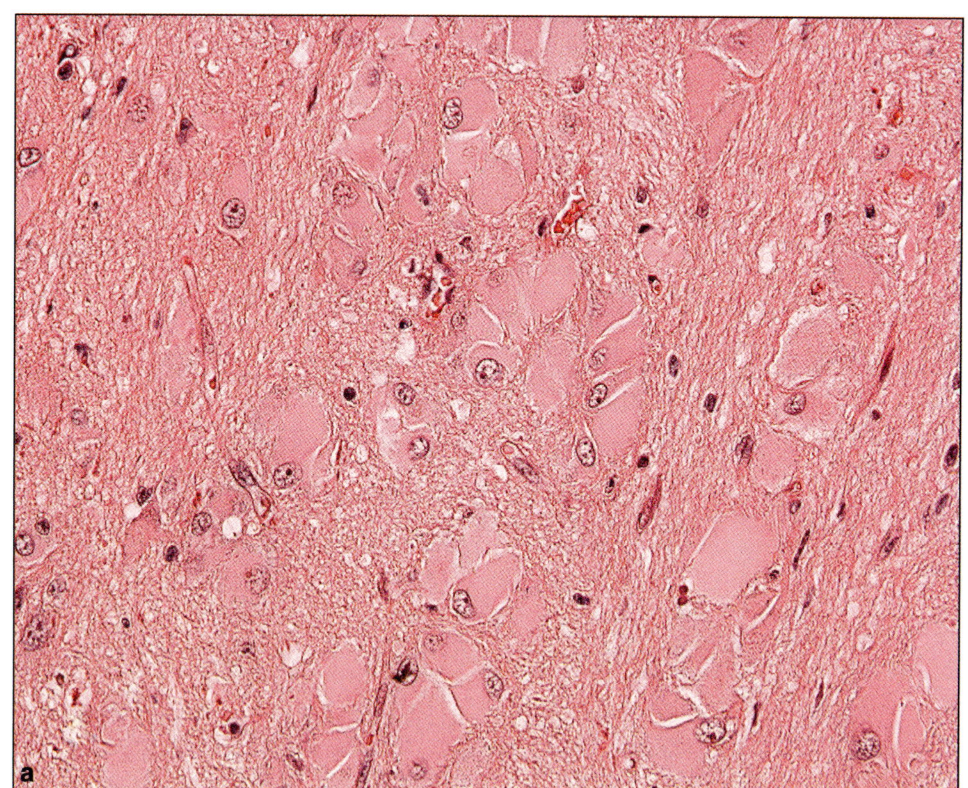

Figure 7.18. Tuberous sclerosis. (a) Giant bizarre cells with abundant eosinophilic cytoplasm in clusters.
(b) Microcalcifications are often encountered in interstitium of tubers.

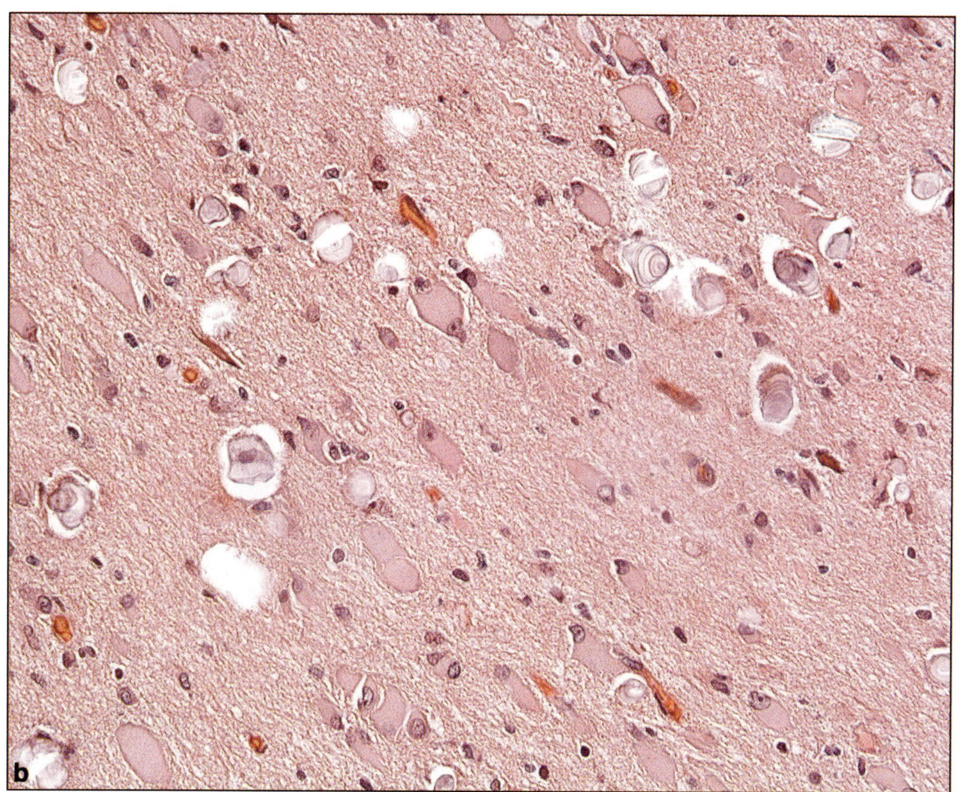

Figure 7.19. Tuberous sclerosis: prominent subpial gliosis with gemistocytic cells.

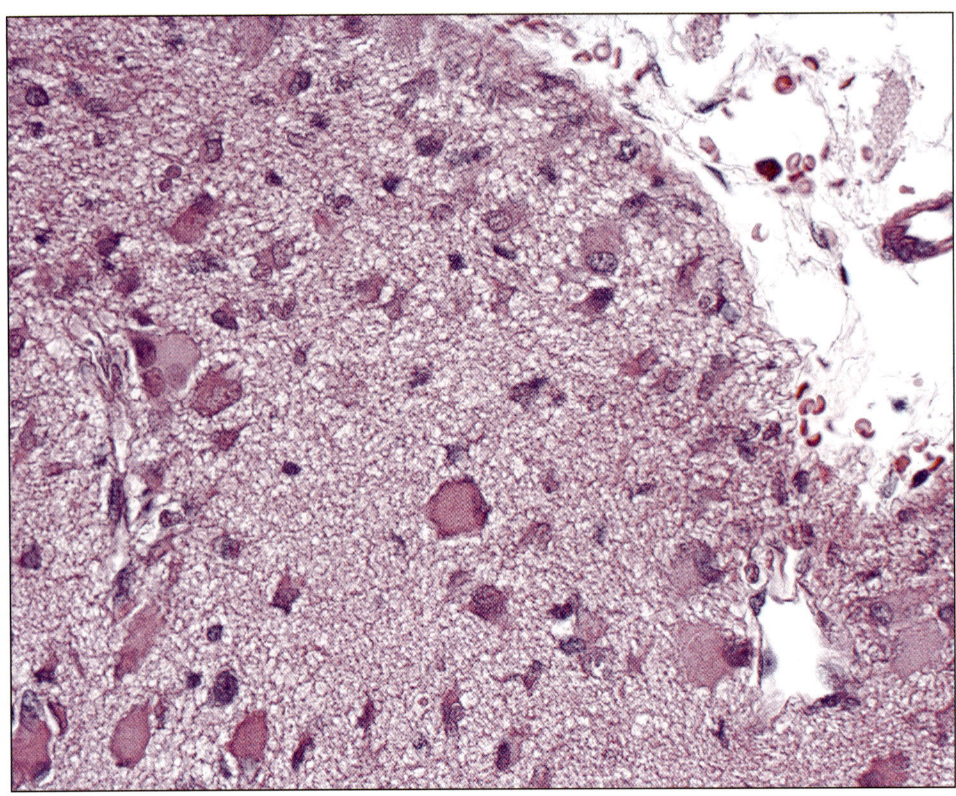

Figure 7.20. Subcortical heterotopic nodules are composed of clustered dysplastic neurons and giant cells. Nissl stain.

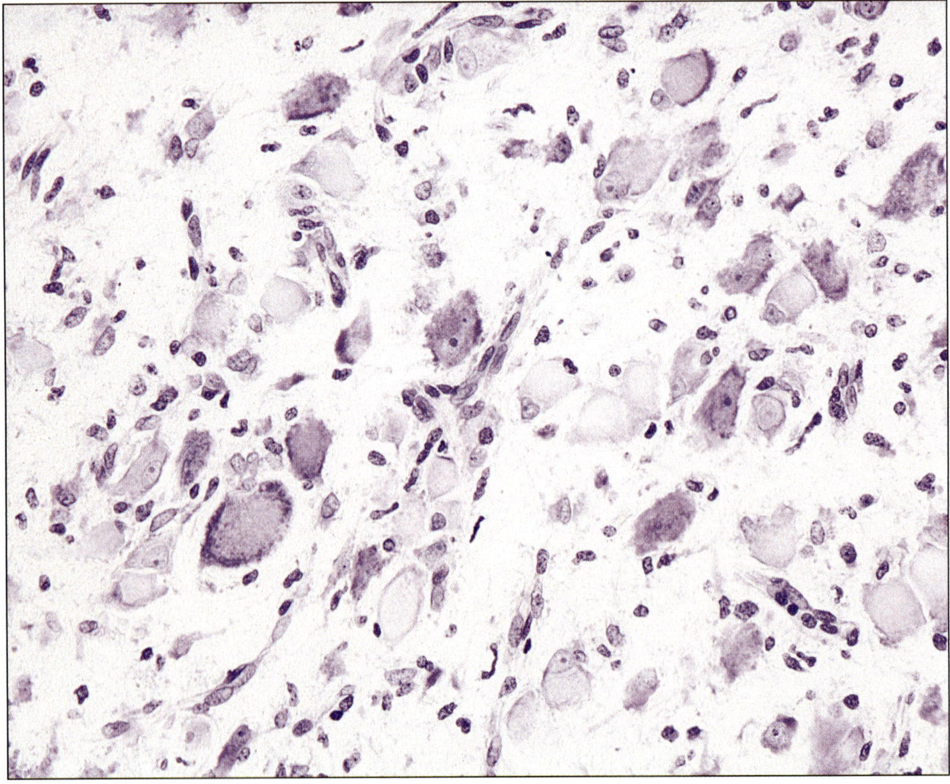

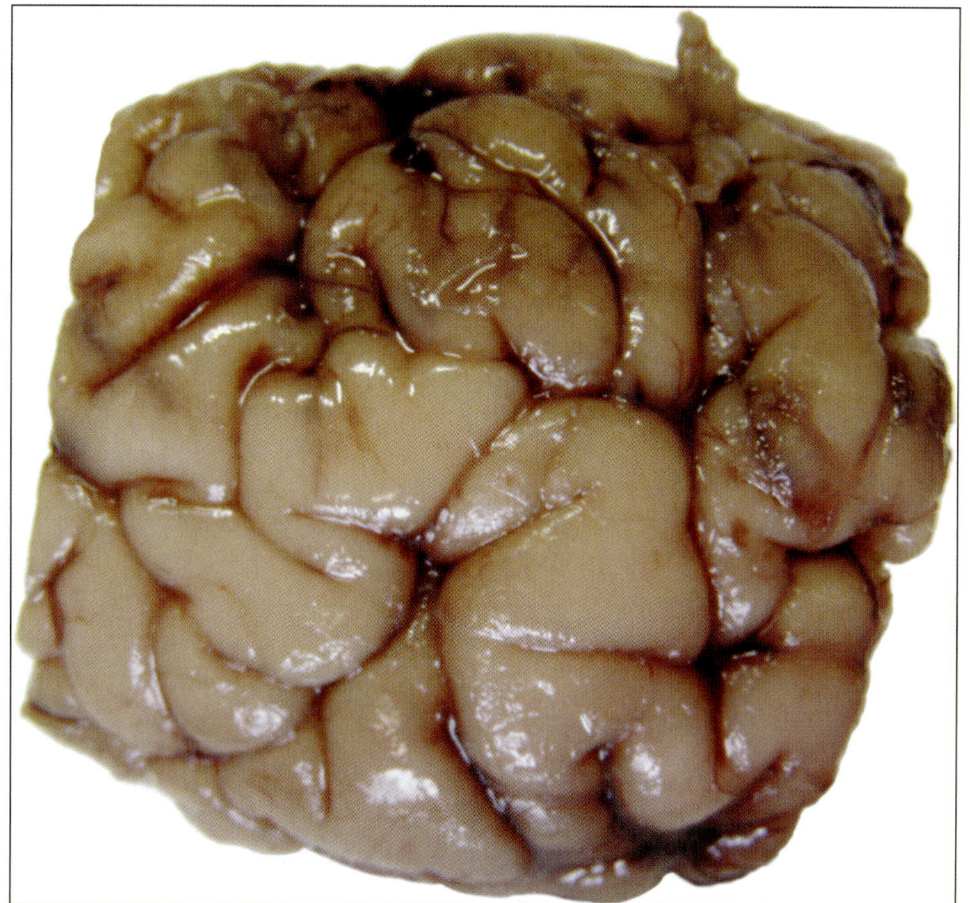

Figure 7.21. Hemimegalencephaly resection specimen.

lesions and cortical tubers, suggesting that acquisition of GFAP may occur in association with migration. Similar cells may also stain for neurofilament indicating neuronal differentiation, or for nestin, vimentin, and other intermediate filaments specific for immature neuroglial cells.

Hemimegalencephaly

HMC is a disease that is characterized by a dysgenetic unilateral enlargement of the cerebrum and it presents with thick cortex, wide convolutions, and reduced sulci and with an increase in the volume of the white matter, which is diagnostic for HMC and easily detectable by computed tomography (CT) imaging as well as MRI techniques (Yagishita et al., 1998).

Neuropathologically, the affected hemisphere is almost invariably enlarged and exhibits an increased consistency, a malformed surface (agyria, polymicrogyria, pachygyria, lissencephaly) (Figure 7.21), and an increase in vascularity.

Microscopically, HMC shows different features from FCD (Di Rocco et al., 2006). The major histological change in HMC is the presence of a number of giant dysplastic oval neurons (up to 80 μm in diameter) in the cerebral cortex and the white matter having relatively large nuclei with prominent nucleoli (Figure 7.22). Laminar organization of the cortex is absent (Figure 7.23) or occasionally shows polymicrogyria, and gray–white matter demarcation is poor.

Figure 7.22.
Hemimegalencephaly:
numerous giant dysplastic
oval neurons having large
nuclei with prominent
nucleoli.

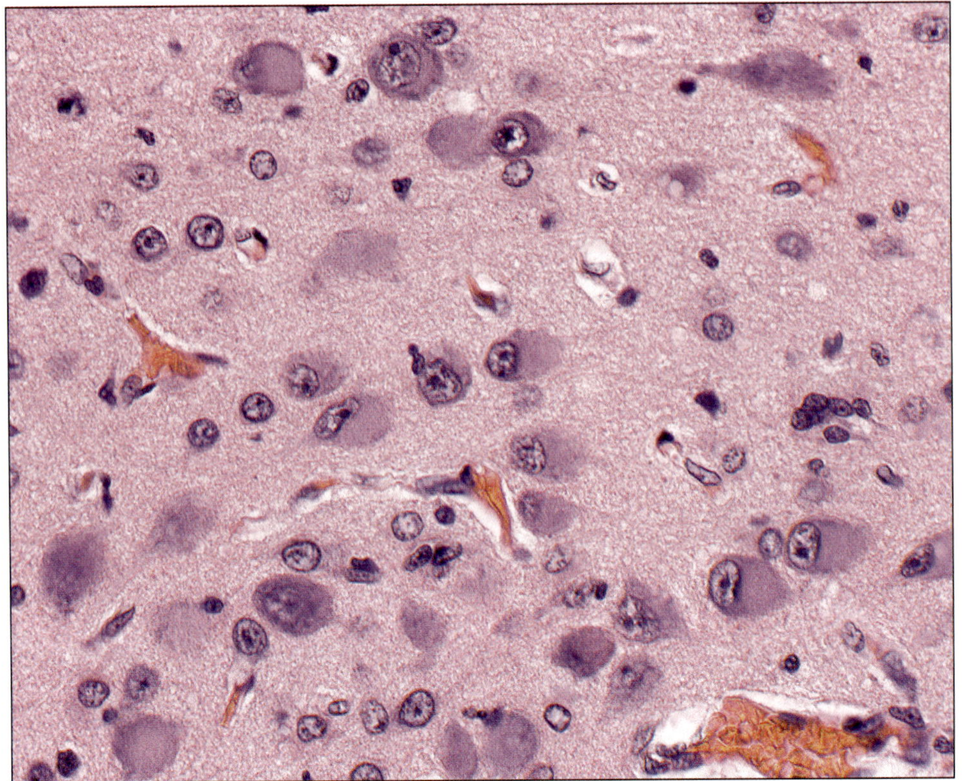

Figure 7.23.
Hemimegalencephaly:
laminar disorganization of
the cortex.

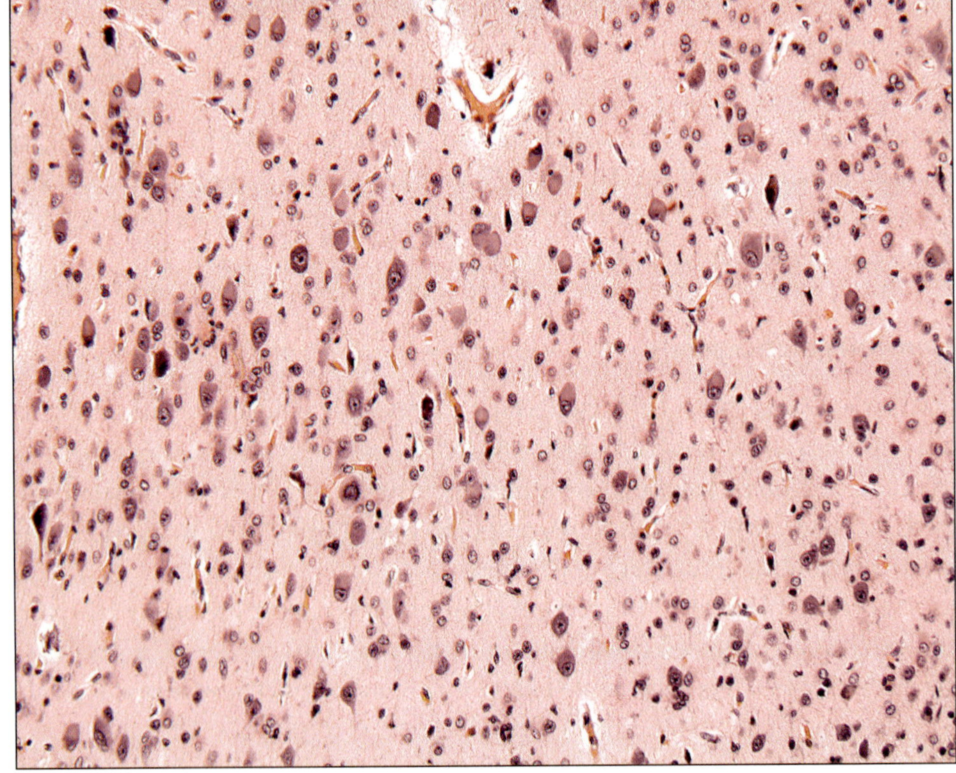

While the neuronal alterations are constant, the glial anomalies are evident only in about 50% of the cases and involve astrocytes more than oligodendrocytes (Flores-Sarnat et al., 2003). They include the presence of anomalous cells, such as balloon cells that are immunopositive for GFAP and vimentin within either the gray or the white matter, multinucleate glial cells involving the molecular layer of the cortex, Rosenthal fibers and areas of demyelination.

REFERENCES

Arai N, Takahashi T, Komori T, Yagishita A, Shimizu H. Diagnostic surgical neuro-pathology of intractable epilepsy. *Neuropathology* 2007; 27: 594–600.

Barkovich AJ, Kuzniecky RI, Jackson GD, Guerrini R, Dobyns WB. Classification system for malformations of cortical development: update 2001. *Neurology* 2001; 57: 2168–78.

Barkovich AJ, Kuzniecky RI, Jackson GD, Guerrini R, Dobyns WB. A developmental and genetic classification for malformations of cortical development. *Neurology* 2005; 65: 1873–87.

Beck H, Goussakov IV, Lie A, Helmstaedter C, Elger CE. Synaptic plasticity in the human dentate gyrus. *J Neurosci* 2000; 20: 7080–6.

Becker AJ, Chen J, Paus S, Normann S, Beck H, Elger CE, et al. Transcriptional profiling in human epilepsy: expression array and single cell real-time qRT-PCR analysis reveal distinct cellular gene regulation. *Neuroreport* 2002; 13: 1327–33.

Blümcke I, Thom M, Wiestler OD. Ammon's horn sclerosis: a maldevelopmental disorder associated with temporal lobe epilepsy. *Brain Pathol* 2002; 12: 199–211.

Camacho DL, Castillo M. MR imaging of temporal lobe epilepsy. *Semin Ultrasound CT MR* 2007; 28: 424–36.

Chung MH, Horoupian DS. Corpora amylacea: a marker for mesial temporal sclerosis. *J Neuropathol Exp Neurol* 1996; 55: 403–8.

Crino PB. Molecular pathogenesis of focal cortical dysplasia and hemimegalencephaly. *J Child Neurol* 2005; 20: 330–6.

Crino PB, Miyata H, Vinters HV. Neurodevelopmental disorders as a cause of seizures: neuropathologic, genetic, and mechanistic considerations. *Brain Pathol* 2002; 12: 212–33.

Daumas-Duport C, Varlet P, Bacha S, Beuvon F, Cervera-Pierot P, Chodkiewicz JP. Dysembryoplastic neuroepithelial tumors: nonspecific histological forms – a study of 40 cases. *J Neurooncol* 1999; 41: 267–80.

Di Rocco C, Battaglia D, Pietrini D, Piastra M, Massimi L. Hemimegalencephaly: clinical implications and surgical treatment. *Childs Nerv Syst* 2006; 22: 852–66.

Flores-Sarnat L, Sarnat HB, Davila-Gutierrez G, Alvarez A. Hemimegalencephaly: part 2. Neuropathology suggests a disorder of cellular lineage. *J Child Neurol* 2003; 18: 776–85.

Hua Y, Crino PB. Single cell lineage analysis in human focal cortical dysplasia. *Cereb Cortex* 2003; 13: 693–9.

Jozwiak J, Jozwiak S, Skopinski P. Immunohistochemical and microscopic studies on giant cells in tuberous sclerosis. *Histol Histopathol* 2005; 20: 1321–6.

Jozwiak J, Jozwiak S, Wlodarski P. Possible mechanisms of disease development in tuberous sclerosis. *Lancet Oncol* 2008; 9: 73–9.

Kasper BS. Mild forms of focal cortical dysplasia: how certain are we? *Brain* 2005; 128: E22; author reply E23.

Kasper BS, Stefan H, Buchfelder M, Paulus W. Temporal lobe microdysgenesis in epilepsy versus control brains. *J Neuropathol Exp Neurol* 1999; 58: 22–8.

Luat AF, Makki M, Chugani HT. Neuroimaging in tuberous sclerosis complex. *Curr Opin Neurol* 2007; 20: 142–50.

Lurton D, Sundstrom L, Brana C, Bloch B, Rougier A. Possible mechanisms inducing granule cell dispersion in humans with temporal lobe epilepsy. *Epilepsy Res* 1997; 26: 351–61.

Maehara T. Neuroimaging of epilepsy. *Neuropathology* 2007; 27: 585–93.

Mathern GW, Kuhlman PA, Mendoza D, Pretorius JK. Human fascia dentata anatomy and hippocampal neuron densities differ depending on the epileptic syndrome and age at first seizure. *J Neuropathol Exp Neurol* 1997; 56: 199–212.

Mizuguchi M, Takashima S. Neuropathology of tuberous sclerosis. *Brain Dev* 2001; 23: 508–15.

Palmini A, Najm I, Avanzini G, Babb T, Guerrini R, Foldvary-Schaefer N, et al. Terminology and classification of the cortical dysplasias. *Neurology* 2004; 62: S2–8.

Prayson RA, Spreafico R, Vinters HV. Pathologic characteristics of the cortical dysplasias. *Neurosurg Clin N Am* 2002; 13: 17–25, vii.

Proper EA, Jansen GH, van Veelen CW, van Rijen PC, Gispen WH, de Graan PN. A grading system for hippocampal sclerosis based on the degree of hippocampal mossy fiber sprouting. *Acta Neuropathol* 2001; 101: 405–9.

Richardson EP, Jr. Pathology of tuberous sclerosis. Neuropathologic aspects. *Ann N Y Acad Sci* 1991; 615: 128–39.

Rickert CH. Cortical dysplasia: neuropathological aspects. *Childs Nerv Syst* 2006; 22: 821–6.

Serrano-Castro PJ, Sanchez-Alvarez JC, Garcia-Gomez T. [Mesial temporal sclerosis (II): clinical features and complementary studies]. *Rev Neurol* 1998; 26: 592–7.

Tassi L, Colombo N, Garbelli R, Francione S, Lo Russo G, Mai R, et al. Focal cortical dysplasia: neuropathological subtypes, EEG, neuroimaging and surgical outcome. *Brain* 2002; 125: 1719–32.

Taylor DC, Falconer MA, Bruton CJ, Corsellis JA. Focal dysplasia of the cerebral cortex in epilepsy. *J Neurol Neurosurg Psychiatry* 1971; 34: 369–87.

Thom M, Holton JL, D'Arrigo C, Griffin B, Beckett A, Sisodiya S, et al. Microdysgenesis with abnormal cortical myelinated fibres in temporal lobe epilepsy: a histopathological study with calbindin D-28-K immunohistochemistry. *Neuropathol Appl Neurobiol* 2000; 26: 251–7.

Thom M, Martinian L, Sen A, Cross JH, Harding BN, Sisodiya SM. Cortical neuronal densities and lamination in focal cortical dysplasia. *Acta Neuropathol* 2005; 110: 383–92.

Urbach H, Scheffler B, Heinrichsmeier T, von Oertzen J, Kral T, Wellmer J, et al. Focal cortical dysplasia of Taylor's balloon cell type: a clinicopathological entity with characteristic neuroimaging and histopathological features, and favorable postsurgical outcome. *Epilepsia* 2002; 43: 33–40.

Watson CNS, Cobb C, Burgerman R, Williamson B. Pathological grading system for hippocampal sclerosis: correlation with magnetic resonance imaging-based volume measurements for the hippocampus. *J Epilepsy* 1996; 9: 56–64.

Yagishita A, Arai N, Tamagawa K, Oda M. Hemimegalencephaly: signal changes suggesting abnormal myelination on MRI. *Neuroradiology* 1998; 40: 734–8.

Yilmazer-Hanke DM, Wolf HK, Schramm J, Elger CE, Wiestler OD, Blumcke I. Subregional pathology of the amygdala complex and entorhinal region in surgical specimens from patients with pharmacoresistant temporal lobe epilepsy. *J Neuropathol Exp Neurol* 2000; 59: 907–20.

8 CYTOPATHOLOGY OF CEREBROSPINAL FLUID

Gregory Moes and Hannes Vogel

CLINICAL INDICATIONS

Examination of cerebrospinal fluid (CSF) specimens is a routine component of most neurological evaluations and includes cell count, biochemical analysis, and cytological examination. Samples may be obtained by lumbar puncture or from the lateral ventricles or cisterna magna either at the time of surgery or from indwelling ventricular shunts. CSF analysis is not only useful for diagnosis of new neoplastic processes, but is routinely used for monitoring the efficacy of central nervous system (CNS) chemotherapy such as recurrence of lymphoma or leukemia and or in the evaluation of infections in immunocompromised patients. As with other aspects of cytology, the cytological findings must be correlated with the clinical, biochemical, and radiographic findings to ensure diagnostic accuracy.

SPECIMEN PREPARATION (CYTOPREPARATION)

CSF specimens are unique in cytology with respect to the small sample size, lack of cellular abundance, and susceptibility of the sample to undergo rapid degeneration. With this in mind, processing of CSF specimens for cell count, biochemical analysis, cytological preparation, and additional tests such as flow cytometric analysis in cases of suspected hematopoietic malignancies should be done as soon as possible. The specimen is collected in plastic tubes and divided among several divisions within the laboratory for specific testing.

Cytological diagnosis should be performed from the third or last tube since it will have less blood contamination in cases of traumatic tap.

The most common stain employed in CSF cytology is the Wright–Giemsa preparation, which is most useful for classification of hematopoietic cells and cytoplasmic detail while the Papanicolaou stain, best for nuclear detail, is the standard used for filter and cytocentrifugation preparations. Cytocentrifugation technique is used by most laboratories since it is easier and faster to prepare slides in comparison with the filter preparation technique.

NORMAL AND REACTIVE CELLULAR CONSTITUENTS SEEN IN CSF CYTOLOGY

CSF specimens are most commonly used to diagnose secondary malignancies including metastatic carcinoma, lymphoma/leukemias, primary brain tumors such as medulloblastomas, and meningitis. Generally speaking, a caveat of CSF specimen analysis is that diagnostic cells will not usually be identified from lesions that do not shed cells readily or lack access to the CSF. Since some tumors shed few cells and CSF specimens tend to be of scant cellularity, it is important to recognize that a single abnormal or foreign cell may be considered a significant finding. Tumors can also be associated with an inflammatory reaction; therefore, recognition of normal cellular constituents in CSF specimens, particularly in reactive conditions, is important in rendering an accurate diagnosis.

There are normally only a few cells in CSF specimens and they almost exclusively consist of *white blood cells* (WBCs) with *lymphocytes* normally accounting for most of the WBCs. While normal counts in adults range from 0 to 5/μl, in neonates counts of up to 30/μl may be encountered. Most of the lymphocytes are small, mature-appearing lymphocytes although a few scattered reactive lymphocytes with larger nuclei, cleaved nuclei with conspicuous nucleoli, and more abundant cytoplasm may be present. *Red blood cells* are not typically present in CSF specimens, but a few are commonly observed due to microtrauma while obtaining the specimen and when numerous, the differential diagnosis includes traumatic tap versus a pathologic process.

Monocytes usually accompany lymphocytes in CSF specimens, usually representing about one third of the cell population, but may be the majority of cells in infectious, autoimmmune or neoplastic conditions. *Macrophages* or *histiocytes* are associated with destructive processes of the CNS including infections, infarction, trauma, postsurgery, benign cysts, tumors, and histiocytosis.

Cytoplasmic inclusions may help in the differential diagnosis and such cells including *lipophages*, also known as "gitter" cells and are associated with intrathecal chemotherapy and causes of parenchymal destruction, *siderophages* seen after hemorrhage, and *melanophages*, which do not necessarily indicate melanoma as they can be seen in other tumors and melanosis cerebri.

Plasma cells are not normally present in CSF, although they may be seen in many chronic inflammatory processes and the presence of plasma cells in CSF specimens of adults should raise the suspicion of plasma cell dyscrasia involving the CSF. *Eosinophils* are found in the CSF usually after traumatic taps. Their presence otherwise suggests hypersensitivity reactions, parasitic infections, or less commonly Hodgkin disease.

Cells derived from the CNS may occasionally be seen in CSF specimens, findings that are highly contingent upon specimen acquisition. For example, shunt specimens are more likely to contain ependymal and choroid cells and neurons and glial cells as a result of physical disruption of the ventricular lining or brain parenchyma by the shunt, while normal neurons or glia are almost never found in lumbar puncture specimens.

Ependymal cells are relatively uniform, small cuboidal to columnar cells that are usually present as a few loosely cohesive clusters (Figure 8.1). The nuclei are single, oval to round, and centrally placed within moderately abundant, basophilic cytoplasm with indistinct cell borders. Cytoplasmic vacuolization and terminal bars or cilia are particularly characteristic of ependymal cells.

Choroid plexus cells, considered specialized ependyma, may be difficult to distinguish from ependymal cells. They share similar cytological features with ependymal cells being present in loosely cohesive clusters. They may also display microacinar arrangements or papillary configurations, raising the differential of well-differentiated adenocarcinoma. The nuclear features are similar to ependymal cells; however, the cytoplasm of choroid plexus cells is usually denser and may contain yellow or brown pigment or appear oncocytic. Cilia are not typically present, especially in specimens from adults.

Specimens from neonates and infants may contain cells of *germinal matrix* origin, often following intraventricular brain hemorrhage associated with prematurity. Molded clusters of immature blastlike cells with round to oval nuclei containing even chromatin and a single small nucleolus may be identified. Hemosiderin-laden macrophages are often present in the background. They are smaller and lack the nuclear pleomorphism and chromatin abnormalities of embryonal tumors or lymphoblasts.

Normal *astrocytes* and *oligodendrocytes* are less commonly identified in CSF specimens, but may be seen in patients with encephalitis, seizure activity, or bleeding. Typically, these cells are identified within fragments of neuroglial tissue seen after shunt placement or third ventriculostomy specimens (Figure 8.2). Astrocytes are large, pale cells with spindled or oval shapes and multiple fibrillar cytoplasmic branches. The nuclei are round to oval and hyperchromatic. Oligodendroglial cells may be seen as single cells or in small sheets and display clear cytoplasm with a small, round hyperchromatic central nucleus. The largest nonneoplastic cells that may be seen in CSF specimens are *neurons* (Figure 8.3). They retain their shape seen in histologic sections, typically demonstrating pyramidal cell body with long processes and dense, granular cytoplasm, a central irregular, large nuclei, and prominent nucleolus.

Figure 8.1. Ependymal cells. Loose cluster of uniform epithelioid cells revealing eccentrically placed, round to oval nuclei with by lacy blue cytoplasm. Cilia and blepharoplasts are pathognomonic when present.

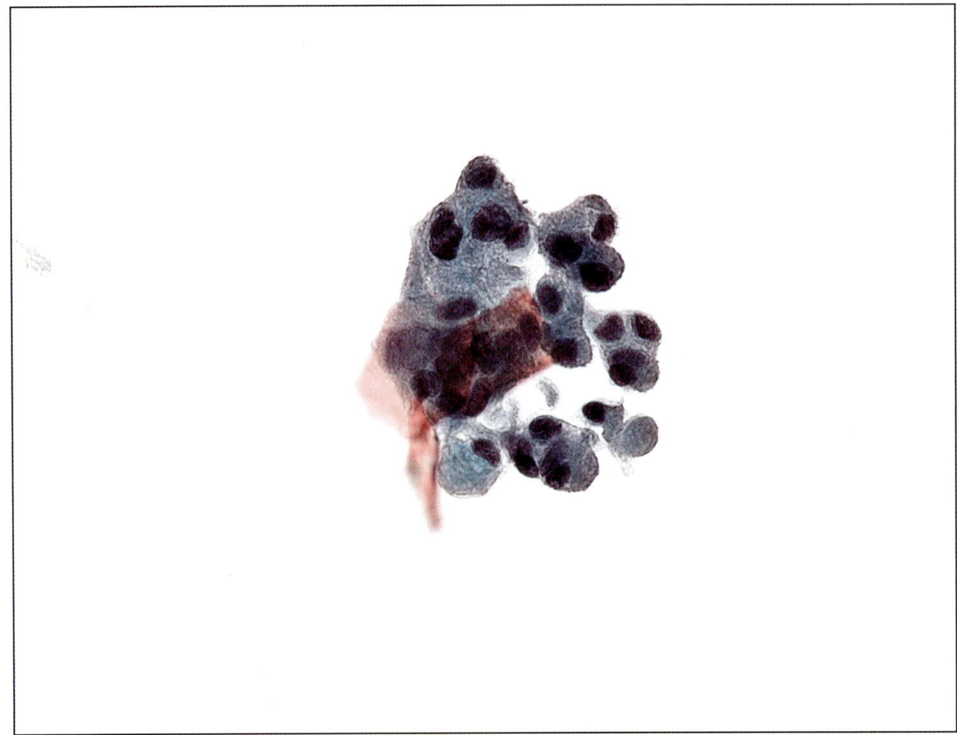

Figure 8.2. Example of shunt specimen. Fragment of rarefied neuropil and bare nuclei. The larger nucleus with a prominent nucleolus (arrow), characteristic of a neuron nucleus, is adjacent to an elongate hyperchromatic nucleus compatible with an astrocyte nucleus. A monocyte nucleus overlies the tissue fragment (arrowhead). The background consists of crenated and intact red blood cells and smaller fragments of acellular neuropil.

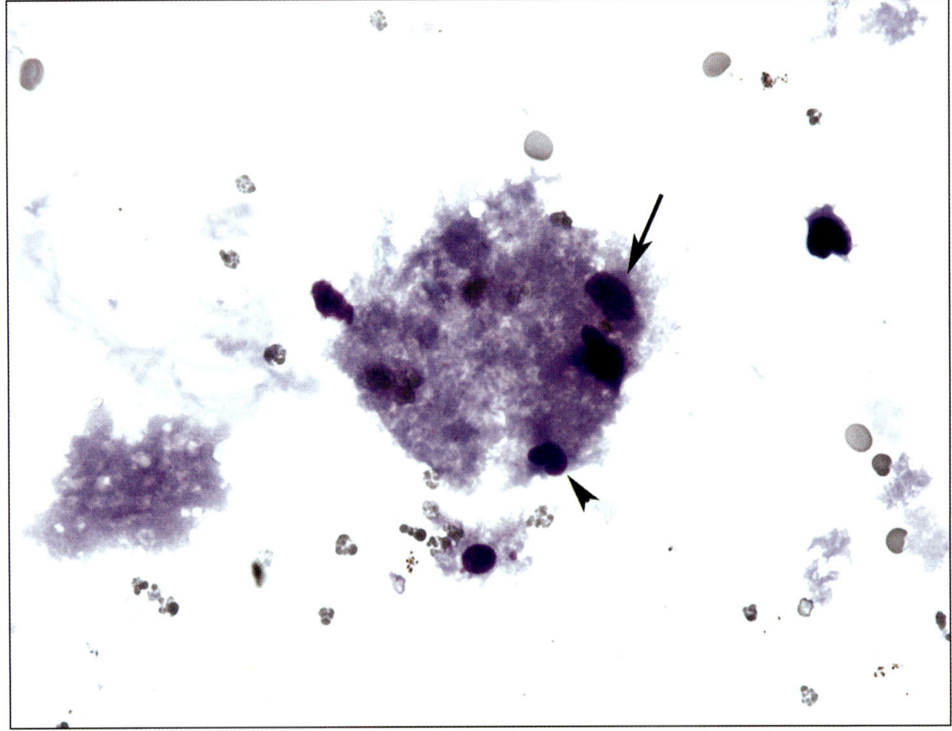

The spectrum of nonneoplastic cells that may be encountered in CSF specimen, including contaminants, is quite broad and should kept in mind in order to avoid a false-positive result. *Squamous cells, skeletal muscle, adipose, fibrous tissue*, and *cartilage* to name of few may be found in CSF specimens as a result of

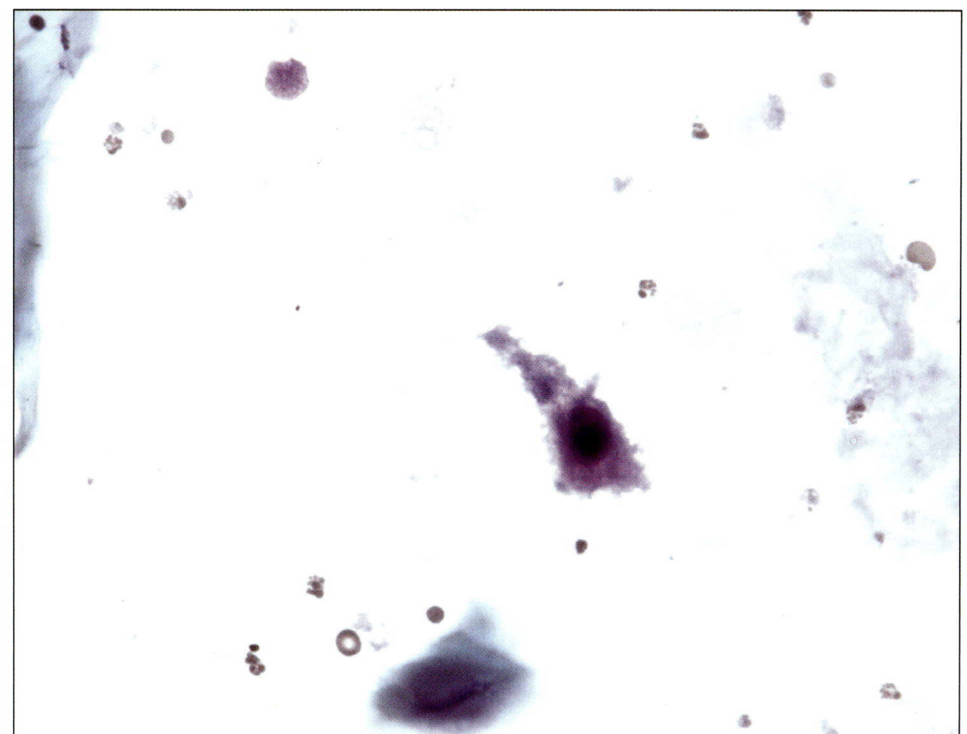

Figure 8.3. Typical cytological appearance of a normal neuron in a CSF specimen. Large polygonal-shaped cell with a large central round nucleus, prominent nucleolus and surrounding pale and granular cytoplasm.

"pick up" in lumbar puncture specimens as the needle passes through the skin and soft tissue. Of particular note, in the event of inadvertently sampling *bone marrow elements* from the vertebral body during a lumbar puncture, immature hematopoietic elements from the bone marrow could lead to a misdiagnosis of lymphoma or leukemia. The key is to identify the different hematopoietic cell lines present in the sample; *megakaryocytes* are particularly reassuring. The few anucleate squamous cells commonly seen in CSF specimens are almost always a result of contamination during the process of specimen preparation. However, when the squamous cells are the predominant cell type, a neoplastic process, such as squamous cell carcinoma, rather than contamination should be considered.

Noncellular elements include *corpora amylacea*. These amorphous round, polysaccharide bodies measuring about 8–25 μm in diameter may be seen in ventricular specimens from elderly patients. *Starch granules*, derived from glove powder, show a refractile Maltese cross polarization pattern and are common contaminants in CSF specimens.

TUMOR DIAGNOSIS IN CSF SPECIMENS

CSF cytology is instrumental in the evaluation of some primary CNS tumors and metastatic malignancies such as carcinoma and lymphoma/leukemia, since certain types of malignancies involve the CNS in a significant percentage of patients with systemic malignancies (Barnholtz-Sloan et al., 2004; Schouten et al., 2002). Detection of neoplasms involving the CNS by CSF cytology is variable, with malignancies involving the leptomeninges, that is, meningeal carcinomatosis, or cases of multiple metastatic foci yielding the most diagnostic specimens.

Lung, breast, and stomach carcinomas are among the most likely to cause malignant meningitis. Although false-negative results are common with CSF cytology, false-positive results are rare and the use of ancillary tests such as immunohistochemistry are useful to increase accuracy (Jorda et al., 1998). The cytological features of metastatic malignancy in CSF are similar to those seen in other body cavity fluid specimens, with a few caveats that adenocarcinoma has a greater tendency to shed as single cells rather than in clusters and malignant cells tend to appear larger than normal cells in the CSF (DeMay, 1996).

Lung cancer, particularly small cell carcinoma, is the most common cancer to metastasize to the CNS (Schouten et al., 2002) (Figures 8.4 and 8.5). In women, *breast carcinoma* is the most common tumor to metastasize to the CNS (Figure 8.6 a,b). The cells are usually present singly or in loose clusters and typical tight clusters and morulae are rare. Intracytoplasmic target vacuoles, although rare, are practically diagnostic for breast carcinoma, particularly lobular carcinoma.

Metastatic melanoma is the third most common tumor after lung and breast to metastasize to the CNS, frequently involving the meninges. In cases where the primary tumor may be occult, primary melanomas should be considered. *Melanoma* is characterized by large single cells with large eccentric nuclei, macronucleoli, and dense eosinophilic cytoplasm. Nuclear pseudoinclusions and brown cytoplasmic pigment are additional diagnostic features of melanoma.

Gastric and pancreatic carcinomas less commonly involve the CNS, but with involvement are likely to spread along the leptomeninges and shed abundant single or small clusters of small- to medium-sized cells with high nuclear to cytoplasmic ratios, coarse nuclear chromatin, and conspicuous nucleoli. The cells will occasionally contain mucin, sometimes dramatically displacing the nucleus to the cytoplasmic rim as in signet ring formation.

Embryonal tumors (*medulloblastoma, CNS primitive neuroectodermal tumor, and retinoblastoma*) are malignant neoplasms of children and young adults. The cells of embryonal tumors all have a similar appearance and the distinction of each is based on the anatomic location of the primary tumor. The propensity of medulloblastoma to infiltrate the subarachnoid space and involve the leptomeninges usually results in shedding numerous tumor cells into the CSF; therefore some cases may be diagnosed by CSF cytology. CSF cytology may also corroborate suspected drop metastases seen in preoperative imaging studies. Despite the term "small round blue cells," medulloblastoma cells often range up to 20 μm in diameter and may actually be very large, particularly in large cell or anaplastic medulloblastoma. The CSF specimen consists of single cells and small cohesive clusters of cells with high nuclear to cytoplasmic ratios, nuclear molding, hyperchromasia, and inconspicuous nucleoli (Figure 8.7). Close examination will reveal moderate nuclear pleomorphism and chromatin that is dark,

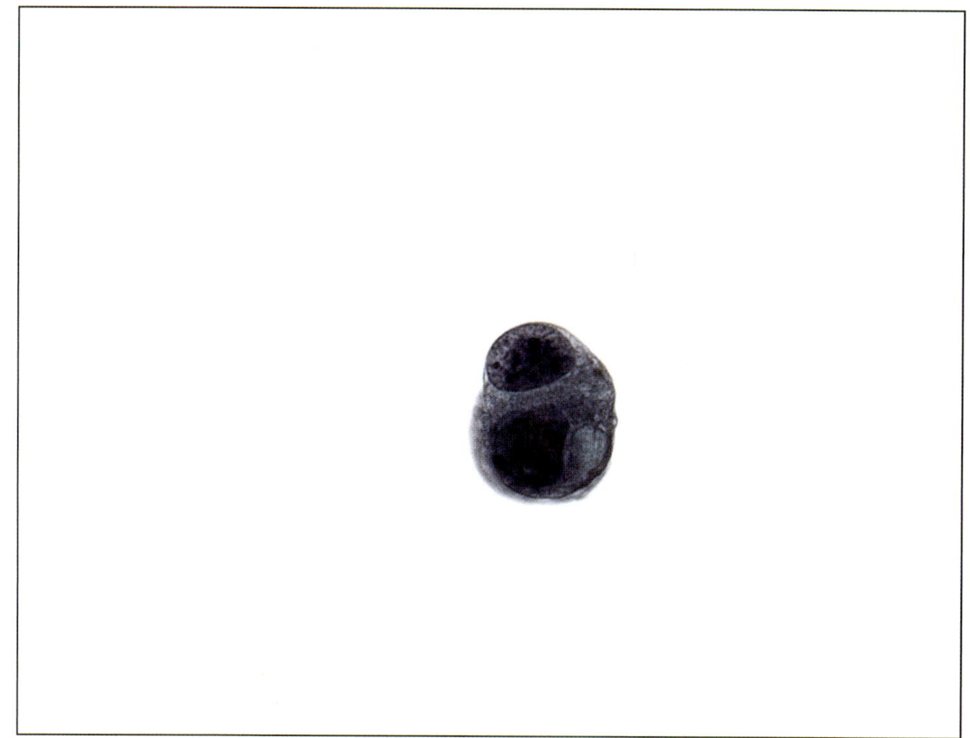

Figure 8.4. Metastatic lung carcinoma. Two cohesive cells revealing indistinct cytoplasmic borders, moderately increase nuclear to cytoplasmic ratios, hyperchromatic, slightly irregular nuclear membranes and lacy, vacuolated cytoplasm.

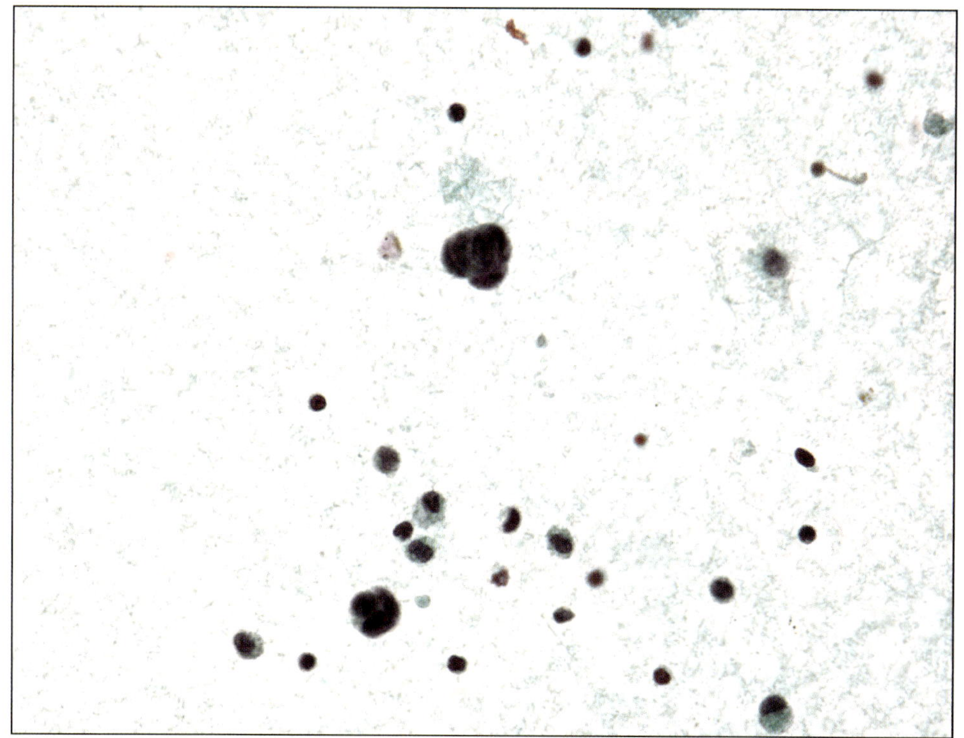

Figure 8.5. Small cell carcinoma of lung. Small tight cohesive groups of cells revealing pronounced nuclear molding, high nuclear to cytoplasmic ratios with a thin rim on basophilic cytoplasm, intensely hyperchromatic nuclei without nucleoli.

dense, or occasionally coarse. If the nucleoli are prominent and multiple, large cell medulloblastoma should be strongly considered. The cytoplasm can be variable ranging form very scanty and transparent to poorly defined. Unfortunately, rosettes so characteristic of embryonal tumors are rarely seen in CSF specimens. Undifferentiated benign cells thought to be of germinal matrix

Figure 8.6. (a) Single intact cells revealing eccentrically placed monomorphic round nuclei with a conspicous nucleolus and abundant moderately dense to delicately vacuolated cytoplasm characteristic of metastatic lobular carcinoma. Intracytoplasmic target vacuoles are highly suggestive of metastatic lobular carcinoma. Some degenerative features are present, an occasional artifact of breast carcinoma in CSF samples. (b) Finely distributed chromatin in a nucleus with a prominent red nucleolus that is eccentrically displaced and indented by cytoplasmic material consistent with mucin.

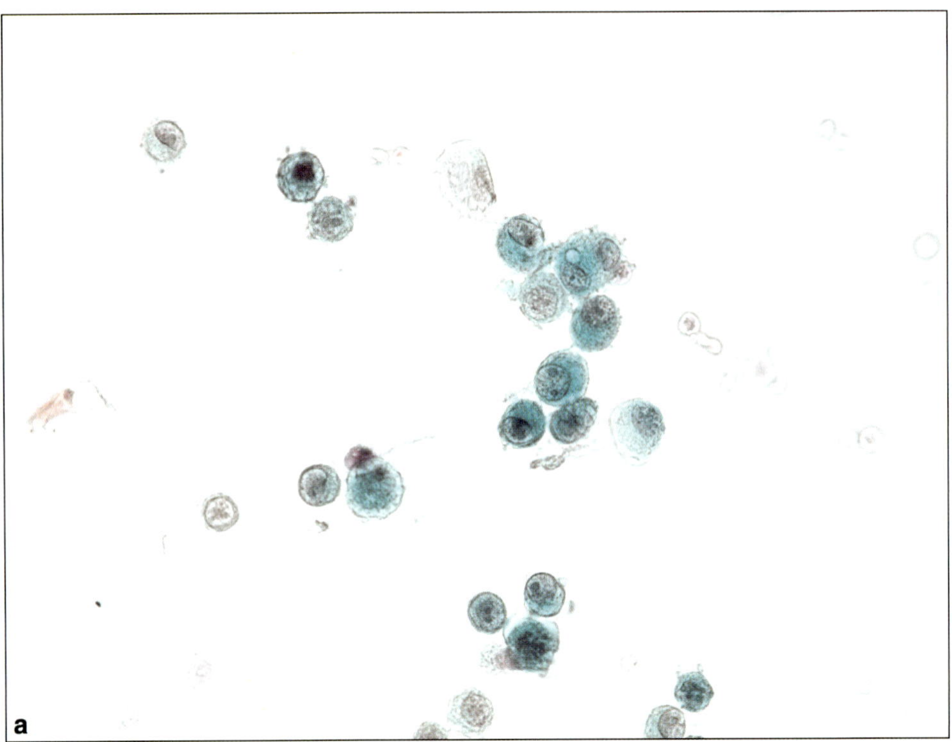

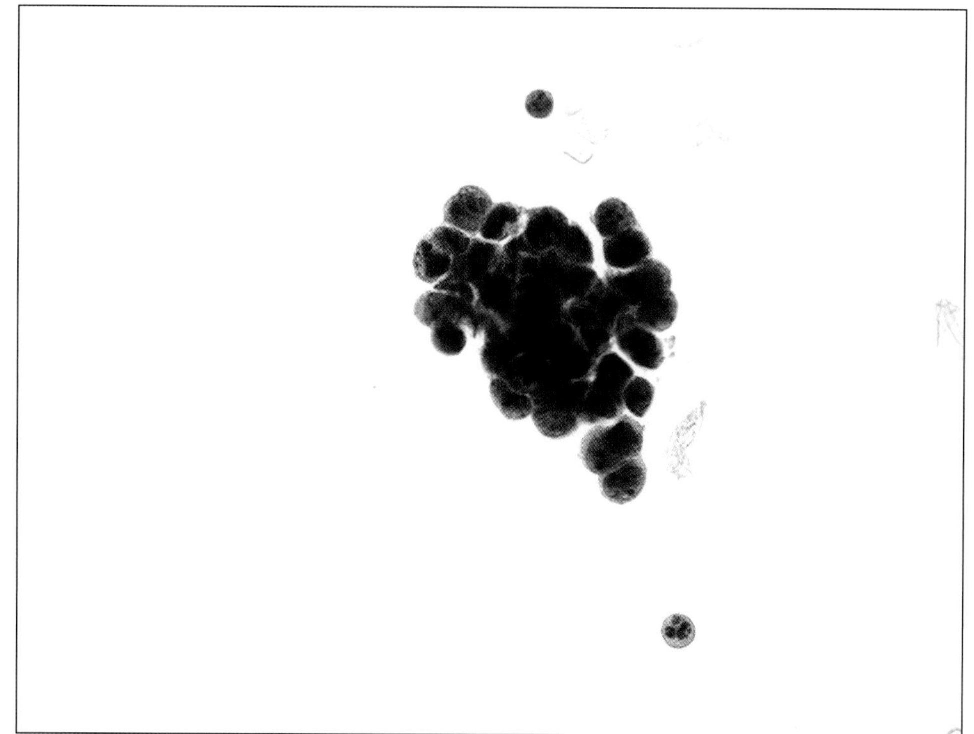

Figure 8.7. Medulloblastoma. Loosely cohesive cluster of primitive appearing cells that display markedly increased nuclear to cytoplasmic ratios, unevenly distributed chromatin, and nuclear molding. Rosette formation is uncommonly seen in cytology specimens, but is extremely useful in the diagnosis of embryonal tumors when present.

origin, which at a glance appear to have similar features, are actually smaller and more uniform with evenly distributed chromatin.

The differential diagnosis includes other small blue cell tumors and metastatic small cell carcinoma of the lung and or lymphoma/leukemia in older individuals. Clinical history and location of the tumor is helpful in the distinction between these entities; however, occasionally ancillary studies such as immunohistochemical studies may be necessary to make the distinction. Lymphoma and leukemia does occur in a similar age group and individual immature blastic cells may closely resemble the cells of embryonal tumors. A key diagnostic feature is cell cohesion and true tissue aggregate and nuclear molding, typically seen in embryonal tumors and dyshesive single cells with nuclear convolutions and membrane irregularities more commonly seen in lymphoma or leukemia (Figure 8.8). Furthermore, embryonal tumor cells tend to be larger and more hyperchromatic than blasts of lymphoma or leukemia. It cannot be stressed enough, however, that occasionally the distinction between these tumor types cannot be made by cytologic inspection alone and in these cases, the clinical history, including history of malignancy, tumor location and adjunctive testing are essential to arrive at the correct diagnosis.

Hematolymphoid Malignancies

The majority of *primary CNS lymphomas* are *large B-cell lymphomas.* A smaller percentage of primary CNS lymphomas are of T-cell origin, whereas primary

Figure 8.8. Leukemia. Dyshesive cells present singly in the background. The cells display moderate to markedly increased nuclear to cytoplasmic ratios, nuclear convolution and indentations, pale immature chromatin, and deep blue cytoplasm. Multiple and prominent nucleoli are seen in several cells.

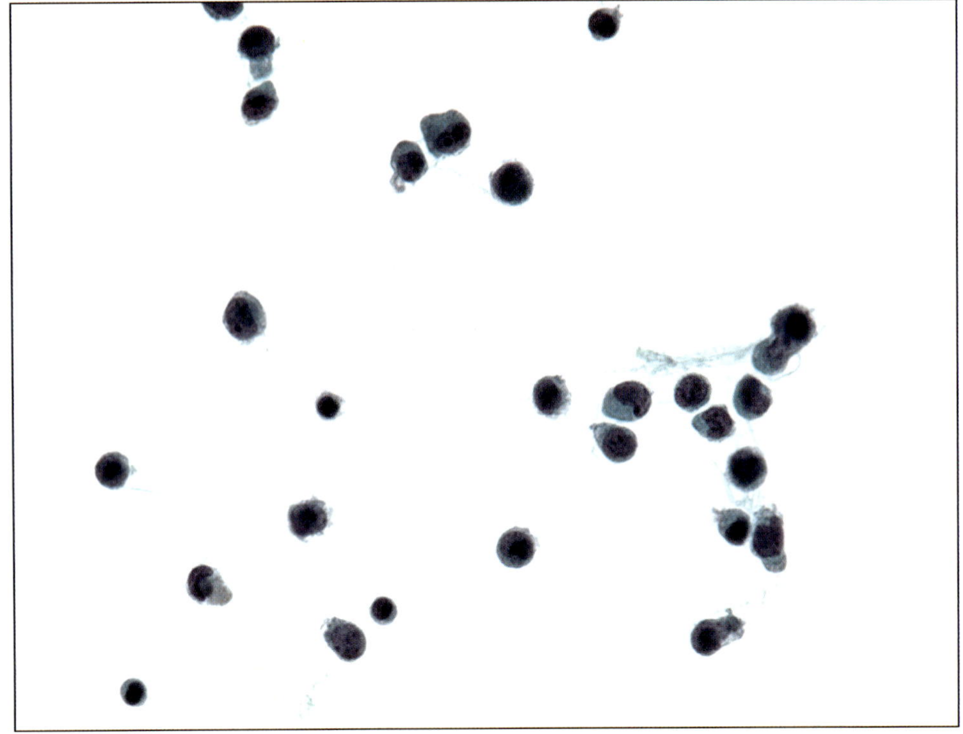

Hodgkin disease is extremely rare. *Acute lymphoblastic lymphoma* (ALL), the most common type of CNS lymphoma in children, is also seen in adults. More commonly, hematopoietic malignancies involving the CNS are secondary to involvement by a systemic lymphoma. Since current chemotherapeutic agents are capable of establishing systemic remissions, but fail to pass the blood–brain barrier, prolonged survival may be contingent upon CNS relapse of lymphoma/leukemia, a particularly common problem with acute lymphoblastic leukemia in which CNS relapses are generally more frequent (DeMay, 1996). Continuous surveillance of CSF specimens is important since the meninges are often the first site of relapse and diagnostic cells are likely to be shed into the CSF. Moreover, patients with CNS disease may be asymptomatic with examination of the CSF specimen remaining an important part of detecting early relapse of lymphoma or leukemia.

Many patients with primary CNS lymphoma are also immunocompromised and thus more susceptible to opportunistic infections and a scenario may arise whereby distinguishing recurrent lymphoma/leukemia from florid reactive inflammatory reactions secondary to infection is problematic. In these situations, a mixed population of small, mature lymphocytes predominating over a few larger forms suggests a reactive process. In cases of uncertainty, reexamination typically establishes the correct diagnosis as benign processes tend to subside. Furthermore, comparison of atypical lymphoid cells with the patient's known malignancy often clarifies the diagnosis. The relative frequency with which certain hematopoietic malignancies involve the CNS is also an important aspect in the process of evaluating any CSF specimen with pleocytosis, remembering that *acute lymphoblastic leukemia* commonly involves the CNS, while *chronic lymphocytic leukemia* is very unlikely, except in blast crisis (DeMay, 1996).

Primary non-Hodgkin lymphomas of the CNS are mostly of large B-cell type. Large B-cell lymphoma is most commonly diagnosed in CSF specimens. Secondary involvement of the CNS by a systemic lymphoma occurs in 5–15% of all patients with non-Hodgkin lymphoma (DeMay, 1996) usually in patients with widespread disease. Cytologic examination of the CSF is useful for the diagnosis of primary or secondary lymphoma and monitoring response to therapy as well as evaluation of CNS relapse. Lymphomatous involvement of the CNS usually reveals abnormalities in the CSF specimen such as an elevated protein or pleocytosis, even in the absence of diagnostic lymphoma cells. For this reason, CSF cytology can be negative even after several examinations before diagnostic cells are identified.

Burkitt lymphoma occurs in children and is occurring with increased frequency in adults as a result of acquired immunodeficiency syndrome (AIDS) (Beral et al., 1991). Many of these patients will have CNS involvement. In Burkitt lymphoma, the cells are typically medium-sized lymphoid cells with moderately increased nuclear to cytoplasmic ratios. The nuclei display slight nuclear membrane irregularities, clumped chromatin with one or more prominent nucleoli, and are surrounded by blue cytoplasm with occasional tiny lipid vacuoles, a finding best appreciated with the Wright–Giemsa stain.

The cytologic features of *large cell lymphoma* can be quite variable, revealing variable amounts cytoplasm and variable nuclear features ranging from smooth to markedly irregular nuclear membranes, varying chromatin patterns, and inconspicuous to prominent nucleoli. The cytomorphology depends on the type of lymphoma or leukemia, but a relatively uniform population of dyshesive small or large hematopoietic cells suggests neoplasia. The monotonous cells display increased nuclear to cytoplasmic ratios, nuclear membrane irregularities, sometimes with protrusions, powdery to coarse chromatin, and occasionally prominent nucleoli. The amount of cytoplasm can be variable, ranging from scant in lymphoblasts to abundant in large cell lymphomas. Mitotic activity is uncommon in CSF specimens, but when present is a finding that should prompt thorough exclusion of a neoplastic process.

The diagnosis of *leukemia* should be based on well-preserved cells and should not be made in the absence of blasts. Atypical lymphocytes, monocytes, and an occasional blast can be present in severe infections such as bacterial viral fungal infections or infected immunosuppressed patients (DeMay, 1996). In this setting, the predominance of blastlike cells is evidence for malignancy rather than reactive changes. However, as stated earlier, diagnostic cells may be sparse in CSF samples, obscured by blood contamination or degenerated and suppressed in numbers by prior corticosteroid therapy.

Lymphoblasts do not form true tissue aggregates, are slightly larger than normal small lymphocytes, and have high nuclear to cytoplasmic ratios with very scant basophilic cytoplasm. The nuclear contours can vary from smooth to convoluted and the chromatin is finer than mature lymphocytes. Single or multiple conspicuous nucleoli are usually identified. The primary differential diagnosis is with reactive lymphocytes. Reactive lymphocytes may have enlarged nuclei with visible nucleoli but contain more cytoplasm and coarser chromatin than lymphoblasts or lymphoma cells. Reactive lymphocytes will usually be seen as part of a spectrum of various cell types.

Germ Cell Malignancies

In cases of suspected germ cell malignancies, CSF specimens are routinely obtained for the measurement of germ cell tumor-related tumor markers and cytological examination. Germ cell tumors typically arise in the suprasellar or pineal gland regions, and the majority resembles gonadal germinoma/seminoma. *Germinoma* cells may be present as a few clusters or singly as uniform, large round to polygonal cells with clear cytoplasm and round nuclei that display fine to coarse chromatin and a characteristic large prominent nucleolus. Germinoma cells are quite fragile, and occasionally a CSF specimen will consist only of a few large atypical bare nuclei with a prominent nucleolus. Although not specific, a background of small mature lymphocytes is a finding typically associated with germinoma. Elements of *immature teratoma* elements may be found in CSF specimens and consist of epithelial cell clusters, scattered squamous cells, or mesenchymal tissue fragments such as small bundles of striated muscle fibers or cartilage.

Primary Tumors of the CNS

The most common primary CNS tumors in both children and adults are *gliomas*. These neoplasms typically are situated in the deep white and gray areas of the brain and tend not to involve the leptomeninges or the ventricular system, thus they are unlikely to shed cells into the CSF. Therefore there is a high negative rate for diagnosis of primary brain tumors by CSF cytology methods and is therefore uncommonly used to diagnose these tumors or monitor recurrence. However, a diagnosis may be possible if a high-grade tumor infiltrates the meninges or the ventricular wall and sheds cells into the CSF.

Astrocytomas may be seen as single cells with angular oval to elongate hyperchromatic nuclei and surrounding eosinophilic cytoplasm or as small clusters of atypical angular nuclei within fragments of neuropil. For all practical purposes, low-grade astrocytomas are extremely difficult to diagnose in CSF specimens, since they shed very few, if any cells, and the cells are typically quite bland and difficult to distinguish from normal or benign reactive cells in the CSF. CSF cytology may allow detection of high-grade astrocytomas as they tend to be distinctive in CSF specimens based on their pleomorphic and epithelioid appearance with well-defined cytoplasm. When present in the CSF, gemistocytic astrocytomas display relatively abundant, finely granular

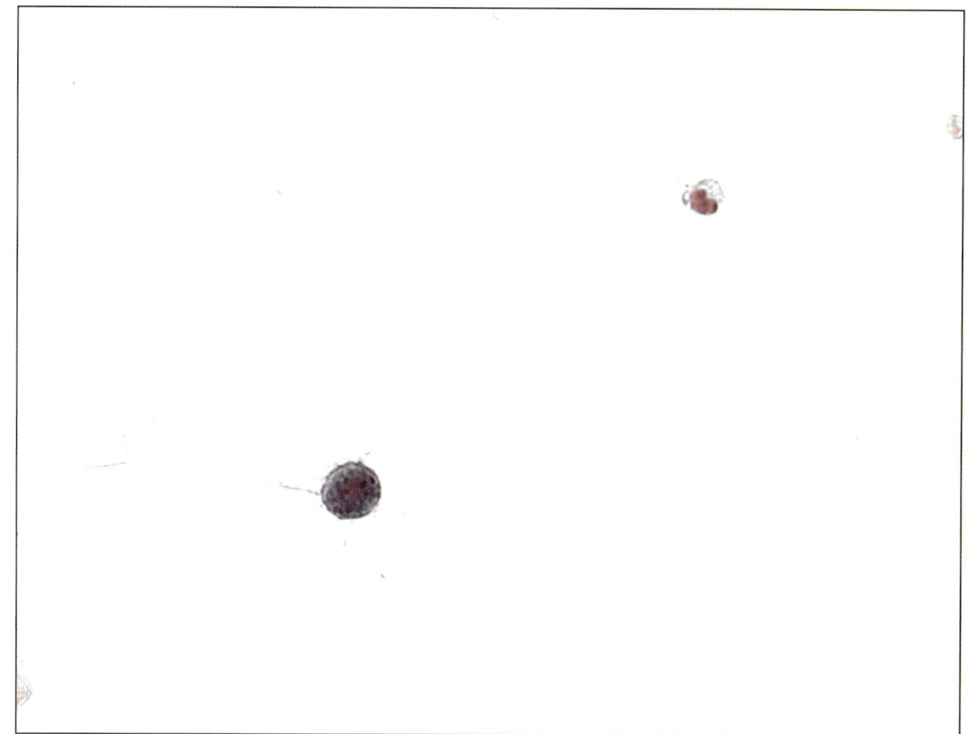

Figure 8.9. Glioblastoma Rare, large highly atypical epithelioid cell with markedly irregular, hyperchromatic nucleus and well-defined scant basophilic cytoplasm. A monocyte is present in the right upper hand corner for size comparison.

densely eosinophilic cytoplasm with an eccentrically placed hyperchromatic round to oval nucleus. *Glioblastoma* most often yields multiple hyperchromatic, large pleomorphic spindled, or bizarre-shaped cells with dense to granular cytoplasm (Figure 8.9). Multinucleate giant cells are rarely found in the CSF specimens and when present are highly suggestive of glioblastoma in the correct clinical setting.

REACTIVE CONDITIONS: INFLAMMATION AND INFECTION

Reactive changes result in increased numbers of normal cells in the CSF including lymphocytes, neutrophils, monocytes, plasma cells, eosinophils, leptomeningeal cell, and rarely glial cells. Cell clusters in CSF are seen only infrequently in benign reactive process, and so the presence of cell clustering in CSF specimens is a finding that is suspicious for malignancy.

In benign reactive conditions, a spectrum of small and transformed lymphocytes will be found. Some conditions, however, may also include "atypical" or immature lymphocytes, such as in cases of severe meningitis in which there may be a marked elevation in the WBC count with a subsequent shift to immature forms including an occasional blast. As always, atypical cells may also be seen in the post chemotherapy/radiation situation, but usually with preservation of the nuclear to cytoplasmic ratios, smudgy, degenerated chromatin, and vacuolated cytoplasm.

Infections

Depending of the stage of *bacterial meningitis*, the CSF cytology specimen may vary from abundant neutrophils in the early phase to residual small lymphocytes in the resolution phase. Cell counts and chemical analysis of the specimen are important factors in cases of infection in the determination of the likely type of infectious agent. For example, although neutrophils may be sparse, they are typically seen in acute bacterial meningitis along with a decreased CSF glucose level while increased numbers of lymphocytes and decreased CSF glucose is classically seen in cases of tuberculous or fungal meningitis.

Viral meningitis is usually a relatively benign disease, but cases of viral encephalitis caused, for example, by enterovirus, mumps, herpes, or cytomegalovirus can be serious illnesses. In these specimens, the most characteristic cytologic features are increased numbers of small, mature lymphocytes, reactive transformed lymphocytes, plasma cells, and histiocytes undergoing phagocytosis. Infection by herpes virus may occasionally reveal cells with viral inclusions; however, characteristic viral inclusions are generally rare. Mollaret meningitis may be associated with viruses such as herpes virus. In these cases the CSF shows marked pleocytosis including lymphocytes neutrophils and large Mollaret cells, which are probably activated monocytes. Mollaret cells have delicate, finally evacuated, pale cytoplasm with the centric irregular reniform nucleus. The chromatin is finely granular with small nucleoli.

The human immunodeficiency virus (HIV-1) is lymphotrophic and neurotrophic and essentially always involves the CNS in AIDS patients. CSF specimens in AIDS patients are nonspecific and similar to that seen primary aseptic meningoencephalitis. Chronic inflammatory cells with reactive changes and histiocytes, including multinucleate giant cells, may be present.

Cryptococcus is the most common fungal organism affecting the CSF (Prayson and Fischler, 1998). It is usually seen in immunosuppressed patients, but it may be seen in otherwise fairly healthy individuals. The yeast forms range from 5 to 15 µm in diameter, revealing a refractile center and a mucoid capsule (Figure 8.10a,b). Special stains such as mucicarmine or Gomorimethenamine silver are useful in the diagnosis. It is important to recognize the lack of an inflammatory response elicited by *Cryptococcus*, and not to overlook the organisms in the Papanicolaou stain as the organisms stain poorly with this stain. Mononuclear pleocytosis with increased CSF protein in the absence of bacterial or fungal infections strongly suggests *Toxoplasma gondii* infection. Cysts and trophozoites are usually identified on the Wright–Giemsa preparations.

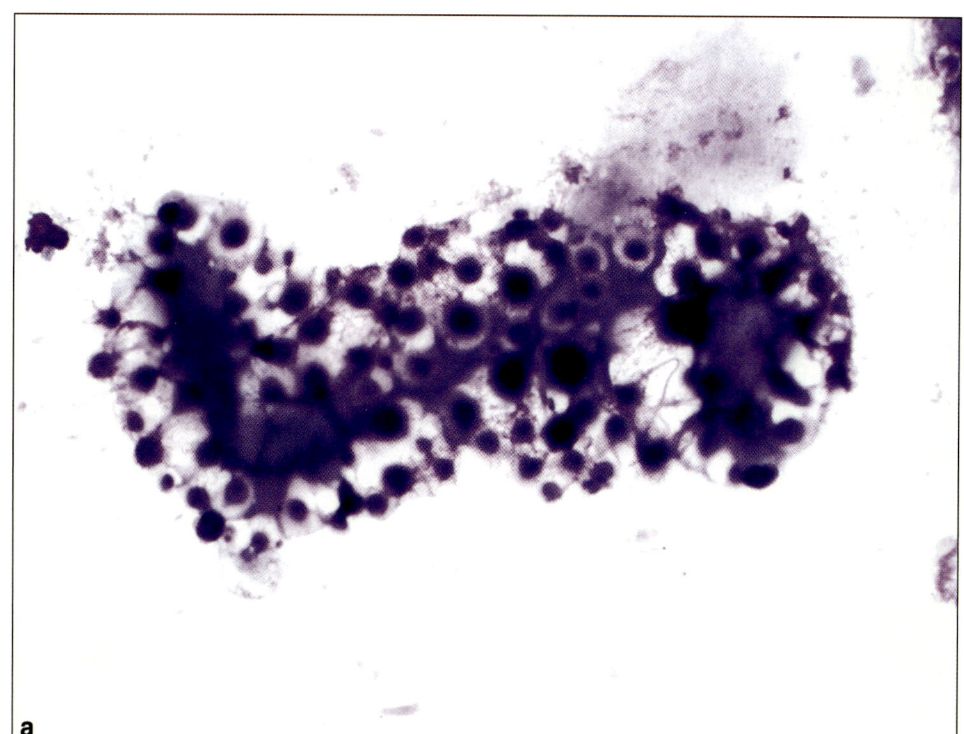

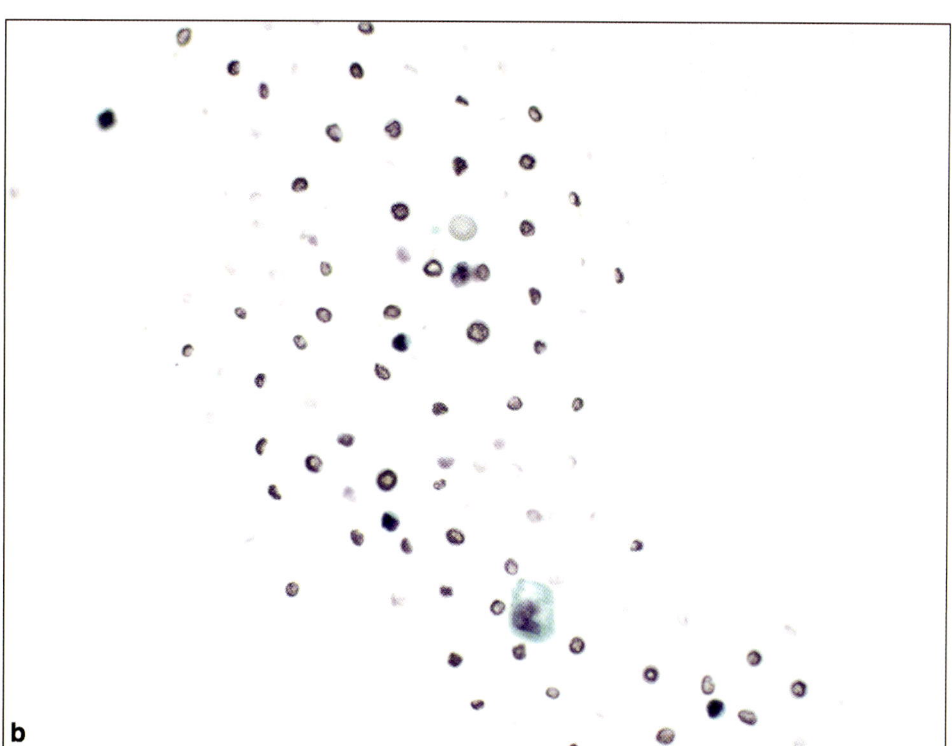

Figure 8.10. *Cryptococcus.* Yeast forms varying between 5 and 15 μm. (a) Modified Wright–Giemsa stain outlines the thick capsule. (b) Cryptococcus stains poorly with Papanicolaou staining and may be missed or interpreted as contaminant.

REFERENCES

Barnholtz-Sloan JS, Sloan AE, Davis FG, Vigneau FD, Lai P, Sawaya RE. Incidence proportions of brain metastases in patients diagnosed (1973 to 2001) in the Metropolitan Detroit Cancer Surveillance System. *J Clin Oncol* 2004; 22: 2865–72.

Beral V, Peterman T, Berkelman R, Jaffe H. AIDS-associated non-Hodgkin lymphoma. *Lancet* 1991; 337: 805–9.

DeMay RM. The art and science of cytopathology. *Exfoliative Cytology*, chap 1. Chicago, IL: ASCP Press, 1996, 427–62.

Jorda M, Ganjei-Azar P, Nadji M. Cytologic characteristics of meningeal carcinomatosis: increased diagnostic accuracy using carcinoembryonic antigen and epithelial membrane antigen immunocytochemistry. *Arch Neurol* 1998; 55: 181–4.

Prayson RA, Fischler DF. Cerebrospinal fluid cytology: an 11-year experience with 5951 specimens. *Arch Pathol Lab Med* 1998; 122: 47–51.

Schouten LJ, Rutten J, Huveneers HA, Twijnstra A. Incidence of brain metastases in a cohort of patients with carcinoma of the breast, colon, kidney, and lung and melanoma. *Cancer* 2002; 94: 2698–705.

INDEX